Therapeutic Potential for Cannabis and Cannabinoids

Therapeutic Potential for Cannabis and Cannabinoids

Editor

Wesley M. Raup-Konsavage

MDPI • Basel • Beijing • Wuhan • Barcelona • Belgrade • Manchester • Tokyo • Cluj • Tianjin

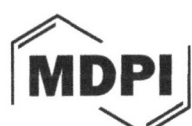

Editor
Wesley M. Raup-Konsavage
Pennsylvania State University
College of Medicine,
Hershey, PA, USA

Editorial Office
MDPI
St. Alban-Anlage 66
4052 Basel, Switzerland

This is a reprint of articles from the Special Issue published online in the open access journal *Biomedicines* (ISSN 2227-9059) (available at: https://www.mdpi.com/journal/biomedicines/special_issues/Cannabis_Cannabinoid).

For citation purposes, cite each article independently as indicated on the article page online and as indicated below:

LastName, A.A.; LastName, B.B.; LastName, C.C. Article Title. *Journal Name* **Year**, *Volume Number*, Page Range.

ISBN 978-3-0365-7582-7 (Hbk)
ISBN 978-3-0365-7583-4 (PDF)

© 2023 by the authors. Articles in this book are Open Access and distributed under the Creative Commons Attribution (CC BY) license, which allows users to download, copy and build upon published articles, as long as the author and publisher are properly credited, which ensures maximum dissemination and a wider impact of our publications.
The book as a whole is distributed by MDPI under the terms and conditions of the Creative Commons license CC BY-NC-ND.

Contents

About the Editor ix

Wesley M. Raup-Konsavage
Special Issue: Therapeutic Potential for Cannabis and Cannabinoids
Reprinted from: *Biomedicines* **2023**, *11*, 902, doi:10.3390/biomedicines11030902 1

Emily R. Hajjar, Allison Herens, Erin L. Kelly, Kayla Madden, Jessica M. Lungen and Brooke K. Worster
A Longitudinal Observational Study of Medical Cannabis Use and Polypharmacy among Patients Presenting to Dispensaries in Pennsylvania
Reprinted from: *Biomedicines* **2023**, *11*, 158, doi:10.3390/biomedicines11010158 5

Karen Mae A. Bacalia, Kevin M. Tveter, Hayley Palmer, Jeffrey Douyere, Savannah Martinez, Ke Sui and Diana E. Roopchand
Cannabidiol Decreases Intestinal Inflammation in the Ovariectomized Murine Model of Postmenopause
Reprinted from: *Biomedicines* **2023**, *11*, 74, doi:10.3390/biomedicines11010074 15

Bettina Greiner, Manuela Sommerfeld, Ulrich Kintscher, Thomas Unger, Kai Kappert and Elena Kaschina
Differential Regulation of MMPs, Apoptosis and Cell Proliferation by the Cannabinoid Receptors CB1 and CB2 in Vascular Smooth Muscle Cells and Cardiac Myocytes
Reprinted from: *Biomedicines* **2022**, *10*, 3271, doi:10.3390/biomedicines10123271 33

Ralph-Sydney Mboumba Bouassa, Judy Needham, Dana Nohynek, Joel Singer, Terry Lee, Florian Bobeuf, et al.
Safety and Tolerability of Oral Cannabinoids in People Living with HIV on Long-Term ART: A Randomized, Open-Label, Interventional Pilot Clinical Trial (CTNPT 028)
Reprinted from: *Biomedicines* **2022**, *10*, 3168, doi:10.3390/biomedicines10123168 51

Guillermo Moreno-Sanz, Alvaro Madiedo, Michael Lynskey and Matthew R. D. Brown
"*Flower Power*": Controlled Inhalation of THC-Predominant Cannabis Flos Improves Health-Related Quality of Life and Symptoms of Chronic Pain and Anxiety in Eligible UK Patients
Reprinted from: *Biomedicines* **2022**, *10*, 2576, doi:10.3390/biomedicines10102576 69

Diana E. Sepulveda, Kent E. Vrana, Nicholas M. Graziane and Wesley M. Raup-Konsavage
Combinations of Cannabidiol and Δ^9-Tetrahydrocannabinol in Reducing Chemotherapeutic Induced Neuropathic Pain
Reprinted from: *Biomedicines* **2022**, *10*, 2548, doi:10.3390/biomedicines10102548 85

Francesca Mottarlini, Marco Fumagalli, Fernando Castillo-Díaz, Stefano Piazza, Giorgia Targa, Enrico Sangiovanni, et al.
Single and Repeated Exposure to Cannabidiol Differently Modulate BDNF Expression and Signaling in the Cortico-Striatal Brain Network
Reprinted from: *Biomedicines* **2022**, *10*, 1853, doi:10.3390/biomedicines10081853 95

Zsolt Gáll, Krisztina Kelemen, Andrea Tolokán, István Zolcseak, István Sável, Réka Bod, et al.
Anticonvulsant Action and Long-Term Effects of Chronic Cannabidiol Treatment in the Rat Pentylenetetrazole-Kindling Model of Epilepsy
Reprinted from: *Biomedicines* **2022**, *10*, 1811, doi:10.3390/biomedicines10081811 111

Zhanna Yekhtin, Iman Khuja, David Meiri, Reuven Or and Osnat Almogi-Hazan
Differential Effects of D9 Tetrahydrocannabinol (THC)- and Cannabidiol (CBD)-Based Cannabinoid Treatments on Macrophage Immune Function In Vitro and on Gastrointestinal Inflammation in a Murine Model
Reprinted from: *Biomedicines* **2022**, *10*, 1793, doi:10.3390/biomedicines10081793 129

Tomer Mizrachi Zer-Aviv, Larglinda Islami, Peter J. Hamilton, Eric M. Parise, Eric J. Nestler, Brenda Sbarski and Irit Akirav
Enhancing Endocannabinoid Signaling via β-Catenin in the Nucleus Accumbens Attenuates PTSD- and Depression-like Behavior of Male Rats
Reprinted from: *Biomedicines* **2022**, *10*, 1789, doi:10.3390/biomedicines10081789 147

Aviad Schnapp, Moria Harel, Dalit Cayam-Rand, Hanoch Cassuto, Lola Polyansky and Adi Aran
A Placebo-Controlled Trial of Cannabinoid Treatment for Disruptive Behavior in Children and Adolescents with Autism Spectrum Disorder: Effects on Sleep Parameters as Measured by the CSHQ
Reprinted from: *Biomedicines* **2022**, *10*, 1685, doi:10.3390/biomedicines10071685 173

Colleen M. Trevino, Cecilia J. Hillard, Aniko Szabo and Terri A. deRoon-Cassini
Serum Concentrations of the Endocannabinoid, 2-Arachidonoylglycerol, in the Peri-Trauma Period Are Positively Associated with Chronic Pain Months Later
Reprinted from: *Biomedicines* **2022**, *10*, 1599, doi:10.3390/biomedicines10071599 187

Hana Golan, Raphael Mechoulam, Reem Smoum, Efrat Cohen-Zada, Sara Pri-Chen, Sapir Wiener, et al.
Anti-Tumorigenic Effect of a Novel Derivative of 2-Hydroxyoleic Acid and the Endocannabinoid Anandamide on Neuroblastoma Cells
Reprinted from: *Biomedicines* **2022**, *10*, 1552, doi:10.3390/biomedicines10071552 199

Torsten Lowin, Christina Kok, Sophie Smutny and Georg Pongratz
Impact of Δ^9-Tetrahydrocannabinol on Rheumatoid Arthritis Synovial Fibroblasts Alone and in Co-Culture with Peripheral Blood Mononuclear Cells
Reprinted from: *Biomedicines* **2022**, *10*, 1118, doi:10.3390/biomedicines10051118 215

Andrea Duranti, Gorane Beldarrain, Antonia Álvarez, Matilde Sbriscia, Silvia Carloni, Walter Balduini and Daniel Alonso-Alconada
The Endocannabinoid System as a Target for Neuroprotection/Neuroregeneration in Perinatal Hypoxic–Ischemic Brain Injury
Reprinted from: *Biomedicines* **2023**, *11*, 28, doi:10.3390/biomedicines11010028 229

Francisco T. Chacon, Wesley M. Raup-Konsavage, Kent E. Vrana and Joshua J. Kellogg
Secondary Terpenes in *Cannabis sativa* L.: Synthesis and Synergy
Reprinted from: *Biomedicines* **2022**, *10*, 3142, doi:10.3390/biomedicines10123142 249

Ivona Maria Tudorancea, Mitică Ciorpac, Gabriela Dumitrița Stanciu, Cătălin Carataşu, Alina Săcărescu, Bogdan Ignat, et al.
The Therapeutic Potential of the Endocannabinoid System in Age-Related Diseases
Reprinted from: *Biomedicines* **2022**, *10*, 2492, doi:10.3390/biomedicines10102492 273

Ronit Vogt Sionov and Doron Steinberg
Anti-Microbial Activity of Phytocannabinoids and Endocannabinoids in the Light of Their Physiological and Pathophysiological Roles
Reprinted from: *Biomedicines* **2022**, *10*, 631, doi:10.3390/biomedicines10030631 323

Matija Sestan-Pesa, Marya Shanabrough, Tamas L. Horvath and Maria Consolata Miletta
Impaired Ghrelin Signaling Does Not Lead to Alterations of Anxiety-like Behaviors in Adult Mice Chronically Exposed to THC during Adolescence
Reprinted from: *Biomedicines* **2023**, *11*, 144, doi:10.3390/biomedicines11010144 . . . . **371**

Rosario Licitra, Maria Marchese, Valentina Naef, Asahi Ogi, Marco Martinelli, Claudia Kiferle, et al.
A Review on the Bioactivity of Cannabinoids on Zebrafish Models: Emphasis on Neurodevelopment
Reprinted from: *Biomedicines* **2022**, *10*, 1820, doi:10.3390/biomedicines10081820 . . . . **385**

About the Editor

Wesley M. Raup-Konsavage

Wesley Raup-Konsavage has over 20 years of research experience in molecular biology. His research is focused on the medicinal properties of cannabis and individual cannabinoid compounds (Δ9-tetrahdyrocannabinol (THC), cannabidiol (CBD), & cannabigerol (CBG)). Currently his lab has two primary focuses:

1. The ability of cannabis/cannabinoids to reduce cancer cell growth.
2. The ability of cannabis/cannabinoids to stimulate epithelial cell growth and the impact of cannabinoid exposure on cell differentiation.

Recently, his laboratory has identified 5-epi CP 55,940, from a screening of over 400 synthetic cannabinoids, as being effective for the reducing growth in colorectal cancer cells. Additionally, his laboratory has shown that CBD is able to reduce colorectal cancer cell growth, and that pure CBD is more efficacious than CBD in botanical extracts. The current work in this area is to identify the mechanism by which cannabinoids are acting to reduce cancer cell growth and to pursue variations of these molecules for improved activity.

The second area of research is focused on exploring the benefits of cannabis/cannabinoids for inflammatory bowel disease (IBD). Previously, he has demonstrated that lithium, which stimulates intestinal epithelial cell growth, also reduced IBD symptoms in a murine model. His current work in this area is examining cannabinoids as potential gastrointestinal therapeutics. The long-term goal is to move successfully identified compounds into an animal model of IBD.

As the scientific director for the Pennsylvania-approved Medical Marijuana Academic Clinical Research Center (ACRC) at Penn State, Dr. Raup-Konsavage works in close collaboration with a number of researchers and clinicians to evaluate the medical efficacy for cannabis across a wide spectrum of diseases and disorders, such as pain, anxiety, and PTSD.

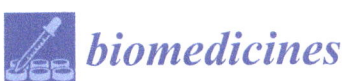

Editorial

Special Issue: Therapeutic Potential for Cannabis and Cannabinoids

Wesley M. Raup-Konsavage

Department of Pharmacology, Penn State College of Medicine, Hershey, PA 17033, USA; wkonsavage@pennstatehealth.psu.edu; Tel.: +717-531-4172

The number of patients reporting the use of cannabis for medical purposes, whether through state-regulated medical marijuana programs or through over-the-counter hemp extracts, continues to grow. The growth in medicinal use of cannabis has in many ways surpassed the scientific data on the benefits and hazards of cannabis, and the scientific community has largely been left playing catch-up. Since 1996, when California became the first jurisdiction to legalize medical cannabis, the number of states following suit has grown and is currently at 37, while nearly 50 countries have legalized medical cannabis (and even more have decriminalized the plant) including Canada, Austria, Uruguay, Australia, South Korea, and Lesotho.

Cannabis sp. produces a number of phytochemicals with potential medical benefits including terpenes, flavonoids, and a unique class of molecules called cannabinoids, of which Δ^9-tetrahydrocannabinol (THC) and cannabidiol (CBD) are the two most studied [1,2]. Amazingly, the plant produces over 100 different cannabinoids with different potential therapeutic targets and activities, and these remain understudied. The therapeutic benefits of cannabinoids are due, in large part, to the endocannabinoid system that exists in the human body, in addition to the ability of cannabinoids to interact and signal through a large number of disparate receptor molecules [3].

The recent growth in cannabis and cannabinoid research is perhaps best highlighted by the establishment of three scholarly journals devoted solely to this topic in the past few years, namely, *Cannabis and Cannabinoid Research*, in 2016, *Medical Cannabis and Cannabinoids*, in 2018, and *The Journal of Cannabis*, in 2019.

1. Original Research Articles

This Special Issue features fourteen original research articles across a wide range of topics and includes 10 reports on phytocannabinoids, 2 studies examining the endocannabinoid system, and 2 papers using synthetic cannabinoids. Three of these studies looked at the role of cannabinoids at mediating pain, two studies examined cannabinoids for treating mental illness, two studies addressed the potential safety of cannabinoids, two looked at cannabinoids as treatment options for gastrointestinal inflammation, and two studies examined the impact of cannabinoids on neurodevelopmental diseases. Other studies examined the impact of cannabinoids on cancer cell growth, anti-inflammatory activity in fibroblasts from patients with rheumatoid arthritis, regulation of matrix metalloproteases and cell proliferation, and regulation of neuroprotective genes in the brain. These various topics highlight the wide-ranging potential benefit of cannabis and cannabinoids to treat an array of human illness and disease.

In a study by Moreno-Sanz and colleagues, the impact of inhaled cannabis to treat pain and anxiety was examined [4]. The authors found that inhalation of pharmaceutical-grade cannabis flower provides patient-reported improvements to pain, mood, anxiety, and sleep. Perhaps most importantly the study reports an overall increased quality of life in a treatment-resistant group of patients. Sepulveda et al. found that pure THC, unlike pure CBD, is capable of reducing hyperalgesia in a murine model of chemotherapeutic-induced peripheral neuropathy [5]. This study also provides support for an "entourage" effect

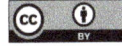

Citation: Raup-Konsavage, W.M. Special Issue: Therapeutic Potential for Cannabis and Cannabinoids. *Biomedicines* 2023, 11, 902. https://doi.org/10.3390/biomedicines11030902

Received: 11 February 2023
Accepted: 23 February 2023
Published: 14 March 2023

Copyright: © 2023 by the author. Licensee MDPI, Basel, Switzerland. This article is an open access article distributed under the terms and conditions of the Creative Commons Attribution (CC BY) license (https://creativecommons.org/licenses/by/4.0/).

because a high CBD hemp extract, unlike the pure CBD, was able to reduce hyperalgesia when normalized to CBD levels; however, high THC extract and pure THC were found to offer the maximum reduction in sensitivity. In a study by Trevino and collaborators, the authors report that levels of the endocannabinoid 2-arachidonoylglcerol (2-AG) in the plasma at time of injury are positively correlated with chronic pain [6]. This suggests that increased activation of the endocannabinoid system can contribute to the development of chronic pain following an injury.

In addition to the Moreno-Sanz study described above, one other study examined cannabinoids in mental illness. A study by Zer-Aviv et al., found that inhibition of the endocannabinoid metabolizing enzyme fatty acid amide hydrolase (FAAH) produces a stress-protective effect through activation of β-catenin in the nucleus accumbens region of the brain [7]. The study also found that the increase in anandamide levels, from inhibition of FAAH, acts through the cannabinoid receptor 1 to increase nuclear levels of β-catenin.

Hajjar and colleagues examined the use of prescription and non-prescription medications in patients using medical cannabis, as self-reported by patients [8]. The study found that patients frequently switch medical cannabis products, which may be due to the need to find a dose and product that work well for the patient. The study also found that despite the use of medical cannabis, the majority of patients taking antidepressants and anxiolytic medications did not change their medications or the dose of these medications. Bouassa et al., found that THC and CBD were well-tolerated by patients with HIV on anti-retroviral therapy [9]. Their study did find that patients on high doses of CBD (800 mg/day) should be monitored for liver pathology.

Bacalia et al. examined the impact of CBD on intestinal inflammation, and they found that in female mice, CBD suppresses inflammation in the absence of estradiol, but it enhances inflammation in animals with estradiol [10]. Yekhtin and colleagues found that both THC and CBD reduced nitric oxide production by lipopolysaccharide (LPS)-stimulated peritoneal macrophages [11]. Interestingly, only CBD was able to reduce cytokine production in LPS-stimulated macrophages, suggesting differences in the anti-inflammatory properties of these two cannabinoids. Both cannabinoids were equally beneficial at improving clinical outcomes in the dextran sodium sulfate murine model of colitis.

Gáll and collaborators found that CBD increases the latency to the first seizure and decreased the mortality associated with the pentylenetetrazol (PTZ)-kindling model of epilepsy in rats [12]. However, no impact was observed for seizure frequency or duration in this model. In a placebo-controlled trial of cannabinoids (CBD and THC at a 20:1 ratio using both extracts and pure compounds), Schnapp et al. found no impact on sleep parameters in patients with autism spectrum disorder [13].

In another study that examined the anti-inflammatory activity of cannabinoids outside of the gastrointestinal tract, Lowin et al. found that the impact of THC on inflammation in synovial fibroblasts from rheumatoid arthritis (RA) patients is dose dependent [14]. Therefore, using THC to treat RA may require titrating the dose to find an effective dose for each patient. Golan and colleagues found that a novel compound (HU-585), a synthetic derivative of anandamide and oleic acid, induces apoptosis and senescence in treatment-resistant neuroblastoma cells [15]. Greiner et al. report that activation of the cannabinoid receptor 2 produces protective effects in vascular smooth muscle cells and cardiac myocytes, and the opposite effect is observed when cannabinoid receptor 1 is activated in these cells [16]. Finally, in a study by Mottarlini and colleagues, it was found that cannabidiol administered via intraperitoneal injection is able to be detected in the prefrontal cortex of the brain, and that CBD treatment modulates the expression of brain-derived neurotropic factor (BDNF) [17]. BDNF plays a role in neurodevelopment, neuroplasticity, and neuroprotection, and the authors propose that CBD may prove beneficial in these areas when taken as a supplement.

2. Review Articles, Brief Reports, and Systematic Reviews

Four review articles in this Special Issue summarize information on a wide array of topics related to cannabinoids. Duranti and collaborators review the current literature on the endocannabinoid system with regard to neuroprotection and neuroregeneration [18]. The focus of their review highlights the potential of modulating the endocannabinoid system to treat hypoxia–ischemia in newborns, which can lead to encephalopathy, a condition for which there are currently limited treatment options. Chacon et al. review some of the less abundant ("secondary") terpenes found in *Cannabis* and the potential therapeutic utility of some of these molecules to treat a number of medical conditions [19]. Tudorancea and colleagues review the evidence that supports targeting the endocannabinoid system to treat age-related conditions such as Alzheimer's disease, osteoarthritis, and hypertension [20]. Finally, Sionov and Steinberg examine the antimicrobial activity of endocannabinoids and phytocannabinoids. This latter review is important because the development of novel antibiotics is an ongoing need as resistance to current drugs is a continually evolving issue [21].

In a brief report by Sestan-Pesa et al. the authors explore the mechanism by which THC may lead to increased risk of schizophrenia, depression, and anxiety by looking at ghrelin signaling [22]. Ghrelin and its receptor, growth hormone secretagogue receptor (GHSR), have previously been found to play a role in anxiety- and depression-related behavior in animal models. However, the authors report no difference in anxiety-like behavior between wild-type and GHSR knockout animals after exposure to THC.

Licitra and colleagues performed a systematic review of the literature on cannabinoids in zebrafish [23]. The authors find that in many ways zebrafish respond similarly to rodents following cannabinoid exposure, and may serve as another useful model for studying the effects of cannabinoids in disease and on humans.

3. Closing Remarks

Cannabis is a complicated plant that produces over 100 cannabinoids in addition to terpenes and flavonoids. Adding to the complexity of trying to address the mechanism of action for cannabis is the fact that the cannabinoids that have been studied have been reported to exhibit activity at a number of different receptors. This makes cannabinoids (and cannabis) a promiscuous drug. While typically viewed as a negative, promiscuous drugs do offer some advantages, most notably the ability to target different pathways of a disease with one medication [24]. The field of medical cannabis is growing rapidly, and as patients continue to use this plant to treat their conditions, there will remain a growing need for the scientific and medical communities to better understand how cannabis can impact the body. Not only is research needed to address the potential benefit and hazards of cannabis and individual cannabinoids, but also we must determine which routes of administration are best for each condition.

Conflicts of Interest: The author declares no conflict of interest.

References

1. Nachnani, R.; Raup-Konsavage, W.M.; Vrana, K.E. The Pharmacological Case for Cannabigerol. *J. Pharmacol. Exp. Ther.* **2021**, *376*, 204–212. [CrossRef] [PubMed]
2. Legare, C.A.; Raup-Konsavage, W.M.; Vrana, K.E. Therapeutic Potential of Cannabis, Cannabidiol, and Cannabinoid-Based Pharmaceuticals. *Pharmacology* **2022**, *107*, 1–19. [CrossRef] [PubMed]
3. Biringer, R.G. Endocannabinoid signaling pathways: Beyond CB1R and CB2R. *J. Cell Commun. Signal.* **2021**, *15*, 335–360. [CrossRef]
4. Moreno-Sanz, G.; Madiedo, A.; Lynskey, M.; Brown, M.R.D. "Flower Power": Controlled Inhalation of THC-Predominant Cannabis Flos Improves Health-Related Quality of Life and Symptoms of Chronic Pain and Anxiety in Eligible UK Patients. *Biomedicines* **2022**, *10*, 2576. [CrossRef]
5. Sepulveda, D.E.; Vrana, K.E.; Graziane, N.M.; Raup-Konsavage, W.M. Combinations of Cannabidiol and Δ^9-Tetrahydrocannabinol in Reducing Chemotherapeutic Induced Neuropathic Pain. *Biomedicines* **2022**, *10*, 2548. [CrossRef] [PubMed]

6. Trevino, C.M.; Hillard, C.J.; Szabo, A.; Deroon-Cassini, T.A. Serum Concentrations of the Endocannabinoid, 2-Arachidonoylglycerol, in the Peri-Trauma Period Are Positively Associated with Chronic Pain Months Later. *Biomedicines* 2022, *10*, 1599. [CrossRef] [PubMed]
7. Zer-Aviv, T.M.; Islami, L.; Hamilton, P.J.; Parise, E.M.; Nestler, E.J.; Sbarski, B.; Akirav, I. Enhancing Endocannabinoid Signaling via β-Catenin in the Nucleus Accumbens Attenuates PTSD- and Depression-like Behavior of Male Rats. *Biomedicines* 2022, *10*, 1789. [CrossRef]
8. Hajjar, E.R.; Herens, A.; Kelly, E.L.; Madden, K.; Lungen, J.M.; Worster, B.K. A Longitudinal Observational Study of Medical Cannabis Use and Polypharmacy among Patients Presenting to Dispensaries in Pennsylvania. *Biomedicines* 2023, *11*, 158. [CrossRef]
9. Bouassa, R.-S.M.; Needham, J.; Nohynek, D.; Singer, J.; Lee, T.; Bobeuf, F.; Samarani, S.; Del Balso, L.; Paisible, N.; Vertzagias, C.; et al. Safety and Tolerability of Oral Cannabinoids in People Living with HIV on Long-Term ART: A Randomized, Open-Label, Interventional Pilot Clinical Trial (CTNPT 028). *Biomedicines* 2022, *10*, 3168. [CrossRef]
10. Bacalia, K.M.A.; Tveter, K.M.; Palmer, H.; Douyere, J.; Martinez, S.; Sui, K.; Roopchand, D.E. Cannabidiol Decreases Intestinal Inflammation in the Ovariectomized Murine Model of Postmenopause. *Biomedicines* 2022, *11*, 74. [CrossRef]
11. Yekhtin, Z.; Khuja, I.; Meiri, D.; Or, R.; Almogi-Hazan, O. Differential Effects of D9 Tetrahydrocannabinol (THC)- and Cannabidiol (CBD)-Based Cannabinoid Treatments on Macrophage Immune Function In Vitro and on Gastrointestinal Inflammation in a Murine Model. *Biomedicines* 2022, *10*, 1793. [CrossRef] [PubMed]
12. Gáll, Z.; Kelemen, K.; Tolokán, A.; Zolcseak, I.; Sável, I.; Bod, R.; Ferencz, E.; Vancea, S.; Urkon, M.; Kolcsár, M. Anticonvulsant Action and Long-Term Effects of Chronic Cannabidiol Treatment in the Rat Pentylenetetrazole-Kindling Model of Epilepsy. *Biomedicines* 2022, *10*, 1811. [CrossRef] [PubMed]
13. Schnapp, A.; Harel, M.; Cayam-Rand, D.; Cassuto, H.; Polyansky, L.; Aran, A. A Placebo-Controlled Trial of Cannabinoid Treatment for Disruptive Behavior in Children and Adolescents with Autism Spectrum Disorder: Effects on Sleep Parameters as Measured by the CSHQ. *Biomedicines* 2022, *10*, 1685. [CrossRef] [PubMed]
14. Lowin, T.; Kok, C.; Smutny, S.; Pongratz, G. Impact of Δ^9-Tetrahydrocannabinol on Rheumatoid Arthritis Synovial Fibroblasts Alone and in Co-Culture with Peripheral Blood Mononuclear Cells. *Biomedicines* 2022, *10*, 1118. [CrossRef]
15. Golan, H.; Mechoulam, R.; Smoum, R.; Cohen-Zada, E.; Pri-Chen, S.; Wiener, S.; Grinberg, I.; Bar-Lev, D.D.; Haj, C.G.; Fisher, T.; et al. Anti-Tumorigenic Effect of a Novel Derivative of 2-Hydroxyoleic Acid and the Endocannabinoid Anandamide on Neuroblastoma Cells. *Biomedicines* 2022, *10*, 1552. [CrossRef]
16. Greiner, B.; Sommerfeld, M.; Kintscher, U.; Unger, T.; Kappert, K.; Kaschina, E. Differential Regulation of MMPs, Apoptosis and Cell Proliferation by the Cannabinoid Receptors CB1 and CB2 in Vascular Smooth Muscle Cells and Cardiac Myocytes. *Biomedicines* 2022, *10*, 3271. [CrossRef]
17. Mottarlini, F.; Fumagalli, M.; Castillo-Díaz, F.; Piazza, S.; Targa, G.; Sangiovanni, E.; Pacchetti, B.; Sodergren, M.H.; Dell'Agli, M.; Fumagalli, F.; et al. Single and Repeated Exposure to Cannabidiol Differently Modulate BDNF Expression and Signaling in the Cortico-Striatal Brain Network. *Biomedicines* 2022, *10*, 1853. [CrossRef]
18. Duranti, A.; Beldarrain, G.; Álvarez, A.; Sbriscia, M.; Carloni, S.; Balduini, W.; Alonso-Alconada, D. The Endocannabinoid System as a Target for Neuroprotection/Neuroregeneration in Perinatal Hypoxic–Ischemic Brain Injury. *Biomedicines* 2022, *11*, 28. [CrossRef]
19. Chacon, F.T.; Raup-Konsavage, W.M.; Vrana, K.E.; Kellogg, J.J. Secondary Terpenes in *Cannabis sativa* L.: Synthesis and Synergy. *Biomedicines* 2022, *10*, 3142. [CrossRef]
20. Tudorancea, I.M.; Ciorpac, M.; Stanciu, G.D.; Caratașu, C.; Săcărescu, A.; Ignat, B.; Burlui, A.; Rezuș, E.; Creangă, I.; Alexa-Stratulat, T.; et al. The Therapeutic Potential of the Endocannabinoid System in Age-Related Diseases. *Biomedicines* 2022, *10*, 2492. [CrossRef]
21. Sionov, R.V.; Steinberg, D. Anti-Microbial Activity of Phytocannabinoids and Endocannabinoids in the Light of Their Physiological and Pathophysiological Roles. *Biomedicines* 2022, *10*, 631. [CrossRef] [PubMed]
22. Sestan-Pesa, M.; Shanabrough, M.; Horvath, T.L.; Miletta, M.C. Impaired Ghrelin Signaling Does Not Lead to Alterations of Anxiety-like Behaviors in Adult Mice Chronically Exposed to THC during Adolescence. *Biomedicines* 2023, *11*, 144. [CrossRef] [PubMed]
23. Licitra, R.; Marchese, M.; Naef, V.; Ogi, A.; Martinelli, M.; Kiferle, C.; Fronte, B.; Santorelli, F.M. A Review on the Bioactivity of Cannabinoids on Zebrafish Models: Emphasis on Neurodevelopment. *Biomedicines* 2022, *10*, 1820. [CrossRef]
24. Espinoza-Fonseca, L.M. The benefits of the multi-target approach in drug design and discovery. *Bioorg. Med. Chem.* 2006, *14*, 896–897. [CrossRef] [PubMed]

Disclaimer/Publisher's Note: The statements, opinions and data contained in all publications are solely those of the individual author(s) and contributor(s) and not of MDPI and/or the editor(s). MDPI and/or the editor(s) disclaim responsibility for any injury to people or property resulting from any ideas, methods, instructions or products referred to in the content.

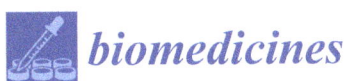

Article

A Longitudinal Observational Study of Medical Cannabis Use and Polypharmacy among Patients Presenting to Dispensaries in Pennsylvania

Emily R. Hajjar [1,*], Allison Herens [2], Erin L. Kelly [3], Kayla Madden [2], Jessica M. Lungen [1] and Brooke K. Worster [2]

1. Jefferson College of Pharmacy, Thomas Jefferson University, Philadelphia, PA 19144, USA
2. Department of Medical Oncology, Sidney Kimmel Cancer Center, Thomas Jefferson University, Philadelphia, PA 19144, USA
3. Department of Family and Community Medicine, Thomas Jefferson University, Philadelphia, PA 19144, USA
* Correspondence: emily.hajjar@jefferson.edu

Abstract: Background: Cannabis use is increasing among adults to treat a variety of health conditions. Given the potential for interactions and adverse events, it is important to assess the use of medical cannabis along with other concomitant medications when assessing for polypharmacy. Methods: The objective of this observational, longitudinal study was to examine medical cannabis (MC) use along with concomitant medications over 12 months in patients with serious medical conditions enrolled in the Pennsylvania (PA) Department of Health's (DOH) Medical Marijuana Program and to collect and catalog which forms of MC patients are taking along with their concomitant medications. Results: There were 213 participants who completed the baseline surveys in full, and 201, 187, and 175 who completed the 1, 6, and 12-month follow-up surveys. The mean age of the participants was 41.3 years, and 54.5% were female. The mean number of MC products taken at baseline was 3.41 and 3.47 at the 12-month survey. Participants took an average of 3.76 (SD 3.15) medications at baseline and 3.65 (SD 3.4) at 12 months. Most commonly used concomitant medications at baseline included vitamins (42.3%), antidepressants (29.1%), analgesics (22.1%), herbal products (19.7%), and anxiolytics (17.8%). Conclusion: Participants used multiple medical cannabis products to treat a number of medication conditions in conjunction with multiple medications.

Keywords: medical cannabis; polypharmacy

Citation: Hajjar, E.R.; Herens, A.; Kelly, E.L.; Madden, K.; Lungen, J.M.; Worster, B.K. A Longitudinal Observational Study of Medical Cannabis Use and Polypharmacy among Patients Presenting to Dispensaries in Pennsylvania. *Biomedicines* **2023**, *11*, 158. https://doi.org/10.3390/biomedicines11010158

Academic Editor: Wesley M. Raup-Konsavage

Received: 30 November 2022
Revised: 5 January 2023
Accepted: 6 January 2023
Published: 8 January 2023

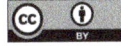

Copyright: © 2023 by the authors. Licensee MDPI, Basel, Switzerland. This article is an open access article distributed under the terms and conditions of the Creative Commons Attribution (CC BY) license (https://creativecommons.org/licenses/by/4.0/).

1. Introduction

Polypharmacy is the use of multiple medications and can be defined in many ways, with the most common definition being the use of five or more medications [1–3]. While polypharmacy is often needed to treat multiple, concomitant medical conditions, it is associated with negative outcomes such as falls, frailty, malnutrition, hospitalization, cognitive impairments, physical impairment, and increased mortality [2,3]. Traditionally, most polypharmacy research has studied prescription, over-the-counter medications, and complementary and alternative medications that patients get from pharmacies and has not included the use of cannabis products.

More states have approved cannabis in medical or recreational capacities, and the use of cannabis among adults is increasing [4–6]. Daily or almost daily use (defined as 300 or more days in a year) has increased to nearly 4% of all US adults reporting use this frequently [7]. However, most clinicians report having infrequent conversations about cannabis use with patients and even less rarely documenting it in the medical record [8]. Commonly reported indications for using medical cannabis include anxiety, pain, appetite stimulation, and insomnia [9]. While more patients are using cannabis, little is known about how often it is used concomitantly with other medications. Use of cannabis has been associated with the risk of adverse events, overdose, cannabis use disorder, and pharmacokinetic and pharmacodynamic drug–drug interactions. [10–12]. With the rise of medical cannabis, it is important to regularly ask patients in all healthcare settings about the use of MC, regardless of medicinal or recreational purposes, when evaluating the potential risks and benefits of MC use for that specific patient. Given the fact that medical cannabis is often used concomitantly to treat conditions that can also be treated with prescription medications, our goal was to evaluate cannabis use patterns over the course of 12 months for patients enrolled in a state medical cannabis program.

2. Materials and Methods

The objective of this observational, longitudinal study was to examine medical cannabis (MC) use over 12 months on polypharmacy in patients with serious medical conditions as defined by the Pennsylvania (PA) Department of Health's (DOH) Medical Marijuana Program, as well as collect and catalog which forms of MC patients are taking and what their concomitant medications are. This study was conducted in partnership with Ethos Cannabis, a state-approved dispensary that has locations across PA. Informed consent, the baseline survey, and the follow-up surveys were administered over the phone and recorded by study staff in Qualtrics. Follow-up surveys occurred after one-, six-, and twelve-month periods.

2.1. Participants

Participants were recruited from dispensaries located throughout PA, through newspaper articles, and in local presentations to community members. Dispensary staff alerted patients to the study by providing flyers with all delivered and in-store purchases, posting information on their website, and verbally asking patients about their interest in participation. If patients agreed to be contacted, dispensary staff securely submitted their contact information to study staff on a weekly basis, or patients could contact study staff directly by phone or email.

Patients were included in the study based on the following criteria: (1) age of at least 18 years old; (2) certification to use MC through the Pennsylvania Medical Marijuana Program, diagnosed by a healthcare provider and self-described as suffering from refractory symptoms or impaired quality of life despite previous medical management; (3) enrollment in the PA DOH Medical Marijuana Program; and (4) reported purchases of cannabis only through state-regulated dispensaries. The rationale for restricting purchases from state-regulated dispensaries was to enable two key aims for the larger, longitudinal study aimed at characterizing information related to MC products available in the PA dispensaries (pills, oils, topical formulations, liquids, and dry leaf or plant formulations for vaporization) and comparing this information to self-reported use [13]. Synthetic and prescription products such as dronabinol (Marinol®), nabilone (Cesamet®), and cannabidiol (Epidiolex®) were not included in this study as they are only available by prescription and are not available in medical marijuana dispensaries in Pennsylvania. Additionally, the rationale for why an individual uses cannabis on any given day may vary between use for medical or recreational purposes. Therefore, it is not practical to require participants to use the products in a strictly 'medical' sense. Exclusion criteria included: (1) known history of ongoing, active substance use disorder (including alcohol) and (2) pregnancy or breastfeeding. Female subjects were asked to sign a waiver attesting to not being pregnant or lactating.

2.2. Measures

2.2.1. Demographics

Demographics were collected at baseline using four items that asked participants their current age, ethnicity (*Latino or Hispanic*), race (*White, Black/African American, American Indian, Alaska Native, Asian, Native Hawaiian or Pacific Islander, or Other*), and gender (*Female, Male, Transgender female, Transgender male, or Other/non-binary*).

2.2.2. Medical Conditions

At baseline, study personnel obtained the certifying medical condition(s) that brought patients to the dispensary. Next, participants were asked to report any other current medical conditions and the number of years since they were first diagnosed with each condition. In addition, the certifying medical condition recorded in the Pennsylvania Medical Marijuana Program database was also obtained through record review.

2.2.3. Medications

At baseline, participants self-reported any medications, supplements, or vitamins that they were actively using. For each follow-up, participants were asked if they were still taking each medication listed in their prior survey and to list any new medications that they were taking. For previously reported medications, participants were asked if the medication had been discontinued and if there had been any dosing changes. For each medication, participants were asked to report the corresponding medical condition and if the medication was related to their certifying condition.

The medications were categorized and recoded by a pharmacist and a pharmacy student on the study team and were then reviewed by a physician and a psychologist for any further clarification, with any discrepancies resolved through consensus among the three team members. The total number of medications used was calculated for each time point. For all follow-up surveys, the number of medications that were pre-existing, new, or stopped were calculated. For pre-specified medication categories (antidepressants, anxiolytics, benzodiazepines, opioids, sedatives/hypnotics, and stimulants; pre-existing medications), dosage changes were calculated as well (unchanged, increased, decreased, or discontinued).

2.2.4. Medical Cannabis Use and Products

At baseline, participants self-reported their MC use patterns and detailed what products they were currently using, if any. For each product, participants were asked to report the manufacturer, brand, formulation (*vaporization cartridge, flower, capsules, tincture, topical, patch, extract, suppository, RSO/edible oil, other*), route of administration (*oral, topical, inhaled, rectal*), CBD and THC percentages and ratios, and type (*indica, sativa, hybrid*). Participants were also asked to report the dosage (*number of inhalations, drops,* etc.) and frequency of use of each product. Participants were asked to report their daily use of each product (1 = *1 time per day* up to 7 = *7 or more times per day*) and how many days per week they used each product (1 = *less than once a week* up to 8 = *seven days a week*).

In each follow-up survey, participants were asked if they were still using any of the products listed in the previous survey and, if so, for updated information on dosage and frequency. If participants reported they were no longer using a specific product, the reason for discontinuation was collected (*did not work, prefer other meds, too expensive, side effects, dispensary too far, availability, other*). Participants were asked to report any new products and all corresponding information about them and the participants' use of them (brand, strain, formulation, route, CBD/THC percentages and ratios, type, dosage, and frequency). A count of total products was calculated as well as counts of discontinued and new products.

During follow-up surveys, participants were asked if they had been using MC since their last survey (*yes—in the last week, yes—but not in the last week, yes—but not in the last month, no*). If participants reported that they had not used MC in the last month or since the last survey, the reason for discontinuation was collected (*did not work, prefer other meds, too expensive, side effects, dispensary too far, availability, other*). If participants responded that they used MC in the last week, it was followed by asking about the frequency of use in the last week (*never, sometimes, regularly*). Next, participants were asked if they had sought guidance about their MC products from their certifying physician or dispensary staff since the last survey (*yes, no*). If participants responded *no*, they were asked if they would be willing to talk to their certifying physician or dispensary staff about trying a different MC product (*yes, maybe, no*).

2.2.5. Side Effects

In all follow-up surveys, participants self-reported any side effects they experienced from MC since the last survey and rated each side effect on an intensity scale (1 = *mild* to 3 = *severe*). In all subsequent surveys, participants were asked if previously reported side effects continued and, if yes, to rate their severity. The counts of total current and discontinued side effects were calculated, as well as the average side effect severity.

2.2.6. Symptoms and Quality of Life

Information on quality of life and the impact of MC on symptoms was collected. This information is reported in other publications.

3. Results

There were initially 215 participants enrolled who were certified to use MC in PA for a serious medical condition between May and October 2020. A total of 594 individuals contacted research staff regarding their interest in participating in the study, of these 594 potential participants, 213 enrolled (2 did not complete the baseline), for a 35% response rate. Of the 379 individuals who did not enroll, reasons included: not meeting criteria (n = 18), declining or withdrawing once the study procedures were reviewed (n = 27), or losing contact after an initial response/no response to our initial outreach (n = 334). An additional 2 participants were not able to complete the baseline survey after initiating the consent process with study staff, and their data were not included in the final sample of 213 participants.

Of the 213 participants who enrolled and completed the baseline surveys in full, 201 participants were retained at their one-month follow-up, 187 were retained at their six-month follow-up, and 175 were retained at their one-year follow-up. Of those who did not complete the study, 35 were lost to follow-up, and 5 declined to participate further.

The mean age of the participants was 41.3 years, with 54.5% being female (Table 1). The mean number of self-reported cannabis products taken at baseline was 3.41 and 3.47 during the 12-month survey (Table 2). Additionally, 55.4% of participants reported using MC via 1 route with 44.6% using MC in 2 or more routes (Table 2). The most common self-reported routes of administration were inhalation (93% at baseline, 86% at 12 months) and oral (44% at baseline, 37.7% at 12 months) (Table 2). A vast majority of patients continued to use cannabis throughout the study period in some form or another, as only 5 patients (2.9%) stopped using cannabis altogether at the 12-month survey. When looking at specific cannabis products, usage varied across the time points, with 55–78% of participants using a product previously reported at an earlier time point. In addition, 43–64% of participants reported using a new medical cannabis product compared to the survey before, and 69–78% of participants reported discontinuing a product.

Table 1. Participant Characteristics.

Variable		Total (N = 213)
Gender	Male	94 (44.1%)
	Female	116 (54.5%)
	Other/Non-binary	3 (1.4%)
Age	Mean (SD)	41.3 (13.3)
	Range	18–78
Race	White	149 (70%)
	Black/African-American	33 (15.5%)
	Asian	6 (2.8%)
	Other/Prefer not to answer	24 (9.4%)
Ethnicity	Hispanic or Latino	20 (9.4%)
	Non-Hispanic/Latino	183 (85.9%)
	Prefer not to answer	10 (4.7%)
Already using cannabis for certifying condition	Yes (n, %)	165 (77.5%)
Use of benzodiazepine, opioid, or sedative	Yes (n, %)	51 (23.9%)
Certifying conditions via PA state database [1]	Chronic Pain/Neuropathy	105 (49.3%)
	Anxiety	78 (36.6%)
	PTSD	33 (15.5%)
	Opioid Use Disorder	10 (4.7%)
	GI disorder (IBD, IBS, Crohn's)	6 (2.8%)
	Cancer	3 (1.4%)
	HIV	2 (0.9%)
	Parkinson's disease	1 (0.5%)
	Epilepsy/Seizure disorder	2 (0.9%)
Self-reported reason for use [1]	Chronic Pain/Neuropathy	108 (50.7%)
	Anxiety	95 (44.6%)
	PTSD	45 (21.1%)
	Opioid Use Disorder	11 (5.2%)
	GI disorder (IBD, IBS, Crohn's)	8 (3.8%)
	Depression	7 (3.3%)
	Arthritis	6 (2.8%)
	Insomnia	5 (2.3%)
	Seizure disorder	4 (1.9%)
	Fibromyalgia	2 (0.9%)
	HIV	2 (0.9%)
	Migraines	1 (0.5%)
	Cancer	1 (0.5%)
	ADHD	1 (0.5%)
	Multiple Sclerosis	1 (0.5%)
	Neurocognitive	1 (0.5%)
Symptom count	Median (Range)	4 (1–14)
Number of medical conditions reported [2]	Median (Range)	3 (1–12)

Note. [1] Participants could list more than one condition; [2] Medical conditions related and unrelated to cannabis certification.

Table 2. Medical Cannabis Usage.

	Baseline (N = 213)	1 Month (N = 201)	6 Months (N = 187)	12 Months (N = 175)
	N (%)	N (%)	N (%)	N (%)
Number of Participants taking a MC product				
Existing Product (reported at a previous survey)	213 (100%)	157 (78.1%)	103 (55.0%)	116 (66.3%)
New Products		87 (43.3%)	121 (64.7%)	90 (51.4%)
Discontinued Products		140 (69.7%)	146 (78.1%)	125 (71.4%)
Number of Self-Reported MC Products				
		Mean (SD)		
Existing		1.82 (1.53)	1.13 (1.36)	1.48 (1.63)
New Products		1.53 (1.44)	2.35 (1.62)	1.99 (1.94)
Discontinued Products		1.55 (1.40)	2.01 (1.63)	1.80 (1.53)
Total Current Products	3.41 (1.52)	3.35 (1.81)	3.48 (1.89)	3.47 (2.45)
Self-Reported MC Formulations				
Inhalation	198 (93%)	185 (92%)	161 (86.1%)	151 (86.3%)
Oral	94 (44.1%)	81 (40.3%)	75 (40.1%)	66 (37.7%)
Topical	35 (16.4%)	36 (17.9%)	24 (12.8%)	20 (11.4%)
Suppository	1 (0.5%)	3 (1.5%)	4 (2.1%)	4 (2.3%)
Number of Self-Reported Routes of Administration				
1 route	118 (55.4%)	114 (56.7%)	109 (58.3%)	101 (57.7%)
2 routes	75 (35.2%)	64 (31.8%)	59 (31.6%)	57 (32.6%)
3 routes	20 (9.4%)	21 (10.4%)	11 (5.9%)	9 (5.1%)
4 routes	0	0	1 (0.5%)	0

Participants took an average of 3.76 (SD 3.15; range of 0–10) medications in addition to their medical cannabis at baseline and 3.65 (SD 3.4; range 0–15) at 12 months. Additionally, 35.2% of patients at baseline and 31.4% of patients at the 12-month survey were taking five or more medications. The most commonly used concomitant medications at baseline included vitamins (42.3%), antidepressants (29.1%), analgesics (22.1%), herbal products (19.7%), and anxiolytics (17.8%) (Table 3). Those medication classes stayed consistent in terms of prevalence at the 12-month mark as well.

Table 3. Most Commonly Used Medications.

Medication Class	Baseline (N = 213)	1 Month (N = 201)	6 Months (N = 187)	12 Months (N = 175)
Vitamins	90 (42.3%)	80 (39.8%)	68 (36.4%)	62 (35.4%)
Antidepressant	62 (29.1%)	58 (28.9%)	54 (28.9%)	45 (25.7%)
Analgesic	47 (22.1%)	43 (21.4%)	31 (16.6%)	31 (17.7%)
Herbal product	42 (19.7%)	38 (18.9%)	31 (16.6%)	27 (15.4%)
Anxiolytic	38 (17.8%)	31 (15.4%)	25 (13.4%)	22 (12.6%)
Antihypertensive	36 (16.9%)	34 (16.9%)	27 (14.4%)	25 (14.3%)
Antihistamine	35 (16.4%)	34 (16.9%)	27 (14.4%)	25 (14.3%)
Anticonvulsant	30 (14.1%)	29 (14.4%)	24 (12.8%)	23 (13.1%)
Asthma/COPD medication	23 (10.8%)	21 (10.4%)	21 (11.2%)	22 (12.6%)

Medications used to treat the same common indications as medical cannabis were analyzed to see if there was a potential change in usage over time. Those taking antidepressants and anxiolytics remained relatively stable on their medications and doses. In those taking an antidepressant, 69% remained on their original antidepressant, and 66.7% remained on the same dose at the 12-month mark, with 10% of the participants discontinuing their antidepressant at 12 months (Table 4). In those taking an anxiolytic, 71.4% remained on their original medication at 12 months, with 64% taking the same dose. This trend stayed consistent with opioids and sedative-hypnotics as well (Table 4). Of those taking a sedative/hypnotic, 80% remained on the same medication throughout the 12 months, with 92.3% staying on the same dose. Of those taking an opioid, 76.9% remained on their original medication, with 81.8% remaining on the same dose. 9.1% of participants were able to decrease their opioids dose, and 7.7% were able to discontinue their opioids at 12 months (Table 4).

Table 4. Concomitant Medication Dosage Changes.

	1 Month	6 Months	12 Months
Antidepressant Dosing Changes	N = 62	N = 58	N = 54
Increased dosage	4 (4.8%)	7 (12.1%)	2 (3.7%)
Same dosage	58 (93.5%)	41 (70.7%)	36 (66.7%)
Decreased dosage	2 (1%)	3 (5.2%)	4 (7.4%)
Anxiolytic Dosage Changes	N = 38	N = 31	N = 25
Increased dosage	0	0	0
Same dosage	29 (76.3%)	19 (61.3%)	16 (64.0%)
Decreased dosage	2 (5.3%)	2 (6.5%)	3 (12.0%)
Sedative/Hypnotic Dosage Changes	N = 13	N = 13	N = 13
Increased dosage	0	1 (7.7%)	0
Same dosage	13 (100%)	8 (61.5%)	12 (92.3%)
Decreased dosage	0	0	0
Opioid Dosage Changes	N = 14	N = 14	N = 11
Increased dosage	0	1 (7.1%)	0
Same dosage	11 (78.6%)	5 (35.7%)	9 (81.8%)
Decreased dosage	2 (14.3%)	2 (14.3%)	1 (9.1%)

The most commonly reported side effects of MC usage included dry mouth, increased appetite, and drowsiness/fatigue (Table 5). Those remained relatively constant across all time points. The most commonly reported reason for discontinuation of an MC product include availability, the MC product not being effect, and the preference to use another medication (Table 6).

Table 5. Most Common Self-Reported Side Effects.

Side Effect	1 Month N (%)	6 Months N (%)	12 Months N (%)
Dry mouth	24 (11.9%)	21 (11.2%)	18 (10.3%)
Increased appetite	21 (10.4%)	33 (17.6%)	20 (11.4%)
Drowsiness/fatigue	19 (9.5%)	27 (14.4%)	16 (9.1%)
Anxiety	8 (4%)	12 (6.4%)	12 (6.9%)
Impaired mentation	7 (3.5%)	15 (8%)	9 (5.1%)
Cough	4 (2%)	7 (3.7%)	10 (5.7%)
Headaches/migraines	4 (2%)	6 (3.2%)	5 (2.9%)
Nausea/vomiting	4 (2%)	2 (1.1%)	1 (0.6%)
Dry eyes	3 (1.5%)	3 (1.6%)	2 (1.1%)
Lung/breathing problems	3 (1.5%)	3 (1.6%)	4 (2.3%)

Table 6. Reasons for discontinuation of a MC product.

	1 Month N (%)	6 Months N (%)	12 Months N (%)
Availability	95 (47.3%)	113 (60.4%)	74 (42.4%)
Not effective	15 (7.5%)	36 (19.2%)	12 (6.9%)
Prefer other medications	8 (4.0%)	4 (2.1%)	20 (11.5%)
Cost	8 (4.0%)	5 (2.6%)	3 (1.7%)
Side effects	5 (2.5%)	1 (0.5%)	3 (1.7%)

4. Discussion

The purpose of this survey was to assess participants' medical cannabis usage within the Pennsylvania Medical Marijuana Program. The data collected in this survey provide needed information about the demographics, numbers of cannabis products used over time, routes of administration, and concomitant medication use of patients enrolled in a state-run medical cannabis program over the course of the year.

This study highlights the fact that patients take multiple medical cannabis products along with multiple other medications. While the average number of concomitant medications was low, it is important to recognize that patients reported using up to 15 additional medications along with cannabis, and approximately 30% were taking 5 or more medications. Some patients may choose to use cannabis as a sole agent or as an adjunctive treatment to other medications, as evidenced by the proportion of patients concomitantly using opioids, benzodiazepines, and antidepressants. The use of medical cannabis can impact the levels of other medications and may have synergistic effects with patients also taking benzodiazepines, sedative-hypnotics, and opioids [14].

Approximately 40% of study participants did report using vitamins, and nearly 20% reported using complementary and alternative medications along with their cannabis. This may be an indication that some people are seeking more natural ways to treat conditions in addition to or as a replacement for prescription medications [15,16].

Another important aspect of the data is that participants exhibited high rates of starting new cannabis products and discontinuing others at each of the follow-up survey time periods. This could be due to patients needing to experiment with various products to find the one that works best for them, as patients exhibit different sensitivities to cannabis depending on the dose, dosage form, and prior use history [8]. This could also be due to product availability, as cannabis products may or may not be available over time depending on demand or crop production [8].

This study has several limitations. First, this study did attempt to look at the specific information for each MC product that participants reported taking. Unfortunately, it was evident during data collection that patient recall of specific information such as THC/CBD percent or ratios was hard to gather for each individual product. This may be due to the fact that people used various products at different times of the day and had a hard time recalling each one individually and the fact that MC products are often interchanged due to varied product availability over time. Patients were able to express that they use certain forms a certain number of times per day, but they may have had multiple products within the same dosage form. For example, patients could verbalize that they used a tincture multiple times per day, but they may have used one type of tincture in the morning and another later in the day depending on therapeutic effects they were looking to achieve or what types of adverse effects they were trying to avoid. For future studies, the challenge of self-reported data will impact how questions are asked with regard to getting accurate information on the types and composition of MC products used. The lack of participant recall also highlights the challenges of using MC in a clinical sense, in that patients could say they were using MC but did not know much more about the individual products. This also underscores the fact that clinicians who are trying to guide the patient's choice of product may prefer to reference documented objective data (dispensing data) as opposed to self-report if small details are needed to help inform therapy decisions.

Another limitation was that study participants were recruited from dispensaries, which may have led to a sample bias toward those that heavily rely on cannabis for symptom management. This may have also impacted the number of people that stopped using cannabis altogether due to lack of efficacy or intolerable side effects, as a majority of patients continued to use MC products throughout the study. Data from a meta-analysis on the efficacy of cannabis in the treatment of pain found that 10% of participants withdrew due to adverse effects [17]. Other meta-analyses on cannabis in multiple sclerosis and chemotherapy-associated nausea and vomiting also found that study withdrawal rates were higher in those taking cannabis as opposed to a placebo [18,19].

Furthermore, the sample was mostly comprised of individuals who identified as white. This may be due to known differences in cannabis use by race [20]. Future surveys should focus on recruiting more diverse participants from both cannabis dispensaries and non-dispensary locations to get a sample more indicative of general use. Lastly, this study was conducted during the COVID-19 pandemic, which may have impacted patients' MC and medication use due to potential social, economic, behavioral, physical, and mental health changes incurred as a result of this world-wide event [21,22].

5. Conclusions

Participants used multiple medical cannabis products to treat a number of medical conditions in conjunction with multiple prescription, over-the-counter, complementary, and alternative products. There is a high rate of variability from time point to time point as to what products people are using, so it is best to continually reassess patient use of medical cannabis products.

Author Contributions: Conceptualization, E.R.H., E.L.K. and B.K.W.; methodology, E.R.H., E.L.K. and B.K.W.; software, E.L.K. and A.H.; validation, E.L.K. and A.H.; formal analysis, A.H. and E.L.K.; investigation, A.H. and K.M.; resources, B.K.W. and E.L.K.; data curation, E.R.H., A.H., K.M., J.M.L. and B.K.W.; writing—original draft preparation, E.R.H.; writing—review and editing, E.R.H., A.H., E.L.K., K.M., J.M.L. and B.K.W.; visualization, E.R.H., A.H. and E.L.K.; supervision, B.K.W.; project administration, E.L.K., A.H., K.M. and B.K.W.; funding acquisition. B.K.W. All authors have read and agreed to the published version of the manuscript.

Funding: MLH Explorations, LLC.

Institutional Review Board Statement: The study was conducted according to the guidelines of the Declaration of Helsinki and approved by the Institutional Review Board of Thomas Jefferson University (IRB# 17C.478 approved 12/18/19).

Informed Consent Statement: Informed consent was obtained from all subjects involved in the study.

Conflicts of Interest: The authors declare no conflict of interest.

References

1. Masnoon, N.; Shakib, S.; Kalisch-Ellett, L.; Caughey, G.E. What is polypharmacy? A systematic review of definitions. *BMC Geriatr.* **2017**, *17*, 230. [CrossRef] [PubMed]
2. Pazan, F.; Wehling, M. Polypharmacy in older adults: A narrative review of definitions, epidemiology and consequences. *Eur. Geriatr. Med.* **2021**, *12*, 443–452. [CrossRef] [PubMed]
3. Khezrian, M.; McNeil, C.J.; Murray, A.D.; Myint, P.K. An overview of prevalence, determinants and health outcomes of polypharmacy. *Ther. Adv. Drug Saf.* **2020**, *11*, 2042098620933741. [CrossRef] [PubMed]
4. Grigorian, A.; Lester, E.; Lekawa, M.; Figueroa, C.; Kuza, C.M.; Dolich, M.; Schubl, S.D.; Barrios, C., Jr.; Nahmias, J. Marijuana use and outcomes in adult and pediatric trauma patients after legalization in California. *Am. J. Surg.* **2019**, *218*, 1189–1194. [CrossRef] [PubMed]
5. Levine, M.; Jontz, A.; Dabrowski, P.; Claudius, I.A.; Kreisler, R.; Yee, N.; LoVecchio, F. Prevalence of marijuana use among trauma patients before and after legalization of medical marijuana: The Arizona experience. *Subst. Abus.* **2021**, *42*, 366–371. [CrossRef] [PubMed]
6. Smart, R.; Pacula, R.L. Early evidence of the impact of cannabis legalization on cannabis use, cannabis use disorder, and the use of other substances: Findings from state policy evaluations. *Am. J. Drug Alcohol Abus.* **2019**, *45*, 644–663. [CrossRef] [PubMed]
7. Substance Abuse and Mental Health Services Administration, Center for Behavioral Health Statistics and Quality. 2019 National Survey on Drug Use and Health: Detailed Tables. 11 September 2020. Available online: https://www.samhsa.gov/data/report/2019-nsduh-detailed-tables (accessed on 11 November 2022).
8. Worster, B.; Ashare, R.L.; Hajjar, E.; Garber, G.; Smith, K.; Kelly, E.L. Clinician Attitudes, Training, and Beliefs About Cannabis: An Interprofessional Assessment. *Cannabis Cannabinoid Res*; 2021; *ahead of print*. [CrossRef]
9. Kimless, D.; Caloura, M.; Markos, V.; Ryan, J.; Abbonizio, S.; Janicki, S. An Observational Cross-Sectional Survey Exploring the Indications for and Responses to Medical Marijuana Use in Certified Patients in Pennsylvania. *J. Prim. Care Community Health* **2022**, *13*, 21501319221129734. [CrossRef] [PubMed]
10. Doohan, P.T.; Oldfield, L.D.; Arnold, J.C.; Anderson, L.L. Cannabinoid Interactions with Cytochrome P450 Drug Metabolism: A Full-Spectrum Characterization. *AAPS J.* **2021**, *23*, 91. [CrossRef] [PubMed]
11. Alsherbiny, M.A.; Li, C.G. Medicinal Cannabis-Potential Drug Interactions. *Medicines* **2018**, *6*, 3. [CrossRef] [PubMed]
12. Hill, K.P.; Gold, M.S.; Nemeroff, C.B.; McDonald, W.; Grzenda, A.; Widge, A.S.; Rodriguez, C.; Kraguljac, N.V.; Krystal, J.H.; Carpenter, L.L. Risks and Benefits of Cannabis and Cannabinoids in Psychiatry. *Am. J. Psychiatry* **2022**, *179*, 98–109. [CrossRef] [PubMed]
13. Pennsylvania General Assembly. 2016 Act 16. Medical Marijuans Act-Enactment. Available online: https://www.legis.state.pa.us/cfdocs/legis/li/uconsCheck.cfm?yr=2016&sessInd=0&act=16 (accessed on 19 December 2022).
14. Brown, J.D.; Winterstein, A.G. Potential Adverse Drug Events and Drug-Drug Interactions with Medical and Consumer Cannabidiol (CBD) Use. *J. Clin. Med.* **2019**, *8*, 989. [CrossRef] [PubMed]
15. Deuel, L.M.; Seeberger, L.C. Complementary Therapies in Parkinson Disease: A Review of Acupuncture, Tai Chi, Qi Gong, Yoga, and Cannabis. *Neurotherapeutics* **2020**, *17*, 1434–1455. [CrossRef] [PubMed]
16. Ingram, G.; Pearson, O.R. Cannabis and multiple sclerosis. *Pract. Neurol.* **2019**, *19*, 310–315. [CrossRef] [PubMed]
17. Mücke, M.; Phillips, T.; Radbruch, L.; Petzke, F.; Häuser, W. Cannabis-based medicines for chronic neuropathic pain in adults. *Cochrane Database Syst. Rev.* **2018**, *3*, CD012182. [CrossRef] [PubMed]
18. Smith, L.A.; Azariah, F.; Lavender, V.T.; Stoner, N.S.; Bettiol, S. Cannabinoids for nausea and vomiting in adults with cancer receiving chemotherapy. *Cochrane Database Syst. Rev.* **2015**, *2015*, CD009464. [CrossRef] [PubMed]
19. Filippini, G.; Minozzi, S.; Borrelli, F.; Cinquini, M.; Dwan, K. Cannabis and cannabinoids for symptomatic treatment for people with multiple sclerosis. *Cochrane Database Syst. Rev.* **2022**, *5*, CD013444. [CrossRef] [PubMed]
20. Pacek, L.R.; Mauro, P.M.; Martins, S.S. Perceived risk of regular cannabis use in the United States from 2002 to 2012: Differences by sex, age, and race/ethnicity. *Drug Alcohol Depend.* **2015**, *149*, 232–244. [CrossRef] [PubMed]
21. Caroppo, E.; Mazza, M.; Sannella, A.; Marano, G.; Avallone, C.; Claro, A.E.; Janiri, D.; Moccia, L.; Janiri, L.; Sani, G. Will Nothing Be the Same Again? Changes in Lifestyle during COVID-19 Pandemic and Consequences on Mental Health. *Int. J. Environ. Res. Public Health* **2021**, *18*, 8433. [CrossRef] [PubMed]
22. Di Renzo, L.; Gualtieri, P.; Pivari, F.; Soldati, L.; Attinà, A.; Cinelli, G.; Leggeri, C.; Caparello, G.; Barrea, L.; Scerbo, F.; et al. Eating habits and lifestyle changes during COVID-19 lockdown: An Italian survey. *J. Transl. Med.* **2020**, *18*, 229. [CrossRef] [PubMed]

Disclaimer/Publisher's Note: The statements, opinions and data contained in all publications are solely those of the individual author(s) and contributor(s) and not of MDPI and/or the editor(s). MDPI and/or the editor(s) disclaim responsibility for any injury to people or property resulting from any ideas, methods, instructions or products referred to in the content.

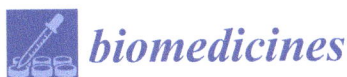

Article

Cannabidiol Decreases Intestinal Inflammation in the Ovariectomized Murine Model of Postmenopause

Karen Mae A. Bacalia [1,2], Kevin M. Tveter [1], Hayley Palmer [1], Jeffrey Douyere [1], Savannah Martinez [1], Ke Sui [1] and Diana E. Roopchand [1,*]

1 Department of Food Science, NJ Institute of Food Nutrition and Health New Brunswick, Rutgers University, New Brunswick, NJ 08901, USA
2 Graduate Program, Department of Nutritional Sciences, Rutgers University, New Brunswick, NJ 08901, USA
* Correspondence: roopchand@sebs.rutgers.edu

Abstract: Cannabidiol (CBD) (25 mg/kg peroral) treatment was shown to improve metabolic outcomes in ovariectomized (OVX) mice deficient in 17β-estradiol (E2). Herein, CBD effects on intestinal and hepatic bile acids (BAs) and inflammation were investigated. Following RNA sequencing of colon tissues from vehicle (VEH)- or CBD-treated sham surgery (SS) or OVX mice (n = 4 per group), differentially expressed genes (DEGs) were sorted in ShinyGO. Inflammatory response and bile secretion pathways were further analyzed. Colon content and hepatic BAs were quantified by LC-MS (n = 8–10 samples/group). Gut organoids were treated with CBD (100, 250, 500 μM) with or without TNFα and lipopolysaccharide (LPS) followed by mRNA extraction and qPCR to assess CBD-induced changes to inflammatory markers. The expression of 78 out of 114 inflammatory response pathway genes were reduced in CBD-treated OVX mice relative to vehicle (VEH)-treated OVX mice. In contrast, 63 of 111 inflammatory response pathway genes were increased in CBD-treated sham surgery (SS) mice compared to VEH-treated SS group and 71 of 121 genes were increased due to ovariectomy. CBD did not alter BA profiles in colon content or liver. CBD repressed *Tnf* and *Nos2* expression in intestinal organoids in a dose-dependent manner. In conclusion, CBD suppressed colonic inflammatory gene expression in E2-deficient mice but was pro-inflammatory in E2-sufficient mice suggesting CBD activity in the intestine is E2-dependent.

Keywords: cannabidiol; inflammation; bile acids; transcriptomics; estrogen deficiency; ovariectomized mice; postmenopause; gut organoids

Citation: Bacalia, K.M.A.; Tveter, K.M.; Palmer, H.; Douyere, J.; Martinez, S.; Sui, K.; Roopchand, D.E. Cannabidiol Decreases Intestinal Inflammation in the Ovariectomized Murine Model of Postmenopause. *Biomedicines* **2023**, *11*, 74. https://doi.org/10.3390/biomedicines11010074

Academic Editor: Wesley M. Raup-Konsavage

Received: 1 December 2022
Revised: 21 December 2022
Accepted: 23 December 2022
Published: 28 December 2022

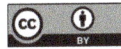

Copyright: © 2022 by the authors. Licensee MDPI, Basel, Switzerland. This article is an open access article distributed under the terms and conditions of the Creative Commons Attribution (CC BY) license (https://creativecommons.org/licenses/by/4.0/).

1. Introduction

In the United States, women typically enter perimenopause in their mid-to-late forties and reach menopause at the average age of 51 [1]. Decline in ovarian 17β-estradiol (E2) levels during the menopause transition results in uncomfortable vasomotor symptoms (e.g., hot flushes) that affect up to 80% of women and can persist for 5–13 years [2–7]. In humans and rodents, the loss of E2 has also been associated with cardiometabolic disease and bone loss [5,6,8] due to reduced gut barrier integrity leading to chronic low-grade inflammation [5,6,9,10]. During the menopause transition, hormone replacement therapy (HRT) is typically prescribed to relieve vasomotor symptoms and HRT was initially believed to mitigate chronic disease [11]. After several clinical studies, HRT appears to be most useful for management of vasomotor symptoms in women under 60 with reported benefits for the cognitive function and decreased risk of bone fracture from osteoporosis [12]. HRT dose and treatment regimen should be individualized according to medical history [13] and the lowest effective dose is generally recommended for no more than 5 years to reduce chronic disease risk [12]. HRT use in women over 60 is associated with increased risk of cancer, heart disease, and stroke [12] leaving this population with few options for symptom management and chronic disease prevention.

Cannabidiol (CBD) is a non-psychotropic phytocannabinoid derived from the industrial hemp plant (*Cannabis sativa* L.). In preclinical studies, CBD was shown to reduce inflammation [14–16], improve gut barrier integrity [17], and protect against bone loss [18–20]. Currently, CBD (i.e., Epidiolex®) is a FDA-approved for treatment of epilepsy-related disorders in both children and adults [21–24]. Although there are currently no studies for the effectiveness of CBD for menopausal or postmenopausal symptoms, a recent survey of 258 perimenopausal and postmenopausal women reported that 86% used medical cannabis and 79% endorsed its use to relieve menopause symptoms [25]. The effects of perorally administered CBD (25 mg/kg/day, 5 days/week for 18 weeks) or vehicle (VEH) treatment (i.e., sesame oil and peanut powder) in the ovariectomized (OVX) mouse model of postmenopause along with sham surgery (SS) controls were recently investigated [26]. Compared to VEH-treated OVX mice, the CBD-treated OVX group had improved oral glucose tolerance, increased energy expenditure, improved bone phenotypes, and the decreased markers of inflammation in bone and intestinal tissues [26]. CBD-treated OVX and SS mice had altered gut microbial communities and BA profiles [26]. Notably, the CBD-treated OVX group, but not the CBD-treated SS group, developed a bloom in *Lactobacillus* species [26]. Studies suggest that probiotic *Lactobacilli* bacteria improve gut barrier integrity leading to the lower levels of inflammatory cytokines in the gut, circulation, and bone [27–31]. A recent meta-analysis of randomized controlled clinical studies cautiously concluded that supplementation with probiotics could increase lumbar bone mineral density in postmenopausal women [32]. BAs modulate gut bacteria [33], inflammation [34], glucose metabolism [35], and bone turnover [36]. Compared to SS groups, several ileal BAs were increased in the VEH-treated OVX group while in CBD-treated OVX mice these BAs were normalized to levels comparable to the SS groups [26].

Oral CBD bioavailability is 6% and increases 4-fold if consumed with fat [37]. Since most ingested CBD would be in the intestinal tract, CBD may improve metabolic health by directly modulating the gut microbiota and/or decreasing intestinal inflammation. In this present study, samples collected from a previously described murine study [26] was used to investigate the response of the colonic transcriptome to CBD or VEH treatment in OVX and SS mice. Targeted metabolomics was performed in order to profile BAs in colon content and liver tissue. Finally, the direct effect of CBD on intestinal inflammation was tested in ileal gut organoids.

2. Materials and Methods

2.1. Chemicals and Materials

Experiments were performed using Optima LC-MS grade formic acid, methanol, acetonitrile, and water purchased from Fisher Scientific (Hampton, NH, USA). Oasis Prime HLB 1cc Cartridges (30 mg) were purchased from Waters (Milford, MA, USA) for filtration of phospholipids from liver samples. Corning Costar Spin-X centrifuge tubes with 0.22 µm nylon membrane (Corning, NY, USA) were used to filter BA extracts prior to injecting. CBD isolate was purchased from Bluebird Botanicals (Louisville, CO, USA). Twelve unconjugated, 9 taurine conjugated, and 6 glycine conjugated BAs were ordered from Sigma-Aldrich Inc. (St. Louis, MO, USA), Cayman Chemical (Ann Arbor, MI, USA), or Steraloids Inc. (Newport, RI, USA). Deuterated internal standards of BAs were purchased from Cayman Chemical. BA and CBD information are detailed in Table S1.

2.2. Animals and Treatment

Animal study protocols were approved by Rutgers institutional animal care and use committee under protocol# PROTO201900041. The details of the mouse study were previously described [26]. Briefly, at age 12 weeks, female wild-type C57BL/6J mice were ovariectomized (OVX) or underwent sham-surgery (SS). After recovery, at age 14 weeks, OVX and SS mice were subdivided to receive either CBD isolate or vehicle (VEH) treatment ($n = 10$ mice/group) for 18 weeks (5 days per week excluding weekends). A calculated volume of VEH (sesame oil) or CBD (25 mg/kg, dissolved in sesame oil, 10 mg/mL) was mixed with 100 mg of powdered peanut butter to prepare individual peroral doses, which were consumed within 1 min of offering. Mice were euthanized by CO_2 asphyxiation and liver, and intestinal tissues were collected as previously described [26]. Individual colon segments were flushed with ice-cold, sterile PBS (pH 7.4) to collect luminal contents. Samples were placed in cryogenic tubes, snap frozen in liquid nitrogen, and stored at −80 °C until analysis.

2.3. Ribonucleic Acid Sequencing (RNA-Seq)

Total ribonucleic acid (RNA) from colon tissue (n = 4 mice/group) was extracted using RNeasy Plus Universal Mini Kit (Catalog#73404, QIAGEN, Germantown, MD, USA). The concentration, quality, and integrity of total RNA was determined using a Nano Drop 2000 spectrophotometer (Thermo Scientific, Wilmington, DE, USA) and RNA samples were provided to Azenta (South Plainfield, NJ, USA) for Standard RNA-Seq processing. Paired-end sequencing was performed using Illumina HiSeq 2 × 150 bp paired-end configuration yielding 124,739 Mbases and 415,802,210 reads.

2.4. RNA Sequencing Data Analysis

Raw reads were pre-processed using FastQC 0.11.9 and Java 14.0.1 software. Phred quality scores of individual sequences were checked before merging paired-end sequences with 20 bp overlap. Trimmomatic-0.39 data analysis software was used to trim adapters of paired-end sequences and assess sequence quality. HISAT2 2.1.0 was used to map reads to a reference mouse genome (grcm38 with Ensembl annotation v38.102) [38]. Differentially expressed genes (DEGs) were analyzed using DESeq2 in R (R Studio v4.2.0) [39]. Gene ontology (GO) enrichment analysis was performed using ShinyGO v0.76.3 (South Dakota State University, Brookings, SD, USA) [40] with the application of FDR correction to generate the list of pathways affected using gene ontology biological processes (GOBP) and Kyoto Encyclopedia of Genes and Genomes (KEGG) databases. The FDR q-value cut-off criteria were assigned as 0.05. The inflammatory response pathway genes were identified in the GOBP network while the bile secretion pathway genes were found in the KEGG network.

PCA plots to compare similarity/difference among RNA-Seq datasets for biological replicates within group and between groups were generated using Metaboanalyst 5.0 [41]. The fold change of DEGs was converted to logCPM (Z-score) values and heat maps of DEGs for each pathway were generated using Euclidean clustering between samples and genes using Origin Pro 2023 software (Origin Lab Corp., Northampton, MA, USA). Venn diagrams were also generated using Origin Pro.

2.5. LC-MS Analysis of Bile Acids

2.5.1. Preparation of Liver and Colon Samples

BAs were extracted from individual liver samples (n = 9–10/group). Frozen liver tissue was sectioned on dry ice and 50–60 mg of median lobe was transferred into 2 mL bead beating tubes with 4 stainless steel beads (2.8 mm, GBSS 089-5000-11, OPS Diagnostics, Lebanon, NJ, USA) and 300 µL of water. Samples were homogenized using a 1600 MiniG® (SPEX SamplePrep, Metuchen, NJ, USA) for 4 min. Homogenized tissue was transferred to microcentrifuge tubes with 300 µL of pre-dried deuterated internal standards (TCA-d4, DCA-d4, CDCA-d4, and GCDCA-d4 at 1 µg/mL each). Protein was precipitated with 99.9% acetonitrile and 1% formic acid (800 µL) and vortexed for 30 s and then placed on an orbital shaker for 1 h at 4 °C. Samples were centrifuged at 13,000× g for 10 min at 4 °C and supernatant was transferred to glass scintillation vials. Pellets remaining after centrifugation was resuspended in 1 mL 80% methanol and sonicated for 1 min with a Qsonica sonicator Q700 with chiller fitted with cuphorn and 8-tube holder (Cole-Palmer, Vernon Hills, IL, USA); 55% AMP, 30 s on, 59 s off, then a final 30 s on). Sonicated samples were centrifuged at 16,000× g for 20 min at 4 °C and supernatants were pooled and dried under speed vacuum at room temperature overnight. Samples were resuspended in 300 µL 50% methanol, placed on orbital shaker for 30 min, vortexed for 2 min, and filtered through Corning® Costar® Spin-X® microcentrifuge tube filters (nylon membrane, pore size 0.22 µm, cat#CLS8169-200ea, Sigma-Aldrich, Darmstadt, Germany) for 5 min at 16,000× g. Samples were transferred into sampler vials (Cat# 6PSV9-1PSS Thermofisher,, Walthm, MA, USA) with 300 µL inserts (9 mm, C4010-630 Thermofisher, Walthm, MA, USA) for HPLC analysis. Concentrations (µg/mg tissue) were determined by dividing final concentrations by tissue weights used for extraction. For each liver sample, the limit of detection (LOD), the limit of quantification (LOQ), and the coefficient of variance (CV) are presented in Table S2. Recoveries ranged from 66–151% for TCA-d4, 35–76% for DCA-d4, 70–102% for GCDCA-d4, and 53–113% for CDCA-d4.

Individual colon content samples (n = 8–9/group) were collected into microfuge tubes by flushing the lumen of the colon with 1× PBS (pH 7.4). The colon content was freeze-dried in a FreeZone 1.0 L Benchtop lyophilizer (model# 7740020, LABCONCO, Kansas City, MO, USA) overnight to evaporate PBS and dry weight (mg) of colon content was recorded. To subtract weight contributed by salts in PBS, 3 tubes containing 1 mL of 1× PBS were freeze-dried and their mean weight was subtracted from dried colon content weights. Deuterated internal standards (TCA-d4, DCA-d4, GCDCA-d4, and CDCA-d4 at 1 µg/mL each) were resuspended in 50% methanol and 300 µL was added to pre-weighed microfuge tubes and dried in speed vacuum (CentriVap concentration system with cold trap, Model 7810014 and 7460020 Labconco, Kansas City, MO, USA), after which colon content (15–30 mg) was added. Then 600 µL of 90% acetonitrile/9.9% water/0.1% formic acid ($v/v/v$) was added to internal standards and dry colon content, vortexed for 1 min, and left on a benchtop shaker at 4 °C for 1 h. After extraction, samples were centrifuged at 15,000× g for 10 min and the supernatant was collected into a clean microfuge tube. For the second round of extraction, 700 µL of 50% methanol/50% water (v/v) was added to the pellet, vortexed for 2 min, and extract was placed in QSonica sonicator Q700 (with chiller fitted with cuphorn and 8-tube holder, Cole-Palmer, Vernon Hills, IL, USA) at 65% amplitude for 2 min. Samples were placed on shaker at 4 °C for 45 min and then centrifuged at 12,000× g for 10 min. Supernatants were transferred to microfuge tubes and extraction was repeated with 600 µL of 90% acetonitrile and 0.1% formic acid. Samples were vortexed for 30 sec and placed in QSonica sonicator at 65% amplitude for 1 min. Samples were placed on shaker at 4 °C for 45 min and then centrifuged at 12,000× g for 10 min. Supernatants from first and second extractions were pooled and solvent was evaporated to dryness using a speed vacuum (CentriVap concentration system with cold trap, Model 7810014 and 7460020 Labconco, Kansas City, MO, USA) and resuspended in 300 µL of 50% methanol. Samples were sonicated at 65% amplitude for 1 min and then filtered using 0.2 µm filters (Corning Costar Spin-x centrifuge tube filters, cat#CLS8169-200ea, Sigma-Aldrich, Darmstadt, Germany). Filtrates were centrifuged at 12,000× g for 10 min and transferred to HPLC vials (6PSV9-1PSS, Thermofisher, Waltham, MA, USA) fitted with 300 µL inserts (9 mm, C4010-630, Thermofisher, Waltham, MA, USA).

For each colon content sample, the limit of detection (LOD), the limit of quantification (LOQ), and the coefficient of variance (CV) are presented in Table S2. Recoveries ranged 94–156% for TCA-d4, 63–124% for DCA-d4, 47–131% for GCDCA-d4, and 75–175% for CDCA-d4.

2.5.2. LC-MS Analysis

Data was generated using an Alliance e2695 HPLC system coupled to a 2998 Photodiode array detector and an Acquity QDa detector mass spectrometer equipped with an electrospray interphase (ESI, Waters, Milford, MA, USA), an autosampler, and a Vacuubrand pump (Essex, CT, USA). For each sample, technical duplicates (10 µL) were injected. The instrument and processing methods have been previously described [26]. A Cortecs C18+ column held at 40 °C (4.6 × 150 mm and 2.7 µm particle size, Waters, Milford, MA, USA) was used to separate analytes and held at the temperature of 40 °C. The mobile phase consisted of 0.1% formic acid in acetonitrile (A) and 0.1% formic acid in water (B). The flow rate was 1 mL/min. A linear gradient was used, specifically: 35–50% A over 30 min, a hold at 50% A for 1 min, an immediate transition to 65% A for 9 min, a gradual increase to 90% A over 2 min, and a hold at 90% A for 6 min. This was immediately followed by a washout with 90% A to 10% A for 6 min before returning to the initial 35% A at 54.1 min, which marked the end of each sample run. The column was allowed to equilibrate for 6 min in 35% A before the next injection. Pure compounds were used to produce standard curves for the quantification of BAs and CBD, as detailed in Table S1.

2.6. Ileal Organoid Experiments

Eight-month-old WT C57BL/6J female mice were euthanized by CO_2 asphyxiation and ileal tissue was collected for crypt isolation according to established methods [42]. Crypts were collected in 1× PBS (pH 7.4, Growcells, Irvine, CA, USA), counted manually, and the concentration of 300 crypts per µL was calculated. Culture was centrifuged at 200× g for 3 min, PBS was aspirated, Cultrex was added to obtain a density of 150 crypts per 25 µL volume, and 48-well plates were seeded with 25 µL Cultrex per well. The plate was incubated in a 37 °C, 5% CO_2 incubator (Galaxy 170, Eppendorf Co., New Brunswick, NJ, USA) for 30 min to allow the polymerization of Cultrex then 250 µL of 1× complete growth medium (CGM) [43] was added per well. CGM was replaced every 2 days. Organoids were passaged every 7 days (1:3 ratio). Mature day 4 organoids were treated with 0, 100, 250, or 500 µM CBD in the presence or absence of Tnfα (100 ng/mL; STEMCELL, Vancouver, BC, Canada) + lipopolysaccharide (LPS; 100 µg/mL; Sigma-Alrich, Darmstadt, Germany) to induce inflammation. Six wells were pooled to create one biological sample ($n = 1$) and treatments were performed in triplicate. Organoids from passages 10–11 were used, and the experiment was performed twice.

CBD (1 mg/mL) was dissolved in 100% methanol and then calculated volumes of this stock were used to obtain 100, 250, or 500 µM CBD concentrations (in 250 µL/well) as well as these same CBD concentrations in combination with lipopolysaccharide (LPS 2 mg/mL 0.9% NaCl stock; 10 µg/mL in CGM; Cat#L6143 Sigma-Alrich) and TNFα (100 µg/mL sterile ddH$_2$O stock; 100 ng/mL in CGM; Cat#78069, STEMCELL). TNFα and LPS alone served as a positive control for inflammation. Samples were dried in speed vacuum (CentriVap concentration system with cold trap, Labconco, Kansas City, MO, USA) and resuspended in CGM media the day of treatment. Organoids were treated for 24 h, CGM was removed, and 500 µL Cultrex organoid harvesting solution (Cat# 3700-100-01, R&D Systems, Minneapolis, MN, USA) was added per well. Organoids (6 wells/treatment) were collected into 15 mL conical tubes precoated with 1× PBS and left to incubate on ice for 1 h to dissolve Cultrex. Samples were centrifuged at 500× g for 5 min at 4 °C, washed with 2 mL of 1× PBS, supernatant was removed, 800 µL of Qiazol was added, and samples were transferred to 1.7 mL microfuge tubes with two 2.8 mm stainless steel beads and frozen at −80 °C until RNA extraction. Samples were thawed on ice followed by vortexing for 30 s, then RNA was extracted using RNeasy plus universal mini kit (Catalog#73404, QIAGEN, Germantown, MD, USA).

2.7. MTT Analysis for Cell Viability

MTT, 3-(4,5-dimethylthiazol-2-yl)-2,5-diphenyltetrazolium bromide reagent (M6494, Thermofisher, Waltham, MA, USA) was diluted 5 mg/mL in sterile 1× PBS per manufacturer's instructions. Concurrently, treatments were performed on an additional 48-well plate of organoids for MTT assay to assess viability. Three wells were used per treatment, including 100% DMSO as a positive control for toxicity. At 24 h post-treatment, 27.5 µL of MTT solution was added to the 250 µL of 1× CGM in each well, then placed in an incubator (37 °C, 5% CO_2) for 2 h. After media and MTT solutions were removed, viable organoids appeared purple/black. Then 50 µL of 2% sodium dodecyl sulfate (SDS) was added to each well and the plate was returned to the incubator (37 °C, 5% CO2) for 1 h. After incubation, 150 µL of pure dimethyl sulfoxide (DMSO) was mixed into each well and incubated for 4 h or overnight to solubilize the formazan crystals. Once solubilization was complete,

200 µL from each well was transferred to a microplate and absorbance was measured in a multimode plate reader (CLARIOStar, BMG Labtech, Cary, NC, USA) at 562 nm.

2.7.1. qPCR of Ileal Organoids and Liver Tissue

RNA was extracted from liver tissue (10–20 mg of right median lobe) as previously described [43]. RNA extracted from organoids or liver samples was quantified by nanodrop and 5 mg was used to prepare cDNA followed by RT-qPCR (QuantStudio 3, Thermo) as previously described [26].

TaqMan™ assay primers (Life Technologies, Carlsbad, CA, USA) used were: *Nos2* (Mm00440502_m1), *Tnfα* (Mm00443258_m1), *Il6* (Mm00446190_m1), and *Il1b* (Mm004342228 _m1). *Hmbs* (Mm01143545_m1) was used as the house keeping gene.

2.8. Statistics

Data were analyzed using GraphPad Prism 8 software (GraphPad Software, Inc., La Jolla, CA, USA). The ROUT test was used to detect and remove any outliers. Normality and variance were tested before choosing parametric or non-parametric tests. To detect differences in liver qPCR and BA analysis, two-way ANOVA was used followed by Benjamini–Hochberg post hoc test with FDR adjustment, $q < 0.05$ was considered significant. Non-parametric BA data were analyzed by Kruskal–Wallis test followed Benjamini–Hochberg post hoc test with FDR adjustment. For organoid experiments, one-way ANOVA was performed followed by Tukey post hoc test, and the significance level was $p < 0.05$.

3. Results

3.1. CBD-Induced Inflammatory Response Pathway Changes in E2-Deficient and -Sufficient Female Mice

A whole transcriptomic RNA-Seq analysis of colon tissues ($n = 4$/group) was performed to investigate differential gene expression due to OVX surgery or CBD treatment. The PCA plot showed that samples within surgery and treatment groups clustered together (Figure S1).

Comparing VEH- and CBD-treated OVX groups, there was a total of 2585 differentially expressed genes (DEGs, $q < 0.05$) of which 1334 genes were upregulated and 1255 were downregulated (Table 1). A comparison of VEH- and CBD-treated SS groups revealed 14,508 DEGs ($q < 0.05$) where 964 genes were upregulated and 13,544 were downregulated (Table 1). There were 3162 DEGs ($q < 0.05$), 1552 increased and 1610 decreased, due to a loss of ovarian E2 (SS+VEH vs. OVX+VEH).

Table 1. Differentially Expressed Genes in Total Transcriptome.

	Upregulated	Downregulated	Total Changed
OVX+VEH vs. OVX+CBD	1334	1255	2589
SS+VEH vs. SS+CBD	964	13,544	14,508
SS+VEH vs. OVX+VEH	1552	1610	3162

The number of differentially expressed genes (DEGs) generated from EdgeR analysis of total transcriptome based on surgery or treatment comparison. Significance based on false discovery rate (FDR) correction ($q < 0.05$). OVX: ovariectomized; SS: sham surgery; VEH: vehicle treatment; CBD: cannabidiol treatment.

Gene ontology (GO) enrichment analysis was performed with ShinyGO for OVX+VEH vs. OVX+CBD, SS+VEH vs. SS+CBD, and SS+VEH vs. OVX+VEH using the gene ontology biological process (GOBP) database. For each of these comparisons, 1000 significantly altered GOBP pathways were identified after FDR correction and the top 20 pathways are shown in Figure S2. In a previous study, relative to VEH-treatment, CBD was found to reduce the expression of inflammatory mediators in the colon (*Il1b*, *Il6*, *Tnf*) and ileum (*Il1b*, *Il6*) in SS and/or OVX mice [26]. To find pathways related to inflammation the GOBP pathways were searched using the key word "inflammatory" and the inflammatory response pathway was found for OVX+VEH vs. OVX+CBD (pathway ranked 323), SS+VEH vs. SS+CBD (pathway ranked 219), and SS+VEH vs. OVX+VEH (pathway ranked 729). Inflammatory pathways were not detected when DEGs were mapped using KEGG.

There were 114 DEGs for the OVX+VEH vs. OVX+CBD comparison, 111 DEGs for the SS+VEH vs. SS+CBD comparison, and 121 DEGs for the SS+VEH vs. OVX+VEH comparison (Figure 1A–D). The annotations of DEGs are provided in Supplementary File S1. There were 39 DEGs uniquely altered due to the CBD treatment of OVX mice and 40 DEGs uniquely altered in the CBD-treated SS group (Figure 1A). For the OVX+VEH vs. OVX+CBD and SS+VEH vs. SS+CBD comparisons, 24 DEGs were in common and all but one (*Epha2*) were changed by CBD in the same direction indicating that the changes were independent of E2 status (Figure 1A,B and Supplementary File S1). There were 34 DEGs due to OVX alone. The remaining overlapping DEGs (40, 11, and 36) were due to either OVX or CBD treatment (Figure 1A). Consistent with prior colon tissue qPCR analysis [26], *Tnf* was significantly decreased in CBD-treated OVX mice compared to VEH-treated OVX mice (Figure 1B,D and Supplementary File S1). *Tnf* was increased in the VEH-treated OVX group compared to the VEH-treated SS group but was not detected as a DEG when comparing the VEH- and CBD-treated SS groups (Figure 1C and Supplementary File S1).

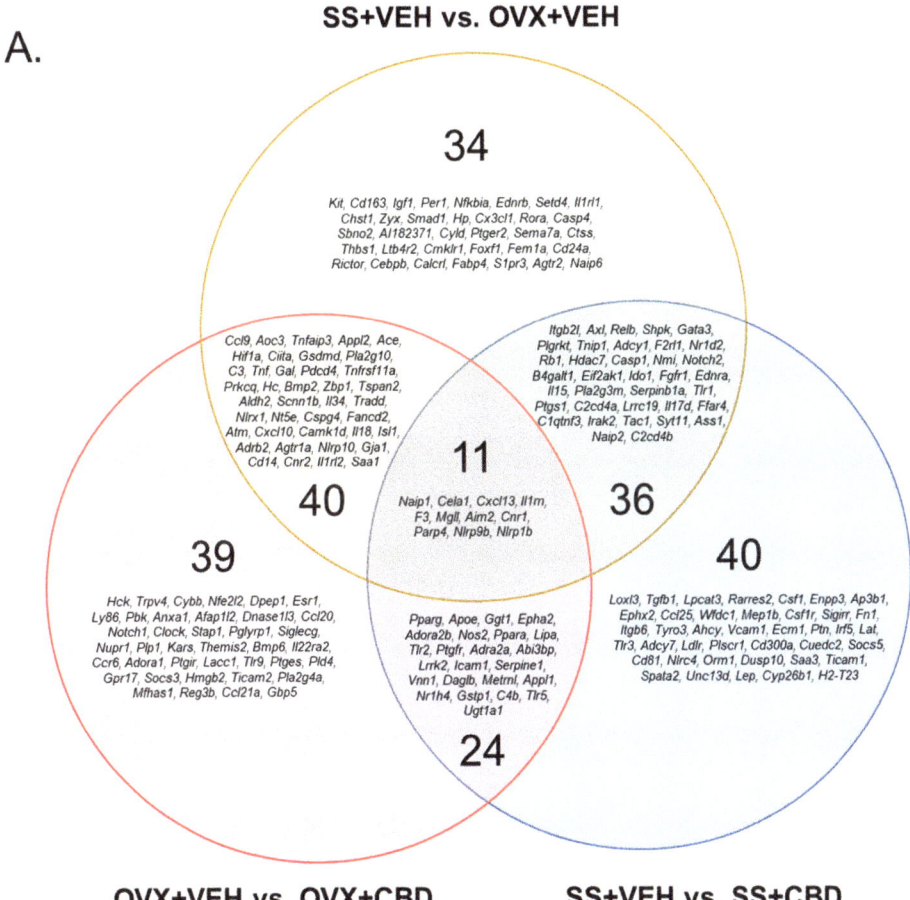

Figure 1. *Cont.*

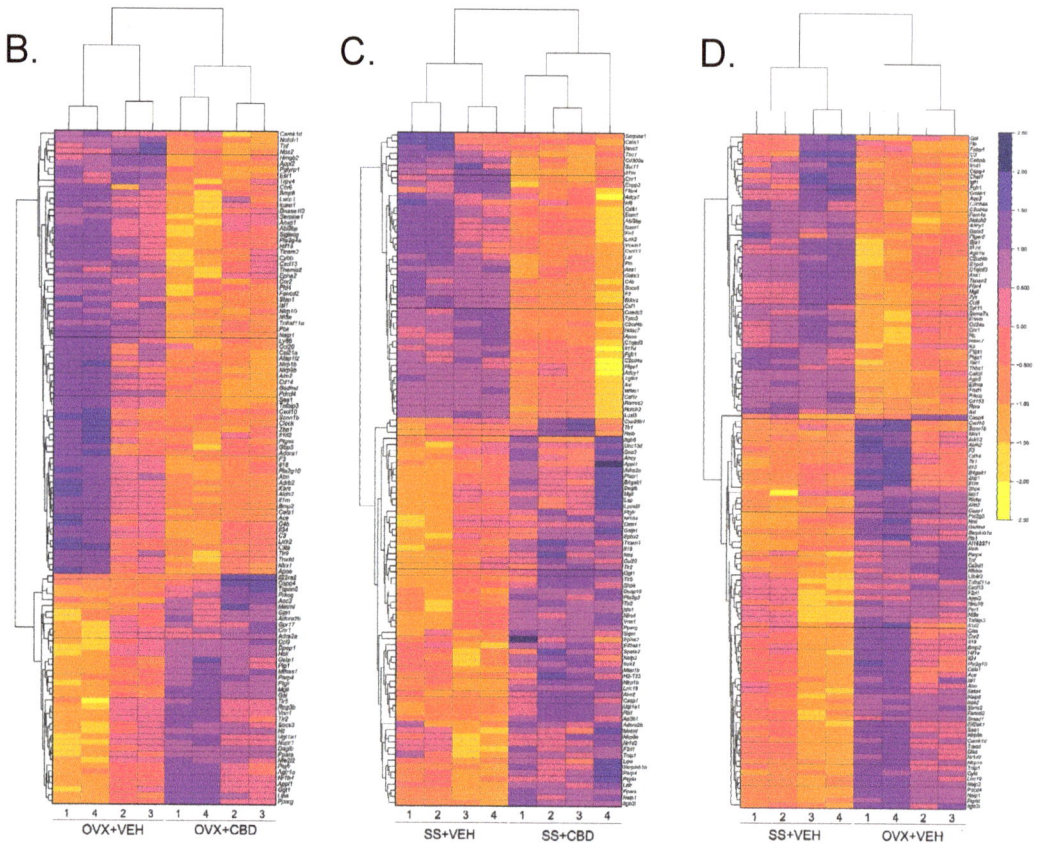

Figure 1. Differentially expressed inflammatory response genes. (**A**) Venn diagram showing the DEGs for each of the indicated comparisons as well as DEGs that are in common between comparisons. DEGs held in common do not necessarily indicate the same direction of change. DEGs for (**B**) OVX+VEH vs. OVX+CBD, (**C**) SS+VEH vs. SS+CBD, and (**D**) SS+VEH vs. OVX+VEH generated based on Euclidean clustering. Z-score scale indicates downregulated genes from 0 to −2.5 (orange to yellow shades) and upregulated genes from 0 to 2.5 (red to purple/navy shades).

For the OVX+VEH vs. OVX+CBD comparison, CBD treatment resulted in the downregulation of 78 of the 114 differentially expressed inflammatory pathway genes (Figure 1B). In contrast, for the SS+VEH vs. SS+CBD comparison, CBD treatment resulted in the upregulation of 63 of the 111 differentially expressed inflammatory pathway genes (Figure 1C). A similar heatmap pattern was observed for the SS+VEH vs. OVX+VEH comparison where 71 of 121 differentially expressed inflammatory pathway genes were increased due to ovarian E2 deficiency (Figure 1D).

3.2. CBD-Induced Bile Secretion Pathway Changes in E2-Deficient and -Sufficient Female Mice

A prior study found that, compared to VEH-treated OVX mice, CBD-treated OVX mice had alterations to serum and ileal content BA profiles [26]. ShinyGO enrichment analysis followed by GOBP pathway enrichment did not uncover any hits using the keyword "bile". Shiny GO enrichment analysis using the KEGG pathway database revealed that CBD significantly altered 134 pathways in OVX mice and 209 pathways in SS mice, while 92 pathways were altered due to ovariectomy. For each of these comparisons, the top 20 KEGG pathways were ranked based on FDR correction (Figure S3). The "Bile secretion" pathway was detected in the top 20 pathways of DEGs for OVX+VEH vs. OVX+CBD and SS+VEH vs. SS+CBD but not for SS+VEH vs. OVX+VEH (Figure S3).

Relative to VEH-treatment, the CBD-treated OVX group had 27 DEGs involved in bile secretion and the CBD-treated SS group had 29 DEGs (Figure 2A and Supplementary File S2). The OVX+VEH vs. OVX+CBD and SS+VEH vs. SS+CBD comparisons had 17 DEGs (*Abcb1a, Abcc3, Abcg2, Abcg5, Adcy3, Adcy5, Nceh1, Nr1h4, Rxra, Sct, Slc10a2, Slc4a2, Slc51b, Ugt1a1, Ugt1a6a, Ugta7c, Ugt2b5*) in common, indicating that these changes to the bile secretion pathway were CBD-induced and unrelated to surgery (Figure 2A and Supplementary File S2). For OVX+VEH vs. OVX+CBD, all 17 DEGs were upregulated due to CBD (Figure 2A,B and Supplementary File S2). For the SS+VEH vs. SS+CBD comparison, 14 DEGs were upregulated and 3 were downregulated by CBD (Figure 2A,C and Supplementary File S2).

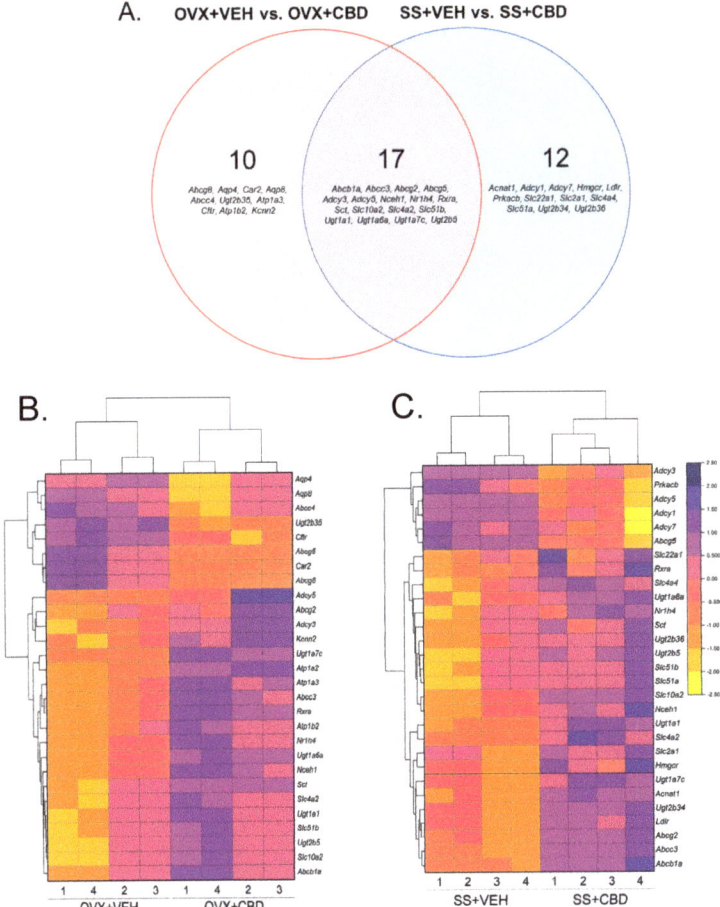

Figure 2. Differentially expressed bile secretion genes. (**A**) Venn diagram showing DEGs for indicated comparisons as well as DEGs that are in common between comparisons. DEGs held in common do not necessarily indicate the same direction of change. DEGs for (**B**) OVX+VEH vs. OVX+CBD and (**C**) SS+VEH vs. SS+CBD were generated based on Euclidean clustering. The Z-score scale indicates downregulated genes from 0 to −2.5 (orange to yellow shades) and upregulated genes from 0 to 2.5 (red to purple/navy shades).

3.3. Colon Content and Hepatic BA Profiles

Due to the upregulation of bile secretion pathway genes in the colon tissue, BAs in colon content were quantified. Hepatic BAs were profiled to investigate potential effects of CBD on hepatic BA production. The hepatic markers of inflammation were also investigated. The concentrations of total BAs (TBAs), primary BAs (PBAs), secondary BAs (SBAs), and conjugated BAs were similar between groups regardless of surgery or CBD treatment (Table S3). CBD did not alter the concentrations of individual BAs in colon content and liver tissue (Table S3). CBD did not induce differences in the hepatic expression of *Tnf*, *Nos2*, *Il1b*, or *Il6* (Figure S4). Compared to SS+VEH group, the OVX+VEH group showed less a hepatic expression of *Il6* (Figure S4).

3.4. CBD Suppressed Inflammation in Ileal Organoids

Compared to vehicle treatment, the combined TNFα and LPS (TL) treatment of ileal organoids induced the gene expression of inflammatory markers *Nos2* and *Tnf* (Figure 3). Organoids treated with CBD concentrations of 100 or 250 μM suppressed the TL-induced expression of *Tnf* and *Nos2* where the latter showed a dose-dependent effect. Organoids treated with 500 μM CBD also appeared to decrease the TL-induced expression of *Tnf* and *Nos2*; however, this reduction may be due to the lower viability of the organoids with the 500 μM CBD dose (Figure S5). The other treatments resulted in organoid viability which was similar to NT (Figure S5). CBD treatments alone did not alter the expression of *Nos2* and *Tnf* (Figure 3). The mRNA levels of *Il1b* and *Il6* were also assessed by qPCR but were not detected.

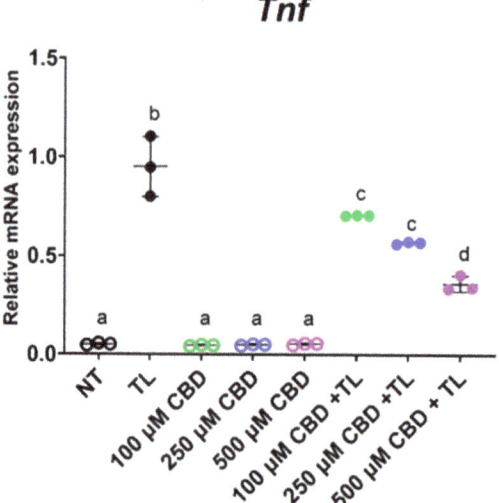

Figure 3. *Cont.*

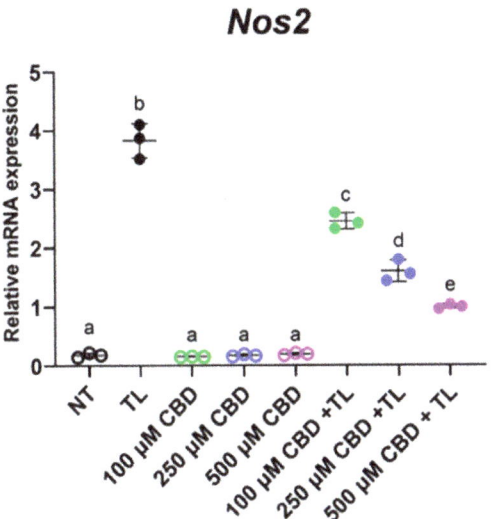

Figure 3. CBD decreased expression of inflammatory markers in intestinal organoids. Mature ileal organoids were treated with Tnfα + LPS (TL) to induce inflammation or treated with increasing concentrations of CBD in the absence or presence of TL. Negative controls consisted of no treatment (NT). On day 4, after organoids were passaged, organoids were incubated with treatments (n = 6 wells per treatment) for 24 h; each well contained approximately 100 mature organoids. Organoids were harvested and RNA was extracted for qPCR and the relative expression of target genes were determined using the 2e-Δct method. Outliers were not detected after ROUT test. Significant differences between treatments were detected using one-way ANOVA followed by a Tukey post hoc test. Different letters indicated significant difference between treatments.

4. Discussion

The anti-inflammatory effects of CBD isolate or CBD-rich extracts have been reported [44], but the differential effects of CBD in female pre- and postmenopausal states remains largely unexplored. The decline in ovarian E2 during perimenopause and after menopause is associated with a pro-inflammatory state which promotes several metabolic disorders, including diabetes, osteoporosis, and neurodegeneration [45]. Due to the drawbacks of HRT use, especially in older postmenopausal women [12], other strategies are needed to address chronic disease burden. CBD products are currently marketed for a variety of indications, including female menopause, but often without adequate evidence [46,47]. Building upon prior work that suggested CBD may have therapeutic application in E2-deficient females [26], in this study, the RNA-Seq analysis of colon tissues revealed that the effect of CBD on inflammatory response pathways depends on E2 status. While CBD decreased the expression of inflammatory response pathway genes in E2-deficient OVX mice (Figure 1B), CBD had the opposite effect in E2-sufficient SS mice (Figure 1C), where the expression of inflammatory response genes was increased. Indeed, the CBD-treated SS and VEH-treated OVX groups showed a similar increase in inflammatory response genes (Figure 1B,D). While the loss of ovarian E2 is known to increase the expression of inflammatory markers in murine tissues [48], the elevated expression of inflammatory response pathway genes in the CBD-treated SS group was unexpected, especially given that the prior qPCR analysis of these tissues showed decreased mRNA levels of selected inflammatory markers (*Il1b*, *Il6*, and *Tnf*) in both CBD-treated OVX and SS groups relative to VEH-treated controls [26]. Notably, compared to VEH-treatment, CBD-treated SS mice had decreased mRNA levels of *Ocln* and *Tjp1*, while the latter was increased in CBD-treated OVX mice, which suggested CBD compromised gut barrier integrity in the E2-sufficient state but was beneficial in E2-deficiency [26]. It remains to be determined whether the induction of the inflammatory response pathway in CBD-treated SS mice is unique to colon tissue or whether this extends to other segments of the intestine or other tissues.

The loss of E2-producing ovary cells with increasing age in perimenopause through postmenopause leads to elevated oxidative stress, which induces inflammation [49]. In young reproductive adult females, ovarian cells have abundant mitochondria that require the high amounts of oxygen for oxidative phosphorylation and optimal cell survival [49]. Reactive oxygen species (ROS), such as superoxide ion and hydrogen peroxide, are created by oxidative phosphorylation and quenched by endogenous glutathione and dietary antioxidants (e.g., vitamins E, C, polyphenols) [49–51]. As aging progresses, ovarian cell membranes and mitochondria are in danger of oxidative damage due to the imperfect detoxification of oxy-radicals and reduced mitochondrial regeneration [49]. Oxidative damage leads to E2 deficiency and subsequent decline in the function and homeostasis of E2-dependent cells throughout the body [49]. CBD reduced ROS production and had a protective effect on Caco-2 monolayer integrity [17]. Together ROS and E2 deficiency may induce systemic inflammation and contribute to menopausal symptoms, such as hot flashes, an increased risk of arteriosclerosis, and decreased gut barrier integrity [17,49].

CBD is a potent antioxidant [14]. Besides its use for patients with epilepsy [21–24], CBD is being investigated for treatment of other neurodegenerative diseases, such as Huntington's disease and schizophrenia [21,50,52,53]. CBD inhibits ROS production and modifies redox balance by activating the redox-sensitive nuclear factor erythroid 2-related factor (Nrf2) in multiple cell types [54,55]. Nrf2 transactivates several antioxidant and cytoprotective genes [55,56]. CBD was shown to reduce ROS production via the inhibition of Tnfα and iNOS [49,50], which is consistent with the CBD suppression of TL-induced inflammation in ileal organoids (Figure 3). CBD is also used for pain relief as it is a cyclooxygenase (COX)-2 inhibitor that reduces glutathione-dependent prostaglandin E2 (PGE2) signaling and subsequent inflammation [49,50]. In the present study, *Ptges*, which encodes PGE2 synthase, was downregulated in the colon tissue of CBD-treated OVX mice compared to VEH-treated OVX mice (Figure 1B and Supplementary File S1).

The presence of ROS species is sensed and monitored by the hypoxia inducible factor (HIF) pathway [57]. In hypoxic conditions, HIF1α is stable and reduces the levels of oxidative phosphorylation and ROS [57]. HIF1α stabilization plays an important role in activating osteoclast activity and bone resorption [58–60]. E2 destabilizes HIF1α, even under hypoxic conditions while E2-deficient OVX mice have stabilized HIF1α, which leads to bone loss [58]. Consistent with these published reports, *Hif1α* was upregulated in VEH-treated OVX mice compared to VEH-treated SS mice (Figure 1D and Supplementary File S1) and exhibited an osteoporotic bone phenotype [26]. The administration of a HIF1α inhibitor was protective against bone loss in OVX mice [58]. In the present study, *Hif1α* was downregulated in CBD-treated OVX mice compared to the VEH-treated mice (Figure 1B and Supplementary File S1) and had improved bone phenotypes [26]. It remains to be determined whether CBD directly or indirectly inhibits HIF1α.

Importantly, a physiologically beneficial level of ROS is required for pathogen resistance and cell signaling [61]. The excessive suppression of ROS was reported to induce inflammation [62], which may be the case in CBD-treated SS mice (Figure 1C). The effects of CBD on ROS in OVX and SS mice remain to be investigated.

While CBD isolate was used in this study, hemp-derived (defined as having <0.3% tetrahydrocannibinol) extract preparations contain other phytocannabinoids as well as terpenes and flavonoids [63,64]. Complex extracts are thought to have superior efficacy compared to CBD isolate preparations due to the synergistic activities of the phytochemical constituents, termed the "entourage effect" [65–67]. Whether other phytochemicals in a CBD-rich extract would temper CBD's stimulation of colonic inflammation in E2-sufficent females remains to be examined. Interestingly, when male C57BL6/J mice were orally administered a CBD-rich cannabis extract (CRCE) for 5 days per week for 2 weeks, they showed a higher colonic expression of pro-inflammatory markers (*Il1β*, *Cxcl1*, and *Cxcl2*) and a decreased expression of *Muc2*, suggesting an induction of intestinal inflammation [68]. Male mice have low circulating E2 levels making them more similar to OVX female mice then SS mice; therefore, the increased expression of colonic markers of inflammation may be due to sex-based difference in profile of hormones other than E2, CBD dose, and/or the presence of other phytochemicals in the CRCE.

The endocannabinoid system functions to maintain the homeostasis of central and peripheral tissues and displays cross-talk with estrogen signaling [69]. Endogenous cannabinoids (i.e., endocannabinoids) arachidonoylethanolamide (anandamide) and 2-arachidonoylglycerol (2-AG) are lipid messengers that signal to CB1 and CB2 endocannabinoid receptors present in central and peripheral tissues [70–72]. CBD activity at endocannabinoid receptors is limited but it can interact with over 65 molecular targets throughout the body [73,74]. The molecular basis of CBD bioactivity in E2-deficient vs. -sufficient states remains to be investigated.

CBD is a partial agonist for CB2, which is mainly expressed in immune cells and peripheral tissues [75]. CB2 is expressed in osteoblasts, osteoclasts, and osteocytes and is an important target for improving bone phenotypes [26,76]. In a previous study, CBD-treated OVX mice had increased femoral mRNA expression of *Cnr2*, which encodes CB2, compared to VEH-treated OVX mice and was associated with decreased bone loss [26]. In the present study, *Cnr2* was upregulated in VEH-treated OVX mice compared to the SS group and CBD treatment lead to a downregulation in the OVX mice (Figure 2B and Supplementary File S1). CBD activity at endocannabinoid receptors is limited, but it has been reported to interact with over 65 molecular targets throughout the body [73,74]. The molecular basis of CBD bioactivity in E2-deficient vs. -sufficient states remains to be investigated.

When *Corynebacterium parvum*-primed and unprimed male mice were treated with CB2 agonist WIN 55212-2 or with CB2 antagonist SR141716A, the levels of pro-inflammatory cytokines in serum was suppressed [77], suggesting that opposing effects on the CB2 receptor can result in the same outcome. Similarly, compared to VEH-treated OVX mice, CBD-treated OVX mice had increased *Cnr2* expression in bone [26] but decreased *Cnr2* expression in the colon (Figure 2B) and in both cases resulted in the reduced expression of inflammatory markers in bone and colon. Further study is needed to explain the mechanism behind these observations.

BAs are synthesized in the liver, stored in the gallbladder, and secreted into the duodenum for the digestion of lipophilic compounds [78]. 95% of Bas are reabsorbed in the ileum and return to the liver via portal circulation, while 5% enter the colon for excretion [78]. Low levels of BAs enter circulation and act as signaling molecules in diverse tissues [78]. Glycine-conjugated BAs have been correlated with increased small intestinal inflammation in rats [79]. Compared to SS groups, VEH-treated OVX mice had increased concentrations of glycine-conjugated Bas, which were reduced in CBD-treated OVX mice [26]. CBD did not alter the BA profiles in colon content (Table S3) but induced the expression of the bile secretion pathway genes in colon tissue independently of E2 status (Figure 2B,C). The CBD-induced increase in bile secretion genes is likely due to it being a lipophilic compound that requires bile-mediated micelle formation for intestinal absorption [80]. An increased BA pool in the liver would be an indicator of hepatic inflammation and damage; however, CBD did not alter hepatic BA profiles in SS or OVX mice (Table S3). OVX has been associated with hepatic tissue inflammation as mice age, becoming apparent 6–7 months after the surgery [48]. There was no observation of OVX-associated increase in the expression of hepatic inflammatory markers (Figure S4), perhaps due to the mice being less than 6 months post-OVX when tissue qPCR analysis was performed.

5. Conclusions

In conclusion, the RNA-Seq analysis of colon tissues allowed a comprehensive investigation of CBD- and OVX-induced transcriptome changes. CBD had a potent anti-inflammatory effect in colon tissues of E2-deficient OVX mice but may contribute to inflammation in intact, E2-sufficient females. To better delineate the CBD mechanisms of action in E2-deficient and -sufficient states, additional experiments are needed to follow up on the extensive gene expression changes. The gut organoid data suggest that CBD may have a direct anti-inflammatory effect on the intestinal epithelium. Future gut organoid studies that test CBD in the absence and presence of E2 treatment would contribute to understanding CBD actions in E2-deficient and -sufficient states. In both the SS and OVX groups, CBD induced similar changes to genes related to bile secretion, indicating changes that were independent of E2 status. OVX or CBD treatment did not alter BA levels in liver or colon content, suggesting that previously observed CBD-induced changes in ileal and serum BAs [26] are more relevant. There is currently widespread use but inadequate investigation of CBD and CBD-rich extracts/products in the menopause and postmenopause [25]. Whether CBD and/or other phytocannabinoids have differential effects in women based on E2 status warrants further study. Given that HRT is not recommended for the prevention of chronic conditions in postmenopausal women, CBD may offer a therapeutic option; however, more research is needed to assist women in making better-informed judgements about individualized CBD risks and benefits.

Supplementary Materials: The following supporting information can be downloaded at: https://www.mdpi.com/article/10.3390/biomedicines11010074/s1, Figure S1: Two-dimensional PCA score plots comparing difference/similarity between collection of DEGs within and between indicated biological samples; Figure S2: Top 20 enriched GOBP pathways generated in ShinyGO; Figure S3: Top 20 enriched KEGG pathways generated in ShinyGO; Figure S4: qPCR of inflammatory markers in liver tissue; Figure S5: Cell viability of ileal organoids. Table S1: Bile acid information, cannabidiol, and HPLC processing method parameters; Table S2: Calibration curves, limit of detection and quantification, and coefficient of variance for bile acid and cannabidiol analysis; Table S3: Bile acid concentrations in colon content and liver. Supplementary File: Gene annotations of DEGs in inflammatory response (S1) and bile secretion (S2) pathways.

Author Contributions: Conceptualization, D.E.R.; methodology, K.M.A.B. and K.M.T.; software, K.M.A.B. and K.M.T.; validation, all authors; formal analysis, K.M.A.B., K.M.T. and H.P.; investigation, all authors; resources, D.E.R. startup funds; data curation, all authors; preparation of figures, tables, and manuscript draft, all authors; writing D.E.R. and K.M.A.B.; editing of manuscript D.E.R. and K.M.A.B.; visualization, K.M.A.B. and K.M.T.; supervision, D.E.R.; project administration, D.E.R.; funding acquisition, D.E.R. All authors have read and agreed to the published version of the manuscript.

Funding: This research was funded by Rutgers University startup funds to D.E.R.

Institutional Review Board Statement: Not applicable.

Informed Consent Statement: Not applicable.

Data Availability Statement: The accession number for deposited RNA sequences is PRJNA908843 and can be found at https://www.ncbi.nlm.nih.gov/bioproject/PRJNA908843. The data can be accessed on 1 January 2023.

Acknowledgments: The authors thank Hung Skyler Hoang for guidance with ShinyGO.

Conflicts of Interest: The authors declare no conflict of interest.

References

1. Peacock, K.; Ketvertis, K.M.; Doerr, C. *Menopause (Nursing)*; StatPearls Publishing: Treasure Island, FL, USA, 2021.
2. Col, N.F.; Guthrie, J.R.; Politi, M.; Dennerstein, L. Duration of vasomotor symptoms in middle-aged women: A longitudinal study. *Menopause* **2009**, *16*, 453–457. [CrossRef] [PubMed]
3. Freeman, E.W.; Sammel, M.D.; Lin, H.; Liu, Z.; Gracia, C.R. Duration of menopausal hot flushes and associated risk factors. *Obstet. Gynecol.* **2011**, *117*, 1095. [CrossRef] [PubMed]
4. Freeman, E.W.; Sammel, M.D.; Sanders, R.J. Risk of long term hot flashes after natural menopause: Evidence from the Penn Ovarian Aging Cohort. *Menopause* **2014**, *21*, 924. [CrossRef] [PubMed]

5. Li, J.-Y.; Chassaing, B.; Tyagi, A.M.; Vaccaro, C.; Luo, T.; Adams, J.; Darby, T.M.; Weitzmann, M.N.; Mulle, J.G.; Gewirtz, A.T. Sex steroid deficiency–associated bone loss is microbiota dependent and prevented by probiotics. *J. Clin. Investig.* **2016**, *126*, 2049–2063. [CrossRef]
6. Shieh, A.; Epeldegui, M.; Karlamangla, A.S.; Greendale, G.A. Gut permeability, inflammation, and bone density across the menopause transition. *JCI Insight* **2020**, *5*, e134092. [CrossRef]
7. Woods, N.F.; Mitchell, E.S. Symptoms during the perimenopause: Prevalence, severity, trajectory, and significance in women's lives. *Am. J. Med.* **2005**, *118*, 14–24. [CrossRef]
8. Mauvais-Jarvis, F.; Clegg, D.J.; Hevener, A.L. The role of estrogens in control of energy balance and glucose homeostasis. *Endocr. Rev.* **2013**, *34*, 309–338. [CrossRef]
9. Collins, F.L.; Rios-Arce, N.D.; Atkinson, S.; Bierhalter, H.; Schoenherr, D.; Bazil, J.N.; McCabe, L.R.; Parameswaran, N. Temporal and regional intestinal changes in permeability, tight junction, and cytokine gene expression following ovariectomy-induced estrogen deficiency. *Physiol. Rep.* **2017**, *5*, e13263. [CrossRef]
10. Yu, M.; Pal, S.; Paterson, C.W.; Li, J.-Y.; Tyagi, A.M.; Adams, J.; Coopersmith, C.M.; Weitzmann, M.N.; Pacifici, R. Ovariectomy induces bone loss via microbial-dependent trafficking of intestinal TNF+ T cells and Th17 cells. *J. Clin. Investig.* **2021**, *131*, e143137. [CrossRef]
11. Harper-Harrison, G.; Shanahan, M.M. Hormone Replacement Therapy. In *StatPearls [Internet]*; StatPearls Publishing: Treasure Island, FL, USA, 2022.
12. Grossman, D.C.; Curry, S.J.; Owens, D.K.; Barry, M.J.; Davidson, K.W.; Doubeni, C.A.; Epling, J.W.; Kemper, A.R.; Krist, A.H.; Kurth, A.E. Hormone therapy for the primary prevention of chronic conditions in postmenopausal women: US Preventive Services Task Force recommendation statement. *JAMA* **2017**, *318*, 2224–2233.
13. Shoupe, D. HRT dosing regimens: Continuous versus cyclic-pros and cons. *Int. J. Fertil. Women's Med.* **2001**, *46*, 7–15.
14. Atalay, S.; Jarocka-Karpowicz, I.; Skrzydlewska, E. Antioxidative and anti-inflammatory properties of cannabidiol. *Antioxidants* **2019**, *9*, 21. [CrossRef] [PubMed]
15. De Filippis, D.; Esposito, G.; Cirillo, C.; Cipriano, M.; De Winter, B.Y.; Scuderi, C.; Sarnelli, G.; Cuomo, R.; Steardo, L.; De Man, J.G. Cannabidiol reduces intestinal inflammation through the control of neuroimmune axis. *PLoS ONE* **2011**, *6*, e28159. [CrossRef] [PubMed]
16. Nichols, J.M.; Kaplan, B.L. Immune responses regulated by cannabidiol. *Cannabis Cannabinoid Res.* **2020**, *5*, 12–31. [CrossRef] [PubMed]
17. Cocetta, V.; Governa, P.; Borgonetti, V.; Tinazzi, M.; Peron, G.; Catanzaro, D.; Berretta, M.; Biagi, M.; Manetti, F.; Dall'Acqua, S. Cannabidiol isolated from *Cannabis sativa* L. protects intestinal barrier from in vitro inflammation and oxidative stress. *Front. Pharmacol.* **2021**, *12*, 641210. [CrossRef]
18. Li, D.; Lin, Z.; Meng, Q.; Wang, K.; Wu, J.; Yan, H. Cannabidiol administration reduces sublesional cancellous bone loss in rats with severe spinal cord injury. *Eur. J. Pharmacol.* **2017**, *809*, 13–19. [CrossRef]
19. Napimoga, M.H.; Benatti, B.B.; Lima, F.O.; Alves, P.M.; Campos, A.C.; Pena-dos-Santos, D.R.; Severino, F.P.; Cunha, F.Q.; Guimarães, F.S. Cannabidiol decreases bone resorption by inhibiting RANK/RANKL expression and pro-inflammatory cytokines during experimental periodontitis in rats. *Int. Immunopharmacol.* **2009**, *9*, 216–222. [CrossRef]
20. Raphael-Mizrahi, B.; Gabet, Y. The cannabinoids effect on bone formation and bone healing. *Curr. Osteoporos. Rep.* **2020**, *18*, 433–438. [CrossRef]
21. Gaston, T.E.; Ampah, S.B.; Bebin, E.M.; Grayson, L.P.; Cutter, G.R.; Hernando, K.; Szaflarski, J.P. Long-term safety and efficacy of highly purified cannabidiol for treatment refractory epilepsy. *Epilepsy Behav.* **2021**, *117*, 107862. [CrossRef]
22. Iffland, K.; Grotenhermen, F. An update on safety and side effects of cannabidiol: A review of clinical data and relevant animal studies. *Cannabis Cannabinoid Res.* **2017**, *2*, 139–154. [CrossRef]
23. Larsen, C.; Shahinas, J. Dosage, efficacy and safety of cannabidiol administration in adults: A systematic review of human trials. *J. Clin. Med. Res.* **2020**, *12*, 129. [CrossRef]
24. Machado Bergamaschi, M.; Helena Costa Queiroz, R.; Waldo Zuardi, A.; Crippa, A.S. Safety and side effects of cannabidiol, a *Cannabis sativa* constituent. *Curr. Drug Saf.* **2011**, *6*, 237–249. [CrossRef]
25. Dahlgren, M.K.; El-Abboud, C.; Lambros, A.M.; Sagar, K.A.; Smith, R.T.; Gruber, S.A. A survey of medical cannabis use during perimenopause and postmenopause. *Menopause* **2022**, *29*, 1028–1036. [CrossRef]
26. Sui, K.; Tveter, K.M.; Bawagan, F.G.; Buckendahl, P.; Martinez, S.A.; Jaffri, Z.H.; MacDonell, A.T.; Wu, Y.; Duran, R.M.; Shapses, S.A. Cannabidiol-Treated Ovariectomized Mice Show Improved Glucose, Energy, and Bone Metabolism with a Bloom in *Lactobacillus*. *Front. Pharmacol.* **2022**, 2282. [CrossRef]
27. Jansson, P.-A.; Curiac, D.; Ahrén, I.L.; Hansson, F.; Niskanen, T.M.; Sjögren, K.; Ohlsson, C. Probiotic treatment using a mix of three *Lactobacillus* strains for lumbar spine bone loss in postmenopausal women: A randomised, double-blind, placebo-controlled, multicentre trial. *Lancet Rheumatol.* **2019**, *1*, e154–e162. [CrossRef]
28. Nilsson, A.; Sundh, D.; Bäckhed, F.; Lorentzon, M. *Lactobacillus reuteri* reduces bone loss in older women with low bone mineral density: A randomized, placebo-controlled, double-blind, clinical trial. *J. Intern. Med.* **2018**, *284*, 307–317. [CrossRef]
29. Rizzoli, R.; Biver, E. Are probiotics the new calcium and vitamin D for bone health? *Curr. Osteoporos. Rep.* **2020**, *18*, 273–284. [CrossRef]

30. Sapra, L.; Dar, H.Y.; Bhardwaj, A.; Pandey, A.; Kumari, S.; Azam, Z.; Upmanyu, V.; Anwar, A.; Shukla, P.; Mishra, P.K. *Lactobacillus rhamnosus* attenuates bone loss and maintains bone health by skewing Treg-Th17 cell balance in Ovx mice. *Sci. Rep.* **2021**, *11*, 1807. [CrossRef]
31. Yang, L.-C.; Lin, S.-W.; Li, I.-C.; Chen, Y.-P.; Tzu, S.-Y.; Chou, W.; Chen, C.-C.; Lin, W.-C.; Chen, Y.-L.; Lin, W.-H. *Lactobacillus plantarum* GKM3 and *Lactobacillus paracasei* GKS6 supplementation ameliorates bone loss in ovariectomized mice by promoting osteoblast differentiation and inhibiting osteoclast formation. *Nutrients* **2020**, *12*, 1914. [CrossRef]
32. Yu, J.; Cao, G.; Yuan, S.; Luo, C.; Yu, J.; Cai, M. Probiotic supplements and bone health in postmenopausal women: A meta-analysis of randomised controlled trials. *BMJ Open* **2021**, *11*, e041393. [CrossRef]
33. Ridlon, J.M.; Kang, D.J.; Hylemon, P.B.; Bajaj, J.S. Bile acids and the gut microbiome. *Curr. Opin. Gastroenterol.* **2014**, *30*, 332. [CrossRef] [PubMed]
34. Chen, M.L.; Takeda, K.; Sundrud, M.S. Emerging roles of bile acids in mucosal immunity and inflammation. *Mucosal Immunol.* **2019**, *12*, 851–861. [CrossRef] [PubMed]
35. Ahmad, T.R.; Haeusler, R.A. Bile acids in glucose metabolism and insulin signalling—Mechanisms and research needs. *Nat. Rev. Endocrinol.* **2019**, *15*, 701–712. [CrossRef] [PubMed]
36. Cho, S.W.; An, J.H.; Park, H.; Yang, J.Y.; Choi, H.J.; Kim, S.W.; Park, Y.J.; Kim, S.Y.; Yim, M.; Baek, W.Y. Positive regulation of osteogenesis by bile acid through FXR. *J. Bone Miner. Res.* **2013**, *28*, 2109–2121. [CrossRef] [PubMed]
37. Perucca, E.; Bialer, M. Critical aspects affecting cannabidiol oral bioavailability and metabolic elimination, and related clinical implications. *CNS Drugs* **2020**, *34*, 795–800. [CrossRef]
38. Kim, D.; Paggi, J.M.; Park, C.; Bennett, C.; Salzberg, S.L. Graph-based genome alignment and genotyping with HISAT2 and HISAT-genotype. *Nat. Biotechnol.* **2019**, *37*, 907–915. [CrossRef]
39. Love, M.I.; Huber, W.; Anders, S. Moderated estimation of fold change and dispersion for RNA-seq data with DESeq2. *Genome Biol.* **2014**, *15*, 550. [CrossRef]
40. Ge, S.X.; Jung, D.; Yao, R. ShinyGO: A graphical gene-set enrichment tool for animals and plants. *Bioinformatics* **2020**, *36*, 2628–2629. [CrossRef]
41. Pang, Z.; Zhou, G.; Ewald, J.; Chang, L.; Hacariz, O.; Basu, N.; Xia, J. Using MetaboAnalyst 5.0 for LC–HRMS spectra processing, multi-omics integration and covariate adjustment of global metabolomics data. *Nat. Protoc.* **2022**, *17*, 1735–1761. [CrossRef]
42. Mahe, M.M.; Aihara, E.; Schumacher, M.A.; Zavros, Y.; Montrose, M.H.; Helmrath, M.A.; Sato, T.; Shroyer, N.F. Establishment of gastrointestinal epithelial organoids. *Curr. Protoc. Mouse Biol.* **2013**, *3*, 217–240. [CrossRef]
43. Tveter, K.M.; Villa-Rodriguez, J.A.; Cabales, A.J.; Zhang, L.; Bawagan, F.G.; Duran, R.M.; Roopchand, D.E. Polyphenol-induced improvements in glucose metabolism are associated with bile acid signaling to intestinal farnesoid X receptor. *BMJ Open Diabetes Res Care* **2020**, *8*, e001386. [CrossRef]
44. Aziz, A.I.; Nguyen, L.C.; Oumeslakht, L.; Bensussan, A.; Ben Mkaddem, S. Cannabinoids as Immune System Modulators: Cannabidiol Potential Therapeutic Approaches and Limitations. *Cannabis Cannabinoid Res.* **2022**. [CrossRef]
45. Della Torre, S.; Benedusi, V.; Fontana, R.; Maggi, A. Energy metabolism and fertility: A balance preserved for female health. *Nat. Rev. Endocrinol.* **2014**, *10*, 13–23. [CrossRef]
46. Zenone, M.A.; Snyder, J.; Crooks, V.A. What are the informational pathways that shape people's use of cannabidiol for medical purposes? *J. Cannabis Res.* **2021**, *3*. [CrossRef]
47. Soleymanpour, M.; Saderholm, S.; Kavuluru, R. Therapeutic Claims in Cannabidiol (CBD) Marketing Messages on Twitter. In Proceedings of the IEEE International Conference on Bioinformatics and Biomedicine (BIBM), Houston, TX, USA, 9–12 December 2021; pp. 3083–3088. [CrossRef]
48. Benedusi, V.; Martini, E.; Kallikourdis, M.; Villa, A.; Meda, C.; Maggi, A. Ovariectomy shortens the life span of female mice. *Oncotarget* **2015**, *6*, 10801–10811. [CrossRef]
49. Miquel, J.; Ramírez-Boscá, A.; Ramírez-Bosca, J.V.; Alperi, J.D. Menopause: A review on the role of oxygen stress and favorable effects of dietary antioxidants. *Arch. Gerontol. Geriatr.* **2006**, *42*, 289–306. [CrossRef]
50. Pereira, S.R.; Hackett, B.; O'Driscoll, D.N.; Sun, M.C.; Downer, E.J. Cannabidiol modulation of oxidative stress and signalling. *Neuronal Signal.* **2021**, *5*, NS20200080. [CrossRef]
51. Pérez, L.M.; Hooshmand, B.; Mangialasche, F.; Mecocci, P.; Smith, A.D.; Refsum, H.; Inzitari, M.; Fratiglioni, L.; Rizzuto, D.; Calderón-Larrañaga, A. Glutathione serum levels and rate of multimorbidity development in older adults. *J. Gerontol. Ser. A* **2020**, *75*, 1089–1094. [CrossRef]
52. McGuire, P.; Robson, P.; Cubala, W.J.; Vasile, D.; Morrison, P.D.; Barron, R.; Taylor, A.; Wright, S. Cannabidiol (CBD) as an adjunctive therapy in schizophrenia: A multicenter randomized controlled trial. *Am. J. Psychiatry* **2018**, *175*, 225–231. [CrossRef]
53. Saft, C.; von Hein, S.M.; Lücke, T.; Thiels, C.; Peball, M.; Djamshidian, A.; Heim, B.; Seppi, K. Cannabinoids for treatment of dystonia in Huntington's disease. *J. Hunting. Dis.* **2018**, *7*, 167–173. [CrossRef]
54. Singer, E.; Judkins, J.; Salomonis, N.; Matlaf, L.; Soteropoulos, P.; McAllister, S.; Soroceanu, L. Reactive oxygen species-mediated therapeutic response and resistance in glioblastoma. *Cell Death Dis.* **2015**, *6*, e1601. [CrossRef] [PubMed]
55. Vomhof-DeKrey, E.E.; Picklo Sr, M.J. The Nrf2-antioxidant response element pathway: A target for regulating energy metabolism. *J. Nutr. Biochem.* **2012**, *23*, 1201–1206. [CrossRef] [PubMed]
56. Vargas, M.R.; Johnson, J.A. The Nrf2–ARE cytoprotective pathway in astrocytes. *Expert Rev. Mol. Med.* **2009**, *11*, e17. [CrossRef] [PubMed]

57. Janbandhu, V.; Tallapragada, V.; Patrick, R.; Li, Y.; Abeygunawardena, D.; Humphreys, D.T.; Martin, E.M.; Ward, A.O.; Contreras, O.; Farbehi, N. Hif-1a suppresses ROS-induced proliferation of cardiac fibroblasts following myocardial infarction. *Cell Stem Cell* **2022**, *29*, 281–297.e12. [CrossRef] [PubMed]
58. Miyauchi, Y.; Sato, Y.; Kobayashi, T.; Yoshida, S.; Mori, T.; Kanagawa, H.; Katsuyama, E.; Fujie, A.; Hao, W.; Miyamoto, K. HIF1α is required for osteoclast activation by estrogen deficiency in postmenopausal osteoporosis. *Proc. Natl. Acad. Sci. USA* **2013**, *110*, 16568–16573. [CrossRef] [PubMed]
59. Shao, J.; Zhang, Y.; Yang, T.; Qi, J.; Zhang, L.; Deng, L. HIF-1α disturbs osteoblasts and osteoclasts coupling in bone remodeling by up-regulating OPG expression. *In Vitro Cell. Dev. Biol.-Anim.* **2015**, *51*, 808–814. [CrossRef] [PubMed]
60. Meng, X.; Lin, Z.; Cao, S.; Janowska, I.; Sonomoto, K.; Andreev, D.; Katharina, K.; Wen, J.; Knaup, K.X.; Wiesener, M.S. Estrogen-mediated downregulation of HIF-1α signaling in B lymphocytes influences postmenopausal bone loss. *Bone Res.* **2022**, *10*, 15. [CrossRef]
61. Ray, P.D.; Huang, B.-W.; Tsuji, Y. Reactive oxygen species (ROS) homeostasis and redox regulation in cellular signaling. *Cell. Signal.* **2012**, *24*, 981–990. [CrossRef]
62. Yang, S.; Lian, G. ROS and diseases: Role in metabolism and energy supply. *Mol. Cell. Biochem.* **2020**, *467*, 1–12. [CrossRef]
63. Silva Sofrás, F.M.; Desimone, M.F. Entourage Effect And Analytical Chemistry: Chromatography As A Tool In The Analysis Of The Secondary Metabolism of *Cannabis sativa* L. *Curr. Pharm. Des.* **2022**. *online ahead of print*. [CrossRef]
64. Bautista, J.L.; Yu, S.; Tian, L. Flavonoids in *Cannabis sativa*: Biosynthesis, Bioactivities, and Biotechnology. *ACS Omega* **2021**, *6*, 5119–5123. [CrossRef]
65. LaVigne, J.E.; Hecksel, R.; Keresztes, A.; Streicher, J.M. *Cannabis sativa* terpenes are cannabimimetic and selectively enhance cannabinoid activity. *Sci. Rep.* **2021**, *11*, 8232. [CrossRef]
66. Anderson, L.L.; Etchart, M.G.; Bahceci, D.; Golembiewski, T.A.; Arnold, J.C. Cannabis constituents interact at the drug efflux pump BCRP to markedly increase plasma cannabidiolic acid concentrations. *Sci. Rep.* **2021**, *11*, 14948. [CrossRef]
67. Pamplona, F.A.; da Silva, L.R.; Coan, A.C. Potential Clinical Benefits of CBD-Rich Cannabis Extracts Over Purified CBD in Treatment-Resistant Epilepsy: Observational Data Meta-analysis. *Front. Neurol.* **2018**, *9*, 759. [CrossRef]
68. Skinner, C.M.; Nookaew, I.; Ewing, L.E.; Wongsurawat, T.; Jenjaroenpun, P.; Quick, C.M.; Yee, E.U.; Piccolo, B.D.; ElSohly, M.; Walker, L.A.; et al. Potential Probiotic or Trigger of Gut Inflammation—The Janus-Faced Nature of Cannabidiol-Rich Cannabis Extract. *J. Diet. Suppl.* **2020**, *17*, 543–560. [CrossRef]
69. Santoro, A.; Mele, E.; Marino, M.; Viggiano, A.; Nori, S.L.; Meccariello, R. The Complex Interplay between Endocannabinoid System and the Estrogen System in Central Nervous System and Periphery. *Int. J. Mol. Sci.* **2021**, *22*, 972. [CrossRef]
70. Di Marzo, V.; Piscitelli, F. The Endocannabinoid System and its Modulation by Phytocannabinoids. *Neurotherapeutics* **2015**, *12*, 692–698. [CrossRef]
71. Joshi, N.; Onaivi, E.S. Endocannabinoid System Components: Overview and Tissue Distribution. In *Recent Advances in Cannabinoid Physiology and Pathology*; Advances in Experimental Medicine and Biology; Springer: Cham, Switzerland, 2019; Volume 1162, pp. 1–12. [CrossRef]
72. Britch, S.C.; Babalonis, S.; Walsh, S.L. Cannabidiol: Pharmacology and therapeutic targets. *Psychopharmacology* **2021**, *238*, 9–28. [CrossRef]
73. Ibeas Bih, C.; Chen, T.; Nunn, A.V.; Bazelot, M.; Dallas, M.; Whalley, B.J. Molecular Targets of Cannabidiol in Neurological Disorders. *Neurotherapeutics* **2015**, *12*, 699–730. [CrossRef]
74. Bab, I.; Zimmer, A. Cannabinoid receptors and the regulation of bone mass. *Br. J. Pharmacol.* **2008**, *153*, 182–188. [CrossRef] [PubMed]
75. Li, L.; Feng, J.; Sun, L.; Xuan, Y.-W.; Wen, L.; Li, Y.-x.; Yang, S.; Zhu, B.; Tian, X.-Y.; Li, S. Cannabidiol Promotes Osteogenic Differentiation of Bone Marrow Mesenchymal Stem Cells in the Inflammatory Microenvironment via the CB2-dependent p38 MAPK Signaling Pathway. *Int. J. Stem Cells* **2022**, *15*, 405–414. [CrossRef] [PubMed]
76. Benamar, K.; Yondorf, M.; Meissler, J.J.; Geller, E.B.; Tallarida, R.J.; Eisenstein, T.K.; Adler, M.W. A novel role of cannabinoids: Implication in the fever induced by bacterial lipopolysaccharide. *J. Pharmacol. Exp. Ther.* **2007**, *320*, 1127–1133. [CrossRef] [PubMed]
77. Marin, J.J.G. Bile Acids in Physiology, Pathology and Pharmacology. *Curr. Drug Metab.* **2015**, *17*, 4–29. [CrossRef]
78. Lázár, B.; László, S.B.; Hutka, B.; Tóth, A.S.; Mohammadzadeh, A.; Berekméri, E.; Ágg, B.; Balogh, M.; Sajtos, V.; Király, K. A comprehensive time course and correlation analysis of indomethacin-induced inflammation, bile acid alterations and dysbiosis in the rat small intestine. *Biochem. Pharmacol.* **2021**, *190*, 114590. [CrossRef] [PubMed]
79. Nakano, Y.; Tajima, M.; Sugiyama, E.; Sato, V.H.; Sato, H. Development of a Novel Nano-emulsion Formulation to Improve Intestinal Absorption of Cannabidiol. *Med. Cannabis Cannabinoids* **2019**, *2*, 35–42. [CrossRef] [PubMed]
80. Bertolini, A. Bile acids and their receptors: Modulators and therapeutic targets in liver inflammation. *Semin. Immunopathol.* **2022**, *44*, 547–564. [CrossRef]

Disclaimer/Publisher's Note: The statements, opinions and data contained in all publications are solely those of the individual author(s) and contributor(s) and not of MDPI and/or the editor(s). MDPI and/or the editor(s) disclaim responsibility for any injury to people or property resulting from any ideas, methods, instructions or products referred to in the content.

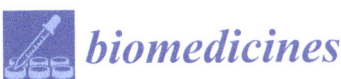

Article

Differential Regulation of MMPs, Apoptosis and Cell Proliferation by the Cannabinoid Receptors CB1 and CB2 in Vascular Smooth Muscle Cells and Cardiac Myocytes

Bettina Greiner [1], Manuela Sommerfeld [1], Ulrich Kintscher [1,2], Thomas Unger [3], Kai Kappert [2,4] and Elena Kaschina [1,2,*]

[1] Cardiovascular–Metabolic–Renal (CMR)-Research Center, Institute of Pharmacology, Corporate Member of Freie Universität Berlin, Humboldt-Universität zu Berlin, Charité—Universitätsmedizin Berlin, 10115 Berlin, Germany
[2] DZHK (German Centre for Cardiovascular Research), Partner Site Berlin, 10115 Berlin, Germany
[3] CARIM School for Cardiovascular Diseases, Maastricht University, 6211 LK Maastricht, The Netherlands
[4] Clinical Chemistry and Pathobiochemistry, Institute of Diagnostic Laboratory Medicine, Corporate Member of Freie Universität Berlin, Humboldt-Universität zu Berlin, Charité—Universitätsmedizin Berlin, 10117 Berlin, Germany
* Correspondence: elena.kaschina@charite.de; Tel.: +49-304-505-250-24

Abstract: Cannabinoids (CB) are implicated in cardiovascular diseases via the two main receptor subtypes CB_1R and CB_2R. This study investigated whether cannabinoids regulate the activity of matrix metalloproteases (MMP-2, MMP-9) in vascular smooth muscle cells (VSMCs) and in cells of cardiac origin (H9c2 cell line). The influence of CB_1- and CB_2 receptor stimulation or inhibition on cell proliferation, apoptosis and glucose uptake was also evaluated. We used four compounds that activate or block CB receptors: arachidonyl-2-chloroethylamide (ACEA)—CB_1R agonist, rimonabant—CB_1R antagonist, John W. Huffman (JWH133)—CB_2R agonist and CB_2R antagonist—6-Iodopravadoline (AM630). Treatment of cells with the CB_2R agonist JWH133 decreased cytokine activated secretion of proMMP-2, MMP-2 and MMP-9, reduced Fas ligand and caspase-3-mediated apoptosis, normalized the expression of TGF-beta1 and prevented cytokine-induced increase in glucose uptake into the cell. CB_1R inhibition with rimonabant showed similar protective properties as the CB_2R agonist JWH133, but to a lesser extent. In conclusion, CB_1R and CB_2R exert opposite effects on cell glucose uptake, proteolysis and apoptosis in both VSMCs and H9c2 cells. The CB_2R agonist JWH133 demonstrated the highest protective properties. These findings may pave the way to a new treatment of cardiovascular diseases, especially those associated with extracellular matrix degradation.

Keywords: cannabinoid receptors; MMP-2; MMP-9; VSMC; H9c2 cells; glucose; cell proliferation; apoptosis; cardiovascular disease

1. Introduction

Recent studies have demonstrated hemodynamic and cardiometabolic effects of cannabinoids [1–5]. The cannabinoid system modulates the extracellular matrix turnover in the heart and blood vessels [6,7]. These findings have led to interest in the biochemical bases of their action. Endocannabinoids exert their effects, at least in part, by stimulating two main receptor subtypes, CB_1 and CB_2 (CB_1R and CB_2R), which belong to a group of seven transmembrane-spanning receptors. They are coupled to Gi/o-proteins and act via an inhibition of adenylylcyclase and subsequently the reduction of cAMP [8,9]. Other than the adenylylcyclase/cAMP pathways, several other intracellular pathways are influenced, such as p38, JNK and ERK [10]. Cannabinoid receptor ligands are divided into endogenous cannabinoids, such as 2-AG and AEA, and exogenous cannabinoids, such as derivatives from the cannabis sativa plant or synthetic cannabinoids [10]. Currently, novel modulators of the cannabinoid system are under investigations. New compounds

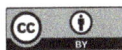

are able to bind to CB receptors in the low nanomolar range with a marked selectivity towards the receptors [11]. Moreover, multitargeting G-protein-coupled receptors is also a promising strategy, as shown for antinociception by bivalent agonists for the opioid and cannabinoid receptors [12,13]. CB_1R stimulation elicits bradycardia, negative inotropy and hypotension [14]. The CB_1R is also implicated in inflammation, apoptosis and oxidative stress in the heart [15], whereas the CB_2R may play a protective anti-inflammatory, antioxidative and antiatherogenic role [15–17]. We have previously shown that blockade of the CB_1R with rimonabant decreased collagen accumulation and prevented upregulation of the profibrotic protein TGF-β1 in the heart and aorta in a myocardial infarction model [7]. Moreover, CB_1R blockade also reduced the activity of the matrix metalloprotease 9 (MMP-9) in cardiac fibroblasts [7]. On the other hand, genetic deletion of the CB_2R increased TGF-β1 and collagen production in a heart failure model [18], pointing to opposite effects of CB_1R and CB_2R. Recent studies provided further findings on extracellular matrix regulation by cannabinoids in the heart and vessels. For example, CB_2R knockout models showed an increase in atherosclerotic vascular changes as well as an increase in MMP-9 expression [19]. In patients with high plaque instability of the carotid artery, decreased CB_2R expression was correlated with a MMP-9 increase [20]. Based on these findings, we hypothesized that cannabinoids may influence proteolytic processes in the vessels directly *via* CB_1R and CB_2R, which are known to be localized on vascular smooth muscle cells (VSMCs) [21,22]. Therefore, we aimed to investigate whether cannabinoids regulate the activity of MMPs in the cells of rat vascular (VSMCs) and cardiac origin (H9c2). Given that the gelatinase A (MMP2) and gelatinase B (MMP9) are capable of degrading components of the extracellular matrix [23], we have focused on their regulation. By using various cannabinoid receptor ligands, we also intended to explore which receptor subtype is implicated in proteolysis. In our study, we used four different synthetic compounds that activate or block cannabinoid receptors: arachidonyl-2-chloroethylamide (ACEA), a CB_1R agonist; rimonabant, a CB_1R antagonist; John W. Huffman (JWH133), a CB_2R agonist; and 6-Iodopravadoline (AM630), a CB_2R antagonist. Since MMPs secretion is closely connected to cell proliferation, apoptosis and glucose metabolism, we analyzed their regulation.

2. Materials and Methods

2.1. Cell Cultures

Primary vascular smooth muscle cells (VSMCs) were isolated from the aorta of male normotensive Wistar rats (200 to 220 g; Charles River Laboratories Germany GmbH) as previously described [24]. Briefly, under dissecting microscope fat, connective tissue and outgoing arteries were removed from the aorta. The vessel was cut longitudinally, and the endothelium was removed with a cell scraper by gentle scraping along the luminal face. VSMCs were isolated by using digestion method, cultured and frozen in liquid nitrogen.

The cells were identified by "hill and valley" growth pattern and immunofluorescence staining with an anti-smooth muscle actin monoclonal antibody (Merk KGaA, Darmstadt, Germany). VSMCs were cultured in Dulbecco's modified Eagle's medium (4.5 g/L glucose) supplemented with 10% fetal bovine serum. Experiments were performed with cultures from passages 4 to 12.

This study was carried out in strict accordance with national and European guidelines for animal experiments with approval by the ethics commission of the regulatory authorities of the City of Berlin, Germany, the "Landesamt für Gesundheit und Soziales" (registration number G0002/16).

Neonatal rat cardiomyocytes (H9c2 cell line, 88092904, Sigmaaldrich, Merk, Germany) are a subclone of the original clonal cell line derived from embryonic BD1X rat heart tissue that exhibit many of the properties of skeletal muscle. The cells were incubated in high-glucose Dulbecco's modified Eagle's medium with 10% fetal bovine serum. Cell splitting was performed when H9c2 cells reached confluence.

2.2. Cell Culture Experiments

Confluent cells were serum-deprived for 24 h. The cells were exposed to recombinant interleukin-1α (IL-1α) 1.0 ng/mL (Sigma-Aldrich, Taufkirchen, Germany) to induce secretion of MMPs. Incubation was performed with or without added compounds for 48 h. The following CB_1R and CB_2R agonists and antagonists were used: CB_1R agonist arachidonyl-2-chloroethylamide (ACEA) (0.5 µM), CB_1R antagonist rimonabant (1.0 µM), CB_2R agonist JWH133 (0.5 µM) and CB_2R antagonist 6-Iodopravadoline (AM630) (1.0 µM). Epigallocatechin gallate (ECEG) (5 µg/mL), an inhibitor of MMPs, was used as a positive control. Conditioned media were obtained by collecting the culture media at the end of the experiment. Proteins were extracted from the cells and processed for Western blot analysis.

2.3. Chemical Compounds

Arachidonyl-2-chloroethylamide (ACEA), JWH133, and 6-Iodopravadoline (AM630) were purchased from Tocris (Bristol, UK). Rimonabant was purchased from Sanofi Aventis Deutschland GmbH (Frankfurt, Germany) and epigallocatechin gallate (ECEG) from Enzo Life Science (Lörrach, Germany).

2.4. Gelatin Zymography

Cultured media harvested from cells were analyzed for MMP2 and MMP9 by gelatin zymography, as described previously [25]. Briefly, conditioned media aliquots were resuspended in nonreducing sample buffer and applied to 10% SDS-PAGE copolymerized with gelatin (1 mg/mL). After electrophoresis, the gels were washed for 1 h in Triton-X-100 (2.5% v/m), incubated overnight in an enzyme buffer (developing buffer) at 37 °C, stained in Coomassie solution for 1.5 h and subsequently destained for 1 h in a destaining solution. By that, the enzymatic active areas became visible as a transparent band on the blue-stained gel. The zymograms were analyzed with Scion ImageJ software.

2.5. Western Blot Analysis

Protein samples were separated via SDS-PAGE and transferred to Amersham Hybond PVDF membranes (VWR International, LLC, Radnor, PENN, USA). Membranes were probed with antibodies against MMP-9, caspase-3 (1:1000 in 1× TBST with 5% *w/v* nonfat dry milk) (Abcam, Hiddenhausen, Germany), FasL, TGF-beta1 (1:500 in 1× TBST with 5% *w/v* nonfat dry milk) (Santa Cruz Biotechnology Inc, Heidelberg, Germany) and then incubated with peroxidase-conjugated secondary antibodies anti-mouse antibody/anti-goat antibody (1:2000 in 1× TBST with 5% *w/v* nonfat dry milk) (Agilent Dako, Santa Clara, CA, USA). Protein expression was normalized to glyceraldehyde-3-phosphate dehydrogenase (GAPDH) (Abcam, Hiddenhausen, Germany). Immunoreactive bands were detected by enhanced chemiluminescence (GE Health Care, Solingen, Germany) and quantified with ImageJ Fiji software.

2.6. Immunofluorescence

Protein expression of FasL, caspase-3 and TGF-beta1 were studied by fluorescence microscopy (Biorevo BZ-9000, Keyence, Japan) on cover slips with cells after stimulation with IL-1α (1.0 ng/mL) in the presence or absence of compounds after 48 h. After treatment, cell permeability was increased by Triton-x (5%). Afterwards the primary antibody was added (1:100 in 5% donkey serum), caspase-3, FasL and TGF-beta1 overnight. After washing, the secondary antibody was added (1:100; FITC/Cy3, Agilent Dako, Santa Clara, CA, USA). Nuclei were stained with Hoechst (1:4000) (Merck Sigma-Aldrich, Darmstadt, Germany).

2.7. IncuCyte Live-Cell Analysis

IncuCyte Live-Cell Analysis System (IncuCyte® S3, Sartorius, Göttingen, Germany) was used to observe cell death and proliferation. The experiments were performed with VSMCs and H9c2 cells. Cells were transferred into 96-well plates and treated with the compounds or vehicle under same conditions (medium with 1% or 10% FBS) for 48 h (up to 5 days). Cell proliferation was monitored by analyzing the occupied area (% confluence) of cell images over time. Analysis of the IncuCyte images was performed with Incucyte® Analysis Software.

2.8. Glucose, Lactate, Electrolytes Concentrations

The concentrations of glucose, lactate, sodium, calcium and potassium were measured in cell supernatant 48 h after treatments. Na, K and Cl were quantified by an indirect ion selective electrode (ISE, Gen. 2 Roche® Diagnostics GmbH) on a Roche® cobas ISE module. Lactate dehydrogenase activity was determined applying Roche® cobas lactate dehydrogenase according to IFCC version 2 (LDHI2, #05169330 190). Glucose and lactate were quantified photometrically on a Roche® cobas analyzer.

2.9. Statistical Analysis

Results are expressed as the mean ± (SD) standard deviation in the graphics unless declared otherwise in the figure legends. Two-group comparisons were analyzed by the 2-tailed Student unpaired *t*-test for independent samples. Welch's correction was used when results in relation to IL-1α were compared, as declared in the figure legends. Pearson R statistical test was used for measuring the strength between glucose and lactate variables and their relationship. Statistical analysis was performed using GraphPad Prism 6 (GraphPad Software Inc., La Jolla, CA, USA).

3. Results

3.1. Regulation of MMP-2 and MMP-9

MMPs' enzymatic activity levels in conditioned media were demonstrated by gelatin zymography. Experiments were performed in different passages of VSMC (P4-P12, $n = 10–16$). The results are presented in Figure 1.

MMP-9 showed a greater upregulation by IL-1α stimulation (Figure 1a; 92.1%, $p < 0.0001$) than proMMP-2 (Figure 1b; 39.7%, $p < 0.001$) and MMP-2 (Figure 1c; 13.6%, n.s.). In comparison to the IL-1α group, treatment with JWH-133 reduced MMP-9 activity by 30.4% (Figure 1a; $p < 0.0001$). Rimonabant, ACEA and AM630 reduced MMP-9 activity slightly but not significantly. Even though less upregulated by IL-1α, proMMP-2 was also reduced by JWH-133 treatment (Figure 1b; 27.6%; $p < 0.05$). Rimonabant reduced proMMP-2 by 14.2%, while AM 630 and ACEA decreased proMMP-2 only by 7.7% and 7.9%, respectively. These changes were statistically not significant.

MMP-2, while showing only a minor upregulation after IL-1α stimulation, was also reduced by JWH-133 treatment (Figure 1c; 13.2%; $p < 0{,}05$). Rimonabant reduced MMP-2 by 10.1%, AM 630 by 11.2% and ACEA only by 6.3%, showing no significant effects. Representative zymographies are shown in Figure 1d,e.

The same experimental setup was used to evaluate MMP activity in H9c2 cardiac cells after treatment with the cannabinoid receptor agonists and antagonists after IL-1α stimulation. Similar to VSMC, MMP activity was more affected by the treatment with the CB_2R agonist JWH-133, which decreased MMP-9 by 12.6% and proMMP-2 by 29.9% (n.s., Figure S1).

MMP-2,9 protein expression analysis is presented in Figure 2. Apart from the proMMP-9 (92 kDa) and MMP-9 (72 kDa) bands, three bands in the area of 45 to 60 kDa were detected (Figure 2a). ProMMP-9 expression increased by 48.4% after stimulation with IL-1α compared to control (Figure 2b), and the CB_2R agonist JWH-133 augmented the increase by 35.5%, whereas the CB_2R antagonist AM 630 increased the expression of proMMP-9 by 50.8%. Moreover, proMMP-9 expression was increased by rimonabant (+4.5%) and CB_1R agonist ACEA (+13.0%). The bands in the area of 45–60 kDa, which were not expressed in the control group, showed a higher degree of regulation than the proMMP-9 and MMP-9 bands (Figure 2b). The CB_2R agonist JWH-133 reduced the MMP expression of the three bands by 60.7%, and the CB_1R antagonist rimonabant reduced MMP expression by 25.7%.

The correlating agonists/antagonists increased MMP activity at this molecular weight, AM630 by (+46.2%) and ACEA by (+40.9%).

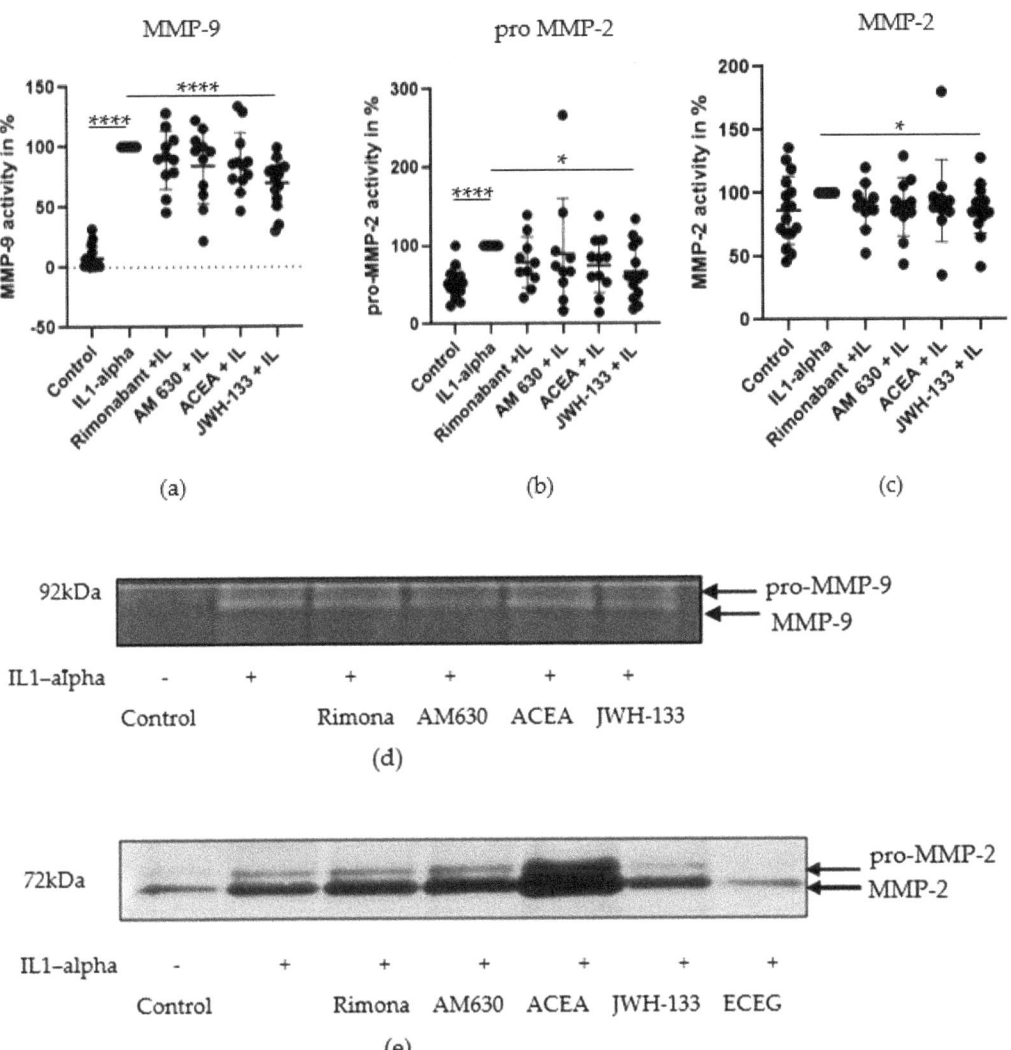

Figure 1. Effect of rimonabant (Rimona), AM630, ACEA and JWH-133 on IL-1α-induced secretion of MMP-9 (**a**), proMMP-2 (**b**) and MMP-2 (**c**) in VSMCs, 48 h after treatment. The *graphs* represent the *densitometric* analysis (mean ± SD; n = 11). Statistical analysis performed with *t*-test with Welch's correction, * $p < 0.05$; **** $p < 0.0001$. (**d**) MMP-9 activity, gelatin zymography, VSMCs, representative zymogram. (**e**) ProMMP-2, MMP-2 activity VSMCs, representative zymogram.

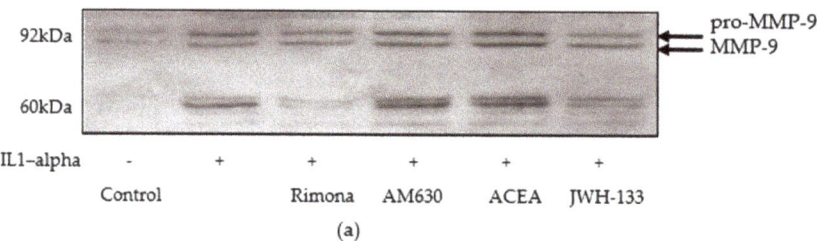

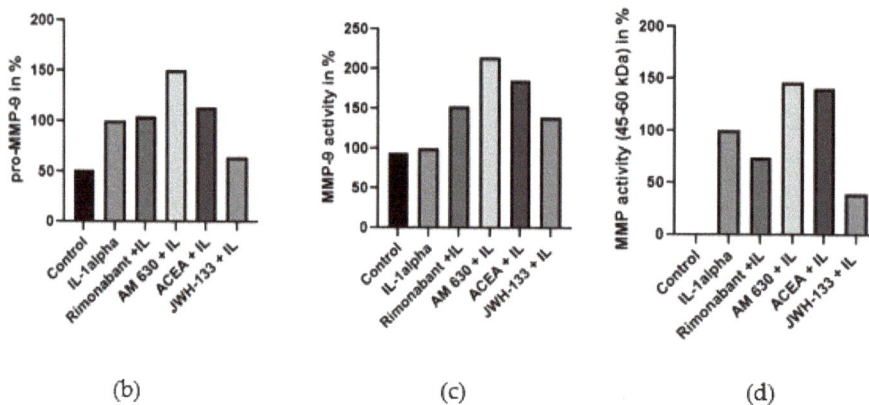

Figure 2. (a) Representative Western blots of MMP-9 in VSMCs, 48 h after stimulation with IL-1α. (b) Densiometric analysis of proMMP-9. (c) Densiometric analysis of MMP-9. (d) Densiometric analysis of MMP (45–60 kDa).

3.2. Regulation of Apoptosis

3.2.1. Apoptosis Ratio

MMP secretion is closely connected with cell death mechanisms. Therefore, the experimental setup used for zymography was also used to perform cell nuclei staining to evaluate apoptosis. The cells were treated with different compounds and cultivated on cover slips. After stimulation of VSMC with IL-1α for 48 h, apoptosis was increased, as demonstrated by an apoptotic ratio (Figure 3). More condensed small cell nuclei with irregular form (blebbing) as well as more disintegrating cells were detected (Figure 3A). IL-1α stimulation increased the number of apoptotic cell nuclei as compared with control. JWH-133 and rimonabant partially mitigated this effect. Rimonabant increased the ratio of normal cell nuclei to apoptotic cell nuclei by 2.5-fold and JWH-133 by 2.0-fold compared to IL-1α-treated cells (Figure 3B). Treatment with ACEA and AM630 did not have a similar effect; apoptosis levels in those two groups were comparable to that after IL-1α stimulation (Figure 3B; IL-1α = 1.0).

The same experimental setup was performed in H9c2 cells. The proapoptotic effect of the IL-1α stimulation was less pronounced in comparison to the IL-1α stimulation in VSMC, hence the effect of the treatment also showed smaller effects. IL-1α treatment increased the number of apoptotic cells 1.2-fold as compared to the control. The CB$_2$R agonist JWH-133 ameliorated this increase 1.1-fold and rimonabant 1.3-fold, while AM 630 treatment showed no difference to the IL-1α group and ACEA showed even more apoptotic cell nuclei than the IL-1α-stimulated H9c2 cells (Figure S2).

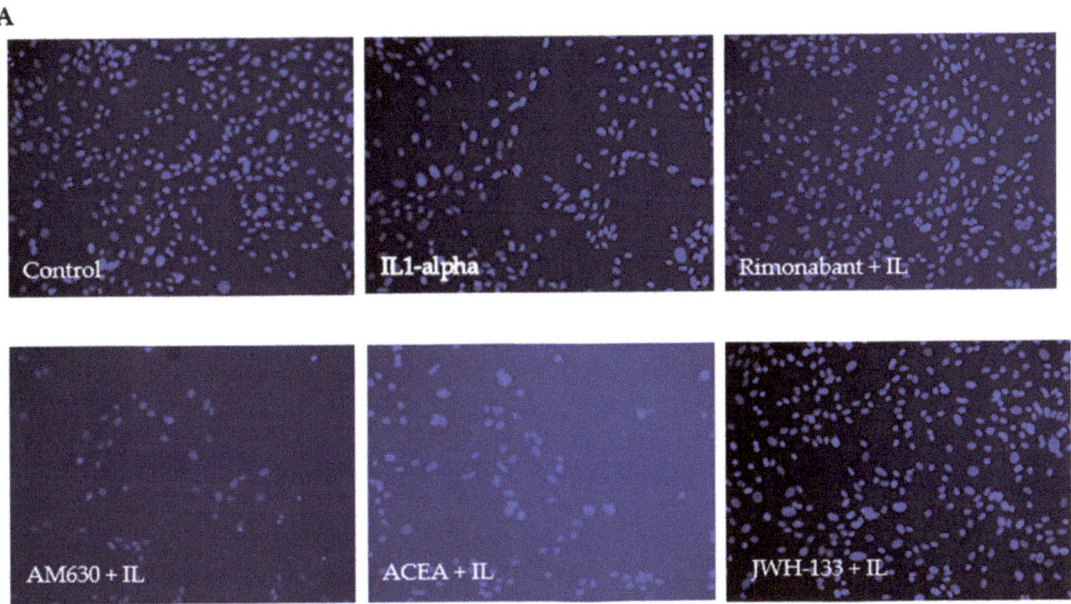

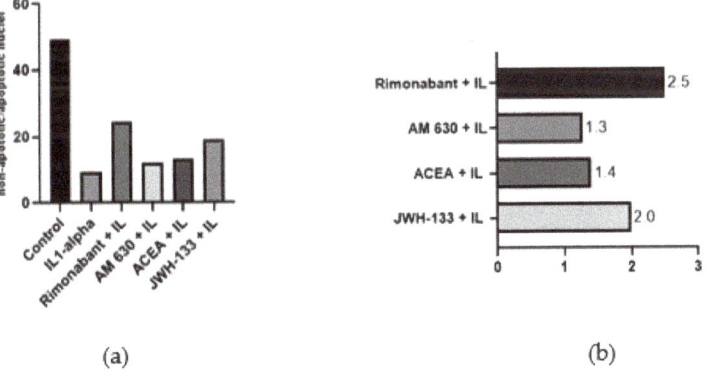

Figure 3. (**A**). Effect of rimonabant, AM630, ACEA and JWH-133 on IL-1α-induced apoptosis in VSMCs. Magnification ×10. More condensed small cell nuclei with irregular form (blebbing) as well as more disintegrating cells were detected after IL-1α stimulation (**B**). (**a**) The ratio of normal cell nuclei to apoptotic cell nuclei in VSMC. The higher the bar, the more normal VSMC could be found in the treatment group. (**b**) The relation of apoptotic ratio in the treatment group to the ratio of the IL-1α-stimulated group. The resulting number expresses the factor of increased normal cell nuclei in comparison to the IL-1α group.

3.2.2. Regulation of Caspase-3, FasL and TGF-Beta1

We further investigated the expression of apoptotic markers caspase-3 and FasL as well TGF-beta1 by fluorescence staining in VSMC. The intensity of caspase-3 expression in different groups is shown in Figure 4A. caspase-3 staining was localized intracellularly in VSMCs. IL-1α showed similar levels of caspase-3 signal compared with the control group. Rimonabant increased caspase-3 expression (2.3-fold), and the CB_1R antagonist ACEA showed an even higher caspase-3 signal (2.8-fold) as compared with IL-1α group. The CB_2R antagonist AM 630 showed an increased caspase-3 signal (1.5-fold), whereas JWH-133 decreased caspase-3 expression under the IL-1α level (by 43.2%) as well as under the control level. Thus, it appears that CB_2R activation reduced apoptosis via caspase-3 signaling.

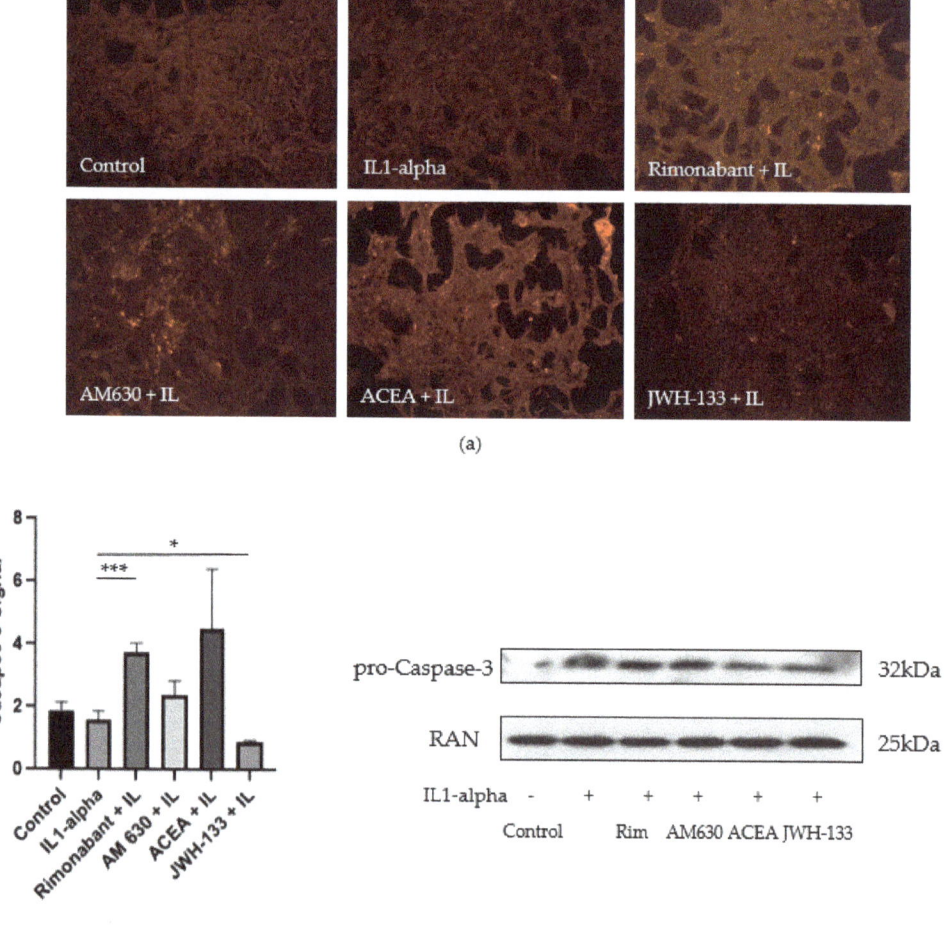

Figure 4. *Cont.*

B

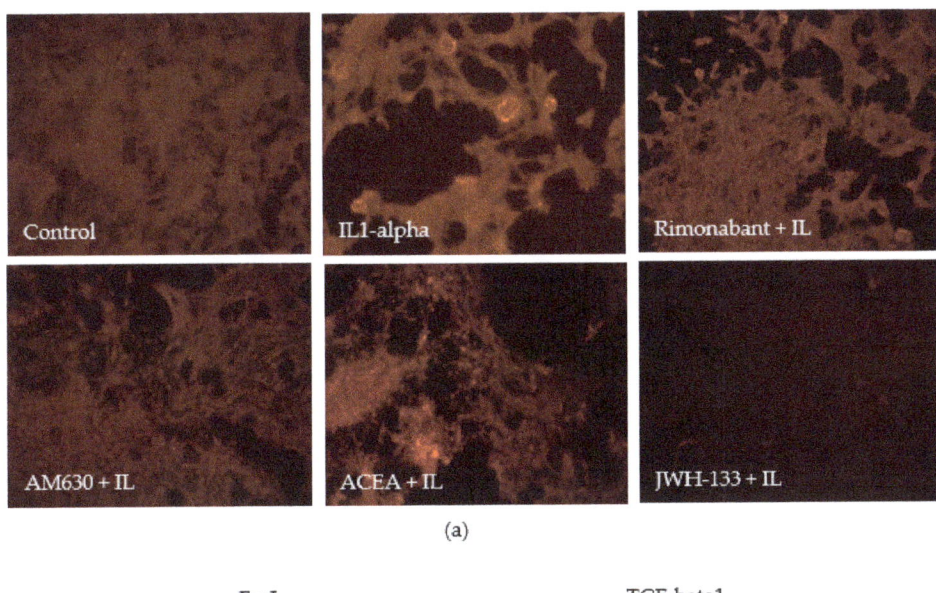

(a)

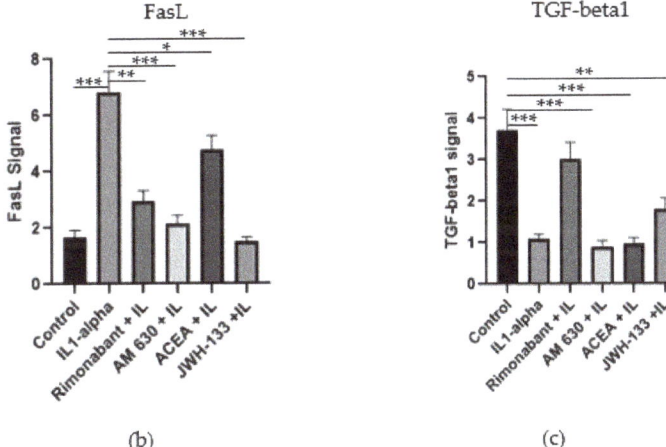

(b)   (c)

Figure 4. (**A**) (**a**) Caspase-3 expression signal in VSMCs, 48 h after treatment with rimonabant, AM 630, ACEA and JWH-133; fluorescent images obtained with Biorevo BZ 900 Microscope using 10× magnification. Exposure time was equal in all observed groups. (**b**) Intensity of caspase-3 expression signal. The results were attained by measuring three areas of interest of the fluorescent image and subtracting the background signal (n = 3). (**c**) Representative Western blots of caspase-3 in VSMCs, 48 h after stimulation with IL-1α. (**B**) (**a**) FasL expression signal in VSMCs, 48 h after treatment with rimonabant, AM 630, ACEA and JWH-133; fluorescent images obtained with Biorevo BZ 900 Microscope using 10× magnification. Exposure time was equal in all observed groups. (**b**) Intensity of FasL expression signal. The results were attained by measuring three areas of interest of the fluorescent image and subtracting the background signal (n = 3). (**c**) Intensity of TGF-beta1 expression signal in VSMCs, 48 h after treatment with rimonabant, AM 630, ACEA, and JWH-133, attained by measuring three areas of interest of the fluorescent image and subtracting the background signal. The measurements were repeated three times per image. Statistical testing was performed using unpaired t-tests. Significance was expressed when $p < 0.05$; (* $p < 0.05$; ** $p < 0.01$; *** $p < 0.001$).

FasL staining was strongly increased by 75.5% after IL-1α stimulation compared with the control (Figure 4B). CB_1R blockage with rimonabant showed a decrease of 57.0% in FasL signal compared to IL-1α, while IL-1α plus ACEA showed the highest expression of all treatment compounds (Figure 4B(a,b)). Treatment with JWH-133 decreased FasL fluorescence signal, 4.5-fold compared to IL-1α, even under control group levels (Figure 4B(a,b)). This result suggests an antiapoptotic effect mitigated via CB_2R activation.

Interestingly, TGF-beta1-expression staining showed opposing results compared to FasL expression (Figure 4C). The involvement of TGF-beta1 in the regulation of cell apoptosis has long been a point of discussion, since it contributes to a plethora of processes in the cell. Our results showed a 3.4-fold downregulation of TGF-beta1 in the IL-1α group compared to control ($p < 0.001$) (Figure 4C). Rimonabant and JWH-133 ($p < 0.005$) reduced this decrease (Figure 4C), while treatment with AM 630 and ACEA even decreased TGF-beta1 as compared to the IL-1α-stimulated group (19.1%, and 11.0%, respectively, $p < 0.001$).

3.3. Regulation of Cell Proliferation: IncuCyte Live-Cell Analysis

IncuCyte live-cell analysis enables the visualization and quantification of cell behavior over time, thus providing insight into cell proliferation and cell death dynamics.

We performed live-cell analysis using a DMEM cell medium containing either 1% FBS or 10% FBS. In line with our previous experiments for zymography analysis, 1% FBS cell medium was used initially. However, such experimental conditions provoked stagnating confluence due to cell death in all groups including the control. Growth rates without IL-1α stimulation in the first 24 h and 48 h were extremely low in all treatment groups (0.1–5.6%). A minimal cell growth rate was observed in the ACEA group (+0% in 24 h, + 3% after 48 h), being in line with the results obtained in the apoptosis analysis.

In order to improve growth conditions, repeated experiments were performed using 10% FBS medium (Figure 5A). A 10% FBS medium increased the growth rates of the control cells in comparison with 1% FBS (14.1% vs. 5.6% after 24 h and 28.0% vs. 5.1% after 48 h). The growth rate of the VSMC after 24 h and 48 h after using 10% FBS DMEM are presented in Figure 5A(a). IL-1α increased the growth rate in comparison to the control in 24 h ($p < 0.001$). Growth rates equalized after 48 h and showed no significant differences between cannabinoid treatment groups without IL-1α stimulation and the control group (Figure S3).

A

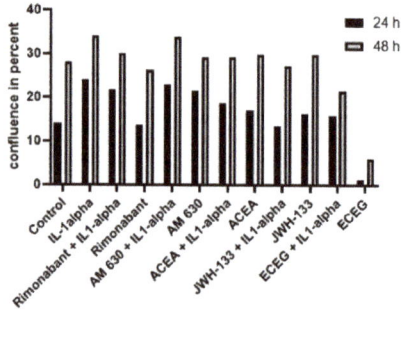

(a)

Figure 5. *Cont.*

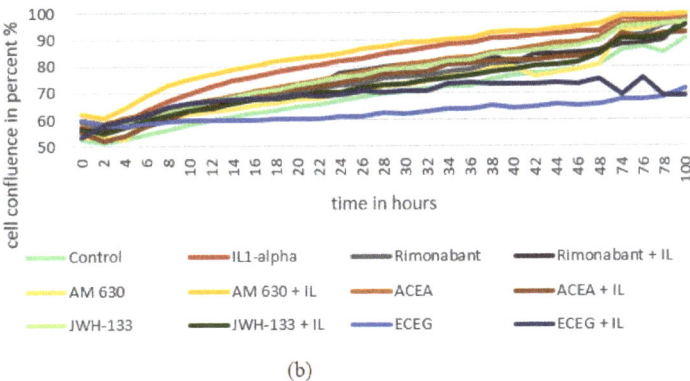

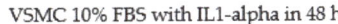

(b)

B

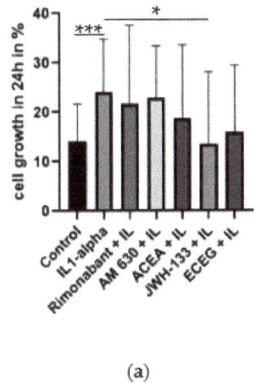 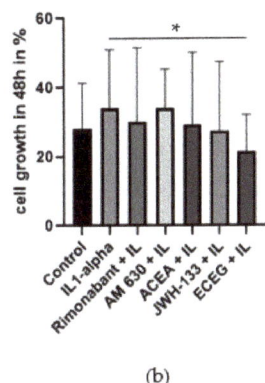

(a) (b)

Figure 5. (**A**) (**a**) VSMC, cell confluence difference (cell growth) at 24 h (confluence at 24 h-confluence at 0 h) and the confluence at 48 h (confluence at 48 h-confluence at 0 h) in the treatment groups. The experiment was performed using 10% FBS medium with and without IL-1α stimulation in all treatment groups. (**b**) VSMC, cell growth in dynamic. Representative graph obtained from IncuCyte Live-Cell Analysis System. Cell proliferation was monitored by analyzing the occupied area (% confluence) of cell images over 100 h. Analysis of the IncuCyte images was performed with Incucyte® Analysis Software. The experiment was performed using 10% FBS medium with and without IL-1α stimulation in all treatment groups. (**B**) The growth rate (confluence difference) of VSMCs estimated by IncuCyte live-cell analysis after treatment with compounds after IL-1α stimulation in 24 h (**a**) and 48 h (**b**). Statistical testing was performed using unpaired t-tests. Significance was expressed when $p < 0.05$; $n = 6$–32 (* $p < 0.05$; *** $p < 0.001$).

We repeated the experiment using IL-1α stimulation in cannabinoid treatment groups. IL-1α increased cell growth rate after 24 h compared to the control group (Figure 5B(b)), and JWH-133 mitigated this increase (Figure 5B(b); $p < 0.05$). After 48 h, only the control compound ECEG decreased the cell growth (Figure 5B(b); $p < 0.05$) as compared with IL-1α.

Repeating the experimental setup using the cardiac H9c2 cell line, we achieved differing results. H9c2 as a secondary cell line showed an increased growth rate. After treatment, similar growth rates leading to full confluence in all groups were observed with and without IL-1α stimulation (Figure S4).

3.4. Regulation of Glucose, Lactate and Electrolytes

In order to ascertain if the treatment compounds influenced cell metabolics, we measured glucose, lactate and electrolytes concentrations in the supernatant. IL-1α stimulation decreased glucose concentration in the supernatant of VSMCs (Figure 6a; $p < 0.01$). JWH-133 and rimonabant normalized glucose levels, as compared to IL-1α stimulation, up to the control levels (Figure 6a; $p < 0.05$). ACEA and AM 630, in contrast, showed no significant effects (Figure 6a).

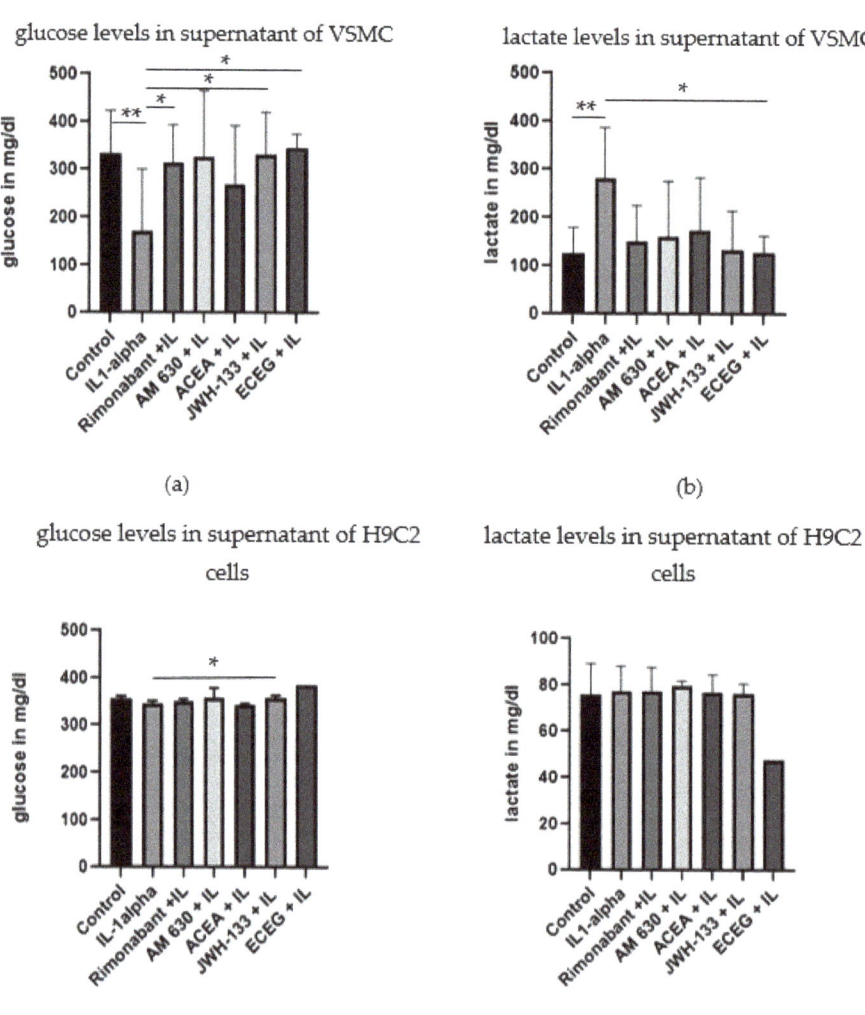

Figure 6. Concentration of glucose (**a**) and lactate (**b**) in the supernatant of VSMC after 48 h of treatment with compounds and IL-1α stimulation. Concentration of glucose (**c**) and lactate (**d**) in the supernatant of H9c2 cells after 48 h of treatment with compounds and IL-1α stimulation. The values are expressed as mean ± SD (VSMC, n = 3–9; H9C2 cells, n = 3). Statistical testing was performed using unpaired t-tests. (* $p < 0.05$; ** $p < 0.01$).

Concomitantly, lactate concentration was increased after the IL-1α stimulation (Figure 6b; 2.2-fold). Rimonabant (by 46.5%) and JWH-133 (by 52.7%) reduced this increase (Figure 6b). The correlation analysis confirmed a negative correlation between glucose levels and lactate levels in the JWH-133 group (r = −0.99; $p < 0.05$) and AM630 group (r = −0.99; $p < 0.01$).

Similar measurements were performed in the supernatant of treated H9c2 cells (Figure 6c,d). JWH-133 also reduced the decrease in glucose concentration after IL-1α stimulation (Figure 6c; $p < 0.05$). In H9c2 cells, lactate levels showed less scattering and similar levels in all treatment groups (Figure 6d). The electrolytes Na, K and Cl were not affected by the different treatments, neither in VSMCs (Figure 7a–c) nor in H9c2 (Figure S5).

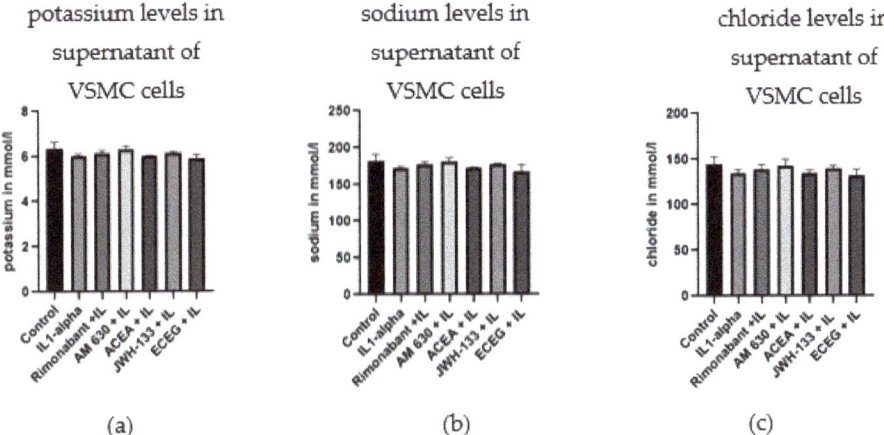

(a)   (b)   (c)

Figure 7. The concentrations of potassium (**a**), sodium (**b**) and chloride (**c**), measured in cell supernatant of VSMCs 48 h after treatments with compounds and IL-1α stimulation.

A comparison of the CB1 and CB2 receptor agonists and antagonists on cytokine-induced MMPs secretion, apoptosis, glucose uptake and cell proliferation in VSMCs and cardiac H9c2 cells is presented in Table 1.

Table 1. Comparison of the effects of the CB1 and CB2 receptor agonists and antagonists on cytokine-induced MMPs secretion, apoptosis, glucose uptake and cell proliferation in VSMCs and cardiac H9c2 cells. ↑—increase; ↓—decrease.

Compound	IL-1α	ACEA	Rimonabant	JWH-133	AM 630	ECEG
CB receptor binding	none	CB1 agonist	CB1 antagonist	CB2 agonist	CB2 antagonist	uncertain
MMP activity VSMC	↑	no effect	↓ MMP-9 ↓ proMMP-2 by tendency	↓↓↓ MMP-9 ↓↓ proMMP-2 ↓↓ MMP-2	no effect	↓↓ MMP-9 ↓↓ proMMP-2 ↓↓ MMP-2
MMP activity H9c2	↑	↑ MMP-9	↑ MMP-9	↓ MMP-9 (13%) ↓ proMMP-2 (30%)	↑ MMP-9 (30%)	↓↓ MMP9
Apoptosis VSMC	↑	no effect	↓↓ 2.5-fold	↓↓ 2.0-fold	no effect	—

Table 1. Cont.

Compound	IL-1α	ACEA	Rimonabant	JWH-133	AM 630	ECEG
Apoptosis H9c2	↑	no effect	↓ 1.3-fold	↓ 1.1-fold	no effect	↓↓ 1.4-fold
Fas L VSMC	↑	↑	↓↓	↓↓	↓	———
Caspase-3 VSMC	↑	↑↑	no effect	↓↓	↑	———
TGF-beta1 VSMC	↓	no effect	↑	↑	no effect	———
Cell proliferation VSMC (10% FBS, 48h)	↑	no effect	no effect	no effect	no effect	↓
Glucose in cell supernatant VSMC	↓↓↓	↑(1.8-fold, n.s.)	↑ 2.1-fold vs. IL1α	↑ 2.2-fold vs. IL1α	↑(2.2-fold, n.s.)	↑ 2.4-fold vs. IL1α
Glucose in cell supernatant H9c2 cells	↓	no effect	no effect	↑ vs. IL1α	no effect	↑ n.s.

4. Discussion

CB receptors are implicated in cardiovascular patho/physiological processes [1–3,5], in particular, in the degradation of the extracellular matrix (ECM) [6,7]. The vascular and cardiac cells could be regulated by these receptors, affecting cell metabolism, proteolytic processes, cell death and proliferation.

In the present study, by using various CB receptor ligands, we intended to find out which receptor subtype is implicated in proteolysis in VSMC. We demonstrated that both CB receptors are involved in the regulation of MMPs, although the CB_2R subtype plays a more important role. In our study, the stimulation of the CB_2R in the VSMCs by the agonist JWH-133 reduced MMP-9 secretion in the supernatant and decreased proMMP-9 protein expression in the cells. In contrast, the CB_2R antagonist AM630 increased MMP-9 expression.

Gelatinase MMP-2 is known to be involved in the degradation of extracellular matrix components and angiogenesis [23]. JWH-133 induced a reduction of both proMMP-2 and MMP-2. The same tendency was demonstrated in H9c2 cells of cardiac origin. Thus, we provide evidence that CB_2R stimulation prevents the cytokine-induced MMP-9 and MMP-2 secretion. Our finding is in line with a study from [20] in neutrophils, which showed that treatment with JWH-133 reduced the release of TNF-α-induced MMP-9 via ERK1/2 phosphorylation. Moreover, JWH-133 exhibited antiproteolytic effects against MMP-1 and MMP-3 in human tenon fibroblasts [26].

CB_1R inhibition with rimonabant in the present study also tended to decrease MMP-9 secretion, confirming our previous data obtained in cardiac fibroblasts [7]. Despite this, an opposite regulation by the CB_1R agonist ACEA could not be shown.

In summary, CB_2R stimulation decreased proteolytic activity in VSMC, mainly by downregulation of MMP-9.

Given the multiple roles of MMPs in cell death and especially in apoptosis, we decided to gain further insights in the effects of the CB agonists and antagonists on apoptosis. The CB_2R agonist JWH-133 as well as the CB_1R antagonist rimonabant mitigated the cell-damaging apoptotic effect of cytokine stimulation in VSMC, as demonstrated by nucleus staining. Further, we could show that the CB_2R agonist JWH-133 reduced the expression of apoptotic markers caspase-3 and FasL, whereas the CB_2R antagonist showed increased caspase-3 expression.

Our results concerning the role of the CB$_2$R in apoptosis are in harmony with studies on cell survival performed in cardiac myocytes and fibroblasts [15] and in the heart ischemia–reperfusion model [27]. Moreover, our data on the CB$_1$R are also in line with the findings that deletion of CB$_1$R or treatment of diabetic mice with CB$_1$R antagonist SR141716 prevented retinal cell death [28].

Nevertheless, the experiments in the H9c2 cell line failed to demonstrate a regulation of apoptosis via CB receptors. Given that these cells showed a decreased reactivity to the IL-1α stimulation, another protocol of apoptosis induction should be tested in future investigations.

TGF-beta1 is an important multifunctional cytokine, which is implied in extracellular matrix remodeling, cell proliferation and cell apoptosis [29]. Interestingly, TGF-beta1 expression was decreased after IL-1α stimulation, in contrast to MMP-9, MMP-2 regulation and the apoptosis rate. These findings are in agreement with Risinger G.M. et al. [30], who showed that TGF-beta1 suppresses the upregulation of MMP-2 by VSMCs. Notably, the CB$_1$R antagonist rimonabant and the CB$_2$R agonist JWH-133 normalized TGF-beta1 expression in the VSMCs up to the control levels.

VSMC proliferation is known to be important for vascular wall remodeling in response to injury. Given that the amount of secreted MMPs depends on cell number, the effect of the treatment protocols on cell proliferation was studied. Therefore, IncuCyte cell life analysis was used to obtain data on the dynamics of cell proliferation and cell death. Neither the CB$_2$R agonist JWH-133 nor the CB$_1$R antagonist rimonabant significantly influenced cell proliferation under the given experimental conditions, suggesting that MMP secretion and apoptosis are regulated by the CB receptors. Nevertheless, at higher FBS concentrations (10%), JWH-133 at one time point 24 h showed antiproliferative properties. Our results may partly explain the controversy from previous studies showing pro-proliferative [22] and antiproliferative [16,31] effects on CB$_2$R stimulation. Interestingly, we also found a strong antiproliferative effect of ECEG that has been used as a control substance in our experimental setting. Thus, further investigations on the role of the CB$_2$R as well as ECEG in the atherosclerosis, angiogenesis and tumor growth would be important.

Since cell metabolism is an essential link between apoptosis and cell proliferation [32], we also addressed the regulation of glucose, lactate and electrolytes after treatment. The electrolytes sodium, potassium and chloride were not affected by treatment with CB$_1$R and CB$_2$R agonists and antagonists. IL-1α stimulation strongly decreased glucose concentration in the supernatant in comparison to the control group. Such decrease can be explained by an increase in glucose uptake into the cell due to activation of glucose transporters GLUT1/4, which are predominant transporters in VSMCs [33,34]. CB$_2$R stimulation with JWH-133 as well as CB$_1$R inhibition with rimonabant reduced the decrease in glucose levels of the supernatant, pointing to a possible interaction of the CB receptors with glucose transporters. Concomitantly, the concentration of lactate was increased after IL-1α stimulation, and rimonabant and JWH-133 also reduced this increase. The effects of JWH-133 on glucose levels were confirmed in cardiac H9c2 cells.

Whether glucose regulation by CB receptors is primary to MMPs secretion requires further investigation. Metabolic changes in VSMC not only contribute to the regulation of cell proliferation, apoptosis and proteolysis but also regulate a switch from the "contractile" phenotype to the proliferative "synthetic" VSMC phenotype [35], thereby influencing the progression of vascular diseases. Therefore, the involvement of the CB receptors in the regulation of glucose metabolism is of relevance in the context of several vascular diseases, including atherosclerosis, diabetes, hypertension and aneurysms.

In summary, the CB$_1$R and the CB$_2$R exert opposite effects on the regulation of cell glucose metabolism, proteolysis and apoptosis in VSMCs and cardiac H9c2 cells.

The stimulation of the CB$_2$R reduced the cytokine-activated secretion of proMMP-2, MMP-2 and MMP-9, reduced FasL and caspase-3 mediated apoptosis, normalized the expression of TGF-beta 1 and prevented cytokine-induced increase in glucose uptake into the cell. CB$_1$R inhibition showed similar protective properties but to a lesser extent. These findings may pave the way to new approaches to treat cardiovascular diseases, especially those associated with extracellular matrix degradation.

Supplementary Materials: The following supporting information can be downloaded at: https://www.mdpi.com/article/10.3390/biomedicines10123271/s1, Figure S1: Effect of Rimonabant, AM630, ACEA and JWH-133 on IL-1α induced secretion of MMP-9 (a), proMMP-2 (b) and MMP-2 (c) in H9c2 cells, 48h after treatment. The graphs represent the densitometric analysis (mean ± SD; n = 5–9 for MMP-9 and MMP-2, pro-MMP-2 (Rimonabant n =1; Control, IL1-alpha n = 2; ACEA, JWH-133, AM 630 n = 3). Statistical analysis performed with t-test with Welchs correction, * p < 0.05; Figure S2: (a) The ratio of non-apoptotic normal cell nuclei to apoptotic cell nuclei in H9c2 cells 48 h after stimulation with IL-1α (b) The non-apoptotic/apoptotic cell nuclei ratio in relation to IL-1α stimulation. Treatment groups with a ratio over 1.0 have more normal cell nuclei than those in the IL-1α group; Figure S3: The growth rate (confluence difference) of VSMCs estimated by IncuCyte live-cell analysis after treatment with compounds without IL-1α stimulation in the treatment groups in 24 h (a) and 48 h (b). Statistical testing was performed using unpaired t-tests between treatment and control group. Significance was expressed when p < 0.05; n = 5–32 (* p < 0.05; *** p < 0,01; **** p < 0.001); Figure S4: The growth rate (confluence difference) of H9c2 cells estimated by IncuCyte live-cell analysis after treatment with compounds without IL-1α stimulation in 24 h (a) and 48 h (b) and with IL1-alpha stimulation in 24 h (c) and 48 h (d). (e) and (f) H9c2, cell growth in dynamic. Representative graph obtained from IncuCyte Live Cell Analysis System. Cell proliferation was monitored by analysing the occupied area (% confluence) of cell images over 48 h. Analysis of the IncuCyte images was performed with Incucyte®Analysis Software. The experiment was performed using 10% FBS medium with (f) and without (e) IL-1α stimulation in all treatment groups; Figure S5: The concentrations of potassium (a), sodium (b) and chloride (c), measured in cell supernatant of H9c2 cells 48 h after treatments with compounds and IL-1α stimulation.

Author Contributions: B.G.: conception and design, performing experiments, collection and assembly of data, data analysis and interpretation, manuscript writing; M.S.: collection and assembly of data; U.K., T.U.: administrative support and advising on manuscript writing; K.K.: conception and design, administrative support, data analysis and interpretation, advising on manuscript writing; E.K.: conception and design, provision of study material, data analysis and interpretation, manuscript writing, final approval of the manuscript. U.K. received research grants/speaker honoraria from Bayer; speaker honoraria from Berlin Chemie, Boehringer Ingelheim, Daiichi Sankyo, Novartis, Sanofi Servier; and participated in advisory boards of Berlin Chemie, Boehringer Ingelheim, Novartis and Sanofi. All authors have read and agreed to the published version of the manuscript.

Funding: This work was supported by Charité Universitätsmedizin Berlin, Germany, and by the "Vascular Network" between CARIM—School for Cardiovascular Diseases, Maastricht University, The Netherlands, and Charité—Universitätsmedizin Berlin, Institute of Pharmacology, Germany. U.K. is supported by the DZHK; BER 5.4 PR, the Deutsche Forschungsgemeinschaft (DFG—KI 712/10-1; SFB-1470-A09); and the Einstein Foundation/Foundation Charité (EVF-BIH-2018-440). K.K. is supported by the Deutsche Forschungsgemeinschaft (DFG—KA 1820/9-1; KA 1820/10-1).

Institutional Review Board Statement: Not applicable.

Informed Consent Statement: Not applicable.

Data Availability Statement: The data presented in this study are available on request from the corresponding author.

Conflicts of Interest: The authors declare no conflict of interest.

References

1. Pacher, P.; Bátkai, S.; Kunos, G. Cardiovascular pharmacology of cannabinoids. *Handb. Exp. Pharmacol.* **2005**, *168*, 599–625. [CrossRef]
2. O'Sullivan, S.E. Endocannabinoids and the Cardiovascular System in Health and Disease. *Handb. Exp. Pharmacol.* **2015**, *231*, 393–422. [CrossRef]
3. Kaschina, E. *Cannabinoid CB1/CB2 Receptors in the Heart: Expression, Regulation, and Function*; Meccariello, C.R.R., Ed.; IntechOpen: London, UK, 2016. [CrossRef]
4. Howlett, A.C.; Abood, M.E. CB1 and CB2 Receptor Pharmacology. *Adv. Pharmacol.* **2017**, *80*, 169–206. [CrossRef]

5. Fulmer, M.L.; Thewke, D.P. The Endocannabinoid System and Heart Disease: The Role of Cannabinoid Receptor Type 2. *Cardiovasc. Hematol. Disord. Drug Targets* **2018**, *18*, 34–51. [CrossRef]
6. Steffens, S.; Pacher, P. Targeting cannabinoid receptor CB(2) in cardiovascular disorders: Promises and controversies. *Br. J. Pharmacol.* **2012**, *167*, 313–323. [CrossRef]
7. Slavic, S.; Lauer, D.; Sommerfeld, M.; Kemnitz, U.R.; Grzesiak, A.; Trappiel, M.; Thöne-Reineke, C.; Baulmann, J.; Paulis, L.; Kappert, K.; et al. Cannabinoid receptor 1 inhibition improves cardiac function and remodelling after myocardial infarction and in experimental metabolic syndrome. *J. Mol. Med.* **2013**, *91*, 811–823. [CrossRef] [PubMed]
8. Matsuda, L.A.; Lolait, S.J.; Brownstein, M.J.; Young, A.C.; Bonner, T.I. Structure of a cannabinoid receptor and functional expression of the cloned cDNA. *Nature* **1990**, *346*, 561–564. [CrossRef] [PubMed]
9. Munro, S.; Thomas, K.L.; Abu-Shaar, M. Molecular characterization of a peripheral receptor for cannabinoids. *Nature* **1993**, *365*, 61–65. [CrossRef] [PubMed]
10. Pertwee, R.G.; Howlett, A.C.; Abood, M.E.; Alexander, S.P.; Di Marzo, V.; Elphick, M.R.; Greasley, P.J.; Hansen, H.S.; Kunos, G.; Mackie, K.; et al. International Union of Basic and Clinical Pharmacology. LXXIX. Cannabinoid receptors and their ligands: Beyond CB_1 and CB_2. *Pharmacol. Rev.* **2010**, *62*, 588–631. [CrossRef]
11. Stefanucci, A.; Macedonio, G.; Dvorácskó, S.; Tömböly, C.; Mollica, A. Novel Fubinaca/Rimonabant hybrids as endocannabinoid system modulators. *Amino Acids* **2018**, *50*, 1595–1605. [CrossRef] [PubMed]
12. Mollica, A.; Pelliccia, S.; Famiglini, V.; Stefanucci, A.; Macedonio, G.; Chiavaroli, A.; Orlando, G.; Brunetti, L.; Ferrante, C.; Pieretti, S.; et al. Exploring the first Rimonabant analog-opioid peptide hybrid compound, as bivalent ligand for CB1 and opioid receptors. *J. Enzyme Inhib. Med. Chem.* **2017**, *32*, 444–451. [CrossRef]
13. Dvorácskó, S.; Keresztes, A.; Mollica, A.; Stefanucci, A.; Macedonio, G.; Pieretti, S.; Zádor, F.; Walter, F.R.; Deli, M.A.; Kékesi, G.; et al. Preparation of bivalent agonists for targeting the mu opioid and cannabinoid receptors. *Eur. J. Med. Chem.* **2019**, *178*, 571–588. [CrossRef]
14. Bátkai, S.; Pacher, P. Endocannabinoids and cardiac contractile function: Pathophysiological implications. *Pharmacol. Res.* **2009**, *60*, 99–106. [CrossRef]
15. Mukhopadhyay, P.; Rajesh, M.; Bátkai, S.; Patel, V.; Kashiwaya, Y.; Liaudet, L.; Evgenov, O.V.; Mackie, K.; Haskó, G.; Pacher, P. CB1 cannabinoid receptors promote oxidative stress and cell death in murine models of doxorubicin-induced cardiomyopathy and in human cardiomyocytes. *Cardiovasc. Res.* **2010**, *85*, 773–784. [CrossRef]
16. Steffens, M.; Zentner, J.; Honegger, J.; Feuerstein, T.J. Binding affinity and agonist activity of putative endogenous cannabinoids at the human neocortical CB1 receptor. *Biochem. Pharmacol.* **2005**, *69*, 169–178. [CrossRef]
17. Hashiesh, H.M.; Sharma, C.; Goyal, S.N.; Jha, N.K.; Ojha, S. Pharmacological Properties, Therapeutic Potential and Molecular Mechanisms of JWH133, a CB2 Receptor-Selective Agonist. *Front. Pharmacol.* **2021**, *12*, 702675. [CrossRef]
18. Defer, N.; Wan, J.; Souktani, R.; Escoubet, B.; Perier, M.; Caramelle, P.; Manin, S.; Deveaux, V.; Bourin, M.C.; Zimmer, A.; et al. The cannabinoid receptor type 2 promotes cardiac myocyte and fibroblast survival and protects against ischemia/reperfusion-induced cardiomyopathy. *FASEB J.* **2009**, *23*, 2120–2130. [CrossRef] [PubMed]
19. Netherland, C.D.; Pickle, T.G.; Bales, A.; Thewke, D.P. Cannabinoid receptor type 2 (CB2) deficiency alters atherosclerotic lesion formation in hyperlipidemic Ldlr-null mice. *Atherosclerosis* **2010**, *213*, 102–108. [CrossRef] [PubMed]
20. Montecucco, F.; Di Marzo, V.; da Silva, R.F.; Vuilleumier, N.; Capettini, L.; Lenglet, S.; Pagano, S.; Piscitelli, F.; Quintao, S.; Bertolotto, M.; et al. The activation of the cannabinoid receptor type 2 reduces neutrophilic protease-mediated vulnerability in atherosclerotic plaques. *Eur. Heart J.* **2012**, *33*, 846–856. [CrossRef] [PubMed]
21. Gebremedhin, D.; Lange, A.R.; Campbell, W.B.; Hillard, C.J.; Harder, D.R. Cannabinoid CB1 receptor of cat cerebral arterial muscle functions to inhibit L-type Ca^{2+} channel current. *Am. J. Physiol.* **1999**, *276*, H2085–H2093. [CrossRef]
22. Rajesh, M.; Mukhopadhyay, P.; Haskó, G.; Huffman, J.W.; Mackie, K.; Pacher, P. CB2 cannabinoid receptor agonists attenuate TNF-alpha-induced human vascular smooth muscle cell proliferation and migration. *Br. J. Pharmacol.* **2008**, *153*, 347–357. [CrossRef]
23. Verma, R.P.; Hansch, C. Matrix metalloproteinases (MMPs): Chemical-biological functions and (Q)SARs. *Bioorg. Med. Chem.* **2007**, *15*, 2223–2268. [CrossRef] [PubMed]
24. Orlandi, A.; Ehrlich, H.P.; Ropraz, P.; Spagnoli, L.G.; Gabbiani, G. Rat aortic smooth muscle cells isolated from different layers and at different times after endothelial denudation show distinct biological features in vitro. *Arterioscler. Thromb.* **1994**, *14*, 982–989. [CrossRef]
25. Vosgerau, U.; Lauer, D.; Unger, T.; Kaschina, E. Cleaved high molecular weight kininogen, a novel factor in the regulation of matrix metalloproteinases in vascular smooth muscle cells. *Biochem. Pharmacol.* **2010**, *79*, 172–179. [CrossRef]
26. Guan, T.; Zhao, G.; Duan, H.; Liu, Y.; Zhao, F. Activation of type 2 cannabinoid receptor (CB2R) by selective agonists regulates the deposition and remodelling of the extracellular matrix. *Biomed. Pharmacother.* **2017**, *95*, 1704–1709. [CrossRef]
27. Li, Q.; Wang, F.; Zhang, Y.M.; Zhou, J.J.; Zhang, Y. Activation of cannabinoid type 2 receptor by JWH133 protects heart against ischemia/reperfusion-induced apoptosis. *Cell Physiol. Biochem.* **2013**, *31*, 693–702. [CrossRef] [PubMed]
28. El-Remessy, A.B.; Rajesh, M.; Mukhopadhyay, P.; Horváth, B.; Patel, V.; Al-Gayyar, M.M.; Pillai, B.A.; Pacher, P. Cannabinoid 1 receptor activation contributes to vascular inflammation and cell death in a mouse model of diabetic retinopathy and a human retinal cell line. *Diabetologia* **2011**, *54*, 1567–1578. [CrossRef] [PubMed]

29. Morikawa, M.; Derynck, R.; Miyazono, K. TGF-β and the TGF-β Family: Context-Dependent Roles in Cell and Tissue Physiology. *Cold Spring Harb. Perspect. Biol.* **2016**, *8*, a021873. [CrossRef] [PubMed]
30. Risinger, G.M.; Updike, D.L.; Bullen, E.C.; Tomasek, J.J.; Howard, E.W. TGF-beta suppresses the upregulation of MMP-2 by vascular smooth muscle cells in response to PDGF-BB. *Am. J. Physiol. Cell Physiol.* **2010**, *298*, C191–C201. [CrossRef]
31. Molica, F.; Matter, C.M.; Burger, F.; Pelli, G.; Lenglet, S.; Zimmer, A.; Pacher, P.; Steffens, S. Cannabinoid receptor CB2 protects against balloon-induced neointima formation. *Am. J. Physiol. Heart Circ. Physiol.* **2012**, *302*, H1064–H1074. [CrossRef]
32. Mason, E.F.; Rathmell, J.C. Cell metabolism: An essential link between cell growth and apoptosis. *Biochim. Biophys. Acta* **2011**, *1813*, 645–654. [CrossRef] [PubMed]
33. Park, J.L.; Loberg, R.D.; Duquaine, D.; Zhang, H.; Deo, B.K.; Ardanaz, N.; Coyle, J.; Atkins, K.B.; Schin, M.; Charron, M.J.; et al. GLUT4 facilitative glucose transporter specifically and differentially contributes to agonist-induced vascular reactivity in mouse aorta. *Arterioscler. Thromb. Vasc. Biol.* **2005**, *25*, 1596–1602. [CrossRef] [PubMed]
34. Buller, C.L.; Loberg, R.D.; Fan, M.H.; Zhu, Q.; Park, J.L.; Vesely, E.; Inoki, K.; Guan, K.L.; Brosius, F.C. A GSK-3/TSC2/mTOR pathway regulates glucose uptake and GLUT1 glucose transporter expression. *Am. J. Physiol. Cell Physiol.* **2008**, *295*, C836–C843. [CrossRef] [PubMed]
35. Shi, J.; Yang, Y.; Cheng, A.; Xu, G.; He, F. Metabolism of vascular smooth muscle cells in vascular diseases. *Am. J. Physiol. Heart Circ. Physiol.* **2020**, *319*, H613–H631. [CrossRef]

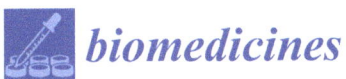

Article

Safety and Tolerability of Oral Cannabinoids in People Living with HIV on Long-Term ART: A Randomized, Open-Label, Interventional Pilot Clinical Trial (CTNPT 028) †

Ralph-Sydney Mboumba Bouassa [1,2], Judy Needham [3,4], Dana Nohynek [3,4], Joel Singer [3,4,5], Terry Lee [3,4], Florian Bobeuf [6], Suzanne Samarani [2,6], Lina Del Balso [6], Natalie Paisible [6], Claude Vertzagias [6], Giada Sebastiani [2,6,7], Shari Margolese [3], Enrico Mandarino [3], Marina Klein [2,6], Bertrand Lebouché [2,6,8,9], Joseph Cox [2,6], Marie-Josée Brouillette [2,6,10], Jean-Pierre Routy [2,6,11], Jason Szabo [6,8,12], Réjean Thomas [12], Emmanuel Huchet [13], Antonio Vigano [14,15], Mohammad-Ali Jenabian [1,16] and Cecilia T Costiniuk [2,6,15,17,*]

1 Department of Biological Sciences and CERMO-FC Research Centre, Université du Québec à Montréal, Montreal, QC H2X 3Y7, Canada
2 Infectious Diseases and Immunity in Global Health Program, Research Institute of McGill University Health Centre, Montreal, QC H4A 3J1, Canada
3 CIHR Canadian HIV Trials Network, Vancouver, BC V6Z 1Y6, Canada
4 Centre for Health Evaluation and Outcome Sciences, St. Paul's Hospital, Vancouver, BC V6Z 1Y6, Canada
5 School of Population and Public Health, University of British Columbia, Vancouver, BC V6T 1Z4, Canada
6 Department of Medicine, Division of Infectious Diseases and Chronic Viral Illnesses Service, McGill University Health Centre, Montreal, QC H4A 3J1, Canada
7 Department of Medicine, Division of Gastroenterology and Hepatology, McGill University Health Centre, Montreal, QC H4A 3J1, Canada
8 Department of Family Medicine, McGill University Health Centre, Montreal, QC H4A 3J1, Canada
9 Canadian Institutes of Health Research Strategy for Patient-Oriented Research Mentorship Chair in Innovative Clinical Trials, Montreal, QC H4A 3J1, Canada
10 Department of Psychiatry, McGill University Health Centre, Montreal, QC H4A 3J1, Canada
11 Department of Medicine, Division of Hematology, McGill University Health Centre, Montreal, QC H4A 3J1, Canada
12 Clinique Médical L'Actuel, Montreal, QC H2L 4P9, Canada
13 Clinique Médical L'Agora, Montreal, QC H2L 4E9, Canada
14 Medical Cannabis Program in Oncology, Cedars Cancer Center, McGill University Health Centre, 1001 Boulevard Decarie, Montreal, QC H4A 3J1, Canada
15 Centre for Cannabis Research, McGill University, Montreal, QC H3A 0G4, Canada
16 Department of Microbiology, Infectiology and Immunology, Université de Montréal, Montreal, QC H3T 1J4, Canada
17 Department of Microbiology and Immunology, McGill University, Montreal, QC H3A 0G4, Canada
* Correspondence: cecilia.costiniuk@mcgill.ca; Tel.: +1-514-934-1934 (ext. 76195); Fax: +1-514-843-2209
† This work was presented at the 3rd Annual Congress on Controversies on Cannabis-Based Medicines (Med-Cannabis 2022), Copenhagen, Denmark, 2–3 November 2022.

Citation: Mboumba Bouassa, R.-S.; Needham, J.; Nohynek, D.; Singer, J.; Lee, T.; Bobeuf, F.; Samarani, S.; Del Balso, L.; Paisible, N.; Vertzagias, C.; et al. Safety and Tolerability of Oral Cannabinoids in People Living with HIV on Long-Term ART: A Randomized, Open-Label, Interventional Pilot Clinical Trial (CTNPT 028). Biomedicines 2022, 10, 3168. https://doi.org/10.3390/biomedicines10123168

Academic Editor: Wesley M. Raup-Konsavage

Received: 31 October 2022
Accepted: 24 November 2022
Published: 7 December 2022

Publisher's Note: MDPI stays neutral with regard to jurisdictional claims in published maps and institutional affiliations.

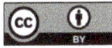

Copyright: © 2022 by the authors. Licensee MDPI, Basel, Switzerland. This article is an open access article distributed under the terms and conditions of the Creative Commons Attribution (CC BY) license (https://creativecommons.org/licenses/by/4.0/).

Abstract: Background: With anti-inflammatory properties, cannabinoids may be a potential strategy to reduce immune activation in people living with HIV (PLWH) but more information on their safety and tolerability is needed. Methods: We conducted an open-label interventional pilot study at the McGill University Health Centre in Montreal, Canada. PLWH were randomized to oral Δ9-tetrahydrocannabinol (THC): cannabidiol (CBD) combination (THC 2.5 mg/CBD 2.5 mg) or CBD-only capsules (CBD 200 mg). Individuals titrated doses as tolerated to a maximum daily dose THC 15 mg/CBD 15 mg or 800 mg CBD, respectively, for 12 weeks. The primary outcome was the percentage of participants without any significant toxicity based on the WHO toxicity scale (Grades 0–2 scores). Results: Out of ten individuals, eight completed the study. Two from the CBD-only arm were withdrawn for safety concerns: phlebotomy aggravating pre-existing anemia and severe hepatitis on 800 mg CBD with newly discovered pancreatic adenocarcinoma, respectively. Seven did not have any significant toxicity. Cannabinoids did not alter hematology/biochemistry profiles. CD4 count, CD4/CD8 ratio, and HIV suppression remained stable. Most adverse effects were mild-moderate. Conclusions: In PLWH, cannabinoids seem generally safe and well-tolerated, though larger studies are needed. Screening for occult liver pathology should be performed and hepatic enzymes monitored, especially with high CBD doses.

Keywords: HIV; cannabinoids; cannabidiol (CBD); tetrahydrocannabinol (THC); chronic liver diseases; quality of life; pilot clinical trial

1. Introduction

People living with HIV (PLWH) experience persistent immune activation and systemic inflammation [1–4]. These processes, in turn, drive development and progression of non-Acquired Immune Deficiency Syndrome (AIDS)-related comorbidities such as cardiovascular diseases, metabolic and neurological disorders, malignancies, and liver fibrosis [1–4]. By attenuating chronic inflammation, one may slow the progression of chronic diseases [5–8].

Historically, cannabis was used by PLWH to alleviate AIDS-related symptoms such as nausea, anorexia and depression [9]. During the modern antiretroviral treatment (ART) era, cannabis use remains common amongst PLWH for both recreational and medicinal reasons, including chronic pain, anxiety and depression [9–13]. The primary phytocannabinoids, delta-9-tetrahydrocannabinol (THC) and cannabidiol (CBD), possess anti-inflammatory and anti-fibrotic properties, as demonstrated in vitro [14–18] and in vivo during animal [19–22] and human observational studies [23–25]. Therefore, cannabinoids might be a potential therapeutic strategy to reduce chronic inflammation in PLWH on ART.

Due to successful advocacy during the early days of the HIV/AIDS epidemic, medical cannabis first became legalized in Canada in 2001 [26]. However, cannabinoid-based medicines (CBM) have not gone through the traditional drug development and formal drug approval process, and formal nonclinical pharmacokinetic and toxicology information are lacking [7]. Consequently, there remains an important lack of safety data for cannabis-based medicines in PLWH in the modern ART era [7]. Moreover, with legalization of recreational cannabis in Canada [27], it is now easier to obtain cannabinoids which may not have been thoroughly evaluated for safety and tolerability [28,29]. Before conducting large scale clinical trials to evaluate the efficacy of CBM for diverse comorbidities and symptomatology experienced by PLWH, a pivotal step will be to determine the safety, tolerability and feasibility, of using oral cannabinoids in this population. Here, we report on the safety and tolerability of oral cannabinoids in PLWH in a randomized, open-label, interventional pilot study. A THC:CBD combination arm was selected as both compounds have therapeutic properties and may function synergistically [30–34]. Furthermore, the use of CBD tends to improve THC tolerability when combined [30–34]. A CBD-only arm was also selected, in part, to observe the effects of CBD monotherapy in addition to feasibility reasons (i.e., capsules availability). Feasibility and effects on immune cell profiles, inflammatory markers, HIV reservoir size and gut microbiome will be reported in separate manuscripts.

2. Methods

2.1. Study Design

This was a randomized, open-label, interventional pilot study (CIHR Canadian HIV Trials Network (CTN) PT028) to assess the safety and tolerability of oral THC:CBD combined or CBD-only capsules consumed daily for 12 weeks [7].

2.2. Enrolment, Selection Criteria and Study Population

Recruitment occurred at the Chronic Viral Illness Service, Royal Victoria Hospital of the McGill University Health Centre in Montreal, Canada. Participants were included if they were 18 years of age or older and had HIV infection with suppressed viral load (VL) <40 copies/mL on ART for at least 3 years. Participants also had to have a negative baseline cannabinoid urine screen. Participants were excluded if they used cannabinoid-containing products outside of the study or within 4 weeks of study commencement. A full list of inclusion/exclusion criteria is included in Supplementary Table S1.

2.3. Study Intervention

Oral capsules, manufactured by Tilray Brands, Inc. (New York City, NY, USA), consisted of highly purified (>98%) cannabinoids in oil. Formulations included TN-TC11M2, a THC:CBD combination in a 1:1 ratio (2.5 mg/2.5 mg), and TN-C200M2, consisting CBD only (200 mg). Capsules were of interest given the potential of orally administered cannabinoids to reduce gut-associated inflammation [35]. Due to person-to-person variability in metabolism and tolerability [36], participants up-titrated cannabinoid doses as tolerated (Table 1), a method which has proven successful in other clinical trials [37]. Dosage ranges for both the THC/CBD combination (2.5 to 15 mg/day) and the CBD-only formulation (200 to 800 mg/day) have been determined based on other clinical trials demonstrating safety, tolerability, and the efficacy of these doses for the management of other pathologies such as chronic pain, epilepsy, schizophrenia, or even multiple sclerosis [38–41].

Table 1. Recommended up-titration schedule for TN-TC11M2 and TN-C200M2 regimens.

Arm 1 (TN-TC11M2: (THC: 2.5 mg/CBD: 2.5 mg))			Arm 2 (TN-C200M2: CBD; 200 mg) Original Titration Schedule *			Arm 2 (TN-C200M2: CBD; 200 mg) Revised Titration Schedule #		
Weeks	Daily Dose	Number of Capsules (Taken Orally and Spaced Out Every 12 h)	Weeks	Daily Dose	Number of Capsules (Taken Orally and Spaced Out Every 12 h)	Weeks	Daily Dose	Number of Capsules (Taken Orally and Spaced Out Every 12 h)
Week 0 and 1 (Day 1–14)	5 mg THC/5 mg CBD	1 capsule twice daily (2 capsules per day)	Week 0 and 1 (Day 1–14)	200 mg CBD	1 capsule once daily	Week 0 and 1 (Day 1–14)	200 mg CBD	1 capsule once daily
Week 2 and 3 (Day 15–28)	10 mg THC/10 mg CBD	2 capsules twice daily, (4 capsules per day)	Week 2 and 3 (Day 15–28)	400 mg CBD	1 capsule twice daily (2 capsules per day)	Week 2–11 (Day 15–84)	400 mg CBD	1 capsule twice daily (2 capsules per day)
Week 4–11 (Day 29–84)	15 mg THC/15 mg CBD	2 capsules three times daily, (6 capsules per day)	Week 4–11 (Day 29–84)	800 mg # CBD	2 capsules twice daily (4 capsules per day)			

* Original titration schedule for arm 2: this titration schedule has been revised because of possible hepatotoxicity of high dose of CBD (800 mg per day); # Revised titration schedule for arm 2.

2.4. Randomization

Participants were randomized in a 1:1 ratio to either TN-TC11M2 (arm 1) or TN-C200M2 (arm 2).

2.5. Safety and Tolerability Assessments and Specimen Collection

The visit schedule is depicted in Figure 1. Participants underwent a physical exam and occurrence of adverse events (AEs), use of concomitant medications and the presence of common symptoms associated with cannabinoids (including dizziness, nausea, headaches, appetite or mood changes) were assessed. Toxicity of TN-TC11M2 and TN-C200M2 was assessed using the World Health Organization (WHO) toxicity scale. All AEs, regardless of grade, were documented, and those possibly related to TN-TC11M2 and TN-C200M2 were managed by dose reduction. Cannabinoids were permanently discontinued when life-threatening AEs occurred. Blood was drawn for CD4 and CD8 T-cells counts, plasma VL, complete blood count, aspartate aminotransferase (AST), alanine aminotransferase (ALT), alkaline phosphatase (ALP), total bilirubin, urea, creatinine and blood glucose, as well as future T-cell activation and inflammatory markers. Nasal swabs and stool specimens were collected at baseline and end of the treatment period for future microbiome analysis. Men had the option of donating a semen specimen collected at baseline and end of the treatment period for future HIV reservoir studies.

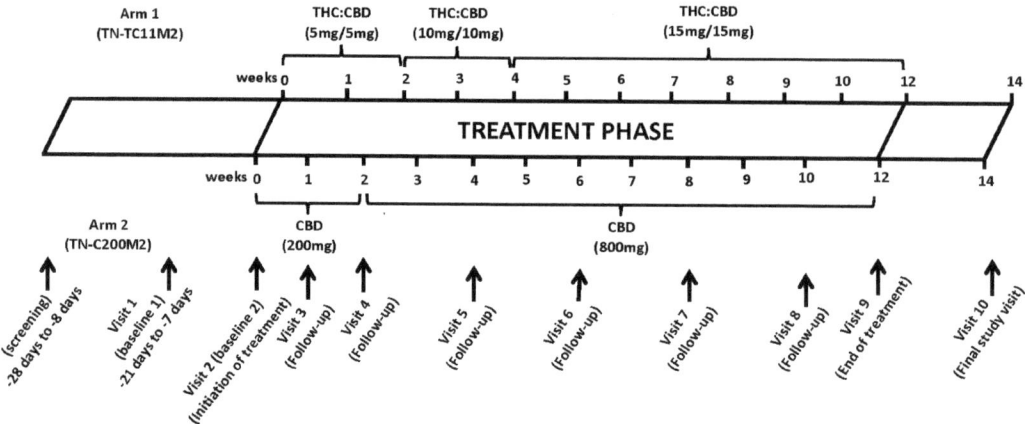

Figure 1. Schedule of visits and procedures. Screening: Up to 4 weeks prior to randomization, during the screening visit, study staff explained the study to the participants and obtained written informed consent prior to initiating any study procedures. Study staff assessed the participant's eligibility by assessing the inclusion and exclusion criteria. Study staff collected the medical history and concomitant medications of the study participants and they underwent a complete physical exam. Blood was collected for hematology, blood chemistry, HIV RNA load and CD4 and CD8 T cells counts. A urine pregnancy test was performed for female participants. Cannabis Use Disorder Identification Test-Revised (CUDIT-R), Drug Use Disorder Identification Test (DUDIT) and Alcohol Use Disorder Identification Test (AUDIT) questionnaires were administrated to the participants and they underwent testing for Hepatitis B and C and syphilis infections. They also underwent urine screen for cannabinoids use. Baseline 1: Up to 3 weeks before the randomization, study staff confirmed eligibility of the candidate and reviewed their medical history. Participants then underwent a second cannabinoids screening test, if his/her initial screen was positive, and answered the CUDIT-R questionnaire in order to identify any problematic cannabis use. The participants underwent a targeted physical exam and blood and semen (from male) were collected to quantify the HIV reservoir size in circulating PBMC from blood and in the semen. Nasal swab and stool specimens were collected from study participants. Antiretroviral Therapy (ART) compliance, alcohol intake and concomitant medication were reviewed by the study staff. Baseline 2 (week 0: Initiation of treatment): Participants confirmed their willingness to participate in the study and eligibility was confirmed, before participants were randomized to either arm 1 or arm 2. Blood was collected from participants. Participants underwent a targeted physical exam. Participants also completed the World Health Organization Quality of Life—HIV Brief Scale (WHOQOLHIV-BREF), Euro-Qol-5Dimension (EQ-5D) questionnaire, and Profile of MoodStates (POMS) questionnaires before receiving a one week supply of the study medication. Follow-up visits (visit 3–8; week 1 to 10): During the follow-up visits, participants underwent a physical examination, and blood was collected to assess the biological study measures. Study drug and ART compliance was assessed. Adverse effects (AEs) were recorded. Pregnancy test was performed on urine of female participants. The participants completed the WHOQOLHIV-BREF, EQ-5D, and POMS questionnaires (Visit 6) and received the study medication until their next visit. End of the treatment (Visit 9; week 12): At Visit 9, participants underwent a physical examination, and blood was collected to assess the biological study measures. Nasal swab and stool specimens were collected from all study participants and semen was collected from male participants. AEs were recorded. A pregnancy test was performed on urine of female participants. Participants then completed the WHOQOLHIV-BREF, EQ-5D, and POMS questionnaires. Final study visit (Visit 10; week 14): At the final visit, participants underwent a physical examination, and blood was collected to assess the biological study measures. AEs were recorded and ART compliance was assessed. A pregnancy test was performed on urine of female participants.

2.6. Quality of Life and Mood Assessment

WHO Quality of Life HIV Brief (WHOQOLHIV-BREF), Euro-Qol-5Dimension (EQ-5D) and Profile of Mood States (POMS) questionnaires were administered at baseline, midway through the study (Visit 6) and at the end of treatment (Visit 9) (Figure 1). WHOQOLHIV-BREF consists of 31 items that measure the following domains: physical health, psychological health, social relationships and environment [42]. EQ-5D is a descriptive questionnaire examining five dimensions: (1) mobility, (2) self-care, (3) usual activities, (4) pain/discomfort and (5) anxiety/depression [43]. Meanwhile, the POMS questionnaire measures the following six factors: (1) tension-anxiety, (2) anger-hostility, (3) fatigue-inertia, (4) depression-dejection, (5) vigour-activity and (6) confusion-bewilderment [44].

2.7. Study Outcome Measures

Endpoints consisted of (1) the proportion of participants in both groups without any sign of significant toxicity as determined by the WHO toxicity scale (i.e., number of participants with grades 0–2 scores on the WHO toxicity scale); (2) the proportions of participants who were able to complete the study and (3) changes in scores on the WHOQOLHIV-BREF scale, EQ-D5 and POMS questionnaires from week 0 to week 12. A description of WHO toxicity scale grades is presented in Supplementary Table S2.

2.8. Ethics

Prior to study enrolment, individuals signed a written informed consent form. This study was approved by the Research Ethics Board of the McGill University Health Centre (#2018-4336) and conducted in conformity with the Declaration of Helsinki.

2.9. Statistical Analyses

Data were recorded onto data collection work sheets and then entered into an InForm collection and trial management online platform. Descriptive statistics were used. Means (standard deviation) and medians (interquartile range) were calculated for quantitative variables and the non-parametric Friedman test was used to assess differences between measures repeated at each visit. Wilcoxon signed-rank test was used to compare paired repeated measurements between two visits. GraphPad Prism Software (version 9.0.0, San Diego, CA, USA) was used for statistical analyses.

3. Results

3.1. Study Participants

Between September 2021–February 2022, 10 PLWH were enrolled. The initial enrollment target was 26 participants, but the study was closed prematurely due to rupture of cannabinoid capsules stock, the impossibility of renewing the stock of capsules with the same manufacturing criteria and enrolment challenges. Baseline characteristics are summarized in Table 2. Median age was 57.5 years (IQR: 54.75–61.75) and most were male (80%). Based on the CUDIT-R results, 7 out of the 10 participants (70%) reported having consumed cannabis during the past 6 months. Study group allocation is depicted in Figure 2.

Table 2. Demographic and biological characteristics of study participants at inclusion ($n = 10$).

	Total Population	THC:CBD Arm ($n = 5$)	CBD Arm ($n = 5$)
Age (Years), median ($\pm$IQR)	57.5 (54.75–61.75)	57.0 (46.5–57.5)	62 (47.0–65.0)
Sex assigned at birth (n (%))			
Male	8 (80%)	5 (100%)	3 (60%)
Female	2 (20%)	0 (0%)	2 (40%)

Table 2. Cont.

	Total Population	THC:CBD Arm (n = 5)	CBD Arm (n = 5)
Ethnicity (n (%))			
White-North American	6 (60%)	3 (60%)	3 (60%)
Black-African	1 (10%)	0 (0%)	1 (20%)
Asian	1 (10%)	1 (20%)	0 (0%)
Mixed ethnicity	2 (20%)	2 (40%)	0 (0%)
Marital status (n (%))			
Single	5 (50%)	2 (40%)	3 (60%)
Living as married	3 (30%)	2 (40%)	1 (20%)
Married	0 (0%)	0 (0%)	0 (0%)
Divorced	2 (20%)	2 (40%)	0 (0%)
Widowed	0 (0%)	0 (0%)	0 (0%)
Highest education level (n (%))			
Elementary (grade) school	0 (0%)	0 (0%)	0 (0%)
Secondary (High) school diploma	3 (30%)	1 (20%)	2 (40%)
College diploma	2 (20%)	1 (20%)	1 (20%)
Apprenticeship or trades certificate or diploma	1 (10%)	1 (20%)	0 (0%)
Bachelor's degree	2 (20%)	1 (20%)	1 (20%)
Professional degree (e.g., MD, PharmD)	0 (0%)	0 (0%)	0 (0%)
Graduate degree (Master or Doctorate)	2 (20%)	2 (40%)	0 (0%)
Cannabis use in the past 6 months (n (%))			
No	3 (30%)	2 (40%)	1 (20%)
Yes	7 (70%)	3 (60%)	4 (80%)
Monthly	5 (72.43%)	2 (40%)	3 (60%)
Weekly	2 (28.57%)	1 (20%)	1 (20%)
Daily	0 (0%)	0 (0%)	0 (0%)
Alcohol use in the past 6 months (n (%))			
No	5 (50%)	2 (40%)	3 (60%)
Yes	5 (50%)	3 (60%)	2 (40%)
Drug use in the past 6 months (n (%))			
No	3 (30%)	2 (40%)	1 (20%)
Yes	7 (70%)	3 (60%)	4 (80%)
History of infectious diseases (n (%))			
Syphilis (treated)	2 (20%)	2 (40%)	0 (0%)
Hepatitis B (Anti-Hepatitis B core antibodies)	4 (40%)	2 (40%)	2 (40%)
Hepatitis C (Anti-Hepatitis C Antibodies)	0 (0%)	0 (0%)	0 (0%)

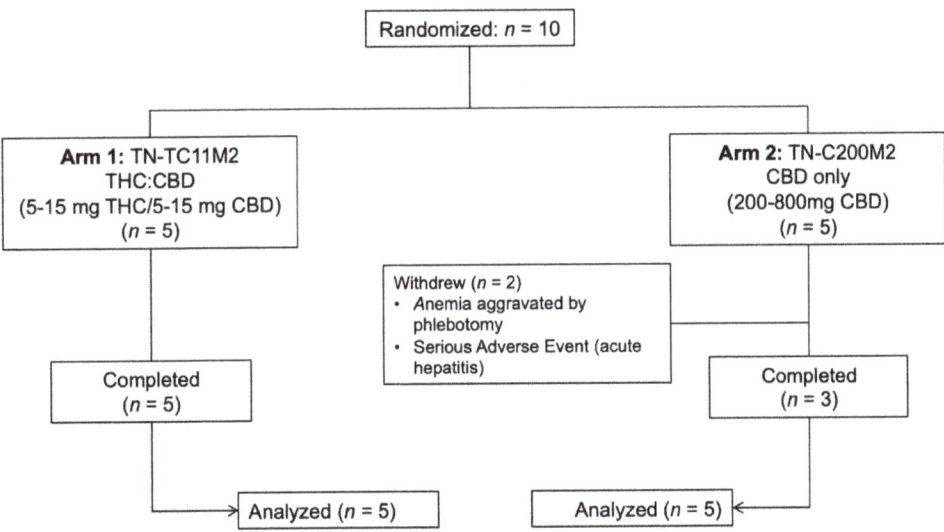

Figure 2. Allocation of participants enrolled in the study (*n* = 10). Distribution of study participants randomized to arm 1 (TN-TC11M2; THC:CBD) or arm 2 (TN-C200M2; CBD-only), to the study.

3.2. Safety and Tolerability

Dosing completion and Adverse Events (AE): Dosing based on participant self-titration is depicted in Figure 3. The majority of participants experienced AEs that were mild or moderate in severity. Eight out of 10 participants completed 12 weeks of treatment. Two participants were withdrawn from the CBD-only arm at 6 weeks for safety concerns. In one case, the 33-year-old female had grade 2 anemia (Hg 83 g/L) at screening, which failed to improve with oral iron supplementation. With frequent phlebotomy, the anemia progressed to grade 3 (lowest Hg 76 g/L) over the course of the study. She was withdrawn to prevent aggravation of her anemia. She also had moderate transaminitis at week 6 which normalized within 1 week following CBD cessation (Figure 4). The second participant withdrawn was a 62-year-old male who developed acute hepatitis at 6 weeks (Figure 4), deemed to be an unexpected, life-threatening serious adverse events (SAE), possibly related to cannabinoid treatment and requiring permanent CBD discontinuation and hepatology evaluation. Imaging revealed a pancreatic head mass, confirmed by pathology as pancreatic adenocarcinoma. Other potential contributors rendering the participant at risk for hepatitis included diabetes type 2, mild hepatic steatosis (diagnosed by abdominal ultrasound), alcohol binging, and possible interaction with ART resulting in increased CBD levels. Due to these two episodes of hepatitis, the protocol was amended and the maximum allowed dose for the CBD-only arm was reduced to 400 mg daily. However, this new protocol amendment only affected one individual.

Eight out the 10 study participants (80%) reported at least one AE, including 4 out of 5 individuals in each arm. The most commonly reported AE was somnolence (50%), followed by diarrhea (20%), difficulty concentrating (20%), transaminitis (20%) and worsened diabetes type 2 (20%). Only somnolence, difficulty concentrating, cognitive impairment and increase appetite were considered definitively related to cannabinoids and resolved with dose reduction. Apart from the SAE, the majority of AEs were of mild-moderate severity. Other AEs, as listed in Table 3, were reported only once and were considered possibly, probably or not related to treatment (10%).

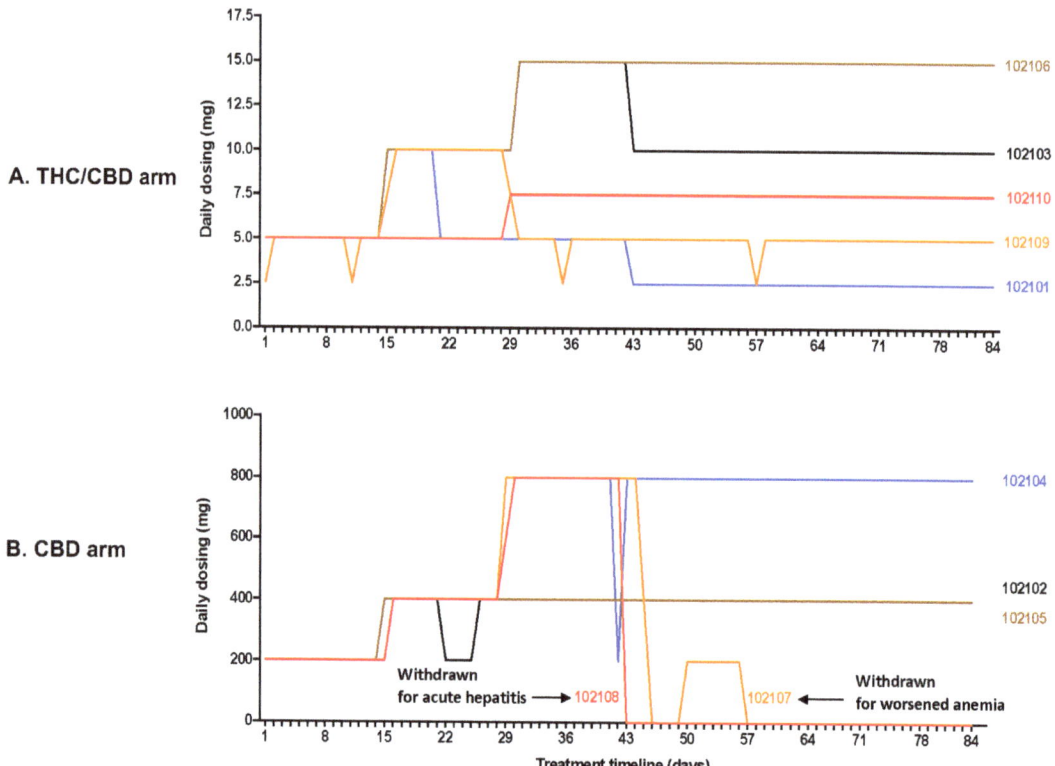

Figure 3. Daily dosage of CBD-only and THC/CBD combination during the 12 weeks of treatment. (**A**) THC/CBD arm: In arm 1 (THC/CBD), two participants were able to reach the maximum daily dose of the study drugs (15 mg THC/15 mg CBD), but only one remained at this dose until the end of the treatment, the other participant reduced his dosing to 10 mg THC/10 mg CBD per day because of the occurrence of AEs (somnolence). Two other participants from arm 1 reached the daily dose 10 mg THC/10 mg CBD, but after 3 weeks of treatment, they reduced their dosing because of the occurrence of AEs, one participant experienced cognitive impairment (#102109), while the other had somnolence, fatigue, difficulty concentrating, nightmares and paranoid thoughts (#102101). One remained at 5 mg THC/5 mg CBD per day and the other one who had multiple AEs reduced his daily dose to 2.5 mg THC/2.5 mg CBD after 5 weeks of treatment. A participant (#102110) from arm 1 who first reduced his daily dosing from 5 mg THC/5 mg CBD after 3 weeks of treatment to 2.5 mg THC:2.5 mg CBD, finally increased his dosing from 2.5 mg THC/2.5 mg CBD per day to reach 7.5 mg THC/7.5 mg CBD per day until the end of treatment. (**B**) CBD arm: 3 participants reached the maximum daily dose of 800 mg CBD after 4 weeks of treatment, but two of them experienced AEs (transient transaminitis for #102107) and SAE (hepatitis with persistent elevated transaminases and worsened diabetes type 2, for #102108) and the treatment was permanently discontinued 1 and 2 weeks after, and they were withdrawn from the study. The other participant who reached the maximum daily dose of 800 mg remained on this daily dose until the end of the study. Finally, two participants from arm 2 gradually increased their daily dosing to reach dose of 400 mg of CBD per day and remained in this range until the end of the study medication.

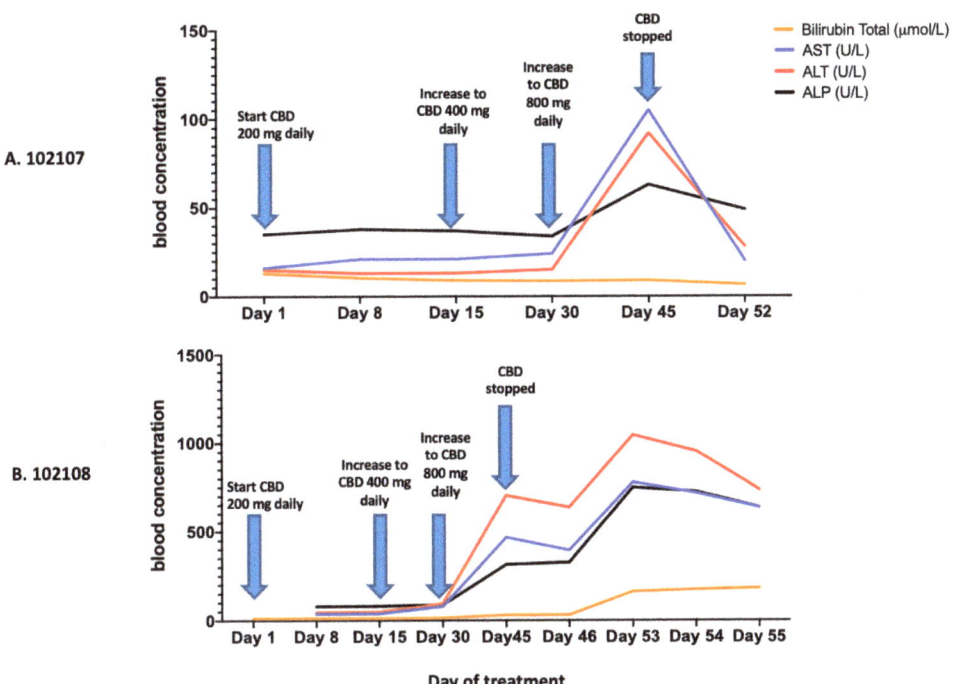

Figure 4. Dynamics of liver enzymes of participant #102107 and #102108 from arm 2 (TN-C200M2: CBD only), during cannabinoid uptake. Evolution of liver enzyme blood levels in (**A**). participant #102107 and (**B**). participant #102108 during the up-titration of CBD dose from the starting of CBD medication to the cessation of the treatment.

Table 3. List of adverse events (AEs) experienced by the participants during the study.

Adverse Events	Total Population (n = 10) (n (%))	THC:CBD Arm (n = 5) (n (%))	CBD Arm (n = 5) (n (%))
Somnolence	5 (50%)	2 (40%)	3 (60)
Diarrhea	2 (20%)	1 (20%)	1 (20%)
Difficulty concentrating	2 (20%)	1 (20%)	1 (20%)
Transaminitis	2 (20%)	0 (0%)	2 (40%)
Worsened diabetes type 2	2 (20%)	1 (20%)	1 (20%)
Abdominal cramps	1 (10%)	1 (20%)	0 (0%)
Acute hepatitis *	1 (10%)	0 (0%)	1 (20%)
Altered perception of peripheral neuropathy of feet bilaterally	1 (10%)	1 (20%)	0 (0%)
Bilateral leg weakness	1 (10%)	0 (0%)	1 (20%)
Cognitive impairment	1 (10%)	1 (20%)	0 (0%)
Constipation	1 (10%)	0 (0%)	1 (20%)

Table 3. Cont.

Adverse Events	Total Population (n = 10) (n (%))	THC:CBD Arm (n = 5) (n (%))	CBD Arm (n = 5) (n (%))
Dental abscess	1 (10%)	1 (20%)	0 (0%)
Dizziness	1 (10%)	0 (0%)	1 (20%)
Dry mouth	1 (10%)	1 (20%)	0 (0%)
Fatigue	1 (10%)	1 (20%)	0 (0%)
Gastroenteritis	1 (10%)	0 (0%)	1 (20%)
Hypocalcemia	1 (10%)	0 (0%)	1 (20%)
Increase appetite	1 (10%)	1 (20%)	0 (0%)
Nausea	1 (10%)	1 (20%)	0 (0%)
Nightmares	1 (10%)	1 (20%)	0 (0%)
Palpitations	1 (10%)	0 (0%)	1 (20%)
Paranoid thoughts	1 (10%)	1 (20%)	0 (0%)
Right sided cramps	1 (10%)	0 (0%)	1 (20%)
Upper tract respiratory infection	1 (10%)	0 (0%)	1 (20%)
Worsened anemia	1 (10%)	0 (0%)	1 (20%)
Worsened renal function	1 (10%)	0 (0%)	1 (20%)

* Life threatening, serious adverse event.

3.3. Hematology, Biochemistry, and HIV Immunology and Virology

As previously indicated, one participant (CBD-only arm) who started the study with a known anemia (83 G/L) of grade 2, progressed to anemia of grade 3 at visit 5 and 6 (Supplementary Table S3). Two diabetic participants developed worsened glucose control. One participant, from the THC/CBD arm, had a glucose which progressively reached, at the end of treatment (Visit 9), a WHO toxicity grade 3 (Supplementary Table S4). The other diabetic was the participant who experienced the SAE. His ALT rise progressed to WHO toxicity grade 4 by Week 6. His blood glucose was of WHO toxicity grade 3 at Weeks 4 and 6 (Figure 4 and Supplemental Table S4). Apart from these diabetic participants, we did not observe any significant changes in glucose control (Table 4). Moreover, cannabinoids did not affect CD4 and CD8 count, nor HIV viral load (Supplementary Table S5). Therefore, in the overall study, 7 out of 10 individuals (70%) did not experience any significant toxicity (Grades 0–2 scores on the WHO toxicity scale).

Table 4. Liver enzyme and kidney function profiles.

(Median (IQR))	Screening Visit	Visit 3	Visit 4	Visit 5	Visit 6	Visit 7	Visit 8	Visit 9	p-Value Friedman Test	p-Value Wilcoxon Matched-Pairs Signed Rank Test (Visit 3 vs. Visit 9)
Creatinine (μmol/L) $	86.0 (70.5–100.0)	87.0 (68.75–105.3)	88.50 (66.50–103.5)	89.00 (71.75–104.5)	92.00 (69.75–104.5)	90.0 (77.0–104.8)	102.0 (76.5–109.5)	80.0 (66.5–103.0)	0.49	0.55
Alanine Aminotransferase (ALT) (U/L) €	19.5 (13.75–37.0)	21.5 (11.5–36.75)	19.5 (12.0–41.25)	19.0 (13.25–34.0)	21.0 (14.25–50.75)	20.5 (9.5–31.25)	20.5 (11.0–25.5)	23.0 (14.0–35.5)	0.31	0.87

Table 4. Cont.

(Median (IQR))	Screening Visit	Visit 3	Visit 4	Visit 5	Visit 6	Visit 7	Visit 8	Visit 9	p-Value Friedman Test	p-Value Wilcoxon Matched-Pairs Signed Rank Test (Visit 3 vs. Visit 9)
Aspartate Amino-transferase (AST) (U/L)	19.0 (13.5–28.0)	18.5 (15.75–26.5)	20.5 (14.75–30.0)	17.0 (14.5–23.5)	19.5 (15.5–48.75)	18.0 (12.0–22.75)	18.0 (10.0–21.0)	20.0 (15.0–28.5)	0.76	>0.99
Alkaline Phosphatase (ALP) (U/L)	68.0 (56.25–83.5)	65.0 (55.5–73.25)	61.0 (52.5–70.5)	58.5 (53.25–78.5)	63.5 (54.75–77.5)	60.0 (51.5–72.5)	60.0 (55.0–62.0)	61.0 (54.0–73.5)	0.0107 *	0.29
Urea (mmol/L) $^£$	6.1 (4.4–7.43)	5.9 (3.87–7.45)	6.3 (4.55–6.83)	6.25 (4.33–7.13)	6.15 (4.95–7.85)	5.95 (4.45–7.67)	6.1 (4.5–8.63)	6.0 (4.4–7.05)	0.38	0.71
Blood Glucose (mmol/L)	5.2 (4.87–6.97)	5.5 (4.57–7.3)	5.3 (4.9–9.4)	5.6 (4.93–9.77)	5.7 (5.1–9.1)	5.0 (4.6–6.13)	5.2 (4.95–5.37)	5.1 (5.0–6.15)	0.38	0.46
Total Bilirubin (mol/L)	10.15 (7.65–12.25)	9.4 (7.87–11.33)	10.0 (7.65–11.53)	8.8 (6.8–15.05)	9.0 (7.67–11.40)	8.05 (7.1–9.57)	9.3 (7.65–10.0)	8.5 (7.05–12.20)	0.98	0.64

$^\$$ µmol/L: Micromolar per liter; $^€$ U/L: Units per liter; * while statistically significant, this was not deemed to be clinically significant. $^£$ mmol/L: Millimolar per liter.

3.4. Quality of Life and Mood Assessment

EQ-5D. Supplementary Figure S1 depicts the distribution of responses to the EQ-5D questionnaire at Baseline 2 (prior to treatment), Visit 6 (during treatment) and Visit 9 (end of treatment). Overall, cannabinoids did not significantly affect QOL.

WHOQOL-HIV BREF. Similar to what was observed with the EQ-5D questionnaire, at baseline and throughout cannabinoid treatment, the majority of participants reported moderate to very good quality of life (100%) and general health (80%, 90% and 100%, at Baseline 2, Visit 6 and Visit 9, respectively) (Supplementary Figure S2). Variations in scores across visits were not significant (Supplementary Figure S2).

POMS. Five out of ten participants (50%) showed a reduction in total mood disturbance (TMD) score over time. Three participants showed a slight increase in their TMD over time, including one in the THC/CBD arm, and 2 in the CBD-only arm who were withdrawn from the study. Variations in scores across visits were not significant (Supplementary Figure S3).

4. Discussion

In this pilot clinical trial, we evaluated the safety and tolerability of oral THC:CBD combination and CBD-only capsules over a 12 week period in PLWH on effective ART. Overall, the capsules were safe and well-tolerated, with AEs mostly mild to moderate in severity. Most participants completed the full 12 weeks of treatment. Importantly, even at the highest dose, capsules did not negatively affect immunological (CD4 and CD8 T cells counts) or virological (HIV viral load) parameters associated with HIV infection.

Highly purified THC:CBD combination and CBD-only capsules demonstrated acceptable safety and tolerability profiles in clinical trials for persons with epilepsy, chronic pain, and symptoms associated with multiple sclerosis and cancers [40,45–56]. In these trials, the common cannabinoid-related AEs were mostly somnolence, diarrhea, abdominal pain, fatigue, nausea, dry mouth, or dizziness, which occurred mainly during the up-titration and were considered mild or moderate in severity and resolved without discontinuation of the cannabinoid [40,45–56]. Similar to these studies, our participants also experienced somnolence and diarrhea as common AEs regardless of study arm. Abdominal pain, fatigue, nausea, dry mouth or dizziness were also reported, but less frequently. All these AEs were mild or moderate in severity and none resulted in treatment discontinuation.

A key observation from this study is the potential risk for transaminitis and hepatotoxicity, particularly for high doses of CBD (800 mg per day) in PLWH. In our study, two participants experienced an abnormal rise in their ALT serum levels above the upper limit of the normal range during the up-titration of CBD from dose 400 to 800 mg. Transient CBD-related elevations of ALT and AST are commonly reported in clinical studies [40,46–48,50,54,56]. Transient transaminase abnormalities do not seem to be of critical long-term clinical significance for the liver as they tend to normalize following dose reduction or treatment discontinuation [57,58]. On the other hand, the second participant who experienced abnormally high elevated transaminases was a 62 years old white man with underling fatty liver disease with elevated levels of transaminases (ALT and AST) and blood glucose before the initiation of CBD treatment, along with alcohol binging which was not openly disclosed to the study team. This participant presented a significant and persistent rise of ALT, AST, ALP and total bilirubin, with an increase in blood glucose levels. In that case, the persistency of the transaminitis, even after treatment discontinuation, prompted us to conduct further liver examinations which revealed a pancreatic adenocarcinoma. The underlying pathological state of this participant with several serious comorbidities and pre-existing elevated transaminases would have facilitated the marked rise of transaminases during the up-titration as shown in another clinical trial where participants having elevated baseline serum ALT had 3 fold greater incidence of significant ALT elevations compared to those starting CBD with normal level of ALT [56]. The likely involvement of high doses of CBD in the aggravation of the pathological state of the participant cannot be excluded [56]. Together, these findings suggest that HIV physicians should consider screening PLWH with risk factors for hepatic steatosis with transient elastography (Fibroscan®, Echosens, Paris, France) before initiating cannabinoid-based medicines given the high number of baseline comorbidities and risks for chronic liver disease in this specific population [59]. Study teams should follow liver enzymes closely to detect any subtle rises in transaminases which may suggest an undiagnosed steatohepatitis. Following the SAE in the later patient, we reduced the maximum dose of CBD to 400 mg po daily in the CBD-only arm. As CBD oils are available for purchase without prescription in Canada and some other jurisdictions, PLWH who use these products should be counselled about their potential hepatotoxicity.

Although two participants in our study had worsened blood glucose control, in one case this was the same participant with the SAE, suggesting that this could have been induced by binge drinking. In the other participant, although less probable, a potential drug interaction between cannabinoid treatment and one of the other medications taken by the participant could not be entirely excluded. Cannabinoids can alter hepatic metabolism of other drugs, making them ineffective or toxic [60,61]. The roles of cannabinoids in glucose metabolism and diabetes have been documented, though mostly in in vitro and animal studies, and suggest beneficial, rather than deleterious effects on diabetic parameters [62–69]. Similarly, observational studies in individuals using cannabis more often suggest a protective effect of cannabis use against metabolic syndrome and diabetes mellitus [70–72]. In another pilot clinical trial assessing the effect of cannabinoids on glycemic parameters in diabetic individuals, although CBD failed to directly improve diabetes parameters, it did not worsen glucose levels [73]. The findings from these other studies suggest that the uncontrolled blood glucose levels observed in two participants in our trial are unlikely due to a direct effect of cannabinoids, but rather to a combination of factors including comorbidities, alcohol consumption and polypharmacy.

Improvement in quality of life and mood are primary reasons why many PLWH use cannabis [74], although cannabinoids did not impact on quality of life or on mood scores throughout the study. However, most participants had good quality of life and mood scores at baseline, perhaps making it difficult to observe significant improvements. Future studies may wish to enroll individuals with poor or moderate mood or quality of life scores at baseline in order to appreciate whether any improvement occurs with treatment. Other studies have shown that cannabis in PLWH [12] or individuals with chronic pain [59] was associated with a marked improvement in quality of life [12,59].

5. Study Limitations

The most important limitation of this pilot study is the small sample size, greatly limiting our ability to generalize these findings to other PLWH. We encountered significant difficulty recruiting participants for this study. The lack of a placebo group and predominance of male participants are other limitations. While THC:CBD capsules were overall well-tolerated in the 5 participants who received them, there was likely a self-selection bias, with individuals participating in the study being more open towards the therapeutic potential of cannabinoids and also more experienced with cannabinoids than those who declined participation.

6. Conclusions

Taken together, our findings suggest that much additional work is needed to understand safety and tolerability in PLWH. Transaminitis in 2/5 participants in the CBD-only group suggests that more work is required to elucidate the best dosages of CBD in this population. Pharmacokinetic studies in this regard could be helpful. We suggest that PLWH should undergo a hepatological screening, ideally with transient elastography or, if unavailable, with simple fibrosis biomarkers like fibrosis-4 score, prior to initiating cannabinoid-based medicine, particularly formulations with high CBD dose, and they should be closely monitored to detect any rise of transaminases reflecting potential hepatotoxicity. Work is also required to better understand the potential benefits and harms of cannabinoids in chronic liver diseases and particularly in the context of HIV. As we recently reviewed [69], the liver contains both CB1 and CB2 receptors and the consequences of administering compounds which target these receptors must be understood. While future studies in PLWH should use a lower maximum dose of CBD, the optimal dose to avoid hepatotoxicity while leveraging anti-inflammatory and immunomodulatory properties of cannabinoids are unknown. Future studies may wish to examine the potential of these compounds to improve specific conditions, such as fatty liver disease, in PLWH. Work is currently ongoing to address whether the treatments in this study had any impact on immune activation, inflammatory markers, HIV reservoir size or gut microbiome, the ultimately goal being a reduction in HIV-associated comorbidities driven by chronic inflammation. Given the small sample size and lack of blinding or use of placebo, we remain cautious in our conclusions regarding the therapeutic benefits until more data is available.

Supplementary Materials: The following supporting information can be downloaded at: https://www.mdpi.com/article/10.3390/biomedicines10123168/s1, Figure S1. Frequency of responses of the EuroQoL-5D (EQ-5D) questionnaire for the quality-of-life assessment during the 12 weeks of treatment. Figure S2. Frequency of responses of the World Health Organization Quality of Life—HIV Brief (WHOQOL-HIV BREF) questionnaire for general quality of life and general health state during the study visits. Figure S3. Total mood disturbance (TMD) score from the Profile of Mood States) (POMS) questionnaire during the study. Table S1. List of exclusion criteria. Table S2. World Health Organization (WHO) Toxicity Scale Grading for Adverse Events. Table S3. Hematological parameters (excel attachment). Table S4. Biochemistry parameters (excel attachment). Table S5. HIV immunological and virological parameters.

Author Contributions: Conceptualization: C.T.C. and M.-A.J.; Participant recruitment and data acquisition: F.B., C.V., L.D.B., N.P., B.L., M.K., M.-J.B., J.C., J.S. (Jason Szabo) J.-P.R., R.T. and E.H.; Methodology, C.T.C., M.-A.J., J.N., J.S. (Joel Singer), T.L., S.M., E.M. and A.V.; Software: J.N., J.S. (Joel Singer) and T.L.; Validation: J.N., J.S. (Joel Singer) and T.L.; Formal Analysis, R.-S.M.B., M.-A.J., C.T.C., J.S. (Joel Singer) and T.L.; Investigation: C.T.C., G.S., M.K., L.D.B., N.P. and M.K.; Resources: C.T.C., M.-A.J., J.N. and D.N.; Data Curation: R.-S.M.B. and C.T.C.; Writing—Original Draft Preparation, R.-S.M.B. and C.T.C.; Writing—Review and Editing, all authors; Supervision, C.T.C., M.-A.J., J.N. and S.S.; Project Administration, C.T.C., J.N., D.N. and M.-A.J.; Funding Acquisition, C.T.C. and M.-A.J.; Manuscript approval: all authors. All authors have read and agreed to the published version of the manuscript.

Funding: This work has been supported by a team grant from the Canadian Institutes of Health Research (CIHR) (# CC1-177334), CIHR Canadian HIV Trials Network and the Lotte & John Hecht Memorial Foundation. Tilray provided study capsules as an in-kind service but did not provide study funding. R.-S.M.B. is supported by a CIHR postdoctoral fellowship. G.S. holds a FRSQ-S Chercheur Boursier Clinicien Senior career award (#296306). M.-A.J. holds the tier 2 CIHR Canada Research Chair in Immuno-Virology. C.T.C. is a recipient of an FRQ-S Junior 2 Chercheur Boursier Clinicien career award.

Institutional Review Board Statement: This study was approved by the McGill University Health Centre (#2018-4336) and conducted in conformity with the Declaration of Helsinki.

Informed Consent Statement: Informed consent was obtained from all subjects involved in the study.

Data Availability Statement: Anonymized data may be available upon reasonable request of the author and the CTN.

Acknowledgments: We thank the participants for their participation in this study. We also thank the staff at the CTN, including Nisha Shewaramani and Elisa Lau (database managers), and Jayamarx Jayaraman (study monitoring) and all CVIS/MUHC research and clinical staff, including Hansi Peiris, Carolina Berini, Sebastien Landry, Benoit Lemire, Jasmine Mian, Kathleen Normandin, Claude Cyr, Yulia Alexandrova, Erik Pavey and Tara Mabanga. We are grateful to the Tilray staff, including Philippe Lucas, Catherine Jacobson and Gosia Grzyb, as well as to Carolyn Baglole and the Research Centre for Cannabis at McGill University.

Conflicts of Interest: G.S. has acted as speaker for Merck, Gilead, Abbvie, Pfizer, Novonordisk, served as an advisory board member for Merck, Novartis, Pfizer, Gilead and Intercept and has received unrestricted research funding from Theratecnologies. C.T.C. has served on advisory boards for Viiv Healthcare and Gilead, and received grant support from Merck, Gilead, Viiv and Tilray Inc. She has also received travel support to attend conferences from Gilead and Viiv Healthcare.

References

1. Cassol, E.; Malfeld, S.; Mahasha, P.; van der Merwe, S.; Cassol, S.; Seebregts, C.; Alfano, M.; Poli, G.; Rossouw, T. Persistent microbial translocation and immune activation in HIV-1-infected South Africans receiving combination antiretroviral therapy. *J. Infect. Dis.* **2010**, *202*, 723–733. [CrossRef] [PubMed]
2. Klatt, N.R.; Funderburg, N.T.; Brenchley, J.M. Microbial translocation, immune activation, and HIV disease. *Trends Microbiol.* **2013**, *21*, 6–13. [CrossRef] [PubMed]
3. Marchetti, G.; Tincati, C.; Silvestri, G. Microbial translocation in the pathogenesis of HIV infection and AIDS. *Clin. Microbiol. Rev.* **2013**, *26*, 2–18. [CrossRef] [PubMed]
4. Zicari, S.; Sessa, L.; Cotugno, N.; Ruggiero, A.; Morrocchi, E.; Concato, C.; Rocca, S.; Zangari, P.; Manno, E.C.; Palma, P. Immune Activation, Inflammation, and Non-AIDS Co-Morbidities in HIV-Infected Patients under Long-Term ART. *Viruses* **2019**, *11*, 200. [CrossRef] [PubMed]
5. Baban, B.; Khodadadi, H.; Salles, É.L.; Costigliola, V.; Morgan, J.C.; Hess, D.C.; Vaibhav, K.; Dhandapani, K.M.; Yu, J.C. Inflammaging and Cannabinoids. *Ageing Res. Rev.* **2021**, *72*, 101487. [CrossRef] [PubMed]
6. Costiniuk, C.T.; Jenabian, M.A. Cannabinoids and inflammation: Implications for people living with HIV. *Aids* **2019**, *33*, 2273–2288. [CrossRef] [PubMed]
7. Costiniuk, C.T.; Saneei, Z.; Routy, J.P.; Margolese, S.; Mandarino, E.; Singer, J.; Lebouché, B.; Cox, J.; Szabo, J.; Brouillette, M.J.; et al. Oral cannabinoids in people living with HIV on effective antiretroviral therapy: CTN PT028-study protocol for a pilot randomised trial to assess safety, tolerability and effect on immune activation. *BMJ Open* **2019**, *9*, e024793. [CrossRef]
8. Hsu, D.C.; Sereti, I. Serious Non-AIDS Events: Therapeutic Targets of Immune Activation and Chronic Inflammation in HIV Infection. *Drugs* **2016**, *76*, 533–549. [CrossRef]
9. Furler, M.D.; Einarson, T.R.; Millson, M.; Walmsley, S.; Bendayan, R. Medicinal and recreational marijuana use by patients infected with HIV. *AIDS Patient Care STDS* **2004**, *18*, 215–228. [CrossRef]
10. Abrams, D.I.; Jay, C.A.; Shade, S.B.; Vizoso, H.; Reda, H.; Press, S.; Kelly, M.E.; Rowbotham, M.C.; Petersen, K.L. Cannabis in painful HIV-associated sensory neuropathy: A randomized placebo-controlled trial. *Neurology* **2007**, *68*, 515–521. [CrossRef]
11. Belle-Isle, L.; Hathaway, A. Barriers to access to medical cannabis for Canadians living with HIV/AIDS. *AIDS Care* **2007**, *19*, 500–506. [CrossRef]
12. Ellis, R.J.; Toperoff, W.; Vaida, F.; van den Brande, G.; Gonzales, J.; Gouaux, B.; Bentley, H.; Atkinson, J.H. Smoked medicinal cannabis for neuropathic pain in HIV: A randomized, crossover clinical trial. *Neuropsychopharmacology* **2009**, *34*, 672–680. [CrossRef]

13. Harris, G.E.; Dupuis, L.; Mugford, G.J.; Johnston, L.; Haase, D.; Page, G.; Haldane, H.; Harris, N.; Midodzi, W.K.; Dow, G. Patterns and correlates of cannabis use among individuals with HIV/AIDS in Maritime Canada. *Can. J. Infect. Dis. Med. Microbiol.* **2014**, *25*, e1–e7. [CrossRef]
14. Anil, S.M.; Shalev, N.; Vinayaka, A.C.; Nadarajan, S.; Namdar, D.; Belausov, E.; Shoval, I.; Mani, K.A.; Mechrez, G.; Koltai, H. Cannabis compounds exhibit anti-inflammatory activity in vitro in COVID-19-related inflammation in lung epithelial cells and pro-inflammatory activity in macrophages. *Sci. Rep.* **2021**, *11*, 1462. [CrossRef]
15. DeMarino, C.; Cowen, M.; Khatkar, P.; Cotto, B.; Branscome, H.; Kim, Y.; Sharif, S.A.; Agbottah, E.T.; Zhou, W.; Costiniuk, C.T.; et al. Cannabinoids Reduce Extracellular Vesicle Release from HIV-1 Infected Myeloid Cells and Inhibit Viral Transcription. *Cells* **2022**, *11*, 723. [CrossRef]
16. Henriquez, J.E.; Rizzo, M.D.; Schulz, M.A.; Crawford, R.B.; Gulick, P.; Kaminski, N.E. Δ9-Tetrahydrocannabinol Suppresses Secretion of IFNα by Plasmacytoid Dendritic Cells From Healthy and HIV-Infected Individuals. *J. Acquir. Immune Defic. Syndr.* **2017**, *75*, 588–596. [CrossRef]
17. Janecki, M.; Graczyk, M.; Lewandowska, A.A.; Pawlak, Ł. Anti-Inflammatory and Antiviral Effects of Cannabinoids in Inhibiting and Preventing SARS-CoV-2 Infection. *Int. J. Mol. Sci.* **2022**, *23*, 4170. [CrossRef]
18. Suryavanshi, S.V.; Zaiachuk, M.; Pryimak, N.; Kovalchuk, I.; Kovalchuk, O. Cannabinoids Alleviate the LPS-Induced Cytokine Storm via Attenuating NLRP3 Inflammasome Signaling and TYK2-Mediated STAT3 Signaling Pathways In Vitro. *Cells* **2022**, *11*, 1391. [CrossRef]
19. Carmona-Hidalgo, B.; González-Mariscal, I.; García-Martín, A.; Prados, M.E.; Ruiz-Pino, F.; Appendino, G.; Tena-Sempere, M.; Muñoz, E. Δ9-Tetrahydrocannabinolic Acid markedly alleviates liver fibrosis and inflammation in mice. *Phytomedicine* **2021**, *81*, 153426. [CrossRef]
20. Chandra, L.C.; Kumar, V.; Torben, W.; Stouwe, C.V.; Winsauer, P.; Amedee, A.; Molina, P.E.; Mohan, M. Chronic administration of Δ9-tetrahydrocannabinol induces intestinal anti-inflammatory microRNA expression during acute simian immunodeficiency virus infection of rhesus macaques. *J. Virol.* **2015**, *89*, 1168–1181. [CrossRef]
21. Kumar, V.; Torben, W.; Mansfield, J.; Alvarez, X.; Stouwe, C.V.; Li, J.; Byrareddy, S.N.; Didier, P.J.; Pahar, B.; Molina, P.E.; et al. Cannabinoid Attenuation of Intestinal Inflammation in Chronic SIV-Infected Rhesus Macaques Involves T Cell Modulation and Differential Expression of Micro-RNAs and Pro-inflammatory Genes. *Front. Immunol.* **2019**, *10*, 914. [CrossRef]
22. McDew-White, M.; Lee, E.; Alvarez, X.; Sestak, K.; Ling, B.J.; Byrareddy, S.N.; Okeoma, C.M.; Mohan, M. Cannabinoid control of gingival immune activation in chronically SIV-infected rhesus macaques involves modulation of the indoleamine-2,3-dioxygenase-1 pathway and salivary microbiome. *EBioMedicine* **2022**, *75*, 103769. [CrossRef] [PubMed]
23. Manuzak, J.A.; Gott, T.M.; Kirkwood, J.S.; Coronado, E.; Hensley-McBain, T.; Miller, C.; Cheu, R.K.; Collier, A.C.; Funderburg, N.T.; Martin, J.N.; et al. Heavy Cannabis Use Associated With Reduction in Activated and Inflammatory Immune Cell Frequencies in Antiretroviral Therapy-Treated Human Immunodeficiency Virus-Infected Individuals. *Clin. Infect. Dis.* **2018**, *66*, 1872–1882. [CrossRef] [PubMed]
24. Rizzo, M.D.; Crawford, R.B.; Henriquez, J.E.; Aldhamen, Y.A.; Gulick, P.; Amalfitano, A.; Kaminski, N.E. HIV-infected cannabis users have lower circulating CD16+ monocytes and IFN-γ-inducible protein 10 levels compared with nonusing HIV patients. *Aids* **2018**, *32*, 419–429. [CrossRef] [PubMed]
25. Yin, L.; Dinasarapu, A.R.; Borkar, S.A.; Chang, K.F.; De Paris, K.; Kim-Chang, J.J.; Sleasman, J.W.; Goodenow, M.M. Anti-inflammatory effects of recreational marijuana in virally suppressed youth with HIV-1 are reversed by use of tobacco products in combination with marijuana. *Retrovirology* **2022**, *19*, 10. [CrossRef] [PubMed]
26. Canada, H. Understanding the New Access to Cannabis for Medical Purposes Regulations. 2016. Available online: https://www.canada.ca/en/health-canada/services/publications/drugs-health-products/understanding-new-access-to-cannabis-for-medical-purposes-regulations.html (accessed on 20 August 2022).
27. Hawke, L.D.; Henderson, J. Legalization of cannabis use in Canada: Impacts on the cannabis use profiles of youth seeking services for substance use. *J. Subst. Abuse Treat* **2021**, *126*, 108340. [CrossRef]
28. Solowij, N.; Broyd, S.; Greenwood, L.M.; van Hell, H.; Martelozzo, D.; Rueb, K.; Todd, J.; Liu, Z.; Galettis, P.; Martin, J.; et al. A randomised controlled trial of vaporised Δ(9)-tetrahydrocannabinol and cannabidiol alone and in combination in frequent and infrequent cannabis users: Acute intoxication effects. *Eur. Arch. Psychiatry Clin. Neurosci.* **2019**, *269*, 17–35. [CrossRef]
29. Windle, S.B.; Wade, K.; Filion, K.B.; Kimmelman, J.; Thombs, B.D.; Eisenberg, M.J. Potential harms from legalization of recreational cannabis use in Canada. *Can. J. Public Health* **2019**, *110*, 222–226. [CrossRef]
30. Bergamaschi, M.M.; Queiroz, R.H.; Zuardi, A.W.; Crippa, J.A. Safety and side effects of cannabidiol, a Cannabis sativa constituent. *Curr. Drug Saf.* **2011**, *6*, 237–249. [CrossRef]
31. Burstein, S. Cannabidiol (CBD) and its analogs: A review of their effects on inflammation. *Bioorg. Med. Chem.* **2015**, *23*, 1377–1385. [CrossRef]
32. Burstein, S.H.; Zurier, R.B. Cannabinoids, endocannabinoids, and related analogs in inflammation. *AAPS J.* **2009**, *11*, 109–119. [CrossRef]
33. Iuvone, T.; Esposito, G.; De Filippis, D.; Scuderi, C.; Steardo, L. Cannabidiol: A promising drug for neurodegenerative disorders? *CNS Neurosci. Ther.* **2009**, *15*, 65–75. [CrossRef]

34. Ribeiro, A.; Ferraz-de-Paula, V.; Pinheiro, M.L.; Vitoretti, L.B.; Mariano-Souza, D.P.; Quinteiro-Filho, W.M.; Akamine, A.T.; Almeida, V.I.; Quevedo, J.; Dal-Pizzol, F.; et al. Cannabidiol, a non-psychotropic plant-derived cannabinoid, decreases inflammation in a murine model of acute lung injury: Role for the adenosine A(2A) receptor. *Eur. J. Pharmacol.* **2012**, *678*, 78–85. [CrossRef]
35. Zgair, A.; Lee, J.B.; Wong, J.C.M.; Taha, D.A.; Aram, J.; Di Virgilio, D.; McArthur, J.W.; Cheng, Y.K.; Hennig, I.M.; Barrett, D.A.; et al. Oral administration of cannabis with lipids leads to high levels of cannabinoids in the intestinal lymphatic system and prominent immunomodulation. *Sci. Rep.* **2017**, *7*, 14542. [CrossRef]
36. Sachse-Seeboth, C.; Pfeil, J.; Sehrt, D.; Meineke, I.; Tzvetkov, M.; Bruns, E.; Poser, W.; Vormfelde, S.V.; Brockmöller, J. Interindividual variation in the pharmacokinetics of Delta9-tetrahydrocannabinol as related to genetic polymorphisms in CYP2C9. *Clin. Pharmacol. Ther.* **2009**, *85*, 273–276. [CrossRef]
37. Ware, M.A.; Wang, T.; Shapiro, S.; Collet, J.P. Cannabis for the Management of Pain: Assessment of Safety Study (COMPASS). *J. Pain* **2015**, *16*, 1233–1242. [CrossRef]
38. Leweke, F.M.; Rohleder, C.; Gerth, C.W.; Hellmich, M.; Pukrop, R.; Koethe, D. Cannabidiol and Amisulpride Improve Cognition in Acute Schizophrenia in an Explorative, Double-Blind, Active-Controlled, Randomized Clinical Trial. *Front. Pharmacol.* **2021**, *12*, 614811. [CrossRef]
39. Leweke, F.M.; Piomelli, D.; Pahlisch, F.; Muhl, D.; Gerth, C.W.; Hoyer, C.; Klosterkötter, J.; Hellmich, M.; Koethe, D. Cannabidiol enhances anandamide signaling and alleviates psychotic symptoms of schizophrenia. *Transl. Psychiatry* **2012**, *2*, e94. [CrossRef]
40. Thiele, E.A.; Marsh, E.D.; French, J.A.; Mazurkiewicz-Beldzinska, M.; Benbadis, S.R.; Joshi, C.; Lyons, P.D.; Taylor, A.; Roberts, C.; Sommerville, K. Cannabidiol in patients with seizures associated with Lennox-Gastaut syndrome (GWPCARE4): A randomised, double-blind, placebo-controlled phase 3 trial. *Lancet* **2018**, *391*, 1085–1096. [CrossRef]
41. Wade, D.T.; Makela, P.; Robson, P.; House, H.; Bateman, C. Do cannabis-based medicinal extracts have general or specific effects on symptoms in multiple sclerosis? A double-blind, randomized, placebo-controlled study on 160 patients. *Mult. Scler.* **2004**, *10*, 434–441. [CrossRef]
42. World Health Organization. *WHOQOL-HIV Bref*; World Health Organization: Geneva, Switzerland, 2002.
43. Herdman, M.; Gudex, C.; Lloyd, A.; Janssen, M.; Kind, P.; Parkin, D.; Bonsel, G.; Badia, X. Development and preliminary testing of the new five-level version of EQ-5D (EQ-5D-5L). *Qual. Life Res.* **2011**, *20*, 1727–1736. [CrossRef] [PubMed]
44. McNair, D.M.; Lorr, M.; Droppleman, L.F. *Manual for the Profile of Mood States*; Educational and Industrial Testing Services: San Diego, CA, USA, 1971.
45. Berman, J.S.; Symonds, C.; Birch, R. Efficacy of two cannabis based medicinal extracts for relief of central neuropathic pain from brachial plexus avulsion: Results of a randomised controlled trial. *Pain* **2004**, *112*, 299–306. [CrossRef] [PubMed]
46. Devinsky, O.; Cross, J.H.; Laux, L.; Marsh, E.; Miller, I.; Nabbout, R.; Scheffer, I.E.; Thiele, E.A.; Wright, S. Trial of Cannabidiol for Drug-Resistant Seizures in the Dravet Syndrome. *N. Engl. J. Med.* **2017**, *376*, 2011–2020. [CrossRef] [PubMed]
47. Devinsky, O.; Patel, A.D.; Cross, J.H.; Villanueva, V.; Wirrell, E.C.; Privitera, M.; Greenwood, S.M.; Roberts, C.; Checketts, D.; VanLandingham, K.E.; et al. Effect of Cannabidiol on Drop Seizures in the Lennox-Gastaut Syndrome. *N. Engl. J. Med.* **2018**, *378*, 1888–1897. [CrossRef] [PubMed]
48. Devinsky, O.; Verducci, C.; Thiele, E.A.; Laux, L.C.; Patel, A.D.; Filloux, F.; Szaflarski, J.P.; Wilfong, A.; Clark, G.D.; Park, Y.D.; et al. Open-label use of highly purified CBD (Epidiolex®) in patients with CDKL5 deficiency disorder and Aicardi, Dup15q, and Doose syndromes. *Epilepsy Behav.* **2018**, *86*, 131–137. [CrossRef]
49. Langford, R.M.; Mares, J.; Novotna, A.; Vachova, M.; Novakova, I.; Notcutt, W.; Ratcliffe, S. A double-blind, randomized, placebo-controlled, parallel-group study of THC/CBD oromucosal spray in combination with the existing treatment regimen, in the relief of central neuropathic pain in patients with multiple sclerosis. *J. Neurol.* **2013**, *260*, 984–997. [CrossRef]
50. Miller, I.; Scheffer, I.E.; Gunning, B.; Sanchez-Carpintero, R.; Gil-Nagel, A.; Perry, M.S.; Saneto, R.P.; Checketts, D.; Dunayevich, E.; Knappertz, V. Dose-Ranging Effect of Adjunctive Oral Cannabidiol vs Placebo on Convulsive Seizure Frequency in Dravet Syndrome: A Randomized Clinical Trial. *JAMA Neurol.* **2020**, *77*, 613–621. [CrossRef]
51. Nurmikko, T.J.; Serpell, M.G.; Hoggart, B.; Toomey, P.J.; Morlion, B.J.; Haines, D. Sativex successfully treats neuropathic pain characterised by allodynia: A randomised, double-blind, placebo-controlled clinical trial. *Pain* **2007**, *133*, 210–220. [CrossRef]
52. Rog, D.J.; Nurmikko, T.J.; Friede, T.; Young, C.A. Randomized, controlled trial of cannabis-based medicine in central pain in multiple sclerosis. *Neurology* **2005**, *65*, 812–819. [CrossRef]
53. Serpell, M.; Ratcliffe, S.; Hovorka, J.; Schofield, M.; Taylor, L.; Lauder, H.; Ehler, E. A double-blind, randomized, placebo-controlled, parallel group study of THC/CBD spray in peripheral neuropathic pain treatment. *Eur. J. Pain* **2014**, *18*, 999–1012. [CrossRef]
54. Thiele, E.A.; Bebin, E.M.; Filloux, F.; Kwan, P.; Loftus, R.; Sahebkar, F.; Sparagana, S.; Wheless, J. Long-term cannabidiol treatment for seizures in patients with tuberous sclerosis complex: An open-label extension trial. *Epilepsia* **2022**, *63*, 426–439. [CrossRef]
55. Ueberall, M.A.; Essner, U.; Mueller-Schwefe, G.H. Effectiveness and tolerability of THC:CBD oromucosal spray as add-on measure in patients with severe chronic pain: Analysis of 12-week open-label real-world data provided by the German Pain e-Registry. *J. Pain Res.* **2019**, *12*, 1577–1604. [CrossRef]
56. Watkins, P.B.; Church, R.J.; Li, J.; Knappertz, V. Cannabidiol and Abnormal Liver Chemistries in Healthy Adults: Results of a Phase I Clinical Trial. *Clin. Pharmacol. Ther.* **2021**, *109*, 1224–1231. [CrossRef]

57. Chesney, E.; Oliver, D.; Green, A.; Sovi, S.; Wilson, J.; Englund, A.; Freeman, T.P.; McGuire, P. Adverse effects of cannabidiol: A systematic review and meta-analysis of randomized clinical trials. *Neuropsychopharmacology* **2020**, *45*, 1799–1806. [CrossRef]
58. Kaufmann, R.; Aqua, K.; Lombardo, J.; Lee, M. Observed Impact of Long-term Consumption of Oral Cannabidiol on Liver Function in Healthy Adults. *Cannabis Cannabinoid Res.* 2021; *ahead of print*. [CrossRef]
59. Abelev, S.; Warne, L.N.; Benson, M.; Hardy, M.; Nayee, S.; Barlow, J. Medicinal Cannabis for the Treatment of Chronic Refractory Pain: An Investigation of the Adverse Event Profile and Health-Related Quality of Life Impact of an Oral Formulation. *Med. Cannabis Cannabinoids* **2022**, *5*, 20–31. [CrossRef]
60. Jiang, R.; Yamaori, S.; Okamoto, Y.; Yamamoto, I.; Watanabe, K. Cannabidiol is a potent inhibitor of the catalytic activity of cytochrome P450 2C19. *Drug Metab. Pharmacokinet.* **2013**, *28*, 332–338. [CrossRef]
61. Stout, S.M.; Cimino, N.M. Exogenous cannabinoids as substrates, inhibitors, and inducers of human drug metabolizing enzymes: A systematic review. *Drug Metab. Rev.* **2014**, *46*, 86–95. [CrossRef]
62. González-Mariscal, I.; Pozo-Morales, M.; Romero-Zerbo, S.Y.; Espinosa-Jimenez, V.; Escamilla-Sánchez, A.; Sánchez-Salido, L.; Cobo-Vuilleumier, N.; Gauthier, B.R.; Bermúdez-Silva, F.J. Abnormal cannabidiol ameliorates inflammation preserving pancreatic beta cells in mouse models of experimental type 1 diabetes and beta cell damage. *Biomed. Pharmacother.* **2022**, *145*, 112361. [CrossRef]
63. González-Mariscal, I.; Krzysik-Walker, S.M.; Doyle, M.E.; Liu, Q.R.; Cimbro, R.; Santa-Cruz Calvo, S.; Ghosh, S.; Cieśla, Ł.; Moaddel, R.; Carlson, O.D.; et al. Human CB1 Receptor Isoforms, present in Hepatocytes and β-cells, are Involved in Regulating Metabolism. *Sci. Rep.* **2016**, *6*, 33302. [CrossRef]
64. Engeli, S. Dysregulation of the endocannabinoid system in obesity. *J. Neuroendocrinol.* **2008**, *20* (Suppl. 1), 110–115. [CrossRef] [PubMed]
65. González-Mariscal, I.; Krzysik-Walker, S.M.; Kim, W.; Rouse, M.; Egan, J.M. Blockade of cannabinoid 1 receptor improves GLP-1R mediated insulin secretion in mice. *Mol. Cell Endocrinol.* **2016**, *423*, 1–10. [CrossRef] [PubMed]
66. Jourdan, T.; Godlewski, G.; Cinar, R.; Bertola, A.; Szanda, G.; Liu, J.; Tam, J.; Han, T.; Mukhopadhyay, B.; Skarulis, M.C.; et al. Activation of the Nlrp3 inflammasome in infiltrating macrophages by endocannabinoids mediates beta cell loss in type 2 diabetes. *Nat. Med.* **2013**, *19*, 1132–1140. [CrossRef]
67. González-Mariscal, I.; Montoro, R.A.; Doyle, M.E.; Liu, Q.R.; Rouse, M.; O'Connell, J.F.; Calvo, S.S.-C.; Krzysik-Walker, S.M.; Ghosh, S.; Carlson, O.D.; et al. Absence of cannabinoid 1 receptor in beta cells protects against high-fat/high-sugar diet-induced beta cell dysfunction and inflammation in murine islets. *Diabetologia* **2018**, *61*, 1470–1483. [CrossRef] [PubMed]
68. Cinar, R.; Godlewski, G.; Liu, J.; Tam, J.; Jourdan, T.; Mukhopadhyay, B.; Harvey-White, J.; Kunos, G. Hepatic cannabinoid-1 receptors mediate diet-induced insulin resistance by increasing de novo synthesis of long-chain ceramides. *Hepatology* **2014**, *59*, 143–153. [CrossRef] [PubMed]
69. Bouassa, R.-S.M.; Sebastiani, G.; Di Marzo, V.; Jenabian, M.-A.; Costiniuk, C.T. Cannabinoids and Chronic Liver Diseases. *Int. J. Mol. Sci.* **2022**, *23*, 9423. [CrossRef]
70. Penner, E.A.; Buettner, H.; Mittleman, M.A. The impact of marijuana use on glucose, insulin, and insulin resistance among US adults. *Am. J. Med.* **2013**, *126*, 583–589. [CrossRef]
71. Rajavashisth, T.B.; Shaheen, M.; Norris, K.C.; Pan, D.; Sinha, S.K.; Ortega, J.; Friedman, T.C. Decreased prevalence of diabetes in marijuana users: Cross-sectional data from the National Health and Nutrition Examination Survey (NHANES) III. *BMJ Open* **2012**, *2*, e000494. [CrossRef]
72. Vidot, D.C.; Prado, G.; Hlaing, W.M.; Florez, H.J.; Arheart, K.L.; Messiah, S.E. Metabolic Syndrome Among Marijuana Users in the United States: An Analysis of National Health and Nutrition Examination Survey Data. *Am. J. Med.* **2016**, *129*, 173–179. [CrossRef]
73. Jadoon, K.A.; Ratcliffe, S.H.; Barrett, D.A.; Thomas, E.L.; Stott, C.; Bell, J.D.; O'Sullivan, S.E.; Tan, G.D. Efficacy and Safety of Cannabidiol and Tetrahydrocannabivarin on Glycemic and Lipid Parameters in Patients with Type 2 Diabetes: A Randomized, Double-Blind, Placebo-Controlled, Parallel Group Pilot Study. *Diabetes Care* **2016**, *39*, 1777–1786. [CrossRef]
74. Costiniuk, C.T.; Saneei, Z.; Salahuddin, S.; Cox, J.; Routy, J.P.; Rueda, S.; Abdallah, S.J.; Jensen, D.; Lebouché, B.; Brouillette, M.J.; et al. Cannabis Consumption in People Living with HIV: Reasons for Use, Secondary Effects, and Opportunities for Health Education. *Cannabis Cannabinoid Res.* **2019**, *4*, 204–213. [CrossRef]

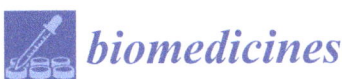

Article

"Flower Power": Controlled Inhalation of THC-Predominant Cannabis Flos Improves Health-Related Quality of Life and Symptoms of Chronic Pain and Anxiety in Eligible UK Patients

Guillermo Moreno-Sanz [1,*], Alvaro Madiedo [2], Michael Lynskey [3] and Matthew R. D. Brown [4,5]

1. Khiron Life Sciences Spain, 28001 Madrid, Spain
2. Khiron Life Sciences, Bogotá 110221, Colombia
3. Drug Sciences, London SW7 2BX, UK
4. Zerenia Clinics, London SW1X 9AE, UK
5. The Royal Marsden Hospital, London SW3 6JU, UK
* Correspondence: gmoreno@khiron.ca

Abstract: In November 2018, the UK's Home Office established a legal route for eligible patients to be prescribed cannabis-based products for medicinal use in humans (CBPMs) as unlicensed medicines. These include liquid cannabis extracts for oral administration ("oils") and dried flowers for inhalation ("flos"). Smoking of CBPMs is expressly prohibited. To date, THC-predominant cannabis flowers remain the most prescribed CBPMs in project Twenty21 (T21), the first multi-center, prospective, observational UK cannabis patient registry. This observational, prospective data review analyzes patient-reported outcome measures (PROMS) collected by T21 associated with the inhalation of KHIRON 20/1, the most prescribed CBPM in the project. PROMS collected at baseline and at subsequent 3-month follow-up included health-related quality of life (HRQoL), general mood, and sleep. Condition-specific measures of illness severity were performed with the Brief Pain Inventory Short Form (BPI-SF) and the Generalized Anxiety Disorder 7-Item Scale (GAD-7). Participants (N = 344) were mostly males (77.6%, average age = 38.3) diagnosed mainly with chronic pain (50.9%) and anxiety-related disorders (25.3%). Inhalation of KHIRON 20/1 was associated with a marked increase in self-reported HRQoL, general mood, and sleep (N = 344; $p < 0.001$). Condition-specific assessments showed significant improvements in pain severity (T = 6.67; $p < 0.001$) and interference (T = 7.19; $p < 0.001$) in patients using KHIRON 20/1 for chronic pain (N = 174). Similar results were found for patients diagnosed with anxiety-related disorders (N = 107; T = 12.9; $p < 0.001$). Our results indicate that controlled inhalation of pharmaceutical grade, THC-predominant cannabis flos is associated with a significant improvement in patient-reported pain scores, mood, anxiety, sleep disturbances and overall HRQoL in a treatment-resistant clinical population.

Keywords: cannabis; chronic pain; anxiety; inhalation; tetrahydrocannabinol; HRQoL

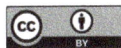

1. Introduction

Cannabis was (re) introduced into British medical practice in the early 1840's by Irish physician Dr. William O'Shaughnessy, an army surgeon serving in Calcutta, India [1]. In the Victorian period, cannabis was widely used for a variety of ailments, including muscle spasms, menstrual cramps, rheumatism, the convulsions of tetanus, rabies, and epilepsy, and as a sedative. Cannabis extracts were typically administered orally in the form of an alcoholic tincture and were commonly incorporated in proprietary medicines [2]. With the introduction of synthetic drugs, herbal remedies were increasingly viewed as unpredictable and many of them, including cannabis extracts and tinctures, were removed from the British Pharmacopoeia of 1932 but retained in the British Pharmaceutical Codex of 1949. Under the Dangerous Drugs Act 1964, which implemented the 1961 UN Single Convention on Narcotic Drugs in the United Kingdom, the prescription of cannabis tinctures continued to be permitted due to a "license of right" received under the Medicines Act 1968. However, this license of right was subsequently not renewed, and the original Misuse of Drugs Regulations of 1973 listed cannabis, cannabis resin, cannabinol and its derivatives in Schedule 4 (now Schedule 1) completely prohibiting medical use [2]. In November 2018, the UK's Home Office (re) established a legal route for the prescription of cannabis-based products for medicinal use in humans (CBPMs) through the amendment of both the Misuse of Drugs Regulations 2001 and Misuse of Drugs Order 2015, rescheduling CBPMs as Schedule 2 drugs [3]. CBPMs remain strictly regulated and include both cannabis extracts for oral administration ("oils") and dried cannabis flowers for inhalation ("flos"). These products may only be prescribed by a specialist medical practitioner as "special" or "bespoke" medications following processes common to all unlicensed medications.

Whilst smoking of cannabis and CBPMs is expressly prohibited in the legislation, cannabis flos remains the most popular cannabis galenic formulation in the UK, a situation similar to that which occurs in other jurisdictions with established medicinal-cannabis access schemes, such as Germany, Canada, and Israel [4]. Qualitative research studies have shown that patients using cannabis for therapeutic purposes tend to choose the inhalation of flos as their preferred method of administration, as it provides a greater control over dosage and speed of onset, as well as a more robust relief of symptoms compared to the oral route [5]. Additionally, the development of vaporizers and inhalers for flos, some of which have attained certification as medical devices, affords patients greater control over administration and dosing of the pharmacologically active molecules present in cannabis, namely cannabinoids Δ9-tetrahydrocannabinol (THC) and cannabidiol (CBD), limiting the occurrence of side effects related to the central nervous system and the inhalation of toxic by-products of combustion [6].

Oral THC has been clinically approved for the treatment of several health conditions, such as chemotherapy-induced nausea and vomiting, wasting syndrome associated with AIDS and cancer, and spasticity in patients with multiple sclerosis, and its ability to treat other neurological conditions is under investigation [7]. A large body of scientific literature indicates that inhalation of chemotype I (THC-predominant) cannabis flos can mitigate symptoms associated with chronic pain, increase relaxation, and facilitate resilience to cope with disability. A series of small placebo-controlled, randomized control trials (RCT) conducted with cannabis flos have shown that this therapy option is efficacious and safe at treating neuropathic pain, whilst also improving mood and daily functioning to a similar extent during treatment periods [8–13]. Analogous results were observed in a placebo-controlled crossover trials investigating patients with multiple sclerosis, in which perception of pain was a secondary outcome [14], or patients with chronic pain of varying etiology [15]. In addition to these RCTs, numerous observational studies contribute to a robust body of real-world evidence (RWE) which suggests that the inhalation of chemotype I cannabis flos could effectively ameliorate other types of chronic pain including pelvic pain [16], migraines [17], or fibromyalgia [18], as well as markedly improve various traumatic psychiatric conditions such as stress, anxiety, or depression [19–21].

A recent single-center, observational study explored the clinical outcomes associated with the use of CBPMs in British patients diagnosed with chronic pain, a condition that affects approximately 28 million people in the UK with an estimated direct and indirect cost of £21.2 billion [22]. To minimize the variability in the formulation, participants were prescribed one single oral cannabis extract normalized in medium-chain triglycerides (MCT) oil. Product composition and route of administration are typically difficult to control for and a frequent confounding factor in observational studies. Authors reported significant improvements in health-related quality of life, pain interference and sleep quality, accompanied by a 30% incidence of side effects of mild or moderate intensity [22]. Following a similar rationale and experimental design, in the present work we aimed at investigating the efficacy and safety of the inhalation of THC-predominant cannabis flowers on a treatment-resistant cohort of patients enrolled in Project Twenty21 (T21), the first multi-center registry of patients receiving bespoke CBPMs in the UK [23,24]. We analyzed clinical outcome measures, collected prospectively through validated questionnaires [25], reported by patients receiving treatment with KHIRON 20/1, the most frequently prescribed chemotype I cannabis flower in T21.

2. Materials and Methods

2.1. Design

We analyzed clinical data collected prospectively between August 2020 and June 2022 to investigate the clinical outcomes associated with the inhalation of THC-predominant flos for therapeutic purposes in a legal and medically supervised setting. Participants were patients registered in Project Twenty21 (T21), the first UK multi-center registry seeking to develop a body of real-world evidence (RWE) to inform on the effectiveness and safety of medical cannabis. Full information relating to T21 procedures is outlined elsewhere [23,25]. In brief, patients receiving CBPMs for a variety of conditions are entered into the registry by invitation and monitored for data collection as part of their standard of care. According to UK regulations, individuals must have an established diagnosis and have failed to respond to at least two treatment options to legally receive CBPMs. Patients provided consent (following Good Clinical Practice guidelines) to the collection of their medical history, past and current treatments, plus a series of symptomatic assessments based on standardized and comprehensively validated self-report questionnaires. Prescribing physicians partnering with T21 use a product formulary that includes a wide range of CBPMs including oral extracts and flos of differing CBD and THC ratios. To date, THC-predominant flos remains the most prescribed CBPM in the project [23]. To reduce the inherent variability associated with the chemical composition of cannabis dried flowers, we decided to include in our data review only those patients receiving at their initial appointment a prescription for KHIRON 20/1, the most frequently prescribed THC-predominant flos in T21. Additional inclusion criterion was that participants had completed health-related quality of life (HRQoL) questionnaires both at the initial appointment (baseline) and at the subsequent 3-month follow up.

2.2. Drugs

KHIRON 20/1 (Pharmadrug Production GmbH, Rostock, Germany) is a chemotype 1 cannabis variety which contains 20% (w/w) of THC and less than 1% (w/w) of CBD in dried weigh. This variety is also referred to by the breeder's name *Hindu Kush* and is classified as an indica-type plant. Indica/sativa terminology relates to structural and botanical features of the cannabis plant and, contrary to what commonly misconstrued, does not provide robust information on the chemical composition nor on the pharmacological characteristics of the flos [26]. The batches of KHIRON 20/1 flos prescribed to T21 participants were produced in full compliance with good manufacturing practices (GMP) requirements and to the standards established in the German monograph for cannabis flos [27].

2.3. CBPM Administration Protocol

The UK´s Misuse of Drugs Regulations 2018 explicitly prohibits smoking of cannabis and CBPMs, therefore, an herbal vaporizer/inhaler is required for the therapeutic administration of cannabis flos. Currently, there are two vaporizers that have attained the EU certification of medical devices for the inhalation of cannabis flowers, both manufactured by the German company Storz&Bickel: the Volcano medic, a tabletop model [28], and the battery-operated, handheld device Mighty Medic [29]. Although most clinical research on vaporizing medicinal cannabis has been performed using the Volcano device, the majority of T21 participants typically prefer a handheld device, such as the Mighty Medic (Figure 1A), both for convenience and economic reasons. Owing to the more rapid effect onset, inhalation allows the experienced patient to easily titrate the dosage to maximize therapeutic benefit and minimize side effects typically related to overt THC-related psychoactivity, by controlling the number, duration, and frequency of inhalations. Figure 1C illustrates the dosing protocol we developed to guide T21 prescribers and cannabis-naïve participants through the process of personalizing cannabis inhalation depending on the needs of each individual patient. In brief, to vaporize THC-predominant flowers, patients are advised to:

1. Fill the Mighty Medic dosing capsules with grounded cannabis flos (Figure 1B). Although the maximum capacity per capsule is 250 mg, dosing is based in both the number and frequency of inhalations rather than the absolute amount of herbal material loaded into the device. This allows an experienced patient to have more control over administration and dosing while, at the same time, adjust and standardize the amount of cannabis flos used to optimize cost–benefit.
2. Turn on the device and set the temperature to 180 °C (Figure 1A). At this temperature, vapor will be composed mainly of steam, most volatile terpenes (e.g., limonene, pinene), and small amounts of THC (boiling point 157 °C) which will start decarboxylating.
3. Once the target temperature is reached, patients are instructed to inhale and exhale naturally. Vapor should not be held in the lungs longer than during regular breathing. The first inhalation is typically less effective since it serves to "prime" the device and warm up the herbal material.
4. After inhaling the indicated number of times (see Figure 1C), patients are advised to wait for 15–20 min and observe for side effects (such as dizziness, tachycardia, nausea, disorientation, euphoria, etc.). After this period, and in absence of side effects, patients can repeat the cycle if symptomatic control has not been achieved, increasing the temperature by 10 °C (Figure 1C).
5. At 190 °C and 200 °C the vapor may feel dryer and less fragrant but will be more concentrated in cannabinoids [30]. Vaporization of cannabinoids continues at high temperatures even if vapor is not visible when exhaling, due to the exhaustion of water in the herbal material.
6. The goal for this 5-day initiation protocol is to provide the prescribing doctor with clear administration instructions to share with patients so that they can experiment with the device and familiarize themselves safely with cannabis inhalation.

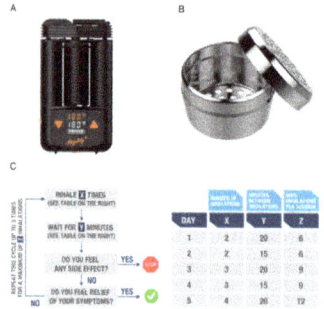

Figure 1. Proposed protocol to initiate naïve patients and prescribing doctors safely into the inhalation of THC-predominant cannabis flos. (**A**) The herbal vaporizer mightly medic is powered by rechargeable batteries and attained EU-mark as a medical device; (**B**) Pharma-grade aluminum dosing capsules holding up to 0.25 g of grinded cannabis flos can be loaded into the mighty heating unit. (**C**) Flowchart depicting a proposed 5-day familiarization plan for naïve users, with daily increases in number and frequency of inhalations to minimize the risk of CNS-related side effects.

2.4. Patient-Reported Outcome Measures (PROMS)

PROMS questionnaires are completed by T21 participants both at baseline/treatment entry and then every 3 months at scheduled follow-ups. The following questionnaires were employed to capture outcome measures that were either common for all participants (HRQoL, Mood and Sleep) or specific for each diagnosed condition (chronic painful conditions or anxiety-related disorders).

2.4.1. Health-Related Quality of Life

The EuroQol 5 Dimensions (EQ-5D-5L) is a widely used, validated, and reliable tool to assess the quality of life of patients in many disease areas through evaluating the severity of each of 5 dimensions (mobility, self-care, usual activities, pain/discomfort, and anxiety/depression) [31]. Two measures of HRQoL were considered:

1. The visual analog score (VAS) of general health (0–100) was interpreted as a patient-reported measure of general health.
2. The sum of ratings for the five dimensions of the EuroQol (5–25) was interpreted as patient-reported measure of HRQoL.

2.4.2. Mood/Depression

The Patient Health Questionnaire (PHQ-9) is a reliable and valid measure of depression severity, which is comprised by a 9-item, self-rated instrument previously validated in general populations, medical populations, and psychiatric samples [32]. Scoring ranges from 0 to 27.

2.4.3. Sleep Disturbances

Quality of sleep was assessed by using four items adapted from the widely used Pittsburgh Sleep Quality Index [33]. Scoring ranges from 4 to 20.

2.4.4. Chronic Pain

Participants diagnosed with chronic pain were asked to complete the Brief Pain Inventory Short Form (BPI-SF). The BPI-SF is validated in patients with both cancer and non-cancer pain and is one of the most used measurement tools for evaluating clinical pain, including both pain severity and the interference of pain on feelings and function [34]. Therefore, items from this scale were used to assess two distinct dimensions of pain: (i) severity of pain; and (ii) the extent to which pain interferes with daily activity. Patients scored both dimensions on a 0–10 scale.

2.4.5. Anxiety

Participants diagnosed with anxiety-related disorders were asked to complete the Generalized Anxiety Disorder 7-Item Scale (GAD-7). The GAD-7 is one of the most frequently used, validated, self-reported questionnaires clinically employed to screen for, diagnose, and assess the severity of generalized anxiety disorder [35]. Each item is scored 0–3 for a composed total range 0–21.

2.5. Statistical Analysis

Demographics are expressed either as percentage or as the mean ± standard deviation. Results of PROMS analysis are represented in box and whisker graphs, which indicate upper and lower extreme values, median, upper quartile, and lower quartile. Statistical analyses were performed by either student's t (comparisons of means at t = 0 and t = 3) or one-way ANOVA (comparisons of means at t = 0, t = 3 and t = 6) followed by Friedman non-parametric test and pair-wise comparisons (Durbin-Conover) using the Jamovi free software V2.2.2 (San Francisco, CA, USA). Post hoc analyses were considered statistically significant if $p < 0.05$.

3. Results

3.1. Participants

A total of 344 patients registered in T21 satisfied the inclusion criteria of (i) having PROMS questionnaires correctly recorded at the initial appointment (t = 0) and, at the least, at the 3-month follow up (t = 3), and (ii) receiving a prescription for KHIRON 20/1 at t = 0. Of those, 140 participants had also reported PROMS at the 6-month follow up (t = 6). Participants enrolled in T21 between August 2020 and June 2022. Demographics and clinical characteristics of the patient cohort are depicted in Table 1. Coherent with the overall patient population of T21, three out of four participants were adult males (77.6%), with an average age of 38.4 ± 10.4 years old. A majority of them were diagnosed with a chronic painful condition (50.8%) or an anxiety-related disorder (25.3%). Other minor qualifying diagnosis were Attention Deficit Hyperactivity Disorder (ADHD) (6.98%), Post Traumatic Stress Disorder (PTSD) (6.1%) or insomnia (2.9%). As required by law, all patients had trialed at the least two standard therapeutic options to treat their condition before accessing medicinal cannabis. Of note, only 16 participants were naïve to cannabis when commencing the T21 process. A vast majority of patients (95.6%) had previously utilized illicitly acquired cannabis, and 3 out of 4 of those consuming cannabis did so with the intention of treating their primary diagnosed condition. Most participants elected to administer CBPM once a day (58.7%).

Table 1. Cohort demographics, previous cannabis use and primary diagnosed conditions.

	Gender			Total
	Male	Female	Non-Binary	
Participants Sample: N (%)	267 (77.6)	76 (22.1)	1 (0.3)	344 (100)
Age: Mean ± SD	38.3 ± 10.6	38.6 ± 9.89	42 ± 0.0	38.4 ± 10.4
Previous Experience with Cannabis: N (%)	259 (97.0)	69 (90.8)	1 (100)	329 (95.6)
Intention of treating their primary condition with cannabis: N (%)	205 (76.8)	56 (73.7)	1 (100)	262 (76.1)
Frequency of cannabis use: N (%)				
Weekly	2 (0.75)	1 (1.32)	0	3 (0.87)
A few times a week	29 (10.9)	12 (15.8)	0	41 (11.9)
Once a day	160 (59.9)	41 (53.9)	1 (100)	202 (58.7)
Multiple times a day	15 (5.62)	3 (3.95)	0	18 (5.23)
Did not answer the question	61 (22.8)	19 (25.0)	0	80 (23.2)
Primary Condition: N (%)				
Chronic painful conditions	134 (50.2)	40 (52.6)	1 (100)	175 (50.8)
Anxiety-related disorders	74 (27.7)	13 (17.1)	0	87 (25.3)
ADHD	19 (7.12)	5 (6.58)	0	24 (6.98)
PTSD	12 (4.49)	9 (11.8)	0	21 (6.10)
Other Mental Health	14 (5.24)	4 (5.26)	0	18 (5.23)
Insomnia	8 (3.00)	2 (2.63)	0	10 (2.91)
Autism Spectrum Disorder	2 (0.75)	0	0	2 (0.58)
Epilepsy	0	1 (2.33)	0	1 (0.52)
Other	4 (1.50)	1 (1.32)	0	5 (1.45)

3.2. General Health Outcome Measures

3.2.1. Health Related Quality of Life (HRQoL)

Inhalation of THC-predominant cannabis flos was associated with a marked improvement both in general health and in health-related quality of life (HRQoL) after 3 months, expressed as the VAS score (Figure 2A, T = 8.80; $p < 0.001$) and the sum of ratings for the 5 dimensions of the EuroQol (Figure 2B T = 10.3; $p < 0.001$), respectively. A similar degree of improvement was reported by participants at the 6-month follow up (Figure 3A,B), which is suggestive of (i) the maximal effect of the treatment being already achieved at the 3-month timepoint which was maintained but not further improved at 6 months, and (ii) no overt tolerance to the treatment developing after 6 months of daily administration. As shown in Table 2, participants diagnosed with chronic pain reported lower baseline levels of HRQoL compared to those diagnosed with anxiety disorders. However, no significant differences in the degree of improvement captured by the EQ-5D were found between these two groups at the 3-month follow up. On the contrary, patients diagnosed with anxiety-related disorders did report a larger improvement in general health compared to chronic pain patients (mean difference 12.4 vs. 6.98; $p < 0.05$), as captured by the VAS of the EuroQoL questionnaire.

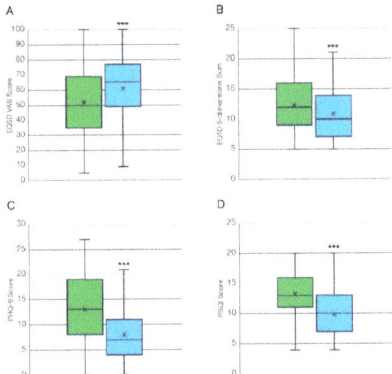

Figure 2. Improvement of general health outcome measures at the 3-month follow-up. Analysis of PROMS shows how the inhalation of KHIRON 20/1 was associated with a marked improvement in self-reported health related QoL (N = 344) measured as (**A**) the scoring of the VAS of the EQ5D, and (**B**) the sum of the 5 dimensions of the EQ5D questionnaire. (**C**) General mood/ clinical depression assessed with the PHQ-9 scale (N = 339) was markedly improved. This effect was mainly driven by patients diagnosed with anxiety-related disorders (Table 2). (**D**) Quality of sleep assessed with the Pittsburgh Sleep Quality Index (N = 344) was improved by the treatment with inhaled chemotype 1 cannabis flos. *** $p < 0.001$.

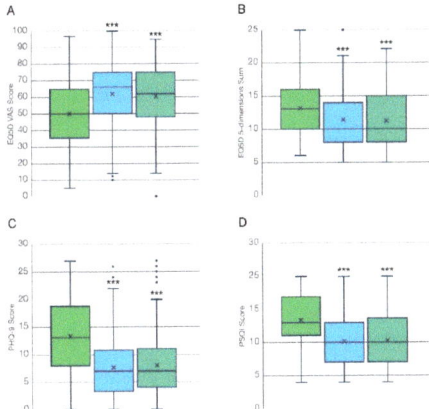

Figure 3. Comparative improvement of general health outcome measures at 3- and 6-month follow-up. Analysis of outcome measures reported by patients that completed the validated questionnaires both at 3- and at 6-month follow-up visits (N = 140). Improvements associated with the inhalation of KHIRON 20/1 in (**A**,**B**) HRQoL, (**C**) General mood/ clinical depression, and (**D**) quality of sleep were maximal at 3 months and maintained, although not further increased, at the 6-month follow-up. *** $p < 0.001$.

Table 2. Comparative analysis on the influence of the two main participants sub-populations by primary indication, chronic painful conditions, and anxiety-related disorders, over the general PROMS: HRQoL, mood/depression and sleep quality. * $p < 0.05$; ** $p < 0.01$.

	General Health EQ5D VAS Score			Health-Related QoL EQ5D 5-Dimensions SUM			Mood/Depression PHQ-9 Score			Quality of Sleep PSQI Score		
	Mean T = 0	Mean T = 3	Mean Diff	Mean T = 0	Mean T = 3	Mean Diff	Mean T = 0	Mean T = 3	Diff Mean	Mean T = 0	Mean T = 3	Mean Diff
Anxiety (N = 107)	57.10	69.55	12.4	10.07	8.31	1.76	13.72	6.58	7.14	12.31	9.16	3.15
Chronic Pain (N = 174)	47.35	54.33	6.98 *	14.24	12.94	1.30	12.78	9.42	3.36 **	13.51	10.79	2.72

3.2.2. General Mood/Depression

Participants reported an improved overall mood associated with the treatment at the 3-month follow-up (Figure 2C, N = 339; T = 15.3; $p < 0.001$), which was maintained up to 6 months (Figure 3C, N = 136; X^2 = 94.0; $p < 0.001$) as indicated by a significant reduction in the PHQ-9 questionnaire scoring. As shown in Table 2, the observed effect was strongly influenced by participants diagnosed with anxiety-related disorders, who reported slightly poorer baseline levels of mood/depression (13.72 vs. 12.78) and a significantly larger average improvement (7.14 vs. 3.36; T= −5.18; $p < 0.01$) in the PHQ-9 scale compared to those participants diagnosed with chronic pain after 3 months.

3.2.3. Sleep Quality

Sleep deprivation is one of the most common comorbidities associated with chronic illness [36]. Quality of sleep, assessed by the Pittsburg sleep quality index (PSQI), was improved following the inhalation of THC-predominant cannabis flowers after 3 months (Figure 2D, N = 344; T = 14.5; $p < 0.001$). This effect was maintained, but not further increased, at the 6-month follow up (Figure 3D, N = 140; X^2 = 74.9; $p < 0.001$). Participants diagnosed with anxiety disorders and chronic pain conditions reported similar basal levels (12.31 vs. 13.51) and no significant differences were found among the average improvement (3.15 vs. 2.72) in the PSQI scores of the two sub-populations (Table 2).

3.3. Indication-Specific Outcome Measures

Besides general outcome measures, which were collected for all patients, T21 participants are asked to complete health questionnaires specific to their primary indication. Here, we report only results from the main two health conditions, which included more than 85% of all participants (Table 1). Results from other less frequent indications, such as ADHD (N = 24) and PTSD (N = 21), will be disclosed in a separated data review once adequate statistical powering is achieved. Participants diagnosed with a chronic painful condition (N = 174) completed the Brief Pain Inventory-Short Form, a 9-item questionnaire used to evaluate (i) the severity of a patient's pain and (ii) the impact of this pain on the patient's daily functioning. Patients diagnosed with anxiety-related disorders or other mental health issues concomitant with anxiety (N = 107) completed the Generalized Anxiety Disorder (GAD-7), which total score for the seven items ranges from 0 to 21.

3.3.1. Pain Severity

Participants reported a 16.2% reduction in pain severity (Figure 4A, N = 174; T = 6.67; $p < 0.001$) from an average baseline value of 5.63 to a mean value of 4.72 at the 3-month follow up, associated with the treatment.

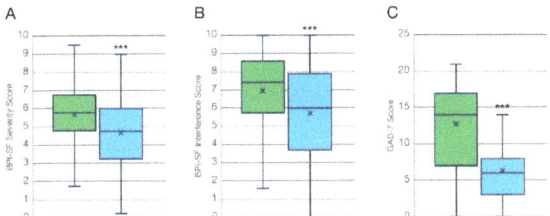

Figure 4. Improvement of indication-specific outcome measures at the 3-month follow-up. Analysis of PROMS shows how the inhalation of KHIRON 20/1 was associated with a marked improvement in self-reported (**A**) pain severity and (**B**) pain interference in patients diagnosed with chronic painful conditions, measured with the Brief Pain Inventory-short form (N = 174). (**C**) Generalized anxiety measured with the GAD-7 questionnaire was markedly decrease after 3 months of treatment with cannabis flos KHIRON 20/1 (N = 107). *** $p < 0.001$.

3.3.2. Pain Interference

Recovery of daily functioning and restoring "their old self" is one of the most recurrent features that chronic, self-medicating, patients associate to their therapeutic use of cannabis. Participants reported a 18.4% reduction in pain interference with their daily activities associated with the treatment from an average baseline value of 6.97 to a mean value of 5.69 at the 3-month follow up (Figure 4B, N = 174; T = 7.19; $p < 0.001$).

3.3.3. Generalized Anxiety Disorder

Participants who completed the GAD-7 questionnaire reported a 50.7% reduction in anxiety symptoms (Figure 4C, N = 107; T = 12.9; $p < 0.001$) from an average baseline value of 12.7 to a mean value of 6.28 at the 3-month follow up.

3.4. Adverse Effects

T21 participants were also encouraged to report any adverse side effects that they considered associated with the treatment with CBPMs. Inhalation of THC-predominant flower was found in general to be safe. Only two participants diagnosed with chronic pain reported minor adverse side effects associated with KHIRON 20/1 from those available in the list: (i) a 42-year-old male with previous experience with cannabis who medicated several times a day reported suffering a "mild headache" which remitted after 1–2 h; and (ii) a 32-year-old female reported suffering "memory loss". This adverse effect was described by the patient as "transient" and "not relevant". Of note, this participant was among the 15 patients (4.4% of total cohort) that were naïve to cannabis prior to enrolling in project T21.

4. Discussion

The presented work investigates the ability of inhaled THC-predominant (chemotype-1) cannabis flos to improve health-related quality of life (HRQoL) and mitigate symptomatology in a treatment-resistant population of patients diagnosed with chronic painful conditions and anxiety-related disorders. Our results indicate that sustained inhalation of cannabis flos KHIRON 20/1 was associated with a robust and long-lasting improvement in HRQoL, mood and quality of sleep. The pharmacokinetics of orally ingested cannabinoids typically display erratic intestinal absorption, high inter- and intra-individual variability, extensive hepatic metabolism, and a delayed onset of effects between 90 and 120 min. In contrast, vaporized cannabinoids are rapidly and reliably absorbed into the bloodstream, achieving peak concentrations in blood generally in under 10 min [37]. These differences in pharmacokinetic properties afford patients a greater degree of control over dosage and speed of onset. Accordingly, both quantitative and qualitative research report on the ability of inhaled cannabis flos to quickly relieve symptoms of depression, stress, and anxiety. Patients describe the bodily sensation of cannabis inhalation as a "sigh of relief", which leads to a state of relaxation promoting a reduction in pain sensation and, subsequently, improved sleep, motility, mood and acceptance [5,38]. For this reason, inhalation of cannabis flos is typically recommended as a rescue medication for acute or "breakthrough" symptoms [39]. However, our results showed sustained reduction in pain severity and interference of chronic pain with daily activities after 3 months of daily administration of KHIRON 20/1, which was maintained at the 6-month follow-up.

This finding is coherent with recent prospective observational studies investigating medical outcomes in chronic pain patients combining different formulations of medicinal cannabis, which also reported significantly lower levels of pain severity and pain interference, improved mood, sleep duration and sleep quality, and overall quality of life at 3 months compared to baseline [40,41]. Besides the 3-month follow up, Wang and collaborators incorporated ecological momentary assessment (EMA) to measure real-time health outcomes once daily for one week before (baseline) and for up to three weeks immediately after starting the treatment. Authors reported a significant reduction in real-time pain intensity (16.5-point reduction in a 0–100 VAS) and anxiety, longer sleep duration and better sleep quality in the first 3 weeks of treatment [40]. In similar studies, chronic pain patients treated exclusively with oral CBPMs also showed maximal improvement 3 months after the treatment initiation, which was sustained for over 6 months [22,42], suggesting that tolerance to the beneficial effects of cannabinoid therapy does not commonly occur. This observation is further supported by results from RCTs leading towards the clinical approval and commercialization of Sativex, in which MS patients showed sustained improvements in pain for more than 12 months without developing tolerance [43].

It is notable that greater than 95% of patients included in our data review were using cannabis illegally to treat their conditions at baseline and yet, we found a marked improvement in all PROMS analyzed. We interpret this finding to indicate that the administration of cannabis flowers in a clinical environment, under the supervision of a trained healthcare provider, further improves the clinical outcomes associated with legally prescribed CBPMs when compared to chronic patients self-medicating with illicit cannabis. This interpretation is further supported by similar findings from different jurisdictions where legally protected access to medical cannabis had recently become available [44,45]. The effect of such regulatory changes may have a greater impact in those experiencing anxiety-related disorders as it eliminates several major concerns for these patients, such as product availability, product reproducibility and the fear of potential legal consequences [5]. Our results indicate indeed that the largest clinical improvements associated with the inhalation of THC-predominant cannabis flos were reported by patients with a primary indication of generalized or social anxiety. First, we found a robust reduction in the GAD-7 scoring, from a baseline value of 12.7 to a value of 6.28 at the 3-month follow up. This remarkable result contrast with those reported by a Canadian group who applied the GAD-7 scale to a large cohort of adults authorized to use cannabis between 2014 and 2019. Although a statistically significant decrease in GAD-7 scoring was noted (from 9.11 to 9.04), it did not meet the threshold to be considered clinically significant [46]. In contrast, participants in our cohort diagnosed with generalized anxiety displayed higher baseline levels of moderate-to-severe anxieties, which could be potentially exacerbated by their illicit use of cannabis. Second, our result show that the cohort of patients diagnosed with anxiety-related disorders had a significantly larger contribution to the improvement in mood captured by the PHQ-9 scale, a measure of clinical depression. It could be postulated that the overall anxiolytic effect of whole flower CBPM could result from the combination of a rapid pharmacological activation of central type-1 cannabinoid (CB1) receptors together with the reassurance of pharmaceutical quality CBPM, legally prescribed by a clinician.

Functional imaging studies in humans have shown a correlation between THC-mediated analgesia and a reduction in neural connectivity between the anterior cingulate cortex (ACC) and cortical areas involved in pain processing, the dorsolateral prefrontal cortex in particular, which are two key brain regions for the modulation of cognitive and emotional inputs [47,48]. Accordingly, results from human lab experiments suggest that

THC prevents the onset of pain sensation by slightly increasing pain threshold but does not effectively reduce the perceived intensity of experimental pain [49]. Instead, THC seems to influence affective processing, thus making pain sensation less unpleasant and more tolerable, which resonates with qualitative assessments made by patients treated with CBPMs [38]. Available evidence also suggests that inhaled THC can potentiate the extinction of fearful and aversive memories in humans and reduce anxiety responses without eliciting psychotic effects [50], although it remains unclear if this effect is mediated by the activation CB1 receptors in the same brain regions. However, significantly increased circuit coupling between the ACC and the amygdala has been described during the processing of fearful stimuli in anxious (but not in healthy) individuals, which also correlated positively with self-reported symptoms of anxiety [51]. The key regulatory role of CB1 receptors in the amygdala, activated by endogenously produced anandamide on fear processing and aversive memory extinction has also been characterized both in preclinical and clinical studies [52,53]. Taken together, this evidence highlights the role of the ACC as a critical mediator in the analgesic and anxiolytic actions of THC, which could also explain why frequent and transient activation of central CB1 receptors could lead to sustained improvement in the emotional processing and a reduction in negative affect and physical symptoms associated with chronic illnesses [19].

The occurrence of adverse side effects experienced by participants was relatively rare, likely because most participants (95.6%) had previous experience with cannabis inhalation. In fact, the one patient reporting transient, mild, memory loss was naïve to cannabis. Adverse CNS-related side effects following cannabis inhalation are typically related to the dose of THC [54]. To counter this we have detailed an administration protocol to guide naïve patients and prescribing doctors following the mantra of "start low and go slow" [39], and based on the number and frequency of inhalations as opposed to the total amount of herbal cannabis loaded in the vaporizer. Pharmacokinetic studies on medically vaporized herbal cannabis have previously been performed with a tabletop model, S&B Volcano, which has a greater capacity to evaporate cannabinoids due to the instrument design and the range of working temperatures [30]. Human pharmacokinetic information for handheld devices is not readily available and it can largely depend on cannabinoid extraction efficiency, which may vary between devices [15]. Therefore, we aimed at providing simple instructions for first-time users to quickly gain control over cannabinoid dosing and speed of onset while minimizing the risk of involuntary overdosing. However, it is worth noticing the relatively safe profile of the inhaled route compared to the sublingual or oral administration. Firstly, due to their lipophilic nature, sublingual absorption of cannabinoids in oily carriers is limited and almost identical to oral ingestion [55]. Secondly, several studies have reported that intoxication, acute psychiatric symptoms, and adverse cardiovascular events are more common in patients following oral ingestion of CBPMs, while hyperemesis syndrome (cycling vomiting) was more likely attributable to inhalation of herbal cannabis [56]. Finally, in response to the clinical requirement of prescribing THC-predominant cannabis flos for extended periods of time in patients experiencing benefit, clinicians should be aware of the relevant contraindications to this substance including psychotic vulnerability and cardiovascular instability, as well as the risks of patients developing cannabis use disorders (CUD).

This work presents several limitations, some of which are inherent to the way real-world data is collected and interpreted [57]. We used a convenience cohort which, while representative of the more than 3,000 patients enrolled by T21 over the last two years, still poses a high risk of selection bias [58]. Additionally, patients were grouped for analysis of PROMS by primary indication, but their diagnosis and etiology could differ. Although a dosing protocol was suggested, it is plausible to assume that each patient established their own individualize dosing regime and that some may not have used an herbal vaporizer to administer their CBPMs, which is also representative of real-world clinical practice [39]. Finally, our research design did not control for placebo effect, which is typically robust in studies using cannabis [58], although this could be partially mitigated by the flexible dosing regimen [10]. Owing to the inherent psychoactivity associated with the central activation of CB1 receptors, complete blinding in studies using THC is virtually impossible. In fact, relief of spontaneous pain typically correlates with high drug-like scores in human lab studies [18]. Therefore, aiming at completely separating the therapeutic properties from the psychoactive properties of THC may be erroneous, as some level of mind alteration may be required for the analgesic effect of cannabis to occur.

5. Conclusions

Our results indicate that controlled inhalation of pharmaceutical grade, THC-predominant cannabis flos was associated with a robust improvement in patient-reported pain scores, general mood, anxiety, sleep, and overall HRQoL in a treatment-resistant clinical population. The effect size, which was larger in patients diagnosed with anxiety disorders compared to chronic pain, appeared to be maximal at 3 months and sustained for at least 6 months. Occurrence of side effects was minimal, probably due to the previous experience of participants with cannabis inhalation. This evidence supports the notion that the administration of cannabis flos in a medicalized environment under the supervision of a trained healthcare provider further improves the clinical outcomes of legally prescribed CBMPs when compared to chronic patients self-medicating with illegal cannabis.

Author Contributions: Conceptualization, G.M.-S. and M.R.D.B.; methodology, G.M.-S. and M.L.; formal analysis, A.M.; investigation, M.L.; resources, M.L.; data curation, A.M. and M.L.; writing—original draft preparation, G.M.-S.; writing—review and editing, G.M.-S. and M.R.D.B.; visualization, G.M.-S.; supervision, G.M.-S.; project administration, G.M.-S. All authors have read and agreed to the published version of the manuscript.

Funding: This research received no external funding.

Institutional Review Board Statement: According to the National Health Service Health Research Authority, Project Twenty21 is classified as research, and the work was conducted in accordance with the Declaration of Helsinki. However, based on the Medical Research Council decision tools, Research Ethics Committee review and approval is not required.

Informed Consent Statement: All subjects involved provided signed informed consent for their data to be used for research purposes.

Data Availability Statement: The data presented in this work are available on request from the corresponding author. The data are not publicly available due to privacy and ethical reasons.

Acknowledgments: Sofia Antonopoulou created the graphical abstract and her assistance with the edition of the figures is gratefully acknowledged.

Conflicts of Interest: G.M.-S. and A.M. are employees of Khiron Life Sciences Corp, a global cannabis company that funded Project T21 and commercializes the CBPM employed in this research, Khiron 20/1. M.R.D.B. is employed by Zerenia Clinics, a subsidiary of Khiron Life Sciences. No other Khiron employee or executive was involved in the design of the work; in the collection, analyses, or interpretation of data; in the writing of the manuscript, or in the decision to publish the results. The authors declare no other conflict of interest.

References

1. O'Shaughnessy, W.B. New remedy for tetanus and other convulsive disorders. *Lancet* **1840**, *34*, 539–541. [CrossRef]
2. House of Lords—Science and Technology—Ninth Report. Available online: https://publications.parliament.uk/pa/ld199798/ldselect/ldsctech/151/15101.htm (accessed on 28 July 2022).
3. Rescheduling of Cannabis-Based Products for Medicinal Use in Humans (Accessible Version)—GOV.UK. Available online: https://www.gov.uk/government/publications/circular-0182018-rescheduling-of-cannabis-based-products-for-medicinal-use-in-humans/rescheduling-of-cannabis-based-products-for-medicinal-use-in-humans-accessible-version (accessed on 28 July 2022).
4. Köstenberger, M.; Nahler, G.; Jones, T.M.; Neuwersch, S.; Likar, R. The Role of Cannabis, Cannabidiol and Other Cannabinoids in Chronic Pain. The Perspective of Physicians. *J. Neuroimmune Pharmacol.* **2021**. [CrossRef] [PubMed]
5. Coomber, R.; Oliver, M.; Morris, C. Using Cannabis Therapeutically in the UK: A Qualitative Analysis. *J. Drug Issues* **2016**, *33*, 325–356. [CrossRef]

6. Abrams, D.I.; Vizoso, H.P.; Shade, S.B.; Jay, C.; Kelly, M.E.; Benowitz, N.L. Vaporization as a Smokeless Cannabis Delivery System: A Pilot Study. *Clin. Pharmacol. Ther.* **2007**, *82*, 572–578. [CrossRef] [PubMed]
7. Fraguas-Sánchez, A.I.; Torres-Suárez, A.I. Medical Use of Cannabinoids. *Drugs* **2018**, *78*, 1665–1703. [CrossRef]
8. Andreae, M.H.; Carter, G.M.; Shaparin, N.; Suslov, K.; Ellis, R.J.; Ware, M.A.; Abrams, D.I.; Prasad, H.; Wilsey, B.; Indyk, D.; et al. Inhaled Cannabis for Chronic Neuropathic Pain: A Meta-Analysis of Individual Patient Data. *J. Pain* **2015**, *16*, 1221–1232. [CrossRef] [PubMed]
9. Wilsey, B.; Marcotte, T.D.; Deutsch, R.; Zhao, H.; Prasad, H.; Phan, A. An Exploratory Human Laboratory Experiment Evaluating Vaporized Cannabis in the Treatment of Neuropathic Pain From Spinal Cord Injury and Disease. *J. Pain* **2016**, *17*, 982–1000. [CrossRef] [PubMed]
10. Wilsey, B.; Marcotte, T.; Deutsch, R.; Gouaux, B.; Sakai, S.; Donaghe, H. Low-Dose Vaporized Cannabis Significantly Improves Neuropathic Pain. *J. Pain* **2013**, *14*, 136–148. [CrossRef]
11. Ellis, R.J.; Toperoff, W.; Vaida, F.; Van Den Brande, G.; Gonzales, J.; Gouaux, B.; Bentley, H.; Atkinson, J.H. Smoked Medicinal Cannabis for Neuropathic Pain in HIV: A Randomized, Crossover Clinical Trial. *Neuropsychopharmacology* **2009**, *34*, 672–680. [CrossRef] [PubMed]
12. Ware, M.A.; Wang, T.; Shapiro, S.; Robinson, A.; Ducruet, T.; Huynh, T.; Gamsa, A.; Bennett, G.J.; Collet, J.P. Smoked Cannabis for Chronic Neuropathic Pain: A Randomized Controlled Trial. *CMAJ* **2010**, *182*, E694–E701. [CrossRef]
13. Ware, M.A.; Wang, T.; Shapiro, S.; Collet, J.P. Cannabis for the Management of Pain: Assessment of Safety Study (COMPASS). *J. Pain* **2015**, *16*, 1233–1242. [CrossRef]
14. Corey-Bloom, J.; Wolfson, T.; Gamst, A.; Jin, S.; Marcotte, T.D.; Bentley, H.; Gouaux, B. Smoked Cannabis for Spasticity in Multiple Sclerosis: A Randomized, Placebo-Controlled Trial. *CMAJ* **2012**, *184*, 1143–1150. [CrossRef]
15. Almog, S.; Aharon-Peretz, J.; Vulfsons, S.; Ogintz, M.; Abalia, H.; Lupo, T.; Hayon, Y.; Eisenberg, E. The Pharmacokinetics, Efficacy, and Safety of a Novel Selective-Dose Cannabis Inhaler in Patients with Chronic Pain: A Randomized, Double-Blinded, Placebo-Controlled Trial. *Eur. J. Pain* **2020**, *24*, 1505–1516. [CrossRef]
16. Carrubba, A.R.; Ebbert, J.O.; Spaulding, A.C.; DeStephano, D.; DeStephano, C.C. Use of Cannabis for Self-Management of Chronic Pelvic Pain. *J. Women's Health* **2020**, *30*, 1344–1351. [CrossRef]
17. Stith, S.S.; Diviant, J.P.; Brockelman, F.; Keeling, K.; Hall, B.; Lucern, S.; Vigil, J.M. Alleviative Effects of Cannabis Flower on Migraine and Headache. *J. Integr. Med.* **2020**, *18*, 416–424. [CrossRef]
18. Van De Donk, T.; Niesters, M.; Kowal, M.A.; Olofsen, E.; Dahan, A.; Van Velzen, M. An Experimental Randomized Study on the Analgesic Effects of Pharmaceutical-Grade Cannabis in Chronic Pain Patients with Fibromyalgia. *Pain* **2019**, *160*, 860–869. [CrossRef]
19. Cuttler, C.; Spradlin, A.; McLaughlin, R.J. A Naturalistic Examination of the Perceived Effects of Cannabis on Negative Affect. *J. Affect. Disord.* **2018**, *235*, 198–205. [CrossRef]
20. Stith, S.S.; Li, X.; Diviant, J.P.; Brockelman, F.C.; Keeling, K.S.; Hall, B.; Vigil, J.M. The Effectiveness of Inhaled Cannabis Flower for the Treatment of Agitation/Irritability, Anxiety, and Common Stress. *J. Cannabis Res.* **2020**, *2*, 47. [CrossRef]
21. Li, X.; Diviant, J.P.; Stith, S.S.; Brockelman, F.; Keeling, K.; Hall, B.; Vigil, J.M. The Effectiveness of Cannabis Flower for Immediate Relief from Symptoms of Depression. *Yale J. Biol. Med.* **2020**, *93*, 251–264.
22. Kawka, M.; Erridge, S.; Holvey, C.; Coomber, R.; Usmani, A.; Sajad, M.; Platt, M.W.; Rucker, J.J.; Sodergren, M.H. Clinical Outcome Data of First Cohort of Chronic Pain Patients Treated with Cannabis-Based Sublingual Oils in the United Kingdom: Analysis From the UK Medical Cannabis Registry. *J. Clin. Pharmacol.* **2021**, *61*, 1545–1554. [CrossRef]
23. Schlag, A.K.; Lynskey, M.; Fayaz, A.; Athanasiou-Fragkouli, A.; Brandner, B.; Haja, B.; Iveson, E.; Nutt, D.J. Characteristics of People Seeking Prescribed Cannabinoids for the Treatment of Chronic Pain: Evidence From Project Twenty 21. *Front. Pain Res.* **2022**, *3*, 85. [CrossRef]
24. Schlag, A.K.; O'Sullivan, S.E.; Zafar, R.R.; Nutt, D.J. Current Controversies in Medical Cannabis: Recent Developments in Human Clinical Applications and Potential Therapeutics. *Neuropharmacology* **2021**, *191*, 108586. [CrossRef]
25. Sakal, C.; Lynskey, M.; Schlag, A.K.; Nutt, D.J. Developing a Real-World Evidence Base for Prescribed Cannabis in the United Kingdom: Preliminary Findings from Project Twenty21. *Psychopharmacology* **2021**, *239*, 1147–1155. [CrossRef]
26. Piomelli, D.; Russo, E.B. The Cannabis Sativa Versus Cannabis Indica Debate: An Interview with Ethan Russo, MD. *Cannabis Cannabinoid Res.* **2016**, *1*, 44–46. [CrossRef]
27. Deutsches Arzneibuch 2018 (DAB). In *Allgemeiner Teil. Monographien Cannabisblüten-Cannabis Flos*; Deutscher Apotheker Verlag: Gerlingen, Germany, 2018.
28. Lanz, C.; Mattsson, J.; Soydaner, U.; Brenneisen, R. Medicinal Cannabis: In Vitro Validation of Vaporizers for the Smoke-Free Inhalation of Cannabis. *PLoS ONE* **2016**, *11*, e0147286. [CrossRef]
29. Carrara, L.; Giroud, C.; Concha-Lozano, N. Development of a Vaping Machine for the Sampling of THC and CBD Aerosols Generated by Two Portable Dry Herb Cannabis Vaporisers. *Med. Cannabis Cannabinoids* **2020**, *3*, 84–94. [CrossRef]
30. Pomahacova, B.; Van Der Kooy, F.; Verpoorte, R. Cannabis Smoke Condensate III: The Cannabinoid Content of Vaporised Cannabis Sativa. *Inhal. Toxicol.* **2009**, *21*, 1108–1112. [CrossRef]
31. Devlin, N.J.; Shah, K.K.; Feng, Y.; Mulhern, B.; van Hout, B. Valuing Health-Related Quality of Life: An EQ-5D-5L Value Set for England. *Health Econ.* **2018**, *27*, 7–22. [CrossRef]

32. Rancans, E.; Trapencieris, M.; Ivanovs, R.; Vrublevska, J. Validity of the PHQ-9 and PHQ-2 to Screen for Depression in Nationwide Primary Care Population in Latvia. *Ann. Gen. Psychiatry* **2018**, *17*, 33. [CrossRef]
33. Buysse, D.J.; Reynolds, C.F.; Monk, T.H.; Berman, S.R.; Kupfer, D.J. The Pittsburgh Sleep Quality Index: A New Instrument for Psychiatric Practice and Research. *Psychiatry Res.* **1989**, *28*, 193–213. [CrossRef]
34. Keller, S.; Bann, C.M.; Dodd, S.L.; Schein, J.; Mendoza, T.R.; Cleeland, C.S. Validity of the Brief Pain Inventory for Use in Documenting the Outcomes of Patients with Noncancer Pain. *Clin. J. Pain* **2004**, *20*, 309–318. [CrossRef] [PubMed]
35. Jordan, P.; Shedden-Mora, M.C.; Löwe, B. Psychometric Analysis of the Generalized Anxiety Disorder Scale (GAD-7) in Primary Care Using Modern Item Response Theory. *PLoS ONE* **2017**, *12*, e0182162. [CrossRef]
36. Smith, M.T.; Haythornthwaite, J.A. How Do Sleep Disturbance and Chronic Pain Inter-Relate? Insights from the Longitudinal and Cognitive-Behavioral Clinical Trials Literature. *Sleep Med. Rev.* **2004**, *8*, 119–132. [CrossRef]
37. Grotenhermen, F. Pharmacokinetics and Pharmacodynamics of Cannabinoids. *Clin. Pharmacokinet.* **2003**, *42*, 327–360. [CrossRef] [PubMed]
38. Lavie-Ajayi, M.; Shvartzman, P. Restored Self: A Phenomenological Study of Pain Relief by Cannabis. *Pain Med.* **2019**, *20*, 2086–2093. [CrossRef]
39. MacCallum, C.A.; Russo, E.B. Practical Considerations in Medical Cannabis Administration and Dosing. *Eur. J. Intern. Med.* **2018**, *49*, 12–19. [CrossRef]
40. Wang, Y.; Jacques, J.; Li, Z.; Sibille, K.; Cook, R. Health Outcomes among Adults Initiating Medical Cannabis for Chronic Pain: A 3-Month Prospective Study Incorporating Ecological Momentary Assessment (EMA). *Cannabis (Res. Soc. Marijuana)* **2021**, *4*, 69–83. [CrossRef]
41. Gruber, S.A.; Smith, R.T.; Dahlgren, M.K.; Lambros, A.M.; Sagar, K.A. No Pain, All Gain? Interim Analyses from a Longitudinal, Observational Study Examining the Impact of Medical Cannabis Treatment on Chronic Pain and Related Symptoms. *Exp. Clin. Psychopharmacol.* **2021**, *29*, 147–156. [CrossRef]
42. Moreno-Sanz, G.; Madiedo, A.; Hernandez, P.; Kratz, J.; Aizpurua-Olaizola, O.; Brown, M.R.D.; López, J.R.; Patiño, J.; Mendivelso, F.O. Sex-Dependent Prescription Patterns and Clinical Outcomes Associated with the Use of Two Oral Cannabis Formulations in the Multimodal Management of Chronic Pain Patients in Colombia. *Front. Pain Res.* **2022**, *3*, 854795. [CrossRef]
43. Wade, D.T.; Makela, P.; Robson, P.; House, H.; Bateman, C. Do Cannabis-Based Medicinal Extracts Have General or Specific Effects on Symptoms in Multiple Sclerosis? A Double-Blind, Randomized, Placebo-Controlled Study on 160 Patients. *Mult. Scler.* **2004**, *10*, 434–441. [CrossRef]
44. Powell, D.; Pacula, R.L.; Jacobson, M. Do Medical Marijuana Laws Reduce Addictions and Deaths Related to Pain Killers? *J. Health Econ.* **2018**, *58*, 29–42. [CrossRef] [PubMed]
45. Bachhuber, M.A.; Arnsten, J.H.; Cunningham, C.O.; Sohler, N. Does Medical Cannabis Use Increase or Decrease the Use of Opioid Analgesics and Other Prescription Drugs? *J. Addict. Med.* **2018**, *12*, 259–261. [CrossRef] [PubMed]
46. Lee, C.; Round, J.M.; Hanlon, J.G.; Hyshka, E.; Dyck, J.R.B.; Eurich, D.T. Generalized Anxiety Disorder 7-Item (GAD-7) Scores in Medically Authorized Cannabis Patients-Ontario and Alberta, Canada. *Can. J. Psychiatry.* **2022**, *67*, 470–480. [CrossRef] [PubMed]
47. Walter, C.; Oertel, B.G.; Felden, L.; Kell, C.A.; Nöth, U.; Vermehren, J.; Kaiser, J.; Deichmann, R.; Lötsch, J. Brain Mapping-Based Model of Δ 9-Tetrahydrocannabinol Effects on Connectivity in the Pain Matrix. *Neuropsychopharmacology* **2016**, *41*, 1659–1669. [CrossRef] [PubMed]
48. Weizman, L.; Dayan, L.; Brill, S.; Nahman-Averbuch, H.; Hendler, T.; Jacob, G.; Sharon, H. Cannabis Analgesia in Chronic Neuropathic Pain Is Associated with Altered Brain Connectivity. *Neurology* **2018**, *91*, E1285–E1294. [CrossRef]
49. De Vita, M.J.; Moskal, D.; Maisto, S.A.; Ansell, E.B. Association of Cannabinoid Administration with Experimental Pain in Healthy Adults: A Systematic Review and Meta-Analysis. *JAMA Psychiatry* **2018**, *75*, 1118–1127. [CrossRef] [PubMed]
50. Raymundi, A.M.; Da Silva, T.R.; Sohn, J.M.B.; Bertoglio, L.J.; Stern, C.A. Effects of Δ 9-Tetrahydrocannabinol on Aversive Memories and Anxiety: A Review from Human Studies. *BMC Psychiatry* **2020**, *20*, 420. [CrossRef] [PubMed]
51. Robinson, O.J.; Krimsky, M.; Lieberman, L.; Allen, P.; Vytal, K.; Grillon, C. The Dorsal Medial Prefrontal (Anterior Cingulate) Cortex—Amygdala Aversive Amplification Circuit in Unmedicated Generalised and Social Anxiety Disorders: An Observational Study. *Lancet Psychiatry* **2014**, *1*, 294–302. [CrossRef]
52. Marsicano, G.; Wotjak, C.T.; Azad, S.C.; Bisogno, T.; Rammes, G.; Cascioll, M.G.; Hermann, H.; Tang, J.; Hofmann, C.; Zieglgänsberger, W.; et al. The Endogenous Cannabinoid System Controls Extinction of Aversive Memories. *Nature* **2002**, *418*, 530–534. [CrossRef] [PubMed]
53. Phan, K.L.; Angstadt, M.; Golden, J.; Onyewuenyi, I.; Popovska, A.; De Wit, H. Cannabinoid Modulation of Amygdala Reactivity to Social Signals of Threat in Humans. *J. Neurosci.* **2008**, *28*, 2313–2319. [CrossRef]
54. Jugl, S.; Sajdeya, R.; Morris, E.J.; Goodin, A.J.; Brown, J.D. Much Ado about Dosing: The Needs and Challenges of Defining a Standardized Cannabis Unit. *Med. Cannabis Cannabinoids* **2021**, *4*, 121–124. [CrossRef] [PubMed]
55. Itin, C.; Domb, A.J.; Hoffman, A. A Meta-Opinion: Cannabinoids Delivered to Oral Mucosa by a Spray for Systemic Absorption Are Rather Ingested into Gastro-Intestinal Tract: The Influences of Fed / Fasting States. *Expert Opin. Drug Deliv.* **2019**, *16*, 1031–1035. [CrossRef]
56. Monte, A.A.; Shelton, S.K.; Mills, E.; Saben, J.; Hopkinson, A.; Sonn, B.; Devivo, M.; Chang, T.; Fox, J.; Brevik, C.; et al. Acute Illness Associated with Cannabis Use, by Route of Exposure: An Observational Study. *Ann. Intern. Med.* **2019**, *170*, 531–537. [CrossRef] [PubMed]

57. Blonde, L.; Khunti, K.; Harris, S.B.; Meizinger, C.; Skolnik, N.S. Interpretation and Impact of Real-World Clinical Data for the Practicing Clinician. *Adv. Ther.* **2018**, *35*, 1763–1774. [CrossRef] [PubMed]
58. Brown, J.D.; Goodin, A.J. Evidence in Context: High Risk of Bias in Medical Cannabis and Cannabinoid Clinical Trials Dictates the Need for Cautious Interpretation. *Med. Cannabis Cannabinoids* **2021**, *4*, 63–66. [CrossRef] [PubMed]

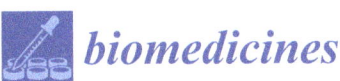

Article

Combinations of Cannabidiol and Δ⁹-Tetrahydrocannabinol in Reducing Chemotherapeutic Induced Neuropathic Pain

Diana E. Sepulveda [1,2], Kent E. Vrana [1], Nicholas M. Graziane [1,2,*] and Wesley M. Raup-Konsavage [1,*]

1. Department of Pharmacology, Penn State College of Medicine, Hershey, PA 17033, USA
2. Department of Anesthesiology & Perioperative Medicine, Penn State College of Medicine, Hershey, PA 17033, USA
* Correspondence: ngraziane@pennstatehealth.psu.edu (N.M.G.); wkonsavage@pennstatehealth.psu.edu (W.M.R.-K.); Tel.: +717-531-8433 (N.M.G.); +717-531-4172 (W.M.R.-K.)

Abstract: Neuropathic pain is a condition that impacts a substantial portion of the population and is expected to affect a larger percentage in the future. This type of pain is poorly managed by current therapies, including opioids and NSAIDS, and novel approaches are needed. We used a cisplatin-induced model of neuropathic pain in mice to assess the effects of the cannabinoids THC and CBD alone or in varying ratios as anti-nociceptive agents. In addition to testing pure compounds, we also tested extracts containing high THC or CBD at the same ratios. We found that pure CBD had little impact on mechanical hypersensitivity, whereas THC reduced mechanical hypersensitivity in both male and female mice (as has been reported in the literature). Interestingly, we found that high CBD cannabis extract, at the same CBD dose as pure CBD, was able to reduce mechanical hypersensitivity, although not to the same level as high THC extract. These data suggest that, at least for CBD-dominant cannabis extracts, there is an increase in the anti-nociceptive activity that may be attributed to other constitutes of the plant. We also found that high THC extract or pure THC is the most efficacious treatment for reducing neuropathic pain in this model.

Keywords: neuropathic pain; tetrahydrocannabinol; cannabidiol; cannabinoids; cannabis

Citation: Sepulveda, D.E.; Vrana, K.E.; Graziane, N.M.; Raup-Konsavage, W.M. Combinations of Cannabidiol and Δ⁹-Tetrahydrocannabinol in Reducing Chemotherapeutic Induced Neuropathic Pain. *Biomedicines* **2022**, *10*, 2548. https://doi.org/10.3390/biomedicines10102548

Academic Editor: Giuseppe Tringali

Received: 1 September 2022
Accepted: 10 October 2022
Published: 12 October 2022

Publisher's Note: MDPI stays neutral with regard to jurisdictional claims in published maps and institutional affiliations.

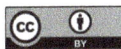

Copyright: © 2022 by the authors. Licensee MDPI, Basel, Switzerland. This article is an open access article distributed under the terms and conditions of the Creative Commons Attribution (CC BY) license (https://creativecommons.org/licenses/by/4.0/).

1. Introduction

Neuropathic pain is a condition that is caused by damage to the nervous system as a result of physical trauma, chemotherapy, infection, metabolic disease, or autoimmune disorders [1,2]. This chronic pain condition affects 7–10% of the population and, unfortunately, current drug treatments have poor efficacy and tolerability [3,4]. Patients are typically unresponsive to analgesics and opioids. In addition to pain, patients also suffer from sleep disturbances, anxiety and depression, and reduced quality of life [5]. The incidence of neuropathic pain is expected to increase in the coming years due in part to the diabetes epidemic, improved cancer survival rates, and age [6]. Therefore, new approaches to treat pain in these patients are clearly needed.

Cannabis has been used for centuries to treat pain, and the plant contains a number of pharmacologically active compounds including cannabinoids and terpenes that might have anti-nociceptive properties [7,8]. The two most abundant and studied cannabinoids in the plant are Δ⁹-tetrahydrocannabinol (THC) and cannabidiol (CBD), and the ratio of these two compounds can vary greatly between cultivars and subtypes of *Cannabis*. Both THC and CBD have been shown to reduce neuropathic pain in animal models [9–13]. However, patients rarely take pure THC or CBD for pain. Additionally, THC and CBD are normally administered together at varying ratios depending on the product consumed. Furthermore, the anti-nociceptive effects of these varying ratios of THC and CBD remain underexplored. Instead, studies have largely focused on THC:CBD co-administered at 1:1 ratios, commonly found in the European-approved Sativex (nabiximols) that has been shown to be effective at treating pain in patients with certain conditions [14–17]. We therefore set out to assess how different combinations of THC and CBD, as both pure compounds and from unfractionated plant extracts, affect mechanical hypersensitivity in a mouse model of chemotherapeutic-induced peripheral neuropathy (CIPN).

2. Materials and Methods

2.1. Animals

All experiments were conducted in a manner approved by the Pennsylvania State University, College of Medicine Institutional Animal Care and Use Committee (IACUC). Male (n = 120) and female (n = 120) age-matched (10–12 weeks) wild-type C57BL/6 mice (The Jackson Laboratory, Bar Harbor, ME) were used in this study. All mice were group-housed with a 12 h light/dark cycle with access to food and water ad libitum.

2.2. Drugs

Cannabidiol (CBD) and Δ^9-tetrahydrocannabinol (THC) were purchased from Cayman Chemical (Ann Arbor, MI, USA). CBD extract was produced through supercritical CO_2 extraction from hemp (Helping Hands Hemp, Womelsdorf, PA, cultivar: YoungSim 10) and THC extract was provided by the NIDA drug program (Research Triangle Institute, Research Triangle Park, NC, USA) the composition of both was verified by an independent laboratory (Keystone State Testing, Harrisburg, PA, USA) Cisplatin was purchased from Acros Organics (Fairlawn, NJ, USA).

2.3. Supercritical CO_2 Extraction

Dried hemp flower, 500 g, was ground and then extracted using supercritical CO_2 in an extractor from Supercritical Fluid Technologies (CannabisSFE, Newark, DE, USA). Extraction was performed at 55 °C, with 413 bars of pressure for 30 min. Extract was collected and dissolved in ethanol to a concentration of 10% extract in 90% ethanol by weight and incubated at −20 °C for 24 h (winterization). The solution was then filtered and ethanol was evaporated. The extract was then resuspended in fractionated coconut oil (Pure Body Naturals, West Chester, OH, USA) at 200 mg/mL and heated to 95 °C for 1 h to decarboxylate the cannabinoids.

2.4. Cisplatin-Induced Neuropathy

Peripheral neuropathy was induced by injecting mice with 5 mg/kg of cisplatin intraperitoneally (IP) once weekly for four weeks, as previously described [13,18]. The mice were co-administered 1 mL of 4% sodium bicarbonate solution subcutaneously prior to the cisplatin injection to reduce nephrotoxicity and to minimize compromised renal functions [13,18]. Mechanical allodynia was assessed using an electronic von Frey anesthesiometer equipped with a semi-flexible polypropylene super-tip (IITC Life Science Inc., Woodland Hills, CA, USA), these assessments were made before and after cisplatin treatment to confirm neuropathic pain state, as described below (Data from the pre and post cisplatin assessments are presented in Supplemental Figures S1–S3).

2.5. Von Frey Testing

Hypersensitivity to mechanical pressure was assessed using an electronic von Frey anesthesiometer (IITC Life Sciences Inc.). For testing, mice were placed in small acrylic chambers on a wire mesh table (IITC Life Sciences Inc.). Animals were allowed to acclimate to the chamber for 20 min prior to testing. The von Frey anesthesiometer was equipped with a semi-flex tip (IITC Life Sciences Inc.), that was applied to the plantar surface of the right hind-paw with increasing force to prompt a withdrawal response. The averages from three tests were calculated with each test being separated by a minimum of 3 min. To measure the effects of test compounds, neuropathic mice were randomly assigned to one of 6 groups and injected intraperitoneally (i.p.) with vehicle (DMSO, Tween 80, saline (1:1:18), i.p.), THC at 6 mg/kg, THC and CBD in combination at 4 mg/kg and 2 mg/kg; 3 mg/kg and 3 mg/kg; 2 mg/kg and 4 mg/kg, respectively, or CBD at 6 mg/kg 1 h prior to tests.

These groups represent THC:CBD ratios of 1:0, 2:1, 1:1, 1:2, or 0:1, as shown in Table 1. All von Frey measurements were performed by experimenters blinded to treatments.

Table 1. Dose of cannabinoid administered at each ratio for pure compounds.

Ratio	THC (mg/kg)	CBD (mg/kg)
0:1	0	6
1:2	2	4
1:1	3	3
2:1	4	2
1:0	6	0

2.6. Statistical Analysis

All results are shown as mean ± standard deviation. Statistical significance was determined using GraphPad Prism Software (9.3.1, San Diego, CA, USA) using a one-way ANOVA with Tukey's correction for multiple comparisons. Two-tailed tests were used for all comparisons.

3. Results

3.1. THC, but Not CBD, Reverses Mechanical Hypersensitivity in Neuropathic Male Mice

To assess the ability of pure CBD or THC to reduce cisplatin-induced neuropathic pain, von Frey tests were conducted to measure mechanical sensitivity in neuropathic male mice treated with varying doses (5, 10, or 20 mg/kg) of pure CBD or THC. Acute CBD treatment, administered 1 h prior to von Frey testing, had no significant impact on mechanical hypersensitivity in neuropathic male mice (Figure 1A). In contrast, there was a dose dependent effect of THC on pain in these animals; with only the lowest dose (5 mg/kg) being unable to reduce pain compared to vehicle treated animals (Figure 1B). Based on these findings, in order to investigate the potential interaction between these two compounds, we used a standard dose of 6 mg/kg of total cannabinoid (THC alone, CBD alone, or a combination of various THC:CBD ratios) for all subsequent experiments, with the knowledge that, at this dose, the THC (THC:CBD ratio of 1:0) would serve as a positive control, based upon previous work [13]. The dose of 6 mg/kg was selected for two reasons, first we wanted to be able to have a dose that limited the cataleptic effects of THC on mice and, second, we wanted a dose of THC that would be responsive to any additive effects of CBD on reducing hyperalgesia.

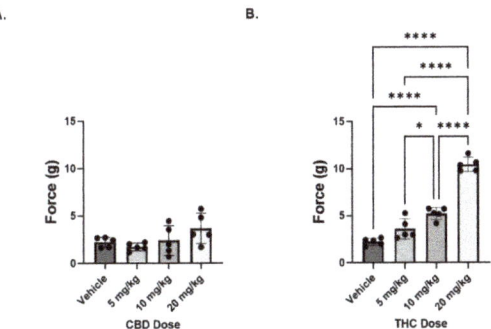

Figure 1. Dose response of cannabinoids on mechanical sensitivity in neuropathic male mice. (**A**) Mice were treated with CBD administered i.p. at 5, 10, or 20 mg/kg 1 h prior to measuring mechanical sensitivity. (**B**) Same as panel A except THC was administered. n = 5 mice per group. * $p < 0.05$, **** $p < 0.001$.

3.2. CBD Does Influence THC-Induced Decreases in Mechanical Hypersensitivity

We next investigated the anti-nociceptive effects of five THC and CBD combinations while maintaining the total cannabinoid administered at 6 mg/kg as shown in Table 1. In neuropathic male mice, we observed a statistically significant decrease in mechanical hypersensitivity after administration of THC:CBD only at the 2:1 ratio (Figure 2A). In contrast, in neuropathic female animals we observed a statistically significant decrease in mechanical hypersensitivity after administration of THC:CBD at ratios of 1:2 and 2:1 (Figure 2B). While the addition of CBD reduces the concentration of THC necessary to reduce hyperalgesia (note that 5 mg/kg pure THC was without effect in Figure 1), no combination of CBD and THC is greater at reducing sensitivity than THC alone.

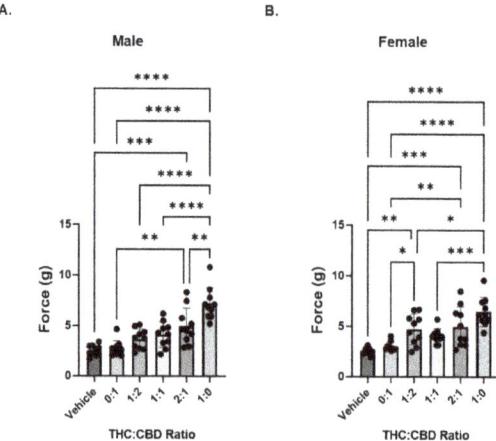

Figure 2. THC reduces mechanical sensitivity in neuropathic mice. (**A**) Neuropathic male mice were treated with 6 mg/kg of total cannabinoid at varying ratios of THC:CBD and mechanical sensitivity was measured by von Frey filament. (**B**) Same as panel A except in female neuropathic mice. n = 10 mice per group. * $p < 0.05$, ** $p < 0.01$, *** $p < 0.005$, **** $p < 0.001$.

3.3. CBD and THC Extracts Are Effective at Attenuating Mechanical Hypersensitivity in Neuropathic Mice

We next compared the anti-nociceptive effects of THC and CBD ratios using CBD-dominant or THC-dominant botanical extracts. Extracts were mixed at varying ratios of THC: CBD. The composition of the extracts (as delivered to the mice) for cannabinoid and most abundant terpene content (Tables S1 and S2), are shown in Tables 2 and 3, respectively.

For full composition of the undiluted extracts please see Supplemental Tables S1 and S2. Using a CBD-dominant botanical extract (containing 40 μg/mL THC; labeled "0:1"), we found a statistical difference between vehicle and treated animals for both sexes (Figure 3A,B).

In neuropathic male mice, we saw a further reduction in mechanical hypersensitivity when THC was added (1:2, 1:1, and 2:1 ratios compared to 0:1, CBD extract), but no change in hypersensitivity as THC concentration increased (Figure 3A). In contrast, in neuropathic female mice, we did not see any further reduction in mechanical hypersensitivity when THC was included in the treatment. That is, the reduction in hypersensitivity was consistent across the tested ratios with what was observed for the CBD extract (0:1 ratio). However, the THC extract alone (1:0 ratio) was significantly better than the CBD extract (Figure 3B). Because the CBD extract contains trace amounts of THC and vice versa; it was not possible to have any extract ratio where the other cannabinoid was exactly zero. Table 4 shows the concentration of THC and CBD delivered at each of the ratios.

Table 2. Cannabinoid composition of extracts as administered to mice; concentrations are in mg/mL. Cells with no values represent assay results below the level of detection.

Cannabinoid	CBD Extract	THC Extract
CBC		0.03
CBD	1.8	0.005
CBDA		0.003
CBDV	0.03	
CBG		0.067
CBGA		0.002
CBN		0.048
THCA		0.002
Δ^9-THC	0.04	1.8
Total Cannabinoid	**1.87**	**1.957**

Table 3. Terpene composition of extracts as administered to mice; concentrations are in ppm. Cells with no values represent assay results below the level of detection.

Terpene	CBD Extract	THC Extract
β-Farnesene		3.13
β-Caryophyllene	191.72	20.97
α-Humulene	55.67	4.11
(−) α-Bisabolol	3.61	2.06
β-Myrcene	0.16	2.51
R(+) Limonene	0.17	1.33
Endo-Fenchyl Alcohol	4.33	1.14
Guaiol		1.4
α-Pinene	0.01	3.58
Linalool	2.87	1.54
(−) Caryophyllene Oxide	37.91	
Trans-Nerolidol	3.91	0.61
Valencene		8.2
β-Pinene		1.74
Total Terpene	**301.63**	**55.27**
Total Terpene (mg/mL)	**0.30**	**0.06**

Table 4. Dose of cannabinoid administered at each ratio for THC and CBD extracts.

Ratio	THC (mg/kg)	CBD (mg/kg)
0:1	0.13	6
1:2	2.09	4.01
1:1	3.07	3.01
2:1	4.04	2.01
1:0	6	0.02

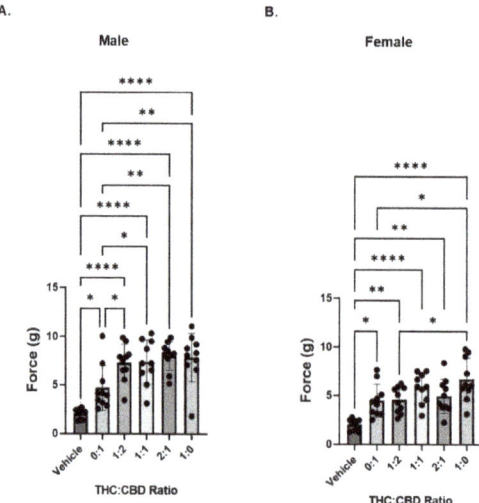

Figure 3. Cannabinoid extracts containing either CBD or THC reduce mechanical sensitivity in neuropathic mice. (**A**) Neuropathic male mice were treated with 6 mg/kg of total cannabinoid at varying ratios of THC:CBD and mechanical sensitivity was measured by von Frey filament. (**B**) Same as panel A except in female neuropathic mice. n = 10 mice per group. * $p < 0.05$, ** $p < 0.01$, **** $p < 0.001$.

4. Discussion

In this study, we examined the effects of CBD and THC on pain associated with chemotherapeutic-induced peripheral neuropathy (CIPN), both as pure compounds and botanical extracts at varying ratios of THC:CBD. These data are important because patients taking medical cannabis or cannabis-based products do not typically take pure CBD or pure THC, but rather are using botanical or botanically derived products. These products typically have varying ratios of THC:CBD but there are few studies that have investigated the optimal ratios of the two primary cannabinoids for treating medical conditions. Most studies that have investigated the interactions between these two cannabinoids have limited their scope to the 1:1 ratio typically found in nabixmols (Sativex®) [14–17]. While our data suggest that a 1:1 ratio of CBD to THC may not be optimal, there is a benefit of including CBD in combination with THC to reduce neuropathic pain, as lower levels of THC produced a reduction in sensitivity when CBD was included, this is especially true for the botanical extracts.

Here, we found that pure CBD alone had little impact on acute pain associated with CIPN. This is in contrast to several other studies that have found that CBD can reduce neuropathic pain in animal models [10,12,19]. An important difference between our study and the previous work is that we are looking at the acute effects of CBD administration as compared to those studies that looked at more prolonged effects of CBD treatment. Interestingly, we did observe that botanically derived CBD mixtures were able to reduce pain in neuropathic animals at a dose where CBD alone was ineffective. While there was a small amount of THC in this extract, the dose administered (0.13 mg/kg) would be too low to account for the observed reduction in pain. A number of the terpenes present in the CBD extract, such as β-caryophyllene and α-humulene, have been found to have antinociceptive properties in their own rights [20,21]. Further studies will need to be conducted to determine which other constituents of the CBD extract contribute to the improved pain tolerance observed in neuropathic mice or if CBD contributes at all.

In contrast, we found that THC, when administered at a dose as low at 2 mg/kg, was able to reduce neuropathic pain when combined with CBD, and the level to which pain was reduced was fairly consistent regardless of the ratio of THC:CBD tested (particularly for botanical extracts). Although, in male mice there is a significantly greater reduction in mechanical sensitivity by pure THC when CBD was excluded. These data are consistent with a recent meta-analysis that found that high THC:CBD ratios were better at reducing pain severity across a wide range of conditions, including diabetic neuropathy, in patients [22]. These data are also consistent with reports that CBD is an antagonist at cannabinoid receptors 1 and 2, and can blunt the effects of THC [23–25]. Based upon the large number of studies that have reported that nabiximols (mixtures of approximately 1:1 THC:CBD) have antinociceptive properties, it was unexpected that we did not see a larger difference in anti-nociceptive potential with different ratios [14–17]. Our data suggest that there is little effect of CBD on reducing neuropathic pain, and that most of the reduction in pain can be attributed to THC, although CBD may help to augment the impact of THC. This is true for not only the pure compounds, but also the botanically derived compounds, particularly in male mice (although the highest concentration of THC also was more effective than the highest concentration of CBD in female mice).

The data comparing the botanical extracts to pure compounds also allows us to examine the controversial "entourage" effect, the idea that the whole plant provides an additive benefit over individual pure compounds [26]. While we are not able to directly compare the responses between the animals that received pure compounds and botanical extracts, the animals that received botanical extracts did show a trend towards increased levels of force compared to those receiving pure compounds. Furthermore, animals, particularly males, receiving the botanical extracts exhibited a greater response at much lower levels of THC when in a botanical extract compared to pure THC.

Another potential reason for looking at combinations of THC:CBD is that the addition of CBD may alter the metabolism or prolong the effectiveness of THC at reducing pain. While our current studies did not directly address this, a recent study in a rat model of neuropathic pain actually found that CBD, when co-administered with THC, reduced the therapeutic window in which THC had an effect [11]. This is in contrast to recent data in humans that has reported that co-administration of THC and CBD can prolong the effects of THC [27]. For this reason, studies in mice or rats may not be optimal for examining the interaction of THC and CBD on the metabolism of cannabinoids, but instead such pharmacokinetic studies might best be conducted in human derived microsomes and ultimately patients.

The mechanism by which THC and CBD reduce neuropathic pain in our model was not examined, but will be the work of future studies. One potential mechanism would be that THC is acting through CB1 receptor to reduce the release of neurotransmitters and neuronal excitability [28]. Both CBD and THC are also known agonists of the TRPV1 receptor and have been shown to reduce pain in murine models through this receptor [29]. CBD and THC have also recently been shown to reduce neuropathic pain through both CB1 and CB2 [30]. Our own recent work on cannabigerol (CBG) and neuropathic pain suggests that it is likely to be a complicated interaction between multiple receptors [31], including α2-adrenergic receptors, of which CBG is a known agonist; however, the role of CBD and THC at this receptor are unknown.

Supplementary Materials: The following supporting information can be downloaded at: https://www.mdpi.com/article/10.3390/biomedicines10102548/s1, The full composition for each extract tested can be found in supplemental Tables S1: Full Cannabinoid Content of Extracts and Table S2: Full Terpene Content of Extracts. Supplemental Figure S1: Pre and Post Cisplatin von Frey assessment for the Dose Response Experiment. Supplemental Figure S2: Pre and Post Cisplatin von Frey Assessment for the Pure Compound Experiment and Supplemental Figure S3: Pre and Post Cisplatin Responses for Extract Experiment.

Author Contributions: Conceptualization, K.E.V., N.M.G. and W.M.R.-K.; Formal analysis, D.E.S., N.M.G. and W.M.R.-K.; Investigation, D.E.S.; Resources, K.E.V.; Data curation, W.M.R.-K.; Writing—original draft preparation, D.E.S. and W.M.R.-K.; Writing—review and editing, K.E.V., N.M.G. and W.M.R.-K.; Visualization, W.M.R.-K.; Project administration, W.M.R.-K.; Funding acquisition, K.E.V. and N.M.G. All authors have read and agreed to the published version of the manuscript.

Funding: This project was supported by a NARSAD Young Investigator Award (27364; NMG) and by the Pennsylvania Department of Health using Tobacco CURE Funds (NMG). KEV (and the Penn State College of Medicine) is the recipient of research support from PA Options for Wellness (a state-approved medical marijuana clinical registrant). The funding sources were not involved in: study design, providing any experimental materials, data collection, analysis and interpretation; writing of the report; or the decision to submit the article for publication.

Institutional Review Board Statement: The animal study protocol was approved by the Institutional Review Board of Penn State College of Medicine (protocol #01327, approved on 5/5/2020).

Informed Consent Statement: Not applicable.

Data Availability Statement: Not applicable.

Acknowledgments: The authors would like to acknowledge members of the state-approved medical marijuana academic clinical research center at Penn State for insights and comments on the data and study design, along with the Drug Discovery, Development, and Delivery (D4) core for assistance with the preparation of the compounds.

Conflicts of Interest: The authors declare no conflict of interest.

References

1. Lee, G.; Grovey, B.; Furnish, T.; Wallace, M. Medical cannabis for neuropathic pain. *Curr. Pain Headache Rep.* **2018**, *22*, 8. [CrossRef]
2. Mitchell, V.A.; Harley, J.; Casey, S.L.; Vaughan, A.C.; Winters, B.L.; Vaughan, C.W. Oral efficacy of Δ(9)-tetrahydrocannabinol and cannabidiol in a mouse neuropathic pain model. *Neuropharmacology* **2021**, *189*, 108529. [CrossRef]
3. Jensen, T.S.; Baron, R.; Haanpää, M.; Kalso, E.; Loeser, J.D.; Rice, A.S.; Treede, R.D. A new definition of neuropathic pain. *Pain* **2011**, *152*, 2204–2205. [CrossRef]
4. Finnerup, N.B.; Attal, N.; Haroutounian, S.; McNicol, E.; Baron, R.; Dworkin, R.H.; Gilron, I.; Haanpää, M.; Hansson, P.; Jensen, T.S.; et al. Pharmacotherapy for neuropathic pain in adults: A systematic review and meta-analysis. *Lancet Neurol.* **2015**, *14*, 162–173. [CrossRef]
5. Nicholson, B.; Verma, S. Comorbidities in chronic neuropathic pain. *Pain Med.* **2004**, *5* (Suppl. S1), S9–S27. [CrossRef]
6. van Hecke, O.A.S.K.R.; Austin, S.K.; Khan, R.A.; Smith, B.H.; Torrance, N. Neuropathic pain in the general population: A systematic review of epidemiological studies. *Pain* **2014**, *155*, 654–662. [CrossRef]
7. Russo, E.B. Cannabinoids in the management of difficult to treat pain. *Ther. Clin. Risk Manag.* **2008**, *ume 4*, 245–259. [CrossRef]
8. Legare, C.A.; Raup-Konsavage, W.M.; Vrana, K.E. Therapeutic potential of cannabis, cannabidiol, and cannabinoid-based pharmaceuticals. *Pharmacology* **2022**, *107*, 131–149. [CrossRef] [PubMed]
9. Ward, S.J.; Ramirez, M.D.; Neelakantan, H.; Walker, E.A. Cannabidiol prevents the development of cold and mechanical allodynia in paclitaxel-treated female C57Bl6 mice. *Anesthesia Analg.* **2011**, *113*, 947–950. [CrossRef]
10. Ward, S.J.; McAllister, S.D.; Kawamura, R.; Murase, R.; Neelakantan, H.; Walker, E.A. Cannabidiol inhibits paclitaxel-induced neuropathic pain through 5-HT(1A) receptors without diminishing nervous system function or chemotherapy efficacy. *Br. J. Pharmacol.* **2014**, *171*, 636–645. [CrossRef] [PubMed]
11. Casey, S.L.; Atwal, N.; Vaughan, C.W. Cannabis constituent synergy in a mouse neuropathic pain model. *Pain* **2017**, *158*, 2452–2460. [CrossRef]
12. King, K.M.; Myers, A.M.; Soroka-Monzo, A.J.; Tuma, R.F.; Tallarida, R.J.; Walker, E.A.; Ward, S.J. Single and combined effects of Δ^9-tetrahydrocannabinol and cannabidiol in a mouse model of chemotherapy-induced neuropathic pain. *J. Cereb. Blood Flow Metab.* **2017**, *174*, 2832–2841. [CrossRef]
13. Henderson-Redmond, A.N.; Crawford, L.C.; Sepulveda, D.E.; Hale, D.E.; Lesperance, J.J.; Morgan, D.J. Sex differences in tolerance to delta-9-tetrahydrocannabinol in mice with cisplatin-evoked chronic neuropathic pain. *Front. Mol. Biosci.* **2021**, *8*, 684115. [CrossRef]
14. Überall, M.A. A review of scientific evidence for THC:CBD oromucosal spray (nabiximols) in the management of chronic pain. *J. Pain Res.* **2020**, *13*, 399–410. [CrossRef]
15. Dykukha, I.; Malessa, R.; Essner, U.; Überall, M.A. Nabiximols in chronic neuropathic pain: A meta-analysis of randomized placebo-controlled trials. *Pain Med.* **2021**, *22*, 861–874. [CrossRef]

16. Sainsbury, B.; Bloxham, J.; Pour, M.H.; Padilla, M.; Enciso, R. Efficacy of cannabis-based medications compared to placebo for the treatment of chronic neuropathic pain: A systematic review with meta-analysis. *J. Dent. Anesthesia Pain Med.* **2021**, *21*, 479–506. [CrossRef]
17. Ueberall, M.A.; Silván, C.V.; Essner, U.; Mueller-Schwefe, G.H.H. Effectiveness, Safety, and Tolerability of Nabiximols Oromucosal Spray vs Typical Oral Long-Acting Opioid Analgesics in Patients with Severe Neuropathic Back Pain: Analysis of 6-Month Real-World Data from the German Pain e-Registry. *Pain Med.* **2022**, *23*, 745–760. [CrossRef]
18. Guindon, J.; Deng, L.; Fan, B.; Wager-Miller, J.; Hohmann, A.G. Optimization of a cisplatin model of chemotherapy-induced peripheral neuropathy in mice: Use of vitamin C and sodium bicarbonate pretreatments to reduce nephrotoxicity and improve animal health status. *Mol. Pain* **2014**, *10*, 56. [CrossRef]
19. Foss, J.D.; Farkas, D.J.; Huynh, L.M.; Kinney, W.A.; Brenneman, D.E.; Ward, S.J. Behavioural and pharmacological effects of cannabidiol (CBD) and the cannabidiol analogue KLS-13019 in mouse models of pain and reinforcement. *J. Cereb. Blood Flow Metab.* **2021**, *178*, 3067–3078. [CrossRef]
20. Somani, S.J.; Modi, K.P.; Majumdar, A.S.; Sadarani, B.N. Phytochemicals and their potential usefulness in inflammatory bowel disease. *Phytother. Res.* **2015**, *29*, 339–350. [CrossRef]
21. Nuutinen, T. Medicinal properties of terpenes found in Cannabis sativa and Humulus lupulus. *Eur. J. Med. Chem.* **2018**, *157*, 198–228. [CrossRef]
22. McDonagh, M.S.; Morasco, B.J.; Wagner, J.; Ahmed, A.Y.; Fu, R.; Kansagara, D.; Chou, R. Cannabis-based products for chronic pain: A systematic review. *Ann. Intern. Med.* **2022**, *175*, 1143–1153. [CrossRef]
23. Russo, E.; Guy, G.W. A tale of two cannabinoids: The therapeutic rationale for combining tetrahydrocannabinol and cannabidiol. *Med. Hypotheses* **2006**, *66*, 234–246. [CrossRef]
24. Russo, E.B. Taming THC: Potential cannabis synergy and phytocannabinoid-terpenoid entourage effects. *Br. J. Pharmacol.* **2011**, *163*, 1344–1364. [CrossRef]
25. Freeman, A.M.; Petrilli, K.; Lees, R.; Hindocha, C.; Mokrysz, C.; Curran, H.V.; Saunders, R.; Freeman, T.P. How does cannabidiol (CBD) influence the acute effects of delta-9-tetrahydrocannabinol (THC) in humans? A systematic review. *Neurosci. Biobehav. Rev.* **2019**, *107*, 696–712. [CrossRef]
26. Russo, E.B. The case for the entourage effect and conventional breeding of clinical cannabis: No "strain," no gain. *Front. Plant Sci.* **2018**, *9*, 1969. [CrossRef] [PubMed]
27. Arkell, T.R.; Lintzeris, N.; Kevin, R.C.; Ramaekers, J.G.; Vandrey, R.; Irwin, C.; Haber, P.S.; McGregor, I.S. Cannabidiol (CBD) content in vaporized cannabis does not prevent tetrahydrocannabinol (THC)-induced impairment of driving and cognition. *Psychopharmacology* **2019**, *236*, 2713–2724. [CrossRef] [PubMed]
28. Vučković, S.; Srebro, D.; Vujović, K.S.; Vučetić, Č.; Prostran, M. Cannabinoids and pain: New insights from old molecules. *Front. Pharmacol.* **2018**, *9*, 1259. [CrossRef]
29. Louis-Gray, K.; Tupal, S.; Premkumar, L.S. TRPV1: A common denominator mediating antinociceptive and antiemetic effects of cannabinoids. *Int. J. Mol. Sci.* **2022**, *23*, 10016. [CrossRef]
30. Casey, S.L.; Mitchell, V.A.; Sokolaj, E.E.; Winters, B.L.; Vaughan, C.W. Intrathecal actions of the cannabis constituents Δ(9)-tetrahydrocannabinol and cannabidiol in a mouse neuropathic pain model. *Int. J. Mol. Sci.* **2022**, *23*, 8649. [CrossRef] [PubMed]
31. Sepulveda, D.E.; Morris, D.P.; Raup-Konsavage, W.M.; Sun, D.; Vrana, K.E.; Graziane, N.M. Cannabigerol (CBG) attenuates mechanical hypersensitivity elicited by chemotherapy-induced peripheral neuropathy. *Eur. J. Pain* **2022**, *26*, 1950–1966. [CrossRef] [PubMed]

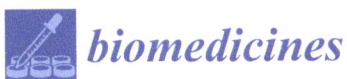

Article

Single and Repeated Exposure to Cannabidiol Differently Modulate BDNF Expression and Signaling in the Cortico-Striatal Brain Network

Francesca Mottarlini [1], Marco Fumagalli [1], Fernando Castillo-Díaz [1], Stefano Piazza [1], Giorgia Targa [1], Enrico Sangiovanni [1], Barbara Pacchetti [2], Mikael H. Sodergren [2,3], Mario Dell'Agli [1], Fabio Fumagalli [1,*] and Lucia Caffino [1]

[1] Department of Pharmacological and Biomolecular Sciences, Università degli Studi di Milano, Via Balzaretti 9, 20133 Milano, Italy; francesca.mottarlini@unimi.it (F.M.); marco.fumagalli3@unimi.it (M.F.); fer.castillo@gmail.com (F.C.-D.); stefano.piazza@unimi.it (S.P.); giorgia.targa@unimi.it (G.T.); enrico.sangiovanni@unimi.it (E.S.); mario.dellagli@unimi.it (M.D.); lucia.caffino@unimi.it (L.C.)

[2] Curaleaf International, London EC2A 2EW, UK; bp@curaleafint.com (B.P.); m.sodergren@imperial.ac.uk (M.H.S.)

[3] Medical Cannabis Research Group, Department of Surgery and Cancer, Imperial College London, London SW7 2AZ, UK

* Correspondence: fabio.fumagalli@unimi.it; Tel.: +39-02-503-18298

Abstract: Cannabidiol (CBD) is a phytocannabinoid contained in the Cannabis sativa plant, devoid of psychotomimetic effects but with a broad-spectrum pharmacological activity. Because of its pharmacological profile and its ability to counteract the psychoactive Δ^9-tetrahydrocannabinol (Δ9THC), CBD may be a potential treatment for several psychiatric and neurodegenerative disorders. In this study, we performed a dose–response evaluation of CBD modulatory effects on BDNF, a neurotrophin subserving pleiotropic effects on the brain, focusing on the cortico-striatal pathway for its unique role in the brain trafficking of BDNF. Male adult rats were exposed to single and repeated CBD treatments at different dosing regimen (5, 15, and 30 mg/kg), to investigate the rapid modulation of the neurotrophin (1 h after the single treatment) as well as a potential drug-free time point (24 h after the repeated treatment). We show here, for the first time, that CBD can be found in the rat brain and, specifically, in the medial prefrontal cortex (mPFC) following single or repeated exposure. In fact, we found that CBD is present in the mPFC of rats treated either acutely or repeatedly with the phytocannabinoid, with a clear dose–response profile. From a molecular standpoint, we found that single, but not repeated, CBD exposure upregulates BDNF in the mPFC, while the repeated exposure increased BDNF only in the striatum, with a slight decrease in the mPFC. Together, these data reveal a CBD dose-dependent and anatomically specific modulation of BDNF, which may be functionally relevant and may represent an added value for CBD as a supplement.

Keywords: cannabidiol; prefrontal cortex; striatum; BDNF

Citation: Mottarlini, F.; Fumagalli, M.; Castillo-Díaz, F.; Piazza, S.; Targa, G.; Sangiovanni, E.; Pacchetti, B.; Sodergren, M.H.; Dell'Agli, M.; Fumagalli, F.; et al. Single and Repeated Exposure to Cannabidiol Differently Modulate BDNF Expression and Signaling in the Cortico-Striatal Brain Network. *Biomedicines* 2022, *10*, 1853. https://doi.org/10.3390/biomedicines10081853

Academic Editor: Wesley M. Raup-Konsavage

Received: 7 July 2022
Accepted: 29 July 2022
Published: 1 August 2022

Publisher's Note: MDPI stays neutral with regard to jurisdictional claims in published maps and institutional affiliations.

Copyright: © 2022 by the authors. Licensee MDPI, Basel, Switzerland. This article is an open access article distributed under the terms and conditions of the Creative Commons Attribution (CC BY) license (https://creativecommons.org/licenses/by/4.0/).

1. Introduction

Cannabidiol (CBD) is one of the most abundant phytocannabinoids present in the Cannabis sativa plant, devoid of psychotomimetic effects [1]. In addition, CBD antagonizes several of the psychoactive effects of the Δ9-tetrahydrocannabinol (Δ9-THC), the major psychoactive compound of Cannabis sativa [2,3]. CBD exhibits a broad-spectrum pharmacological profile that makes it a potential treatment for several psychiatric and neurodegenerative disorders [4,5]. In fact, while CBD displays low affinity for cannabinoid CB1 and CB2 receptors [6], it can act as a negative allosteric modulator at these receptors [7,8]. In addition, its mechanism of action involves, at least, inhibition of anandamide hydrolysis [9], as well as action at the vanilloid receptor 1 (TRPV1) [9], the serotoninergic

5-HT1A receptor [10], and PPARγ receptors [11]. Friedman et al., reviewed the pharmacology of cannabinoids in neurological disorders, underlining the criticisms related to the bioavailability of these highly lipophilic molecules, such as the way of administration. With regards to CBD, the authors concluded that the bioavailability of oral administration in humans is poor (6–19%) and variable, according to several clinical studies [12,13]. For this reason, many in vivo studies concerning the effects of CBD in the central nervous system (CNS), including ours, considered other ways of administration, such as intraperitoneal (i.p.) injection. Regardless of the mode of administration, a clear characterization of the brain distribution of CBD and of its neuroplastic effects is still lacking.

Brain-derived neurotrophic factor (BDNF) belongs to a group of proteins termed neurotrophins, which play a pleiotropic role in the CNS. Besides its role during neurodevelopment and its neuroprotective properties, BDNF and its high affinity receptor TrkB are crucial regulators of neuroplasticity [14]. BDNF-induced activation of downstream signaling cascades regulates different cellular processes including neuroprotection, cognition, and stress coping [15]. Furthermore, modulation of BDNF levels may be critical for treatment of both psychiatric [16] and neurodegenerative disorders [17].

The organization of the BDNF gene is complex, exhibiting several 5' non-coding exons, each with a separate promoter region that triggers the transcription of a common 3' exon and encoding for the same protein [18]. The functions of these multiple variants have not yet been fully clarified but, indeed, specific transcripts may undergo different intracellular targeting. Thus, it appears that BDNF function is controlled in a dynamic manner not only at the transcriptional and translational level, but also via specific mRNA targeting as well as processing and secretion of its protein [19,20]. In fact, the cleavage of the BDNF precursor gives rise to the mature form of the neurotrophin (mBDNF, 14 kDa), which is anterogradely transported to its target neurons [21,22]. This is an important point in the overall regulation of the BDNF system as, for instance, BDNF is not synthesized in the striatum. After its release, BDNF binds to its high-affinity receptor TrkB that, after autophosphorylation, stimulates downstream pathways, primarily phosphoinositide 3-kinase (PI3-K) and mitogen-activated protein kinase (MAPK) pathways. Several botanicals and natural compounds, including CBD, have been shown to modulate neuroplasticity acting on BDNF levels [23] in animal models of several disorders such as depression [24], schizophrenia [25], addiction [26], ischemia [27], and Alzheimer's disease [28]. However, information on the fine-tuned regulation of BDNF in the action of CBD is still fragmentary.

Accordingly, we performed a dose–response study in rats to evaluate the rapid modulation (1 h) of the neurotrophin as well as its downstream signaling following a single injection of CBD. In addition, we exposed rats to repeated CBD treatment (five consecutive injections, once a day) with sacrifice 24 h after the last injection, to investigate a potential drug-free time point, focusing our attention on CBD-induced modulation of BDNF in the cortico-striatal pathway.

2. Materials and Methods

2.1. Animals

Adult male Sprague Dawley rats (Charles River, Calco, Italy) weighing 280 to 300 g on arrival were housed in groups of 2 in standard polycarbonate cages under standard laboratory conditions of temperature (21 ± 1 °C), humidity (50–60%), and artificial light (from 07:00 to 19:00 h). [29]. All animal procedures were conducted at the Department of Pharmacological and Biomolecular Sciences at the University of Milan, and carried out in accordance with the principles set out in the following laws, regulations, and policies governing the care and use of laboratory animals: Italian Governing Law (D.lgs 26/2014; Authorization n.19/2008-A issued 6 March 2008, by Ministry of Health); the NIH Guide for the Care and Use of Laboratory Animals (2011 edition) [30]; and EU directives and guidelines (EEC Council Directive 2010/63/UE). All efforts were made to minimize animal suffering and to keep the lowest number of animals used. The experiments have been reported in compliance with the ARRIVE guidelines.

2.2. Drug Preparation

CBD extracted from Cannabis plants was provided by Curaleaf International, UK, as a purified powder. Purity for CBD was above 95%; HPLC traces are provided as CBD powder was dissolved in a vehicle of Tween-80 (2%) and saline (NaCl 0.9%), protected from light, in agitation at 60 °C (avoiding boiling) until the complete mixing. The dissolved CBD was freshly prepared immediately prior to injection, and it was administered at different concentrations: 5 mg/kg, 15 mg/kg, and 30 mg/kg.

2.3. Experiments

Upon arrival, all the animals were habituated in the facility before starting any procedure for one week. Rats were left undisturbed for two days and then they were handled for 5 days before the injections; such manipulation was performed to avoid any potential bias due to stress-related effects. After this period of acclimation to the facility and the procedures, a total of 48 animals were divided into two separate sets of rats for acute (Experiment 1) and repeated (Experiment 2) treatments with CBD. In Experiment 1, a subset of 32 male Sprague Dawley rats was exposed to acute treatment of different CBD doses and was further subdivided into four experimental groups: (1) control group receiving a single i.p. injection of saline ($n = 8$), (2) single i.p. injection of CBD 5 mg/kg ($n = 8$), (3) single i.p. injection of CBD 15 mg/kg ($n = 8$), and (4) single i.p. injection of CBD 30 mg/kg ($n = 8$). The animals were sacrificed one hour after the acute treatment with saline or CBD. In Experiment 2, a subset of 32 male Sprague Dawley rats was subdivided into four experimental groups: rats exposed to (1) repeated saline ($n = 8$), or CBD treatments at the dose of (2) 5 mg/kg ($n = 8$), (3) 15 mg/kg ($n = 8$), or (4) 30 mg/kg ($n = 8$) for seven consecutive days. Animals were sacrificed twenty-four hours after the last treatment with saline or CBD. After decapitation, brains from Experiment 1 and 2 were rapidly removed, and the medial prefrontal cortices (mPFC, defined as Cg1, PL, and IL subregions, corresponding to plates 5–9) and striatum tissues (caudate putamen, corresponding to plates 10–25) were immediately dissected from 2 mm thick slices following the coordinates of the Rat Brain Atlas of Paxinos and Watson [31], then frozen on dry ice and stored at −80 °C for subsequent molecular analysis.

2.4. Plasma Preparation for CBD Measurements

Trunk blood from each rat was promptly collected after decapitation in tubes containing sodium citrate 3.8% (200 µL × 2 mL of blood collected) as anticoagulant agent. Plasma was separated by centrifugation (6500× g for 20 min) and stored at −20 °C for future molecular analysis. Plasma samples were prepared for CBD quantification as follows: 25 µL of the internal standard [cannabigerol (CBG) 3 ng/µL] was added to 150 µL of each plasma sample. Protein precipitation was performed by adding 100 µL of acetonitrile, while the extraction of CBD was performed with 1 mL of hexane. The samples were mixed by vortex and centrifuged at 10,000 rpm for 10 min, 900 µL of the supernatant was transferred into a new 1.5 mL tube, and the solvent was removed under nitrogen gas flow. The residue was reconstituted in 150 µL of methanol. Each sample was mixed and centrifuged at 10,000 rpm for 5 min. The final supernatant was used for the LC–MS/MS analysis.

2.5. Brain Tissue Preparation for CBD Measurements

The extraction of CBD from the mPFC was performed by using the whole protein homogenate extracted from each sample (see Protein Extracts preparation below). Ten µL of the internal standard (CBG 3 ng/µL) was added to 250 µL of each protein homogenate. The samples were mixed by vortex and centrifuged at 10,000 rpm for 10 min, 900 µL of the supernatant was transferred into a new 1.5 mL tube, and the solvent was removed under nitrogen gas flow. The residue was reconstituted in 150 µL of methanol. Each sample was mixed and centrifuged at 10,000 rpm for 5 min. The final supernatant was used for the LC–MS/MS analysis [32].

2.6. LC–MS/MS Analysis

HPLC was performed through an Exion LCTM AC System (AB Sciex, Foster City, CA, USA) composed of a vacuum degasser, a double plunger pump, a cooled autosampler, and a temperature-controlled column oven. The MS/MS analysis was carried out with a Triple QuadTM 3500 system (AB Sciex, Foster City, CA, USA). The analytes were separated on a Synergi 4 µm Hydro-RP 80 A LC Colum 150 × 4.6 mm (Phenomenex, Torrance, CA, USA) with a mobile phase composed of 0.1% formic acid in water (A) and methanol (B) at a rate flow of 0.800 mL/min. The chromatographic gradient is described below in Table 1.

Table 1. Chromatographic gradient used for analysis by LC-MS/MS. Phase A: 0.1% formic acid in water; phase B: methanol.

Time (min)	Flow (mL/min)	% A	% B
0	0.8	40	60
1	0.8	40	60
10	0.8	0	100
12	0.8	0	100
12.10	0.8	40	60
17	0.8	40	60

The injection volume was 10 µL for each sample. Mass spectrometric detection was done in negative ionization (ESI) mode, and the parameters were set as follows: curtain gas at 30 psi, ionization voltage at −4500 V, source temperature at 500 °C, and nebulization gas 1 and nebulization gas 2 at 50 psi. The optimized compound-dependent MS/MS parameters (declustering potential, entrance potential, collision energy, and collision cell exit potential) were obtained, in multiple-reaction-monitoring (MRM) mode, by a separate infusion of the analyte (CBD) and the internal standard (CBG). The analyte and the internal standard were analyzed by using the following mass transitions: 313/245 (CBD), 315/136 (CBG). The LC–MS/MS system was controlled by AB Sciex Analyst (version 1.7) software.

The Limit of Detection (LOD) of CBD was detected by multiple injections in LC-MS of serial dilutions of the sample. LOD was found 1.2 pg. This can be considered the lowest concentration of CBD that the instrument is able to detect.

2.7. RNA Preparation and Real-Time Polymerase Chain Reaction

Total RNA from mPFC was isolated by single-step guanidinium isothiocyanate/phenol extraction using PureZol RNA isolation reagent (Bio-Rad Laboratories, Segrate, Milan, Italy) according to the manufacturer's instructions and quantified by spectrophotometric analysis. Following total RNA extraction, the samples were processed for real-time reverse transcription polymerase chain reaction (real time RT-PCR) to assess mRNA levels. Briefly, an aliquot of each sample was treated with DNase to avoid DNA contamination. RNA was analyzed by TaqMan qRT-PCR instrument (CFX384 real time system, Bio-Rad Laboratories) using the iScriptTM one-step RT-PCR kit for probes (Bio-Rad Laboratories). Samples were run in 384-well formats in triplicate as multiplexed reactions. Data were analyzed with the comparative threshold cycle ($\Delta\Delta$Ct) method using *36B4* as reference gene [33]. Primers and probe for *Bdnf exon IV* and *VI* were purchased from Applied Biosystems (*Bdnf exon IV*: ID Rn01484927_m1 and *Bdnf exon VI*: ID Rn01484928_m1). Primers and probe for total *Bdnf* and *36B4* were purchased from Eurofins MWG-Operon. Their sequences are shown below:

- total *Bdnf*: forward primer 5′-AAGTCTGCATTACATTCCTCGA-3′, reverse primer 5′-GTTTTCTGAAAGAGGGACAGTTTAT-3′, probe 5′- TGTGGTTTGTTGCCGTTGCCAAG-3′;
- *36B4*: forward primer 5′-TTCCCACTGGCTGAAAAGGT-3′, reverse primer 5′-CGCAG CCGCAAATGC-3′, probe 5′-AAGGCCTTCCTGGCC GATCCATC-3′.

2.8. Protein Extracts Preparation and Western Blot Analyses

Proteins from mPFC and striatum were homogenized in a glass−glass potter in cold 0.32 M sucrose buffer pH 7.4 containing 1 mM HEPES, 0.1 mM PMSF, in presence of commercial cocktails of protease and phosphatase (Sigma-Aldrich, Milan, Italy) inhibitors and then sonicated. Total proteins were measured in the whole homogenate and quantified according to the Bradford Protein Assay procedure (Bio-Rad, Milan, Italy), using bovine serum albumin as calibration standard, and stored at $-20\,°C$ for subsequent molecular analysis. Western blots (WB) were run using sodium dodecyl sulfate -8% polyacrylamide gel under reducing conditions as previously described [34] on the whole homogenate lysate (10 µg) of mPFC and striatum and then electrophoretically transferred (dry transfer) onto nitrocellulose membranes (GE Healthcare). The strips of nitrocellulose membrane close to the molecular weights at which the bands of the protein of interest were expected were cut from the entire squared blot (full areas) as suggested by their specific molecular weight and the information present in the datasheet of the antibody. Blots were blocked for 1 h at room temperature ($25 \pm 2\,°C$) with I-Block solution (Life Technologies, Monza, Italy) in TBS + 0.1% Tween-20 buffer and washed with TBS + 0.1% Tween-20 buffer. The conditions of the primary antibodies were the following: anti mBDNF (1:1000, Icosagen, Tartu, Estonia, cod: 327-100), anti phospho-TrkB Tyr706 (1:500, Novus Biologicals, Littleton, CO, USA, cod: NBP2-54764), anti phospho-Akt Ser473 (1:1000, Cell Signaling Technology, Danvers, MA, USA, cod: 9271), anti phospho-ERK2 Thr185/Tyr187 (1:1000, Cell Signaling Technology, cod: 4370), anti-total TrkB (1:500, Cell Signaling Technology, cod: 4603), Akt (1:1000, Cell Signaling Technology, cod: 9272), ERK2 (1:5000, Cell Signaling Technology, cod: 4695), and anti β-actin (1:10.000, Sigma-Aldrich, cod: A5441). Results were standardized to β-actin control protein, which was detected by evaluating the band density at 43 kDa. Immunocomplexes were visualized by chemiluminescence using the Chemidoc MP Imaging System (Bio-Rad Laboratories) after 2–3 min of enhanced chemiluminescence substrate (ECL) exposure (Cyanagen Srl, Bologna, Italy). Activation of the proteins investigated were expressed as a ratio between the phosphorylated and the respective total forms and analyzed. Gels were run two times each, and the results represent the average from two different runs. We used a correction factor to average the different gels: correction factor gel B = average of (OD protein of interest/OD β-actin for each sample loaded in gel A)/(OD protein of interest/OD β-actin for the same sample loaded in gel B) [35].

2.9. Statistical Analysis

Data were collected in individual animals and are presented in bar graphs as means of 8 independent determinations ± standard errors (SEM). Shapiro−Wilk and the Kolmogorov-Smirnov tests were employed to determine normality of residuals (see Supplementary Tables S1–S4). Molecular results from the single CBD treatment as well as CBD content measurements in plasma and mPFC and mRNA and protein level determinations, normally distributed, were analyzed by ordinary one-way ANOVA followed by Tukey's post-hoc test, or for repeated CBD treatments by unpaired Student's t-test. Data with a non-normal distribution were analyzed by the Kruskal−Wallis one-way ANOVA for ranks followed by Dunn's multiple comparisons test, or by the Wilcoxon−Mann−Whitney test. Outlier calculation was performed with Grubb's test on the free platform GraphPad by Dotmatics. Statistical significance was assumed at $p < 0.05$.

3. Results

Figure 1 shows CBD plasma levels following single (Figure 1a) or repeated injections (Figure 1b) with 5, 15 or 30 mg/kg of CBD. The concentration of CBD in the plasma increased dose-dependently under both experimental conditions (Figure 1a: KW = 18.24, $p = 0.0001$; CBD 5 mg/kg = +32.53 ng/mL; CBD 15 mg/kg = +79.78 ng/mL vs. 5 mg/kg, $p = 0.0327$; CBD 30 mg/kg = +181.998 ng/mL vs. 5 mg/kg, $p < 0.0001$; Figure 1b: $F(2,21) = 102.4$, $p < 0.0001$; CBD 5 mg/kg = +2.04 ng/mL; CBD 15 mg/kg = +10.51 ng/mL vs. 5 mg/kg $p = 0.0010$, CBD 30 mg/kg + 23,96 ng/mL vs. 15 mg/kg, $p < 0.0001$).

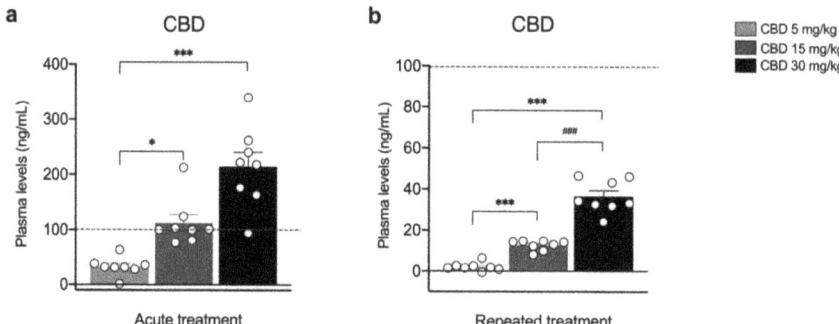

Figure 1. Concentration of CBD in the plasma of rats treated with a single (**a**) or repeated (**b**) CBD administration at the dose of 5 mg/kg, 15 mg/kg, or 30 mg/kg and killed respectively one (**a**) and twenty-four hours (**b**) after the last treatment. Bar graphs represent the mean ± SEM from eight independent determinations for each experimental group. Red dashed line in panel a indicates the y axis limit (100) of the bar chart represented in panel b. Ordinary one-way ANOVA followed by Tukey's multiple comparisons test, or Kruskal−Wallis one-way ANOVA for ranks followed by Dunn's multiple comparisons test for non-normally distributed data. * $p < 0.05$, *** $p < 0.001$ vs. 5 mg/kg, ### $p < 0.001$ vs. 15 mg/kg. CBD 5 mg/kg $n = 8$ CBD 15 mg/kg $n = 8$, CBD 30 mg/kg $n = 8$.

Figure 2 shows CBD cortical levels following single (Figure 2a) or repeated injections (Figure 2b) with 5, 15, or 30 mg/kg of CBD. At variance from plasma CBD levels, it appears that cortical CBD concentration rises significantly over untreated rats only at the highest dose employed (i.e., 30 mg/kg) under both experimental conditions (Figure 2a: KW = 12.89, $p = 0.0016$; CBD 30 mg/kg = +0.31 ng CBD/ng protein vs. 5 mg/kg, $p = 0.0010$; Figure 2b: KW = 17.90, $p = 0.0001$; CBD 30 mg/kg + 0.10 ng CBD/ng protein vs. 5 mg/kg, $p = 0.0001$; CBD 30 mg/kg + 0.09 ng CBD/ng protein vs. 15 mg/kg, $p = 0.0070$). Of note, CBD was undetectable at the 5 mg/kg dose following both single and repeated administrations.

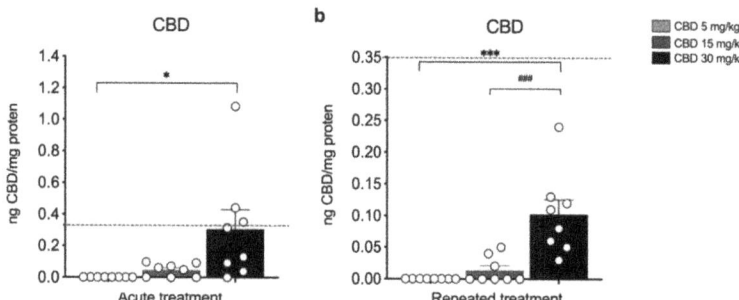

Figure 2. Concentration of CBD in the medial prefrontal cortex (mPFC) of rats treated with a single (**a**) or repeated (**b**) CBD administration at the dose of 5 mg/kg, 15 mg/kg, or 30 mg/kg and killed respectively one (**a**) and twenty-four hours (**b**) after the last treatment. Bar graphs represent the mean ± SEM from eight independent determinations for each experimental group. Red dashed line in panel a indicates the y axis limit (0.35) of the bar chart represented in panel b. Ordinary one-way ANOVA followed by Tukey's multiple comparisons test, or Kruskal−Wallis one-way ANOVA for ranks followed by Dunn's multiple comparisons test for non-normally distributed data. * $p < 0.05$, *** $p < 0.001$ vs. 5 mg/kg, ### $p < 0.001$ vs. 15 mg/kg. CBD 5 mg/kg $n = 8$ CBD 15 mg/kg $n = 8$, CBD 30 mg/kg $n = 8$.

We next evaluated the dose-dependent effects of acute CBD exposure on the gene expression levels of *total Bdnf* and related exons in the mPFC. In particular, we analyzed the main *Bdnf* exons, i.e., *exon IV*, the most abundant exon of somatic origin, and *exon VI*, which is expressed at dendrite level. Figure 3 illustrates the effects of a single injection of 5, 15, and 30 mg/kg of CBD on the gene expression levels of *total Bdnf* and its exons. While *total Bdnf* as well as *exon VI* gene expression levels are unchanged (Figure 3a: $F(3,27) = 1.553$, $p = 0.224$; Figure 3c: $F(3,27) = 1.980$, $p = 0.1407$), the transcription of *exon IV* is significantly upregulated in the mPFC, but only at the highest dose employed (Figure 3b: KW= 10.24, $p = 0.0166$, + 21.14% vs. saline $p = 0.0173$).

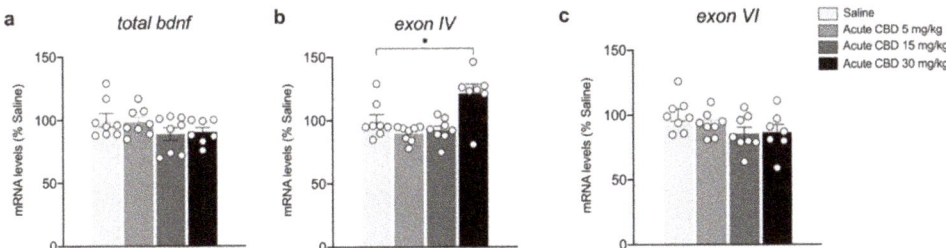

Figure 3. Effects of acute CBD exposure on Bdnf gene expression levels in the mPFC. Rats were treated with a single injection of CBD 5 mg/kg, 15 mg/kg, or 30 mg/kg, and killed one hour after the treatment. *Total Bdnf* (**a**), *Bdnf exon IV* (**b**), and *Bdnf exon VI* (**c**) mRNA levels in mPFC are expressed as percentages of saline-treated rats. Bar graphs represent the mean ± SEM from eight independent determinations for each experimental group. Ordinary one-way ANOVA followed by Tukey's multiple comparisons test, or Kruskal–Wallis one-way ANOVA for ranks followed by Dunn's multiple comparisons test for non-normally distributed data. * $p < 0.01$ vs. saline-treated rats. Saline $n = 8$ CBD 5 mg/kg $n = 8$ CBD 15 mg/kg $n = 8$, CBD 30 mg/kg $n = 7$.

We then analyzed protein levels of the mature form of the neurotrophin BDNF (mBDNF). As shown in Figure 4, acute CBD treatment up-regulates mBDNF levels in the whole homogenate of the mPFC at 30 mg/kg (Figure 4a: $F(3,27) = 3.361$, $p = 0.0333$, + 30.00% vs. saline $p = 0.0230$), but not at the lower doses used. Similarly, we found increased phosphorylation of the BDNF high-affinity receptor TrkB in Tyr(Y)706 (Figure 4b: $F(3,28) = 7.893$, $p = 0.0006$, + 43.63% vs. saline $p = 0.0035$), with no changes in its total expression (Figure 4c: KW 4.440, $p = 0.2177$). Of note, the levels of TrkB receptor activation, expressed as the ratio between the phosphorylated and non-phosphorylated (pTrkB/TrkB), are increased only following the single injection of CBD 30 mg/kg (Figure 4d: KW= 17.82, $p = 0.0005$, + 15.25% vs. saline $p = 0.0220$), with no effect at the lower doses.

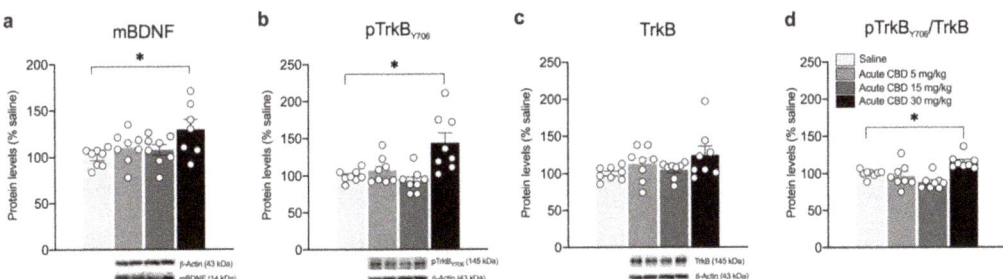

Figure 4. Effects of acute CBD exposure on mBDNF and TrkB receptor protein levels in the mPFC. Rats were treated with a single injection of CBD 5 mg/kg, 15 mg/kg, or 30 mg/kg and killed one hour after treatment. Protein levels of BDNF (**a**), phospho(p)-TrkBY706 (**b**), TrkB (**c**), and of the ratio pTrkB/TrkB (**d**) measured in the homogenate of mPFC are expressed as percentages of saline-treated

rats. Below the graphs representative immunoblots are shown for mBDNF (14 kDa), pTrkB Y706 (145 kDa), TrkB (145 kDa), and β-Actin (43 kDa) proteins. Bar graphs represent the mean ± SEM from eight independent determinations for each experimental group. Ordinary one-way ANOVA followed by Tukey's multiple comparisons test, or Kruskal-Wallis one-way ANOVA for ranks followed by Dunn's multiple comparisons test for non-normally distributed data. * $p < 0.05$ vs. saline-treated rats. Saline $n = 8$, CBD 5 mg/kg $n = 8$ CBD 15 mg/kg $n = 8$, CBD 30 mg/kg $n = 8$ (mBDNF $n = 7$).

Then, to investigate whether alterations in the BDNF-TrkB system induced by a single CBD exposure would engage the recruitment of BDNF downstream pathways, we analyzed the expression and phosphorylation of Akt and ERK2 effectors (Figure 5). As shown in Figure 5, while no significant changes are observed either in the phosphorylated (Ser473) (Figure 5a: $F(3.28) = 2.907$, $p = 0.0521$) or in the total form of Akt (Figure 5b: KW = 6.804, $p = 0.0784$), their ratio expressed as pAkt/Akt is significantly increased following the acute CBD treatment at 30 mg/kg (Figure 5c: $F(3.28) = 2.959$, $p = 0.0494$, + 33.38% vs. saline $p = 0.0328$). Conversely, the analysis of ERK2 phosphorylation (Thr185/Tyr187) does not show any relevant changes (Figure 5d: KW= 8.619, $p = 0.0348$; Figure 5f: KW= 1.054, $p = 0.7882$), whereas, despite that the ANOVA analysis of ERK2 expression is statistically significant, the multiple comparisons test does not show any relevant change (Figure 5e: KW = 4.662, $p = 0.1983$).

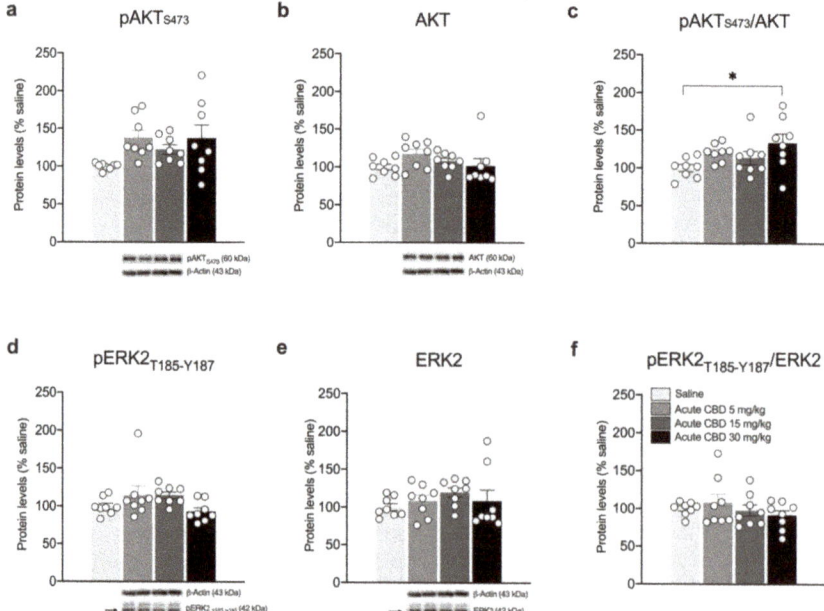

Figure 5. Effects of acute CBD exposure on BDNF-downstream signaling in the mPFC. Rats were treated with a single injection of CBD 5 mg/kg, 15 mg/kg, or 30 mg/kg and killed one hour after treatment. Protein levels of phospho(p)-AktS473 (**a**), Akt (**b**), pAkt/Akt (**c**), pERK2T185-Y187 (**d**), ERK2 (**e**), and pERK2/ERK2 (**f**) measured in the homogenate of mPFC are expressed as percentages of saline-treated rats. Below the graphs, representative immunoblots are shown for pAktS473 (60 kDa), Akt (60 kDa), pERK2T185-Y187 (42 kDa), ERK2 (42 kDa), and β-Actin (43 kDa) proteins. Bar graphs represent the mean ± SEM from eight independent determinations for each experimental group. Ordinary one-way ANOVA followed by Tukey's multiple comparisons test, or Kruskal-Wallis one-way ANOVA for ranks followed by Dunn's multiple comparisons test for non-normally distributed data. * $p < 0.05$ vs. saline-treated rats. Saline $n = 8$, CBD 5 mg/kg $n = 8$ CBD 15 mg/kg $n = 8$, CBD 30 mg/kg $n = 8$.

Based on the results observed following the single exposure of CBD, showing a significant effect on BDNF and its downstream signaling only at the highest dose employed, we decided to further analyze the neuroplastic effect of a repeated treatment with the phytocannabinoid employing only the highest dose. We found that repeated exposure to CBD (30 mg/kg) did not cause any change in the gene expression levels of *total Bdnf*, and *exon IV* and *VI* in the mPFC (Figure 6a: −10.75% vs. saline, t(14) = 1.224, p = 0.2410; Figure 6b: −9% vs. saline, t(14) = 0.8836, p = 0.3918; Figure 6c: −9.75% vs. saline, t(14) = 1.027, p = 0.3219). Of note, despite that no alterations are present in the mRNA levels of Bdnf and related exons, repeated CBD exposure reduces slightly, but significantly, mBDNF protein levels (Figure 7a: −11.75% vs. saline, t(14) = 2.443, p = 0.0284) and pTrkB/TrkB ratio (Figure 7d: −14.25% vs. saline, t(14) = 2.708, p = 0.0170).

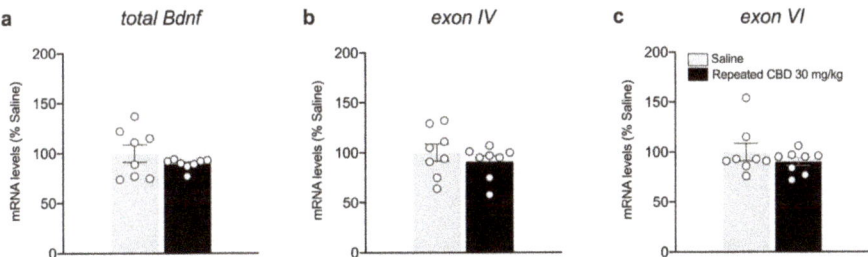

Figure 6. Effects of repeated CBD exposure on Bdnf gene expression levels in the mPFC. Rats were treated with repeated injections of CBD 30 mg/kg for seven days and killed twenty-four hours after the last treatment. *Total Bdnf* (**a**), *exon IV* (**b**), and *exon VI* (**c**) mRNA levels in mPFC are expressed as percentages of saline-treated rats. Bar graphs represent the mean ± SEM from eight independent determinations for each experimental group. Unpaired Student's *t*-test. Saline n = 8, CBD 30 mg/kg n = 8.

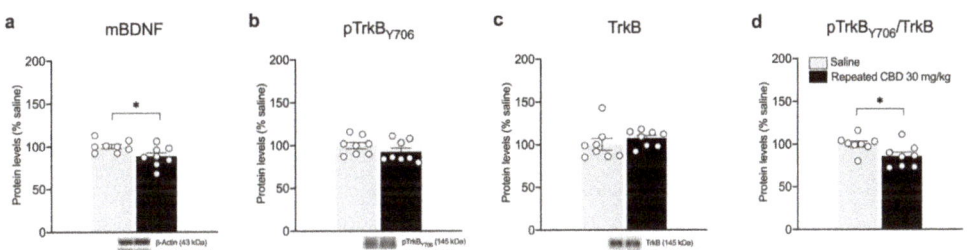

Figure 7. Effects of repeated CBD exposure on mBDNF and TrkB receptor protein levels in the mPFC. Rats were treated with repeated injections of 30 mg/kg for seven days and killed twenty-four hours after the last treatment. Protein levels of BDNF (**a**), phospho(p)-TrkBY706 (**b**), TrkB (**c**), and of the ratio pTrkB/TrkB (**d**) measured in the homogenate of mPFC are expressed as percentages of saline-treated rats. Below the graphs, representative immunoblots are shown for mBDNF (14 kDa), pTrkBY706 (145 kDa), TrkB (145 kDa), and β-Actin (43 kDa) proteins. Bar graphs represent the mean ± SEM from eight independent determinations for each experimental group. Unpaired Student's *t*-test or Wilcoxon−Mann−Whitney test. * p < 0.05 vs. saline-treated rats. Saline n = 8, CBD 30 mg/kg n = 8.

Interestingly, we found that the pAkt/Akt ratio is reduced (Figure 8c: −33.13% vs. saline, t(14) = 2.959, p = 0.0104), in line with reduced levels of Akt phosphorylation in Ser473 (Figure 8a), whereas no changes are observed in total Akt levels (Figure 8b: +9% vs. saline, t(14) = 0.6370, p = 0.5344). As previously shown after a single injection, the analysis of ERK2 does not show any alteration following repeated CBD exposure when compared to saline-treated animals (Figure 8d: −0.88% vs. saline, t(14) = 0.0594, p = 0.9535; Figure 8e: −7% vs. saline, U = 17, p = 0.1304; Figure 8f: +7% vs. saline, t(14) = 0.5305, p = 0.6041).

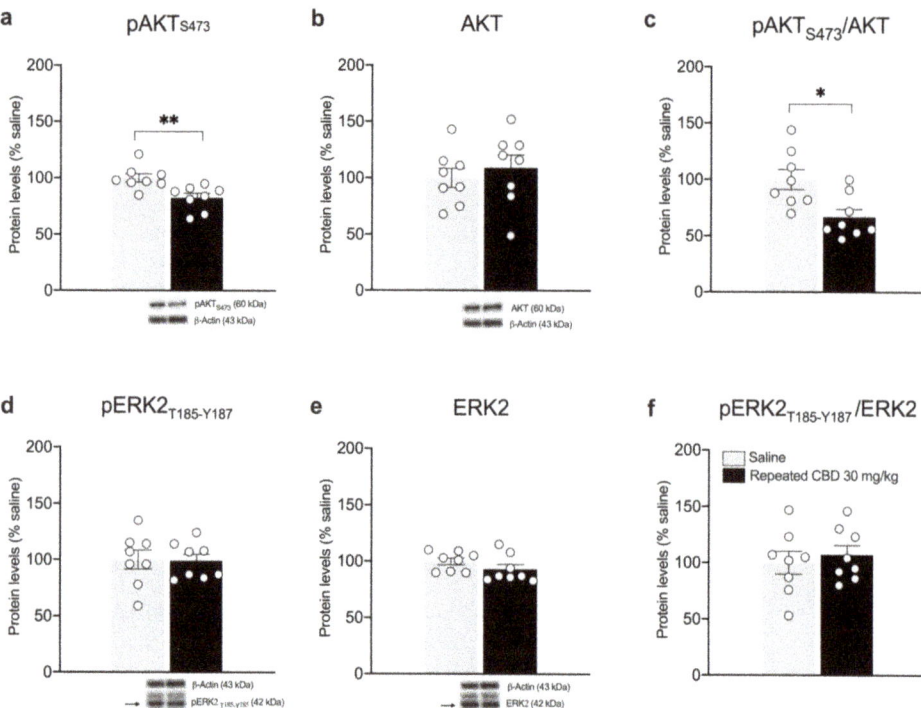

Figure 8. Effects of repeated CBD exposure on BDNF-downstream signaling in the mPFC. Rats were treated with repeated injections of 30 mg/kg for seven days and killed twenty-four hours after the last treatment. Protein levels of phospho(p)-AktS473 (**a**), Akt (**b**), pAkt/Akt (**c**), pERK2T185-Y187 (**d**), ERK2 (**e**), and pERK2/ERK2 (**f**) measured in the homogenate of mPFC are expressed as percentages of saline-treated rats. Below the graphs, representative immunoblots are shown for pAktS473 (60 kDa), Akt (60 kDa), pERK2T185-Y187 (42 kDa), ERK2 (42 kDa), and β-Actin (43 kDa) proteins. Bar graphs represent the mean ± SEM from eight independent determinations for each experimental group. Unpaired Student's *t*-test or Wilcoxon−Mann−Whitney test. * $p < 0.05$, ** $p < 0.01$ vs. saline-treated rats. Saline $n = 8$, CBD 30 mg/kg $n = 8$.

BDNF protein is known to undergo anterograde transport from the mPFC toward striatum [21]. In line with the reduction observed in the mPFC, we analyzed the BDNF-TrkB system in the striatum. Of note, accordingly, mBDNF protein levels are increased following repeated exposure to 30 mg/kg of CBD (Figure 9a: +36.5% vs. saline, U= 0, $p = 0.0002$). No changes are observed in the TrkB receptor levels (Figure 9b–d), either in the phosphorylated (Figure 9b: −12.75% vs. saline, U= 20, $p = 0.3969$) or in the total form of TrkB receptor (Figure 9c: −8.37% vs. saline, t(14) = 1.454, $p = 0.1680$) as well as in the pTrkB/TrkB ratio (Figure 9d: −7.5% vs. saline, U = 19, $p = 0.3357$). The evaluation of BDNF downstream effectors Akt and ERK2 revealed a significant increase in pAkt (Ser473) (+29.13% vs. saline, t(14) = 4.599, $p = 0.0004$) and total Akt (+24.88% vs. saline, t(14) = 5.550, $p < 0.0001$) as shown in Figure 10a,b, respectively, with no changes in the pAkt/Akt ratio (Figure 10c: (+3.75% vs. saline, t(14) = 0.7222, $p = 0.4821$). In line with our previous observations, no changes are detected for ERK2 (Figure 10d: −12.38% vs. saline, t(14) = 1.579, $p = 0.1366$; Figure 10e: +1.38% vs. saline, t(14) = 0.1393, $p = 0.8912$; Figure 10f: −8.13% vs. saline, U= 20, $p = 0.2345$).

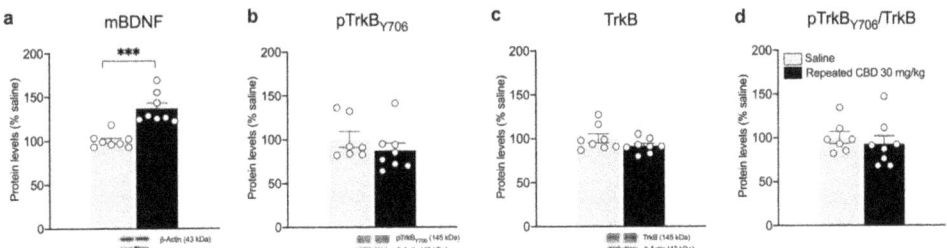

Figure 9. Effects of repeated CBD exposure on mBDNF and TrkB receptor protein levels in the striatum. Rats were treated with repeated injections of 30 mg/kg for seven days and killed twenty-four hours after the last treatment. Protein levels of mBDNF (**a**), phospho(p)-TrkBY706 (**b**), TrkB (**c**), and of the ratio pTrkB/TrkB (**d**) measured in the homogenate of the striatum are expressed as percentages of saline-treated rats. Below the graphs, representative immunoblots are shown for mBDNF (14 kDa), pTrkBY706 (145 kDa), TrkB (145 kDa), and β-Actin (43 kDa) proteins. Bar graphs represent the mean ± SEM from eight independent determinations for each experimental group. Unpaired Student's *t*-test. *** $p < 0.001$ vs. saline-treated rats. Saline $n = 8$ (pTrkB $n = 7$), CBD 30 mg/kg $n = 8$.

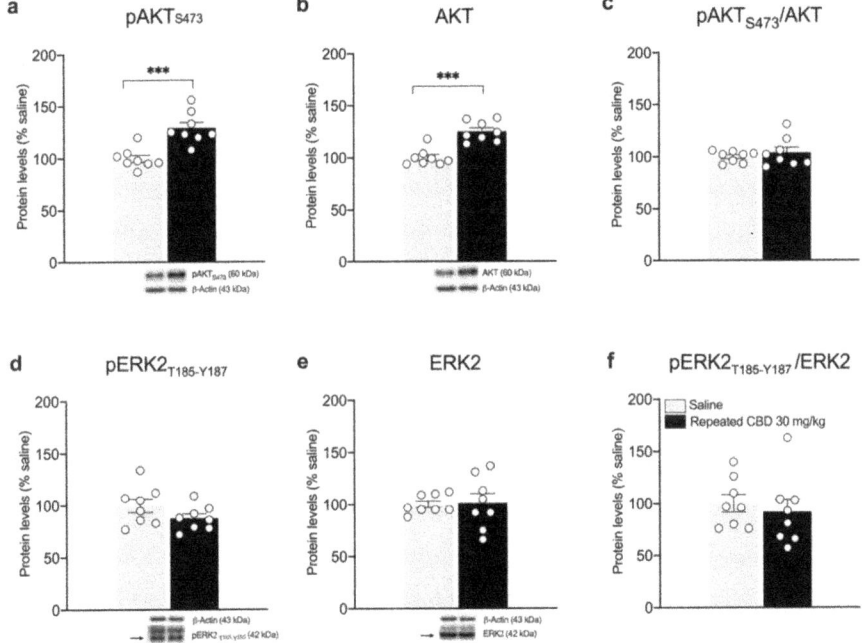

Figure 10. Effects of repeated CBD exposure on BDNF-downstream signaling in the striatum. Rats were treated with repeated injections of 30 mg/kg for seven days and killed twenty-four hours after the last treatment. Protein levels of phospho(p)-AktS473 (**a**), Akt (**b**), pAkt/Akt (**c**), pERK2T185-Y187 (**d**), ERK2 (**e**), and pERK2/ERK2 (**f**) measured in the homogenate of the striatum are expressed as percentages of saline-treated rats. Below the graphs, representative immunoblots are shown for pAktS473 (60 kDa), Akt (60 kDa), pERK2T185-Y187 (42 kDa), ERK2 (42 kDa), and β-Actin (43 kDa) proteins. Bar graphs represent the mean ± SEM from eight independent determinations for each experimental group. Unpaired Student's *t*-test. *** $p < 0.001$ vs. saline-treated rats. Saline $n = 8$, CBD 30 mg/kg $n = 8$.

4. Discussion

We show here, for the first time, that following single or repeated exposure, CBD can be found in the rat brain and, specifically, in the medial prefrontal cortex (mPFC). In fact, we found that CBD is present in the mPFC of rats treated either acutely or repeatedly with the phytocannabinoid, with a clear dose–response profile. In fact, whereas CBD cannot be detected at the lowest dose of CBD, i.e., 5 mg/kg, it is measurable at the dose of 15 mg/kg, reaching its peak at the maximal dose tested (30 mg/kg). Similarly, with the brain, a clear dose–response effect of CBD exposure was observed when measuring its levels in the rat plasma. In fact, it is barely detectable at 5 mg/kg of CBD, whereas its concentration increases dose-dependently at the other doses employed, reaching concentrations that are indeed much higher when compared with the brain levels. Again, we observed a significant reduction in CBD following repeated exposure when comparing plasma concentrations with those of single exposure. Taken together, these results indicate that CBD is already bioavailable within 1 h following the single injection and it is still detectable 24 h after the repeated administration, albeit at much lower concentration. Other authors investigated the impact of different methods (pulmonary, oral, and subcutaneous) and dosage of acute administration, on brain and serum level of CBD in rats. For this reason, the comparison among previous works and ours with respect to brain uptake is hard to perform. Independently of the route of administration, doses comparable to those used in our study (10 mg/kg) led to relevant brain uptake. Hlozek et al., showed a peak of concentration of 200 ng/g at 2 h after oral administration that was enhanced by the feeding state of the animals [36]. Another study observed a high brain uptake after acute subcutaneous injection of 10 mg/kg of CBD in mice with a peak reached after 1 h [37]. Again, Deiana et al., evaluated the pharmacokinetics of a high acute dose of CBD (120 mg/Kg) in rats (i. p.), thus measuring a Tmax of 60–120 min and relevant amount of CBD still after 24 h at brain level [38]. To the best of our knowledge, no previous studies regarding repeated exposure to CBD were conducted.

In line with the presence of the phytocannabinoid in the mPFC following a single exposure, we found that a single dose (30 mg/kg) of CBD is sufficient to upregulate Bdnf exon IV, the most abundant variant of the BDNF gene, which is paralleled by a similar increase in cortical mBDNF and TrkB. Such up-regulation drives the selective activation of the PI3K pathway (i.e., Akt). These effects might be beneficial for the overall regulation of cell homeostasis, potentially fostering the ability to promote synaptic transmission and plasticity, neuroprotection, and activity-dependent structural remodeling [14].

Conversely, a slight decrease was observed in the levels of mBDNF paralleled by reduction in TrkB and Akt activation following repeated exposure to CBD in the mPFC. Such a variable profile is not surprising when examining the neurotrophin expression [39,40]. To further strengthen this concept, we have also shown that an opposite modulation of BDNF can dissect the antidepressant from the reinforcing properties of ketamine [41]. These lines of evidence suggest that a more prolonged treatment with CBD should be performed to cause BDNF up-regulation.

As already revised by Lucas et al. [42] and Ujvàry et al. [43], CBD is mainly metabolized by iso-enzymes CYP2C19 and CYP3A4 at hepatic level. Several studies involving rodent models showed that CBD is mainly excreted in the intact or glucuronide form, while the major metabolites are hydroxylated derivatives and their glucuronide conjugates. For this reason, hepatic passage could be involved in the reduction in CBD plasmatic concentration during repeated exposure. However, the pharmacology of hydroxylated metabolites is still poorly investigated.

Overall, these data indicate that a single dose of 30 mg/kg is sufficient to trigger the activation of BDNF and its downstream signaling in the mPFC, whereas repeated exposure to the same dosing regimen downregulates the neurotrophin system. These data highlight the tight dependence of BDNF modulation upon CBD levels in the mPFC. In fact, it appears that when CBD is available in the mPFC in appreciable concentrations, the BDNF system is activated, such as after the single treatment. This finding may also suggest that, at least at the 30 mg/kg dose, which is indeed not the highest used in the literature, CBD may mediate, through BDNF, some short-term benefits for the brain by facilitating synaptic transmission, rather than long-term benefits. One potential outcome of the increase observed following a single exposure to BDNF relies on the possibility that it may contribute toward setting up a proper adaptive response of neural cells in response to environmental challenges, be they positive or adverse. For instance, we have demonstrated that exposure to stress prevents the ability to mount a neuroadaptive response to adverse external stimuli via up-regulation of cortical BDNF expression [44]. However, it is interesting to note that a single stress also favored the performance in a single cognitive test through transient up-regulation of cortical Bdnf mRNA levels [45]. Based on these lines of evidence, there is the possibility that CBD-induced up-regulation of cortical BDNF expression may favor cell coping under similar situations.

Another interesting finding of our experiments derives from the evidence that BDNF expression is elevated in the rat striatum following repeated exposure. It is well established that the striatum lacks Bdnf messenger RNA and that the neurotrophin is supplied to the striatum through anterograde transport from the mPFC [21]. Notably, we found a reduction in mBDNF in the mPFC and a significant increase in the striatum, potentially supporting an increased anterograde trafficking of BDNF, mediated by CBD. Interestingly, it appears that CBD has also activated the downstream BDNF pathway mediated by Akt, thus mediating the intracellular signaling cascade promoted by the neurotrophin. Notably, it has been previously shown that CBD leads to stronger connectivity between prefrontal cortex and striatum in humans, an effect that may perhaps be due to BDNF trafficking [46]. Evidence also exists that BDNF is critical for the survival of striatal neurons in animal models of Huntington's disease [47]; therefore, repeated treatment with CBD, through BDNF up-regulation, may represent a potential strategy to rescue, at least partially, striatal neurons from degeneration. BDNF is also important for the survival of striatal GABA neurons [48]. This is crucial in view of the notion that dysfunction in cortical and subcortical GABAergic pathways characterize, among others, the pathophysiology of schizophrenia [49]. It is in fact established that, in the striatum, GABA is pivotal for the regulation of overactivity of excitatory neurotransmissions as well as memory functions, which are perturbed in schizophrenic patients [50,51]. Taken together, these data suggest that CBD-induced increase in striatal BDNF may be functionally relevant and may represent an added value for CBD as supplement.

5. Conclusions

In conclusion, we have demonstrated that CBD can be detected in the plasma and mPFC, following single or repeated injections. In both districts, CBD is detected following a specific dose−response profile. Further, we showed that CBD can modulate BDNF expression in a manner that depends upon the length of the treatment and following a specific anatomical pattern. Accordingly, our data are likely to reflect the targeting of specific neuroplastic processes in the cortico-striatal pathway rather than an interference with specific neurotrophic responses.

Supplementary Materials: The following supporting information can be downloaded at: https://www.mdpi.com/article/10.3390/biomedicines10081853/s1, Figures S1–S4: Western blot uncropped immunoblot representative images of the data shown in Figures 4, 5 and 7–10. Supplementary Tables S1–S4 show the normality of residuals calculation of data shown in Figures 1–10.

Author Contributions: Conceptualization, M.D., F.F. and L.C.; methodology, F.M., M.F., F.C.-D., S.P., G.T., E.S. and B.P.; software, F.M. and E.S.; investigation, F.M., M.F., F.C.-D., S.P., G.T. and E.S.; writing—original draft preparation, F.M. and M.F.; writing—review and editing, B.P., M.H.S. and M.D., F.F. and L.C.; supervision, M.D., F.F. and L.C.; funding acquisition, F.F. All authors have read and agreed to the published version of the manuscript.

Funding: This research was funded by Curaleaf International, UK and by grants from MIUR Progetto Eccellenza.

Institutional Review Board Statement: All animal procedures were conducted in accordance with the ethical standards and according to national and international guidelines and were revised and approved by the authors' institutional review board (Organism for Animal Wellbeing—OPBA) and conducted at the Department of Pharmacological and Biomolecular Sciences at the University of Milan. The animal study protocol was approved and carried out in accordance with the principles set out in the following laws, regulations, and policies governing the care and use of laboratory animals: Italian Governing Law (D.lgs 26/2014; Authorization n.19/2008-A issued March 6, 2008, by Ministry of Health); the NIH Guide for the Care and Use of Laboratory Animals (2011 edition) [30]; and EU directives and guidelines (EEC Council Directive 2010/63/UE).

Informed Consent Statement: Not applicable.

Data Availability Statement: Not applicable.

Acknowledgments: Francesca Mottarlini is the recipient of a postdoc fellowship from Zardi Gori Foundation.

Conflicts of Interest: Mikael Sodergren is a Clinical Senior Lecturer at Imperial College and Chief Medical Officer at Curaleaf International, from whom he receives payments as a consultant. The other authors declare no conflict of interests.

References

1. Russo, E.B.; Marcu, J. Cannabis Pharmacology: The Usual Suspects and a Few Promising Leads. *Adv. Pharmacol.* **2017**, *80*, 67–134. [CrossRef] [PubMed]
2. Zuardi, A.W.; Shirakawa, I.; Finkelfarb, E.; Karniol, I.G. Action of cannabidiol on the anxiety and other effects produced by delta 9-THC in normal subjects. *Psychopharmacology* **1982**, *76*, 245–250. [CrossRef] [PubMed]
3. Zuardi, A.W.; Morais, S.L.; Guimaraes, F.S.; Mechoulam, R. Antipsychotic effect of cannabidiol. *J. Clin. Psychiatry* **1995**, *56*, 485–486. [PubMed]
4. Izzo, A.A.; Borrelli, F.; Capasso, R.; Di Marzo, V.; Mechoulam, R. Non-psychotropic plant cannabinoids: New therapeutic opportunities from an ancient herb. *Trends Pharmacol. Sci.* **2009**, *30*, 515–527. [CrossRef]
5. Campos, A.C.; Moreira, F.A.; Gomes, F.V.; Del Bel, E.A.; Guimaraes, F.S. Multiple mechanisms involved in the large-spectrum therapeutic potential of cannabidiol in psychiatric disorders. *Philos. Trans. R. Soc. B Biol. Sci.* **2012**, *367*, 3364–3378. [CrossRef]
6. Thomas, B.F.; Gilliam, A.F.; Burch, D.F.; Roche, M.J.; Seltzman, H.H. Comparative receptor binding analyses of cannabinoid agonists and antagonists. *J. Pharmacol. Exp. Ther.* **1998**, *285*, 285–292.
7. Laprairie, R.B.; Bagher, A.M.; Kelly, M.E.; Denovan-Wright, E.M. Cannabidiol is a negative allosteric modulator of the cannabinoid CB1 receptor. *Br. J. Pharmacol.* **2015**, *172*, 4790–4805. [CrossRef]
8. Martinez-Pinilla, E.; Varani, K.; Reyes-Resina, I.; Angelats, E.; Vincenzi, F.; Ferreiro-Vera, C.; Oyarzabal, J.; Canela, E.I.; Lanciego, J.L.; Nadal, X.; et al. Binding and Signaling Studies Disclose a Potential Allosteric Site for Cannabidiol in Cannabinoid CB2 Receptors. *Front. Pharmacol.* **2017**, *8*, 744. [CrossRef]
9. Bisogno, T.; Hanus, L.; De Petrocellis, L.; Tchilibon, S.; Ponde, D.E.; Brandi, I.; Moriello, A.S.; Davis, J.B.; Mechoulam, R.; Di Marzo, V. Molecular targets for cannabidiol and its synthetic analogues: Effect on vanilloid VR1 receptors and on the cellular uptake and enzymatic hydrolysis of anandamide. *Br. J. Pharmacol.* **2001**, *134*, 845–852. [CrossRef]
10. Russo, E.B.; Burnett, A.; Hall, B.; Parker, K.K. Agonistic properties of cannabidiol at 5-HT1a receptors. *Neurochem. Res.* **2005**, *30*, 1037–1043. [CrossRef]
11. O'Sullivan, S.E. An update on PPAR activation by cannabinoids. *Br. J. Pharmacol.* **2016**, *173*, 1899–1910. [CrossRef]
12. Friedman, D.; French, J.A.; Maccarrone, M. Safety, efficacy, and mechanisms of action of cannabinoids in neurological disorders. *Lancet Neurol.* **2019**, *18*, 504–512. [CrossRef]
13. Gaston, T.E.; Friedman, D. Pharmacology of cannabinoids in the treatment of epilepsy. *Epilepsy Behav.* **2017**, *70*, 313–318. [CrossRef]
14. Bramham, C.R.; Messaoudi, E. BDNF function in adult synaptic plasticity: The synaptic consolidation hypothesis. *Prog. Neurobiol.* **2005**, *76*, 99–125. [CrossRef]
15. Nagappan, G.; Lu, B. Activity-dependent modulation of the BDNF receptor TrkB: Mechanisms and implications. *Trends Neurosci.* **2005**, *28*, 464–471. [CrossRef]
16. Wang, C.S.; Kavalali, E.T.; Monteggia, L.M. BDNF signaling in context: From synaptic regulation to psychiatric disorders. *Cell* **2022**, *185*, 62–76. [CrossRef]
17. Caffino, L.; Mottarlini, F.; Fumagalli, F. Born to Protect: Leveraging BDNF Against Cognitive Deficit in Alzheimer's Disease. *CNS Drugs* **2020**, *34*, 281–297. [CrossRef]
18. Aid, T.; Kazantseva, A.; Piirsoo, M.; Palm, K.; Timmusk, T. Mouse and rat BDNF gene structure and expression revisited. *J. Neurosci. Res.* **2007**, *85*, 525–535. [CrossRef]
19. Santi, S.; Cappello, S.; Riccio, M.; Bergami, M.; Aicardi, G.; Schenk, U.; Matteoli, M.; Canossa, M. Hippocampal neurons recycle BDNF for activity-dependent secretion and LTP maintenance. *EMBO J.* **2006**, *25*, 4372–4380. [CrossRef]

20. Simonato, M.; Tongiorgi, E.; Kokaia, M. Angels and demons: Neurotrophic factors and epilepsy. *Trends Pharmacol. Sci.* **2006**, *27*, 631–638. [CrossRef]
21. Altar, C.A.; Cai, N.; Bliven, T.; Juhasz, M.; Conner, J.M.; Acheson, A.L.; Lindsay, R.M.; Wiegand, S.J. Anterograde transport of brain-derived neurotrophic factor and its role in the brain. *Nature* **1997**, *389*, 856–860. [CrossRef]
22. Conner, J.M.; Lauterborn, J.C.; Yan, Q.; Gall, C.M.; Varon, S. Distribution of brain-derived neurotrophic factor (BDNF) protein and mRNA in the normal adult rat CNS: Evidence for anterograde axonal transport. *J. Neurosci.* **1997**, *17*, 2295–2313. [CrossRef]
23. Sangiovanni, E.; Brivio, P.; Dell'Agli, M.; Calabrese, F. Botanicals as Modulators of Neuroplasticity: Focus on BDNF. *Neural Plast.* **2017**, *2017*, 5965371. [CrossRef]
24. Sales, A.J.; Fogaca, M.V.; Sartim, A.G.; Pereira, V.S.; Wegener, G.; Guimaraes, F.S.; Joca, S.R.L. Cannabidiol Induces Rapid and Sustained Antidepressant-Like Effects Through Increased BDNF Signaling and Synaptogenesis in the Prefrontal Cortex. *Mol. Neurobiol.* **2019**, *56*, 1070–1081. [CrossRef]
25. Peres, F.F.; Diana, M.C.; Levin, R.; Suiama, M.A.; Almeida, V.; Vendramini, A.M.; Santos, C.M.; Zuardi, A.W.; Hallak, J.E.C.; Crippa, J.A.; et al. Cannabidiol Administered During Peri-Adolescence Prevents Behavioral Abnormalities in an Animal Model of Schizophrenia. *Front. Pharmacol.* **2018**, *9*, 901. [CrossRef]
26. Galaj, E.; Xi, Z.X. Possible Receptor Mechanisms Underlying Cannabidiol Effects on Addictive-like Behaviors in Experimental Animals. *Int. J. Mol. Sci.* **2020**, *22*, 134. [CrossRef]
27. Mori, M.A.; Meyer, E.; Soares, L.M.; Milani, H.; Guimaraes, F.S.; de Oliveira, R.M.W. Cannabidiol reduces neuroinflammation and promotes neuroplasticity and functional recovery after brain ischemia. *Prog. Neuropsychopharmacol. Biol. Psychiatry* **2017**, *75*, 94–105. [CrossRef] [PubMed]
28. Watt, G.; Shang, K.; Zieba, J.; Olaya, J.; Li, H.; Garner, B.; Karl, T. Chronic Treatment with 50 mg/kg Cannabidiol Improves Cognition and Moderately Reduces Abeta40 Levels in 12-Month-Old Male AbetaPPswe/PS1DeltaE9 Transgenic Mice. *J. Alzheimers Dis.* **2020**, *74*, 937–950. [CrossRef] [PubMed]
29. Chapman, R.H.; Stern, J.M. Maternal stress and pituitary-adrenal manipulations during pregnancy in rats: Effects on morphology and sexual behavior of male offspring. *J. Comp. Physiol. Psychol.* **1978**, *92*, 1074–1083. [CrossRef] [PubMed]
30. National Research Council (US) Committee for the Update of the Guide for the Care and Use of Laboratory Animals. *Guide for the Care and Use of Laboratory Animals*, 8th ed.; National Academy of Sciences: Washington, DC, USA, 2011. [CrossRef]
31. Paxinos, G.; Watson, C. *The Rat Brain in Stereotaxic Coordinates*, 7th ed.; Eselvier: Amsterdam, The Netherlands, 2013; p. 472.
32. Ravula, A.; Chandasana, H.; Setlow, B.; Febo, M.; Bruijnzeel, A.W.; Derendorf, H. Simultaneous quantification of cannabinoids tetrahydrocannabinol, cannabidiol and CB1 receptor antagonist in rat plasma: An application to characterize pharmacokinetics after passive cannabis smoke inhalation and co-administration of rimonabant. *J. Pharm. Biomed. Anal.* **2018**, *160*, 119–125. [CrossRef]
33. Caffino, L.; Giannotti, G.; Malpighi, C.; Racagni, G.; Fumagalli, F. Short-term withdrawal from developmental exposure to cocaine activates the glucocorticoid receptor and alters spine dynamics. *Eur. Neuropsychopharmacol.* **2015**, *25*, 1832–1841. [CrossRef]
34. Caffino, L.; Piva, A.; Giannotti, G.; Di Chio, M.; Mottarlini, F.; Venniro, M.; Yew, D.T.; Chiamulera, C.; Fumagalli, F. Ketamine Self-Administration Reduces the Homeostasis of the Glutamate Synapse in the Rat Brain. *Mol. Neurobiol.* **2017**, *54*, 7186–7193. [CrossRef]
35. Caffino, L.; Verheij, M.M.M.; Roversi, K.; Targa, G.; Mottarlini, F.; Popik, P.; Nikiforuk, A.; Golebiowska, J.; Fumagalli, F.; Homberg, J.R. Hypersensitivity to amphetamine's psychomotor and reinforcing effects in serotonin transporter knockout rats: Glutamate in the nucleus accumbens. *Br. J. Pharmacol.* **2020**, *177*, 4532–4547. [CrossRef]
36. Hlozek, T.; Uttl, L.; Kaderabek, L.; Balikova, M.; Lhotkova, E.; Horsley, R.R.; Novakova, P.; Sichova, K.; Stefkova, K.; Tyls, F.; et al. Pharmacokinetic and behavioural profile of THC, CBD, and THC+CBD combination after pulmonary, oral, and subcutaneous administration in rats and confirmation of conversion in vivo of CBD to THC. *Eur. Neuropsychopharmacol.* **2017**, *27*, 1223–1237. [CrossRef]
37. Brzozowska, N.; Li, K.M.; Wang, X.S.; Booth, J.; Stuart, J.; McGregor, I.S.; Arnold, J.C. ABC transporters P-gp and Bcrp do not limit the brain uptake of the novel antipsychotic and anticonvulsant drug cannabidiol in mice. *PeerJ* **2016**, *4*, e2081. [CrossRef]
38. Deiana, S.; Watanabe, A.; Yamasaki, Y.; Amada, N.; Arthur, M.; Fleming, S.; Woodcock, H.; Dorward, P.; Pigliacampo, B.; Close, S.; et al. Plasma and brain pharmacokinetic profile of cannabidiol (CBD), cannabidivarine (CBDV), Delta(9)-tetrahydrocannabivarin (THCV) and cannabigerol (CBG) in rats and mice following oral and intraperitoneal administration and CBD action on obsessive-compulsive behaviour. *Psychopharmacology* **2012**, *219*, 859–873. [CrossRef]
39. De Foubert, G.; Carney, S.L.; Robinson, C.S.; Destexhe, E.J.; Tomlinson, R.; Hicks, C.A.; Murray, T.K.; Gaillard, J.P.; Deville, C.; Xhenseval, V.; et al. Fluoxetine-induced change in rat brain expression of brain-derived neurotrophic factor varies depending on length of treatment. *Neuroscience* **2004**, *128*, 597–604. [CrossRef]
40. Coppell, A.L.; Pei, Q.; Zetterstrom, T.S. Bi-phasic change in BDNF gene expression following antidepressant drug treatment. *Neuropharmacology* **2003**, *44*, 903–910. [CrossRef]
41. Caffino, L.; Di Chio, M.; Giannotti, G.; Venniro, M.; Mutti, A.; Padovani, L.; Cheung, D.; Fumagalli, G.F.; Yew, D.T.; Fumagalli, F.; et al. The modulation of BDNF expression and signalling dissects the antidepressant from the reinforcing properties of ketamine: Effects of single infusion vs. chronic self-administration in rats. *Pharmacol. Res.* **2016**, *104*, 22–30. [CrossRef]
42. Lucas, C.J.; Galettis, P.; Schneider, J. The pharmacokinetics and the pharmacodynamics of cannabinoids. *Br. J. Clin. Pharmacol.* **2018**, *84*, 2477–2482. [CrossRef]

43. Ujvary, I.; Hanus, L. Human Metabolites of Cannabidiol: A Review on Their Formation, Biological Activity, and Relevance in Therapy. *Cannabis Cannabinoid. Res.* **2016**, *1*, 90–101. [CrossRef]
44. Fumagalli, F.; Caffino, L.; Racagni, G.; Riva, M.A. Repeated stress prevents cocaine-induced activation of BDNF signaling in rat prefrontal cortex. *Eur. Neuropsychopharmacol.* **2009**, *19*, 402–408. [CrossRef]
45. Brivio, P.; Sbrini, G.; Riva, M.A.; Calabrese, F. Acute Stress Induces Cognitive Improvement in the Novel Object Recognition Task by Transiently Modulating Bdnf in the Prefrontal Cortex of Male Rats. *Cell Mol. Neurobiol.* **2020**, *40*, 1037–1047. [CrossRef]
46. Grimm, O.; Loffler, M.; Kamping, S.; Hartmann, A.; Rohleder, C.; Leweke, M.; Flor, H. Probing the endocannabinoid system in healthy volunteers: Cannabidiol alters fronto-striatal resting-state connectivity. *Eur. Neuropsychopharmacol.* **2018**, *28*, 841–849. [CrossRef] [PubMed]
47. Zuccato, C.; Ciammola, A.; Rigamonti, D.; Leavitt, B.R.; Goffredo, D.; Conti, L.; MacDonald, M.E.; Friedlander, R.M.; Silani, V.; Hayden, M.R.; et al. Loss of huntingtin-mediated BDNF gene transcription in Huntington's disease. *Science* **2001**, *293*, 493–498. [CrossRef] [PubMed]
48. Mizuno, K.; Carnahan, J.; Nawa, H. Brain-derived neurotrophic factor promotes differentiation of striatal GABAergic neurons. *Dev. Biol.* **1994**, *165*, 243–256. [CrossRef] [PubMed]
49. Fujihara, K.; Miwa, H.; Kakizaki, T.; Kaneko, R.; Mikuni, M.; Tanahira, C.; Tamamaki, N.; Yanagawa, Y. Glutamate Decarboxylase 67 Deficiency in a Subset of GABAergic Neurons Induces Schizophrenia-Related Phenotypes. *Neuropsychopharmacology* **2015**, *40*, 2475–2486. [CrossRef]
50. Behrens, M.M.; Ali, S.S.; Dao, D.N.; Lucero, J.; Shekhtman, G.; Quick, K.L.; Dugan, L.L. Ketamine-induced loss of phenotype of fast-spiking interneurons is mediated by NADPH-oxidase. *Science* **2007**, *318*, 1645–1647. [CrossRef] [PubMed]
51. Lewis, D.A.; Hashimoto, T.; Volk, D.W. Cortical inhibitory neurons and schizophrenia. *Nat. Rev. Neurosci.* **2005**, *6*, 312–324. [CrossRef] [PubMed]

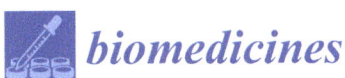

Article

Anticonvulsant Action and Long-Term Effects of Chronic Cannabidiol Treatment in the Rat Pentylenetetrazole-Kindling Model of Epilepsy

Zsolt Gáll [1,*,†], Krisztina Kelemen [2,†], Andrea Tolokán [1], István Zolcseak [1], István Sável [1], Réka Bod [2], Elek Ferencz [3], Szende Vancea [3], Melinda Urkon [1] and Melinda Kolcsár [1]

[1] Department of Pharmacology and Clinical Pharmacy, George Emil Palade University of Medicine, Pharmacy, Science, and Technology of Targu Mures, 540142 Târgu Mureș, Romania; tolokan.andrea@gmail.com (A.T.); istvanzolcseak@gmail.com (I.Z.); savelistvan@gmail.com (I.S.); melinda.urkon@umfst.ro (M.U.); melinda.kolcsar@umfst.ro (M.K.)

[2] Department of Physiology, George Emil Palade University of Medicine, Pharmacy, Science, and Technology of Targu Mures, 540142 Târgu Mureș, Romania; krisztina.kelemen@umfst.ro (K.K.); bod.reka-barbara@stud16.umftgm.ro (R.B.)

[3] Department of Physical Chemistry, George Emil Palade University of Medicine, Pharmacy, Science, and Technology of Targu Mures, 540142 Târgu Mureș, Romania; elek.ferencz@umfst.ro (E.F.); vancsa.szende@gmail.com (S.V.)

* Correspondence: zsolt.gall@umfst.ro; Tel.: +40-265-215-551 (ext. 364)

† The authors contributed equally to this work.

Abstract: Cannabidiol (CBD) showed anticonvulsant action in several preclinical models and is currently approved by regulatory agencies to treat childhood epilepsy syndromes. However, CBD treatment has limited benefits, and its long-term effects on cognition are not fully understood yet. This study aimed to examine the impact of long-term CBD treatment in the pentylenetetrazole (PTZ)-kindling model of epilepsy. Adult male Wistar rats ($N = 24$) received PTZ (35 mg/kg intraperitoneally) every other day until two consecutive generalized seizures occurred. CBD (60 mg/kg body weight) was administered daily by the oral route until the kindled state was achieved ($n = 12$). To confirm that the formulation and administration techniques were not of concern, liquid chromatography–mass spectrometry was performed to test the brain penetration of the CBD formula. As a result of CBD treatment, a lower mortality rate and significantly prolonged generalized seizure latency (925.3 ± 120.0 vs. 550.1 ± 69.62 s) were observed, while the frequency and duration of generalized seizures were not influenced. The CBD-treated group showed a significant decrease in vertical exploration in the open field test and a significant decrease in the discrimination index in the novel object recognition (NOR) test (-0.01 ± 0.17 vs. 0.57 ± 0.15, $p = 0.04$). The observed behavioral characteristics may be connected to the decreased thickness of the stratum pyramidale or the decreased astrogliosis observed in the hippocampus. In conclusion, CBD treatment did not prevent kindling, nor did it affect seizure frequency or duration. However, it did increase the latency to the first seizure and decreased the prolonged status epilepticus-related mortality in PTZ-kindled rats. The cognitive impairment observed in the NOR test may be related to the high dose used in this study, which may warrant further investigation.

Keywords: cannabidiol; epilepsy; animal model; cognitive dysfunction

1. Introduction

Cannabidiol (CBD), the second most important component of *Cannabis sativa*, has no psychotropic effects and holds low toxicity in both humans and experimental animals. Thus, it has been studied in a wide dose range for potential use in various neurological and psychiatric diseases [1–5]. CBD has a weak affinity for cannabinoid receptors CB1 and CB2, acting as a negative allosteric modulator and inverse agonist, respectively [6]. Besides, it

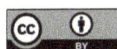

Citation: Gáll, Z.; Kelemen, K.; Tolokán, A.; Zolcseak, I.; Sável, I.; Bod, R.; Ferencz, E.; Vancea, S.; Urkon, M.; Kolcsár, M. Anticonvulsant Action and Long-Term Effects of Chronic Cannabidiol Treatment in the Rat Pentylenetetrazole-Kindling Model of Epilepsy. *Biomedicines* **2022**, *10*, 1811. https://doi.org/10.3390/biomedicines10081811

Academic Editor: Wesley M. Raup-Konsavage

Received: 20 June 2022
Accepted: 26 July 2022
Published: 28 July 2022

Publisher's Note: MDPI stays neutral with regard to jurisdictional claims in published maps and institutional affiliations.

Copyright: © 2022 by the authors. Licensee MDPI, Basel, Switzerland. This article is an open access article distributed under the terms and conditions of the Creative Commons Attribution (CC BY) license (https://creativecommons.org/licenses/by/4.0/).

also has an antagonistic effect on GPR55 receptors, partial agonist action on 5-HT1A, and a negative allosteric modulatory effect on opioid receptors (μ and δ) [7]. Ion channels are also important targets for CBD, the most-studied being the transient receptor potential vanilloid type 1 (TRPV1) and ankyrin type 1 (TRPA1), and T-type voltage-gated calcium channels, which are involved in the regulation of Ca^{2+} signaling in the brain [3,8,9]. Therefore, CBD treatment could have numerous beneficial outcomes in neuropsychiatric illnesses; however, at present, the only approved indication for CBD is to treat seizures associated with childhood epilepsy syndromes like Lennox–Gastaut and Dravet syndromes [10,11].

CBD has a well-described anticonvulsant effect based on in vitro and in vivo models of epilepsy. In vitro, CBD reduced the amplitude and duration of epileptiform activities induced by low concentrations of magnesium and 4-aminopyridine but did not influence signal propagation [12]. CBD administered in a dose range of 40–360 mg/kg body weight ameliorated the seizures induced by electric currents or convulsive agents such as pilocarpine, penicillin, and pentylenetetrazole (PTZ) in rodents [12–17]. It should be noted that, when CBD is administered before seizure induction, in the acute phase, it reduces seizure severity, but there is little information about how CBD affects the processes that take place during the chronic phase or how it might modify the course of the disease [18,19]. It is important to consider that CBD has anti-inflammatory, antiapoptotic, and neuroprotective effects, possibly due to the existence of cannabinoid receptors both in glial cells and on the surface of B, NK, and T lymphocytes, as all of these cells are involved in neuroinflammation. Several studies confirmed that neuroinflammatory processes may play an important role in epileptogenesis, seizure worsening, or developing epilepsy-associated neuropsychiatric comorbidities (e.g., anxiety, depression, cognitive impairment) [20–26].

Epileptogenesis can be triggered by lesions of varying duration and intensity that, after a certain period of time, will cause spontaneous and recurrent seizures [27]. Between the initial insult and the emergence of spontaneous seizures, some adaptive changes occur at both the cellular and molecular levels, but these have not yet been fully elucidated [28,29]. It is known that pentylenetetrazole (PTZ) can cause acute seizures in rats at higher doses, but when used at lower, subconvulsive doses, it can produce a chronic epileptic state characterized by a progressive decrease in the seizure threshold and a continuous increase in seizure severity [30]. Behavioral, biochemical, and structural changes in neural development can all be induced by PTZ kindling. Despite lacking spontaneous seizures, a seizure threshold decrease in kindled animals mimics epilepsy phenotypes through an imbalance between the excitatory and inhibitory neurotransmission systems. [31–33]. In addition, the PTZ-kindling model has been shown to reflect the cognitive impairments [34,35] and the characteristic cellular changes related to epilepsy in rats, such as astrogliosis [18] and microglia activation [36].

This study aimed to evaluate the effects of chronic CBD administration in the PTZ-kindling model of epilepsy in rats using behavioral tests, bioanalytical assay for brain exposure quantification, and immunohistochemistry to assess cellular alterations, and finally, to evaluate the role CBD plays in cognitive performance change.

2. Materials and Methods
2.1. Animals

Experimentally naive, adult male Wistar rats were provided by the Biobase of the George Emil Palade University of Medicine, Pharmacy, Science, and Technology of Targu Mures. Before the experiments, all animals were subjected to a 7-day habituation period, when acclimatization to single housing, daily handling, and standard environmental conditions (12 h light–dark cycle, 20 ± 2 °C temperature, 60% ± 10% humidity) were carried out. Standard rodent pellet chow ("Cantacuzino" National Institute of Research and Development) and tap water were provided ad libitum. Body weight was recorded once weekly, and their health status and well-being were monitored daily. The applied procedures were in accordance with European Directive 2010/63/EU and approved by the

Ethics Committee for Scientific Research of the George Emil Palade University of Medicine, Pharmacy, Science, and Technology of Targu Mures (approval no. 63/2018).

This study was designed to evaluate the long-term effects of CBD in the PTZ-kindling model of epilepsy. Therefore, to study the protective effects of CBD (60 mg/kg, oral), the drug was administered either 24 h before or 1 h after PTZ injections. The PTZ-kindled animals were randomly divided into two groups, a control group (orally received the vehicle, 1 mL/kg, n = 12) and a CBD-treated group (orally administered CBD, 60 mg/kg, n = 12). All 24 animals underwent the PTZ-kindling procedure, i.e., intraperitoneal injection of a subconvulsive dose of 35 mg/kg PTZ every other day for 50 days. Both the control and the CBD-treated group underwent the same care and injection protocol, and they were evaluated equally. The third group of animals (sham, n = 8) was used to compare the eventual cellular alterations observed by immunohistochemistry; these animals were, every other day, administered i.p. injections of the vehicle instead of PTZ, and they were not treated with CBD.

2.2. Drugs and Reagents

Crystalline cannabidiol (99.5% purity from Trigal Pharma GmbH, Wien, Austria), dissolved in extra virgin olive oil (Salov S.p.A., Massarosa, Italy) was administered to the animals. The individually calculated CBD dose based on the previously measured body weight (60 mg/kg body weight) was administered daily by adsorbing CBD oil onto food pellets. Pellets that were not loaded with CBD, but which were coated with olive oil, were administered to the control group. CBD treatment was initiated at day 0, before the first PTZ injection. The dose of CBD was chosen based on previously published results showing that doses below 50 mg/kg body weight did not exhibit anticonvulsant effects [18,37]. An overview of the experimental design is illustrated in Figure 1.

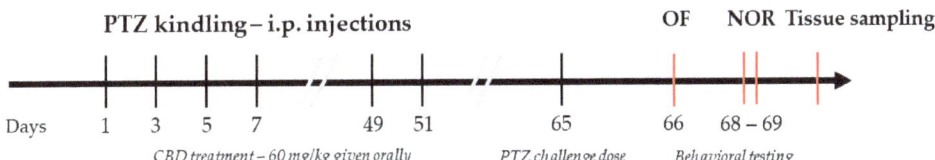

Figure 1. Timeline illustration of the experimental model. Cannabidiol was administered orally in a dose of 60 mg/kg each day, starting from day 0 until achieving a kindled state. Abbreviations: OF, open field test; NOR, novel object recognition test.

The plasma concentration and brain penetration ratio of the formulation (i.e., CBD dissolved in virgin olive oil and adsorbed on food pellets) used in this study was determined using plasma and brain samples obtained from anesthetized animals (ketamine–xylazine 100 mg/kgbw and 10 mg/kgbw, respectively) at two preliminarily determined time points (1 h and 24 h) after administration, corresponding to Cmax and Cmin, respectively. Each interval group consisted of 5 animals. Serum and brains were collected, frozen, and kept at −20 °C until analysis. Ketamin hydrochloride (Bela-Pharm GmbH & Co. KG, Vechta, Germany) and xylazine hydrochloride (Bioveta, Ivanovice na Hané, Czech Republic) were used for anesthesia.

2.3. Determination of Plasma and Brain Levels of CBD

To ensure the proper selectivity accompanied with high sensitivity for the quantification of CBD in rat plasma and homogenized brain tissue samples, liquid chromatography, coupled with mass spectrometric detection (LC–MS), was used. The system was an Agilent 1100 chromatograph equipped with an Agilent Triple Quadrupole MS detector (Agilent G6410A1, Technologies, Santa Clara, CA, USA), realizing the separation by using a Kinetex Polar C18 (100 × 4.6 mm, 2.6 μm, Phenomenex, Torrance, CA, USA) stationary phase with a flowrate of 0.5 mL/min, at 30 °C, with a total runtime of 4.5 min. To support specificity, negative electrospray ionization with multiple-reaction monitoring (MRM) mode was applied, quantifying the ion with 245 m/z, derived from 313 m/z. The potential fragmentation pathway of cannabidiol and the characteristic MRM mass spectrum are presented on Supplementary Figure S1, while the detailed chromatographic conditions are summarized in Supplementary Table S1. The method was partially validated in accordance with the ICH Q2(R2) guideline, demonstrating the specificity, linearity, accuracy, and limit of quantification. The results of the validation procedure are presented in Supplementary Table S2. The obtained chromatograms for the limit of quantification, and representative chromatograms of the plasma and homogenized brain tissue samples are presented on Supplementary Figure S2.

Methanol (Sigma-Aldrich, Steinheim, Germany), acetonitrile (Merck, Darmstadt, Germany), formic acid (Scharlau Chemie, Sentmenat, Spain), and water (Millipore Direct Q10, Merck Millipore, Burlington, MA, USA) used for analytical procedures were of HPLC grade.

Brain and plasma samples were collected on the last day of the experiment (day 70 and day 71, respectively) and underwent the same processing steps as described previously [38]. Briefly, blood obtained via cardiac puncture in K3 EDTA tubes was centrifuged at 3000 g for 10 min at 4 °C within 2 h of collection. The plasma samples were frozen at -20 °C until further pre-analytical processing. Following blood collection, the animals were perfused with approximately 30 mL of normal saline until the entire volume of blood was removed. This technique ensures that the measured concentrations reflect the concentrations in brain tissue by eliminating contributions from brain vasculature. The brains were removed within 7 min of when the thorax was opened. Tissue samples were weighed, homogenized in 5 mL phosphate buffer (PBS) in a grinding ball mill (UltraTurrax Tube Drive, IKA, Königswinter, Germany) for 10 min, and stored at -70 °C until analysis.

Plasma samples were diluted with blank plasma if necessary and mixed with 3 volumes of methanol to induce plasma protein precipitation. The mixture was vortexed for 10 s and then centrifuged (Sigma 2–15 centrifuge, Sigma, Osterode am Harz, Germany) for 10 min at 9167 g. The supernatant was diluted with a mobile phase and injected into the LC-MS/MS system. Homogenized brain tissue samples underwent the same procedures as plasma samples.

2.4. Pentylenetetrazole Induced Kindling Model (PTZ-Kindling)

Pentylenetetrazole (PTZ, Sigma Aldrich, St. Louis, MO, USA) was dissolved in 0.9% saline at a concentration of 35 mg/mL and injected intraperitoneally (i.p.) in a volume of 1.0 mL/kg at a sub-convulsive dose of 35 mg/kg according to the previously published schedule [39,40]. Seizure scoring was performed in real-time, followed by two blinded observers' confirmation of the registered data. Briefly, after each PTZ injection, rats were housed singly in transparent plexiglass cages and monitored for 1 h. Seizure intensities were rated by one experienced observer according to a modified Racine scale as follows: 0 = no response; 1 = ear and facial twitching; 2 = myoclonic jerks without rearing; 3 = myoclonic jerks with rearing; 4 = turning over into side position with tonic-clonic seizures; 5 = turning over into back position, generalized tonic-clonic convulsions, and loss of balance and falling. The same scoring scale was used by the two blinded observers who analyzed the video registrations offline. The final seizure score was established by combining the scores given by each observer.

An animal was considered kindled when it had experienced stage 4 or 5 seizures on two consecutive trials. At the beginning of the experiment, the sensitivity to the convulsant action of PTZ was assessed, and animals having two consecutive stage 5 seizures after the first two PTZ doses were not included in the study.

2.5. Behavioral Assays

For the assessment of the behavioral aspects, open field (OF) and novel object recognition (NOR) tests were performed at days 66 and 68–69, respectively (Figure 1).

2.5.1. Open Field Test

The OF test was performed in a 60 × 60 cm black-based box with transparent walls, with a height of 50 cm, to observe the animals' locomotor and exploratory behavior. The illumination in the testing room was controlled and maintained between 50 and 100 lux. After the animals were placed in the middle of the testing area, their behavior was recorded for five minutes from above. After each test, 70% ethanol was used to disinfect the apparatus. All trials were analyzed offline with EthoVision XT (version 11.5, Noldus IT, Wageningen, The Netherlands), monitoring the distance moved, the number of entries, and the time spent in the center zone (central 30 × 30 cm area), vertical activity (wall climbing, rearing), and grooming activity.

2.5.2. Novel Object Recognition Test

In an empty testing chamber (60 × 60 cm), animals were habituated for 10 min, then returned to their home cage, and the chamber was cleaned as described above. In the familiarization phase, two identical novel objects constructed of wood (10 × 4 × 4 cm) were placed in the chamber (30 cm apart from each other) (Supplementary Figure S3). Object placement was chosen so that animals could walk freely around the arena's edge, as they would have done in an open field. Thus, the animals were required to move into the center of the chamber to interact with the objects rather than unintentionally encountering them as they explored the arena perimeter.

Observations of animal activity were conducted for 5 min. A nose touch was classified as an interaction with an object. For the subsequent memory test, the animals had to interact with each object for at least 2.5 s during the familiarization phase. The animals were returned to their home cages after their five-minute time frame had ended. Before each test, the chamber and objects were cleaned with a 70% ethanol solution.

The inter-trial interval between familiarization and testing was 24 h. One of the familiar objects encountered during the familiarization phase was then replaced with a novel object, which was different in color and configuration but about the same size. Across tests, the position of the novel object (i.e., left or right) was counterbalanced. Following the same procedure as the one during familiarization, animals were reintroduced to the chamber and allowed to explore it for five minutes. Time spent by the animal in exploring individual objects during familiarization phase, total time spent by the animal in exploring both objects during the test and training phase, the total distance moved, the time spent moving, and the number of rears were quantified by a computerized analysis system (EthoVision XT, version 11.5, Noldus IT, Wageningen, The Netherlands).

2.6. Histological Staining

2.6.1. Perfusion and Brain Sectioning

A mixture of ketamine–xylazine (100 mg/kgbw and 10 mg /kgbw) was injected intraperitoneally to induce deep anesthesia. Rats were perfused transcardially with ice-cold normal saline solution (0.9%, for 1.5 min), followed by ice-cold fixative solution containing 4% paraformaldehyde (Sigma Aldrich, St. Louis, MO, USA) and 0.25% picric acid (Sigma Aldrich, St. Louis, MO, USA) in 0.1 M phosphate buffer (PB, pH = 7.4, Sigma Aldrich, St. Louis, MO, USA) for 20 min. After perfusion, the brains were removed from the skull and postfixed overnight in 4% PFA. Then, 60 µm-thick coronal sections were cut with a vibratome (VT 1000S, Leica, Nussloch, Germany) and washed in 0.1 M PB.

2.6.2. Fluorescent Immunohistochemistry

Triple immunofluorescent staining was used to visualize neurons, astrocytes, and microglia. Brain sections were transferred into a 24-well tissue culture plate (TPP, Trasadingen, Switzerland) and were immunostained in a free-floating manner in a 500 µL volume on an orbital shaker (Heidolph Instruments, Schwabach, Germany). After three 10 min washes in 0.1 M PB, sections were washed three times for 10 min in tris-buffered saline (TBS), then blocked in TBS containing 10% normal horse serum (NHS; Vector Laboratories,

Burlingame, CA, USA) and 0.1% Triton-X (Sigma-Aldrich, St. Louis, MO, USA) for 45 min, in order to block nonspecific binding sites and to enhance antibody penetration.

Sections were then incubated with the primary antibodies against NeuN for neurons (NeuN; guinea pig raised-polyclonal, dilution 1:500; product no: 266004, Synaptics Systems GmbH, Goettingen, Germany), GFAP for astrocytes (GFAP; mouse raised-monoclonal dilution 1:500; product no: 173211, Synaptics Systems GmbH, Goettingen, Germany), and IBA1 for microglia (IBA1; rabbit raised-polyclonal, dilution 1:500; HistoSure: HS234013, Synaptics Systems GmbH, Goettingen, Germany) in 0.1% TBS-T overnight at room temperature.

The next day, sections were washed thoroughly in TBS, then fluorescently labeled secondary antibodies made up in TBS were applied at room temperature for 4 h to label the NeuN immunostaining with Alexa488-conjugated donkey anti-guineapig (1:500, Jackson ImmunoResearch Laboratories, West Grove, PA, USA), to label the GFAP immunostaining with Alexa647-conjugated donkey anti-mouse (1:500, Jackson ImmunoResearch Laboratories, West Grove, PA, USA) and to label the IBA1 immunostaining with Alexa594-conjugated donkey anti-rabbit (1:500, Jackson ImmunoResearch Laboratories, West Grove, PA, USA).

Afterwards, stained sections were washed 3 times for 20 min in TBS and 2 times for 10 min in 0.1 M PB, mounted on slides and coverslipped with a mounting medium (Vectashield, Vector Laboratories, Burlingame, CA, USA) and sealed with nail polish.

2.6.3. Confocal Image Acquisition and Analysis of Fluorescent Immunostaining

The digitalization of sections was conducted using confocal microscopy. To obtain high-resolution z-stacks, all images were acquired using a Leica TCS SP8 confocal laser scanning microscope (Leica Microsystems GmbH, Wetzlar, Germany) using HC PL APO CS2 20X/0.75 and HC PL APO CS40X/0.85 dry objectives and unidirectional scanning at 200 Hz. Images were processed and quantified using the Leica Application Suite X (Leica Microsystems GmbH, Wetzlar, Germany) software. High-magnification images of 1024 × 1024 pixels were collected, and regions of interest (ROIs) in individual sections were selected (400 μm × 600 μm). Z-stack deepness was defined as 5 μm, each image comprising of 3 subsequent z-stack layers, resulting in 10 μm-deep recordings. The image of the hippocampal sample was acquired in three different channels. The NeuN staining was used to distinguish hippocampal regions and layers based on the density and relative location of the cells. Light signals from photon scatter around the edges of tissue, tears in the tissue, and vasculature were excluded from analysis.

Fluorescence intensity was measured over ROIs, then corrected for autofluorescence and non-specific signals using a background subtraction. Astrocytes, microglia, and neuronal debris in CA1 and CA3 were consistently counted in the same area in all slices and were expressed as cells/mm^2. Image J software was used for manual cell-counting. Three sections from each slide, four slides per animal, and five to eight animals per group were used for histological assessment.

Custom Cell Counter Algorithm

For the validation of cell-counting procedures, all ROIs previously investigated were cropped and split to separate RGB (red–green–blue) channels using the Image J software. Each immunostaining channel (green for NeuN, cyan for GFAP, and red for IBA1, respectively) were further analyzed by our custom cell-counter algorithm written in the Python programming language (version 3.9.9), implementing the OpenCV library (version 4.5.5). ROIs were preprocessed by Gaussian blurring, in order to reduce background noise. Desirable foreground image objects were evidentiated using adaptive thresholding, which was followed by morphological opening and closing functions, based on the extent of cell clustering and overall image quality. Next, the area and longest diagonal of all cell-like structures were calculated. If any surface detected had an overlap of at least 60% with another in the subsequent layers and its longest diagonal exceeded the value corresponding to 6.5 μm, the element could be considered a cell. Cellular debris was defined as NeuN-positive fragments with dimensions between 2.5 and 6.5 µm, encircled by GFAP-positive astrocyte signals as described previously [41]. Finally, all cell contours were projected on the original ROI, thus enabling a visual inspection of the detected structures (Figure 2).

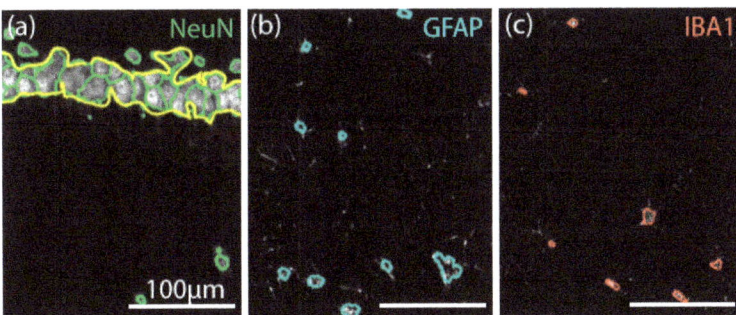

Figure 2. Analysis of different cell types by a cell-counter algorithm. (**a**) NeuN+ cells (green) with an explicitly delimited pyramidal layer (yellow), (**b**) GFAP+ (cyan), and (**c**) IBA1+ (red) cells evidentiated and contoured by our custom cell-counter algorithm. All three immunostainings are superposed in their z-stack maximum-intensity projections.

2.7. Statistical Analysis

Data were analyzed using GraphPad Prism 8 (version 8.0.1, GraphPad Software Inc., San Diego, CA, USA). Differences in survival curves were tested using the log-rank test (Mantel-Cox). Kolmogorov–Smirnov tests were performed on each set of data to determine whether it had a normal distribution. Non-normally distributed data was analyzed with a Mann–Whitney test; otherwise, an unpaired t test was used. For matched observations, a two-way ANOVA with Sidak's multiple comparison test was used. The mixed-effect model with Geisser–Greenhouse correction was used in case of missing values. An alpha value of 0.05 was used as the cutoff for significance.

3. Results

3.1. Seizure Score

Twenty-four rats were used for PTZ kindling, from which 18 ended up reaching a kindled state and, due to this, were each consecutively tested with a challenge dose of PTZ. The remaining six animals ($n = 5$ in the kindled and $n = 1$ in the CBD-treated group) died before completing the study, so the behavioral assessment was performed on $n = 7$ kindled and $n = 11$ CBD-treated animals. The mortality rate tended to decrease following chronic CBD treatment (5/12 vs. 1/12, Chi square = 3.429, $p = 0.064$, Figure 3a), especially in the early phase of the kindling.

Analyzing the parameters characterizing the development of the kindling process, it was observed that the total number of PTZ injections required to achieve a kindled state did not show a significant difference between CBD-treated and control groups (median 15.5 vs. 16, $p = 0.833$, Figure 3b). The seizure scores registered during kindling were analyzed using the mixed-effect model with Geisser–Greenhouse correction, and it was noted that the time factor was significant in the development of generalized seizures (Racine 4 and 5 seizures) for both groups ($F (1.667, 16.39) = 53.63$, $p < 0.001$, Figure 3c). However, treatment and the time x treatment interaction were not significant ($F (1, 15) = 2.397$, $p = 0.142$ and $F (6, 59) = 1.174$, $p = 0.333$, respectively). Furthermore, there was no difference in the duration of generalized seizures between the CBD-treated and control groups (74 ± 25.7 vs. 89 ± 40 s, $p = 0.425$). Conversely, the mean (± SEM) latency to first generalized seizure was significantly longer in the CBD-treated group (925.3 ± 120.0 vs. 550.1 ± 69.62 s, Figure 3d), and the mixed-effects analysis confirmed that treatment had a significant influence on this parameter ($F (1, 15) = 6.3872$, $p = 0.023$).

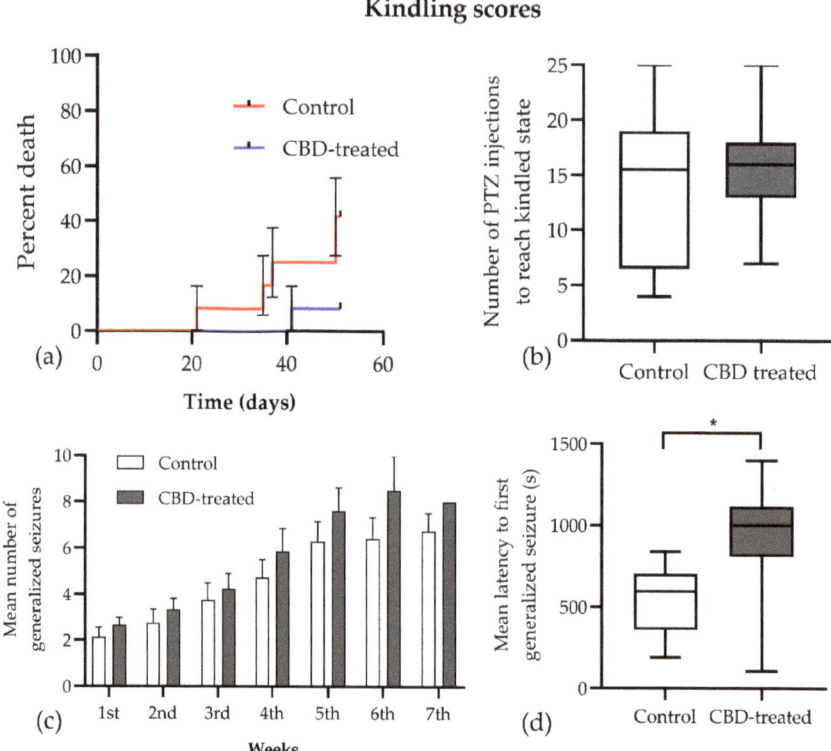

Figure 3. Effects of chronic CBD treatment on the kindling scores induced by pentylenetetrazole in rats. The development of kindling was characterized by the following parameters: (**a**) mortality rate due to generalized seizures, (**b**) the total number of PTZ injections to reach the kindled state, (**c**) the number of generalized seizures, and (**d**) the latency to the first generalized seizure. Data are expressed as mean ± SEM in the bar graph and as mean (solid line) with the range in the floating bar graphs; * $p < 0.05$ vs. control.

The challenge dose of PTZ induced the same seizure pattern in both groups, and all animals had Racine 5 seizures that did not differ in duration between groups (127.4 ± 63.58 vs. 131.2 ± 31.53 s, $p = 0.312$). However, the latency to maximal seizure in the CBD-treated group showed high variability among animals (777.8 ± 228.4 vs. 651.1 ± 220.0 s, Figure 4a) with no significant differences between groups ($t(15) = 0.397$, $p = 0.697$).

3.2. CBD Plasma and Brain Concentrations

To verify whether the in-house-prepared CBD solution administered by the oral route would achieve the desired concentrations at the site of action, serum and brain CBD concentrations were assessed at 1 h and 24 h after administration, corresponding to Cmax and Cmin, respectively. The mean peak concentration was 1976.1 ± 1151.41 ng/mL in serum and 5260 ± 3284 ng/g in brain, while the minimum concentrations were 24.2 ± 3.25 ng/mL and 91.4 ± 20 ng/g, respectively (Table 1). Brain-to-plasma ratios calculated for each animal showed higher values at 24 h compared to 1 h after administration, suggesting a slower brain CBD-elimination rate.

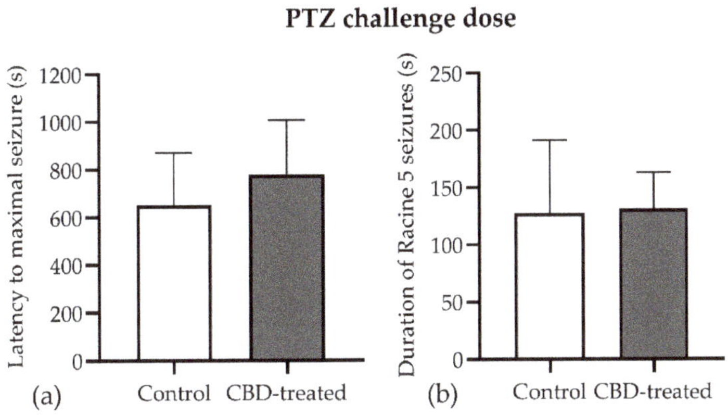

PTZ challenge dose

Figure 4. Lack of long-term effect of CBD (60 mg/kg) in the PTZ-kindling model. (**a**) Latency to maximal seizure observed after PTZ injection. (**b**) Duration of the generalized seizures (clonic convulsion with loss of righting reflex and/or bouncing, two or more clonic convulsions, tonic convulsion or status epilepticus) induced by a challenge dose of PTZ. Data are expressed as mean ± SEM (n = 7–11) for each parameter.

Table 1. Cannabidiol concentrations in plasma and brain at Cmax and Cmin after the oral administration of 60 mg/kg body weight.

CBD Concentrations	Rat #	Plasma Concentration (ng/mL)	Brain Concentration (ng/g)	Brain-to-Plasma Ratio
1 h after administration	1	259.93	1058.50	4.072
	2	6326.57	16,886.61	2.669
	3	800.39	1475.58	1.844
	4	198.69	642.07	3.232
	5	2295.02	2455.34	1.070
	Mean	1976.12	5260.6	2.577
	SEM	1151.41	3284.0	0.524
24 h after administration	6	23.20	111.08	4.788
	7	26.20	79.98	3.053
	8	28.67	105.28	3.672
	9	22.50	- *	-
	10	20.40	69.35	3.400
	Mean	24.19	91.4	3.728
	SEM	3.25	20.0	0.336

* As a result of inadequate tissue perfusion, the brain tissue sample was excluded from analysis. # Data points are labeled by rat number.

3.3. Open Field Test

Chronic CBD treatment had no effect on exploratory and locomotor parameters in the open field test. The control animals apparently entered more times in the center zone of the arena (7.4 ± 15.1 vs. 3.43 ± 5.62, p = 0.77, Figure 5a), but they spent the same amount of time exploring it (17.69 ± 4.48 vs. 18.15 ± 2.49, p = 0.92, Figure 5b). The distance travelled and the vertical exploration expressed as supported rearings did not vary between groups (p > 0.05) (Figure 5c,d).

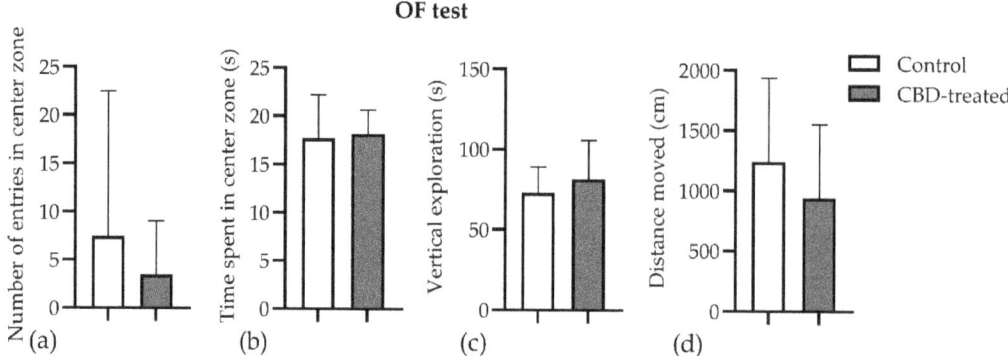

Figure 5. Assessment of locomotor activity in the open field. Rats were submitted to a PTZ-kindling protocol with or without chronic cannabidiol (60 mg/kg body weight) administration (mean ± SEM, n = 18). (**a**) The number of entries in the center zone; (**b**) time spent in the central zone of the arena, defined as a 30 × 30 cm square out of an 60 × 60 cm total surface of the arena; (**c**) the vertical exploration of the animals was expressed as the time spent leaning on the walls of the arena; (**d**) total distance moved during the 5 min testing session. CBD, cannabidiol. Data are expressed as mean ± SEM (n = 7–11) for each parameter.

3.4. Novel Object Recognition Test

There was no effect of CBD treatment on the total distance traveled and on the exploration time of the arena or objects. Conversely, the mean discrimination index was decreased by CBD treatment (0.57 ± 0.15 vs. −0.01 ± 0.17, p = 0.0367, Figure 6). The results indicate that CBD-treated animals were impaired in distinguishing between the novel and familiar objects.

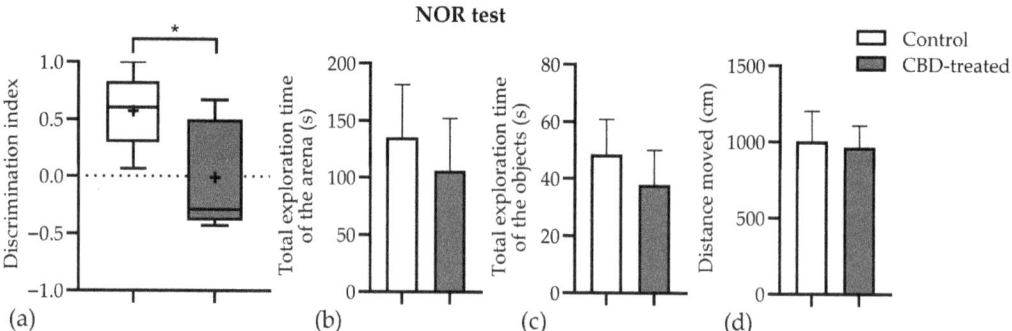

Figure 6. The effects of chronic CBD (60 mg/kg body weight) treatment on cognitive performance of rats subjected to a PTZ-kindling protocol. (**a**) Discrimination index (DI), which shows the discrimination between the novel and familiar objects, i.e., the difference in exploration time for a familiar object, but then dividing this value by the total amount of exploration of the novel and familiar objects [DI = (TN − TF)/(TN + TF)] showed a significant decrease in the CBD-treated group. + sign shows the arithmetic mean, whereas the line represents the median; (**b**) the total exploration time of the arena (mean ± SEM) did not show statistically significant difference between groups; (**c**) the total exploration time of the objects (mean ± SEM) was also similar for both groups; (**d**) the total distance moved by both groups (mean ± SEM) during the 5 min testing session was almost equal, and the results were similar to those found in the OF test. CBD, cannabidiol; * p < 0.05 vs. control. Data are expressed as mean ± SEM (n = 7–11) for each parameter.

3.5. Fluorescent Immunohistochemistry

3.5.1. Validation of Manual and Algorithmic Cell Counter Strategies

Neurons, astrocytes, and microglia were triple-immunostained in the hippocampus, where the CA1 and CA3 regions were analyzed (Figure 7). Sham, i.e., healthy control ($n = 6$), PTZ-kindled control ($n = 5$), and CBD-treated ($n = 8$) groups showed different pattern of immunostaining for astrocytes labeled with anti-GFAP antibody (cyan), for neurons labeled with anti-NeuN antibody (green), and for microglia labeled with anti-IBA1 antibody (red).

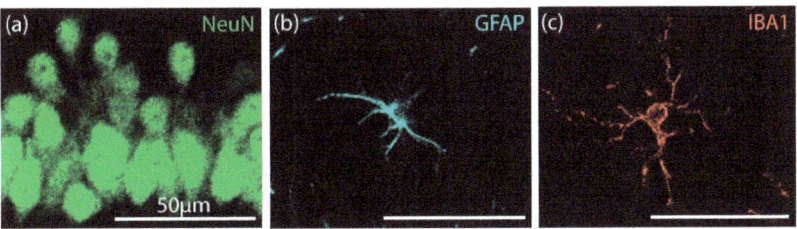

Figure 7. Neuron, astocyte, and microglia triade. Representative confocal microscopy image of the tripple immunostaining of the (**a**) neuron-NeuN, (**b**) astrocyte-GFAP, and (**c**) microglia-IBA1 in the CA3 subfield of the hippocampus.

We used a custom cell-counter algorithm to quantify the cells of interest. The manual counting method was used as the reference method. The mean of the two observers was compared with the values provided by the algorithm. For the statistical analysis the bias, precision and limits of agreement were used as proposed by Bland and Altman to compare two methods of measurement. The methods were considered to be interchangeable if the bias was smaller than ±10% for each cell type and if there was no tendency of the difference to increase with the mean (Supplementary Figure S4).

3.5.2. Effects of CBD on the Neuron–Astrocyte–Microglia Triad in the Hippocampus

The thickness of the stratum pyramidale showed differences between groups, a two-way ANOVA analysis showing a significant impact of CBD treatment (F (2, 119) = 3.963, $p = 0.02$). The PTZ-kindling procedure decreased the stratum pyramidale thickness compared to sham animals, and CBD treatment induced a further significant thinning in the CA3. A similar tendency could be observed in the pyramidal layer of the CA1 region as well, but it did not reach significance (Figure 8a, Supplementary Figure S5).

The cell density of GFAP-positive astrocytes was decreased by CBD treatment (F (2, 119) = 6.546, $p = 0.002$,) both in the CA1 and CA3 regions of the hippocampus (Figure 8b). The post hoc analysis confirmed that the CBD-treated group had significantly decreased astrocyte density in the CA1 region ($p = 0.045$). Conversely, neither the PTZ-kindling nor the CBD treatment had any effect on the total number of IBA1-positive cells (F (2, 119) = 0.2522, $p = 0.78$, Figure 8c).

Neuronal debris, i.e., fragments of NeuN positive cells closely attached to the branches of astrocytes in the stratum radiatum, was observed in both the CA1 and the CA3 regions. Despite the fact that PTZ-kindling did not influence the density of neuronal debris when compared to sham animals, the CBD-treated group had significantly decreased neuronal debris in the CA3 region of the hippocampus when compared to PTZ-kindled controls (Figure 8d, $p = 0.0359$).

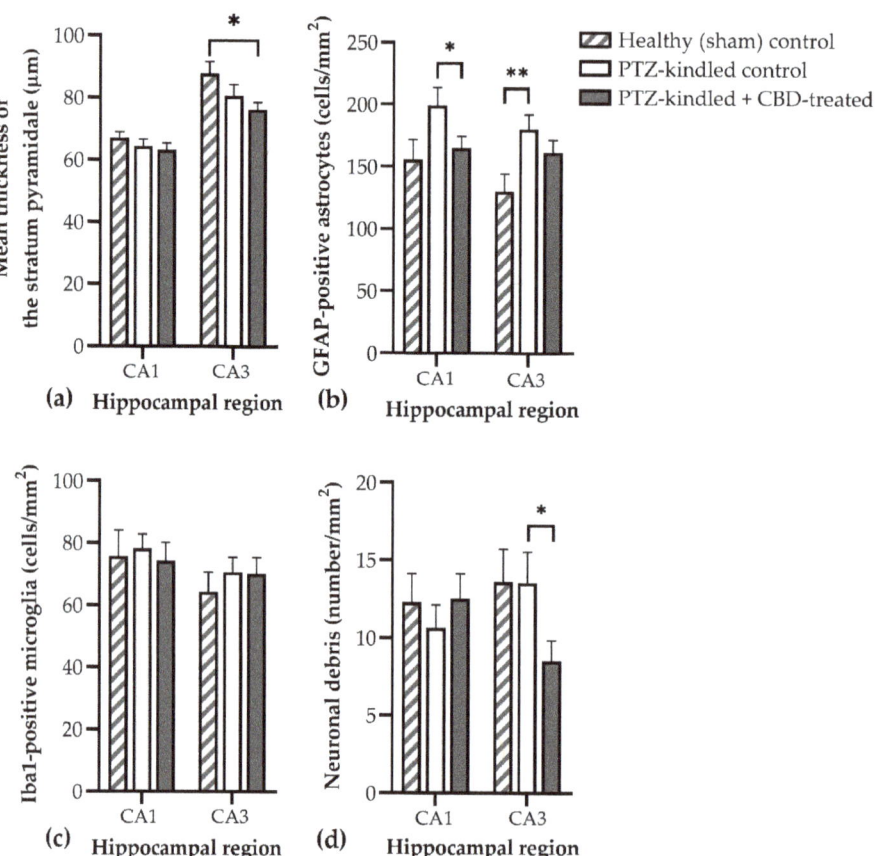

Figure 8. Effects of chronic CBD (60 mg/kg body weight) treatment on the hippocampal reorganization induced by PTZ-kindling in rats. (**a**) Mean thickness of the pyramidal cell layer; (**b**) the density of GFAP-positive astrocytes; (**c**) the density of IBA1-positive microglia; (**d**) the density of neuronal debris, defined as NeuN-positive fragments surrounded by astrocytes. Data are expressed as mean ± SEM (n = 5–8).; CBD, cannabidiol; * $p < 0.05$; ** $p < 0.01$.

4. Discussion

This study revealed that chronic treatment with CBD reduced seizure-related mortality and prolonged the latency for the appearance of generalized seizures in PTZ-kindled rats. However, the development of kindling and the maximum seizure severity were not influenced. Interestingly, CBD treatment decreased the cognitive performance of rats in the NOR test. Furthermore, at the cellular level, the CA3 and CA1 regions of the hippocampal formation of CBD-treated rats showed significant differences compared to PTZ-kindled controls, which may explain the decreased mortality and cognitive performance.

CBD has been demonstrated to affect the central nervous system dose-dependently without any psychoactive action. In low doses, it showed anxiolytic and antidepressive-like effects [4,42–47] like serotonergic drugs [48,49], whereas in higher doses (30–100 mg/kg), its anticonvulsant and antipsychotic actions were proven [1,16,18,19,37]. There are, however, many discrepancies between the previously reported results, which may partly be attributed to the unfavorable pharmacokinetic properties of CBD. It is possible that highly lipophilic drugs such as CBD can precipitate in the stomach when administered orally in the form of suspensions, resulting in prolonged absorbtion, a long time to peak plasma concentration, and low bioavailability [50]. Moreover, the vehicle of administration was shown to significantly influence the Cmax and AUC of CBD [51]. Although this issue is clearly present in laboratory experiments as well, very few studies have provided data about the pharmacokinetics of CBD formulations administered to animals [37,52].

To achieve better bioavailability, CBD was dispersed in olive oil and incorporated into the food pellets. The obtained results showed that brain concentrations correlated well with the plasma concentrations, and the brain-to-plasma ratio was consistently higher 24 h after administration, which indicates the high affinity of CBD to brain tissue. These brain concentrations are very similar to those reported recently by Uttl et al. [37]. However, plasma concentrations obtained at 1 h after administration showed that, in some cases, absorbtion was not complete. So, this study confirmed that CBD, even when dissolved in oil, which is the most common formulation of CBD used in humans, showed significant variations in the absorption phase, making the study of peak-time effects challenging, which could underlie the controversial results published previously. Hence, future studies should relate CBD's effects to its plasma concentration, rather than the dose administered.

The most important finding of this study is that CBD decreased seizure-related mortality and increased the latency to tonic-clonic seizures in the PTZ-kindling model, although it was not tested at peak plasma/brain concentrations. From a translational point-of-view, this result may provide evidence for the long-term protective action of CBD against the progression of epileptic syndromes and the potential prevention of breakthrough seizures. As previously reported, a single administration of CBD at different doses exhibits anticonvulsant effects in several animal models of epilepsy, but it does not necessarily reduce the frequency or the severity of seizures. In contrast, CBD modified the duration of generalized seizures, the latency to seizure onset, and the mortality [1,12,14,16,18,19,53]. In pilocarpine-induced seizures, CBD administered at 100 mg/kg doses did not affect the severity of seizures [14]. However, the same study reported a reduction in mortality and the occurrence of tonic-clonic seizures in the penicillin model of partial seizure [14]. The reduction of seizure duration and the increase of the latency to first seizure by CBD at a dose of 60 mg/kg were also reported after the acute intraperitoneal administration of PTZ [19].

When administered for a longer period, CBD delayed the progression of kindling in PTZ-kindled mice, but it did not prevent generalized seizures [19]. In rats, Mao et al. reported a decrease of the mean seizure score and the kindling rate in the CBD-treated group (50 mg/kg administered intraperitoneally) [18]. However, CBD was administered before PTZ injections in both studies; thus, the observed anticonvulsant action corresponds to the peak-time effect of CBD described after acute administration. In an interesting approach, Hosseinzadeh et al. demonstrated that the intracerebroventricular injection of CBD might have long-term protective effects in the pilocarpine model of epilepsy in rats [16], and the neuroprotective effects of CBD described by in vitro and in vivo studies [1,54] point to the potential benefits of chronic adjunctive treatment with CBD. On the other hand, it is important to differentiate between epileptic seizures and epilepsy syndromes. CBD is currently approved for the treatment of seizures associated with Lennox–Gastaut syndrome or Dravet syndrome based on a favorable benefit–risk profile [10], but there is little evidence about its effectiveness in other types of epileptic seizures. Therefore, the present study proposed to study the effects of CBD on seizures by delivering the seizure-precipitating factor (i.e., PTZ injection) outside of CBD's maximal anticonvulsant protection. The only significant difference between the treatment groups was the prolonged latency to the first generalized seizure; the other parameters related to kindling were not modified by CBD treatment. Interestingly, this led to a reduced mortality rate in the CBD-treated group, which is in agreement with previous studies [12].

The next important finding of this study is the effects of chronic CBD treatment on the cognitive performance of PTZ-kindled rats. CBD has been proposed to exert neuroprotective effects in epilepsy [55] and possesses several mechanisms to protect against memory impairments in various diseases [23]. However, a dose-dependent nature of these neuroprotective effects was also demonstrated, the lower and middle range doses (5–20 mg/kg) showing improvements in memory assessment tasks [56]. In this experiment, the decrease of the discrimination index in the NOR test clearly showed that CBD-treated animals could not recall the familiar object and interacted with both familiar and novel objects more equally. Studies have shown that the hippocampus plays a significant role in object-recognition memory. If this structure is damaged, there will be moderate and reliable changes in anterograde memory [57]. The histological analysis of the hippocampal formation revealed that CBD-treated animals had a reduced thickness of the stratum pyramidale in the CA3 and CA1 regions. As confirmed by others, this measurement of stratum pyramidale thickness is robust and constant, because it does not differ across a series of coronal sections collected around the anteroposterior axis of the same animal [58]. Additionally, stratum pyramidale thickness was shown to reflect the neurodegeneration caused by toxic substances such as cadmium [59] and amyloidbetapeptide 1–40 [60] in rat models with cognitive impairments similar to those observed in this study.

On the other hand, CBD treatment decreased the number of GFAP-positive astrocytes to sham levels. The results of this study confirmed again that PTZ-kindling induces astrogliosis in the CA3 and CA1 regions of the hippocampus [61] and that CBD treatment prevents the proliferation of astrocytes [18]. Astrocytes were demonstrated to play an important role in epileptogenesis by releasing inflammatory cytokines and altering the excitability of the neurons [62]. The reduction in mortality in the CBD-treated group may be due to the long-term antiproliferative effects of CBD on astrocytes, which may be part of a promising novel therapeutic strategy targeting neuroinflammation [63].

Furthermore, it is important to note that the number of microglial cells in the hippocampus was not significantly influenced by CBD; however, a decreasing trend was observed. Microgliosis was also linked with epileptogenesis, especially in the status epilepticus models of epilepsy [64]. Although it seems to play a role in the increased excitability of the neurons, its involvement in cognitive impairment was not demonstrated yet. As a limitation of the study, it should be noted that only one microglia-specific histological marker was used (i.e., IBA1), which did not allow the investigation of microglial activation. Another important cellular marker of neuronal apoptosis may be neuronal debris, as described by Lana et al. [41,65–67]. This study showed that CBD-treated rats had a decreased number of neuronal debris in the stratum radiatum, despite a lower number of astrocytes, which suggests that microglial activity had an important contribution to the clearance of neuronal debris in this group. Further studies using specific microglial activation and apoptosis markers are needed to fully understand the effects of CBD on the interplay between neurons, astrocytes, and microglia.

5. Conclusions

Chronic CBD treatment did not prevent PTZ-induced kindling in rats, but a reduction in mortality associated with prolonged status epilepticus was observed. Analyzing the seizure activities, it was found that the frequency and duration were not influenced by CBD, but the latency to the first generalized seizure was increased. The NOR test showed that CBD treatment impaired recognition memory, which may warrant further investigation. The main findings of the study (i.e., reduced mortality and cognitive dysfunction) may be connected to the observed hippocampal histological changes, such as reduced thickness of the stratum pyramidale or decreased astrogliosis.

Supplementary Materials: The following supporting information can be downloaded at: https://www.mdpi.com/article/10.3390/biomedicines10081811/s1, Figure S1: The potential fragmentation of CBD in negative electrospray ionization and the characteristic MRM mass spectrum of CBD (313 $m/z \rightarrow$ 245 m/z, collision energy: 20 eV); Figure S2: The chromatograms obtained for the quantification limits (A: plasma with 1 ng/mL CBD and B: homogenized brain sample with 1 ng/ml CBD) and the representative chromatograms of the real samples (C: plasma with 47.3 ng/ml CBD and D: homogenized brain sample with 6.0 ng/ml CBD); Figure S3: Schematic illustration of the novel object recognition task; Figure S4: Bland–Altman plots representing the agreement between the cell counter algorithm and human manual counting of NeuN, GFAP, and IBA1 positive cells in the rat hippocampus; Figure S5: Representative image of morphological changes in the CA3 hippocampal pyramidal layer of (a) PTZ kindled controls and (b) CBD treated rats; Table S1: The chromatographic conditions and the MS detector parameters used for the analysis of plasma and homogenized brain tissue samples; Table S2: The summary of the analytical method validation process.

Author Contributions: Conceptualization, Z.G. and K.K.; formal analysis, S.V. and M.K.; funding acquisition, Z.G.; investigation, Z.G., K.K., A.T., R.B. and M.U.; methodology, K.K., A.T., E.F. and S.V.; project administration, Z.G.; software, Z.G., K.K., A.T., I.Z., I.S. and R.B.; supervision, S.V. and M.K.; validation, S.V. and M.K.; visualization, Z.G., K.K. and R.B.; writing—original draft, Z.G., K.K., E.F. and M.U.; writing—review and editing, R.B. and M.K. All authors have read and agreed to the published version of the manuscript.

Funding: This work was supported by the University of Medicine, Pharmacy, Science and Technology "George Emil Palade" of Târgu Mureș Research grant number 293/3/14.01.2020.

Institutional Review Board Statement: The animal study protocol was approved by the Ethics Committee of George Emil Palade University of Medicine, Pharmacy, Science, and Technology of Targu Mures (63/2018).

Informed Consent Statement: Not applicable.

Data Availability Statement: The data presented in this study are available on request from the corresponding author.

Acknowledgments: The authors thank Trigal Pharma GmbH (Wien, Austria) for donating the crystalline cannabidiol used in this study.

Conflicts of Interest: The authors declare no conflict of interest. The funders had no role in the design of the study; in the collection, analyses, or interpretation of data; in the writing of the manuscript, or in the decision to publish the results.

References

1. Devinsky, O.; Roberta Cilio, M.; Cross, H.; Fernandez-Ruiz, J.; French, J.; Hill, C.; Katz, R.; Consultant, I.; Di Marzo, V.; Jutras-Aswad, D.; et al. Cannabidiol: Pharmacology and potential therapeutic role in epilepsy and other neuropsychiatric disorders. CRITICAL REVIEW AND INVITED COMMENTARY. *Epilepsia* **2014**, *55*, 791–802. [CrossRef] [PubMed]
2. Khoury, J.M.; Neves, M.d.C.L.d.; Roque, M.A.V.; Queiroz, D.A.d.B.; Corrêa de Freitas, A.A.; de Fátima, Â.; Moreira, F.A.; Garcia, F.D. Is there a role for cannabidiol in psychiatry? *World J. Biol. Psychiatry* **2019**, *20*, 101–116. [CrossRef]
3. Silvestro, S.; Mammana, S.; Cavalli, E.; Bramanti, P.; Mazzon, E. Use of Cannabidiol in the Treatment of Epilepsy: Efficacy and Security in Clinical Trials. *Molecules* **2019**, *24*, 1459. [CrossRef]
4. Gáll, Z.; Farkas, S.; Albert, Á.; Ferencz, E.; Vancea, S.; Urkon, M.; Kolcsár, M. Effects of Chronic Cannabidiol Treatment in the Rat Chronic Unpredictable Mild Stress Model of Depression. *Biomolecules* **2020**, *10*, 801. [CrossRef] [PubMed]
5. Bonaccorso, S.; Ricciardi, A.; Zangani, C.; Chiappini, S.; Schifano, F. Cannabidiol (CBD) use in psychiatric disorders: A systematic review. *Neurotoxicology* **2019**, *74*, 282–298. [CrossRef]
6. Gonçalves, E.C.D.; Baldasso, G.M.; Bicca, M.A.; Paes, R.S.; Capasso, R.; Dutra, R.C. Terpenoids, Cannabimimetic Ligands, beyond the Cannabis Plant. *Molecules* **2020**, *25*, 1567. [CrossRef]
7. Ibeas Bih, C.; Chen, T.; Nunn, A.V.W.; Bazelot, M.; Dallas, M.; Whalley, B.J. Molecular Targets of Cannabidiol in Neurological Disorders. *Neurotherapeutics* **2015**, *12*, 699–730. [CrossRef] [PubMed]
8. Katona, I. Cannabis and Endocannabinoid Signaling in Epilepsy. In *Endocannabinoids. Handbook of Experimental Pharmacology*; Pertwee, R., Ed.; Springer: Cham, Switzerland, 2015; pp. 285–316.
9. Boczek, T.; Zylinska, L. Receptor-dependent and independent regulation of voltage-gated ca^{2+} channels and ca^{2+}-permeable channels by endocannabinoids in the brain. *Int. J. Mol. Sci.* **2021**, *22*, 8168. [CrossRef] [PubMed]
10. Chen, J.W.; Borgelt, L.M.; Blackmer, A.B. Cannabidiol: A New Hope for Patients With Dravet or Lennox-Gastaut Syndromes. *Ann. Pharmacother.* **2019**, *53*, 603–611. [CrossRef] [PubMed]
11. Wise, J. European drug agency approves cannabis-based medicine for severe forms of epilepsy. *BMJ* **2019**, *366*, l5708. [CrossRef]
12. Jones, N.A.; Hill, A.J.; Smith, I.; Bevan, S.A.; Williams, C.M.; Whalley, B.J.; Stephens, G.J. Cannabidiol Displays Antiepileptiform and Antiseizure Properties In Vitro and In Vivo. *J. Pharmacol. Exp. Ther.* **2010**, *332*, 569–577. [CrossRef]
13. Consroe, P.; Benedito, M.A.C.; Leite, J.R.; Carlini, E.A.; Mechoulam, R. Effects of cannabidiol on behavioral seizures caused by convulsant drugs or current in mice. *Eur. J. Pharmacol.* **1982**, *83*, 293–298. [CrossRef]
14. Jones, N.A.; Glyn, S.E.; Akiyama, S.; Hill, T.D.M.; Hill, A.J.; Weston, S.E.; Burnett, M.D.A.; Yamasaki, Y.; Stephens, G.J.; Whalley, B.J.; et al. Cannabidiol exerts anti-convulsant effects in animal models of temporal lobe and partial seizures. *Seizure* **2012**, *21*, 344–352. [CrossRef] [PubMed]

15. Bialer, M.; Johannessen, S.I.; Levy, R.H.; Perucca, E.; Tomson, T.; White, H.S. Progress report on new antiepileptic drugs: A summary of the Twelfth Eilat Conference (EILAT XII). *Epilepsy Res.* **2015**, *111*, 85–141. [CrossRef] [PubMed]
16. Hosseinzadeh, M.; Nikseresht, S.; Khodagholi, F.; Naderi, N.; Maghsoudi, N. Cannabidiol Post-Treatment Alleviates Rat Epileptic-Related Behaviors and Activates Hippocampal Cell Autophagy Pathway Along with Antioxidant Defense in Chronic Phase of Pilocarpine-Induced Seizure. *J. Mol. Neurosci.* **2016**, *58*, 432–440. [CrossRef]
17. Shirazi-zand, Z.; Ahmad-Molaei, L.; Motamedi, F.; Naderi, N. The role of potassium BK channels in anticonvulsant effect of cannabidiol in pentylenetetrazole and maximal electroshock models of seizure in mice. *Epilepsy Behav.* **2013**, *28*, 1–7. [CrossRef]
18. Mao, K.; You, C.; Lei, D.; Zhang, H. High dosage of cannabidiol (CBD) alleviates pentylenetetrazole-induced epilepsy in rats by exerting an anticonvulsive effect. *Int. J. Clin. Exp. Med.* **2015**, *8*, 8820–8827.
19. Vilela, L.R.; Lima, I.V.; Kunsch, É.B.; Pinto, H.P.P.; de Miranda, A.S.; Vieira, É.L.M.; de Oliveira, A.C.P.; Moraes, M.F.D.; Teixeira, A.L.; Moreira, F.A. Anticonvulsant effect of cannabidiol in the pentylenetetrazole model: Pharmacological mechanisms, electroencephalographic profile, and brain cytokine levels. *Epilepsy Behav.* **2017**, *75*, 29–35. [CrossRef]
20. Miziak, B.; Konarzewska, A.; Ułamek-Kozioł, M.; Dudra-Jastrzębska, M.; Pluta, R.; Czuczwar, S.J. Anti-epileptogenic effects of antiepileptic drugs. *Int. J. Mol. Sci.* **2020**, *21*, 2340. [CrossRef]
21. Walter, L.; Stella, N. Cannabinoids and neuroinflammation. *Br. J. Pharmacol.* **2004**, *141*, 775–785. [CrossRef]
22. Rosenberg, E.C.; Patra, P.H.; Whalley, B.J. Therapeutic effects of cannabinoids in animal models of seizures, epilepsy, epileptogenesis, and epilepsy-related neuroprotection. *Epilepsy Behav.* **2017**, *70*, 319–327. [CrossRef]
23. Mori, M.A.; Meyer, E.; Soares, L.M.; Milani, H.; Guimarães, F.S.; de Oliveira, R.M.W. Cannabidiol reduces neuroinflammation and promotes neuroplasticity and functional recovery after brain ischemia. *Prog. Neuro Psychopharmacol. Biol. Psychiatry* **2017**, *75*, 94–105. [CrossRef] [PubMed]
24. Elliott, D.M.; Singh, N.; Nagarkatti, M.; Nagarkatti, P.S. Cannabidiol attenuates experimental autoimmune encephalomyelitis model of multiple sclerosis through induction of myeloid-derived suppressor cells. *Front. Immunol.* **2018**, *9*, 3. [CrossRef]
25. Dopkins, N.; Miranda, K.; Wilson, K.; Holloman, B.L.; Nagarkatti, P.; Nagarkatti, M. Effects of Orally Administered Cannabidiol on Neuroinflammation and Intestinal Inflammation in the Attenuation of Experimental Autoimmune Encephalomyelitis. *J. Neuroimmune Pharmacol.* **2021**, *1*, 3. [CrossRef] [PubMed]
26. Ożarowski, M.; Karpiński, T.M.; Zielińska, A.; Souto, E.B.; Wielgus, K. Cannabidiol in neurological and neoplastic diseases: Latest developments on the molecular mechanism of action. *Int. J. Mol. Sci.* **2021**, *22*, 4294. [CrossRef] [PubMed]
27. Löscher, W.; Brandt, C. Prevention or modification of epileptogenesis after brain insults: Experimental approaches and translational research. *Pharmacol. Rev.* **2010**, *62*, 668–700. [CrossRef] [PubMed]
28. Dichter, M.A. Posttraumatic epilepsy: The challenge of translating discoveries in the laboratory to pathways to a cure. *Epilepsia* **2009**, *50* (Suppl. 2), 41–45. [CrossRef]
29. Pitkänen, A. Therapeutic approaches to epileptogenesis—hope on the horizon. *Epilepsia* **2010**, *51* (Suppl. 3), 2–17. [CrossRef]
30. Löscher, W. Critical review of current animal models of seizures and epilepsy used in the discovery and development of new antiepileptic drugs. *Seizure* **2011**, *20*, 359–368. [CrossRef]
31. Corda, M.G.; Orlandi, M.; Lecca, D.; Giorgi, O. Decrease in GABAergic function induced by pentylenetetrazol kindling in rats: Antagonism by MK-801. *J. Pharmacol. Exp. Ther.* **1992**, *262*, 792–800. [PubMed]
32. Samokhina, E.; Samokhin, A. Neuropathological profile of the pentylenetetrazol (PTZ) kindling model. *Int. J. Neurosci.* **2018**, *128*, 1086–1096. [CrossRef] [PubMed]
33. Gáll, Z.; Kelemen, K.; Mihály, I.; Salamon, P.; Miklóssy, I.; Zsigmond, B.; Kolcsár, M. Role of Lacosamide in Preventing Pentylenetetrazole Kindling-Induced Alterations in the Expression of the Gamma-2 Subunit of the GABAA Receptor in Rats. *Curr. Mol. Pharmacol.* **2020**, *13*, 251–260. [CrossRef]
34. Grecksch, G.; Becker, A.; Rauca, C. Effect of age on pentylenetetrazol-kindling and kindling-induced impairments of learning performance. *Pharmacol. Biochem. Behav.* **1997**, *56*, 595–601. [CrossRef]
35. Mortazavi, F.; Ericson, M.; Story, D.; Hulce, V.D.; Dunbar, G.L. Spatial learning deficits and emotional impairments in pentylenetetrazole-kindled rats. *Epilepsy Behav.* **2005**, *7*, 629–638. [CrossRef] [PubMed]
36. Gol, M.; Ghorbanian, D.; Hassanzadeh, S.; Javan, M.; Mirnajafi-Zadeh, J.; Ghasemi-Kasman, M. Fingolimod enhances myelin repair of hippocampus in pentylenetetrazol-induced kindling model. *Eur. J. Pharm. Sci.* **2017**, *96*, 72–83. [CrossRef] [PubMed]
37. Uttl, L.; Hložek, T.; Mareš, P.; Páleníček, T.; Kubová, H. Anticonvulsive effects and pharmacokinetic profile of cannabidiol (Cbd) in the pentylenetetrazol (ptz) or n-methyl-d-aspartate (nmda) models of seizures in infantile rats. *Int. J. Mol. Sci.* **2022**, *23*, 94. [CrossRef] [PubMed]
38. Gáll, Z.; Vancea, S.; Szilágyi, T.; Gáll, O.; Kolcsár, M. Dose-dependent pharmacokinetics and brain penetration of rufinamide following intravenous and oral administration to rats. *Eur. J. Pharm. Sci.* **2015**, *68*, 106–113. [CrossRef] [PubMed]
39. Corda, M.G.; Giorgi, O.; Longoni, B.; Orlandi, M.; Biggio, G. Decrease in the function of the gamma-aminobutyric acid-coupled chloride channel produced by the repeated administration of pentylenetetrazol to rats. *J. Neurochem.* **1990**, *55*, 1216–1221. [CrossRef] [PubMed]
40. Davoudi, M.; Shojaei, A.; Palizvan, M.R.; Javan, M.; Mirnajafi-Zadeh, J. Comparison between standard protocol and a novel window protocol for induction of pentylenetetrazol kindled seizures in the rat. *Epilepsy Res.* **2013**, *106*, 54–63. [CrossRef]

41. Lana, D.; Melani, A.; Maria Pugliese, A.; Cipriani, S.; Nosi, D.; Pedata, F.; Grazia Giovannini, M.; Barreto, G.E.; Blalock, E. The neuron-astrocyte-microglia triad in a rat model of chronic cerebral hypoperfusion: Protective effect of dipyridamole. *Front. Aging Neurosci.* **2014**, *6*, 322. [CrossRef]
42. Campos, A.C.; Guimarães, F.S. Involvement of 5HT1A receptors in the anxiolytic-like effects of cannabidiol injected into the dorsolateral periaqueductal gray of rats. *Psychopharmacology* **2008**, *199*, 223–230. [CrossRef]
43. Zanelati, T.V.; Biojone, C.; Moreira, F.A.; Guimarães, F.S.; Joca, S.R.L. Antidepressant-like effects of cannabidiol in mice: Possible involvement of 5-HT 1A receptors. *Br. J. Pharmacol.* **2010**, *159*, 122–128. [CrossRef]
44. Crippa, J.A.S.; Nogueira Derenusson, G.; Borduqui Ferrari, T.; Wichert-Ana, L.; Duran, F.L.S.; Martin-Santos, R.; Vinícius Simões, M.; Bhattacharyya, S.; Fusar-Poli, P.; Atakan, Z.; et al. Neural basis of anxiolytic effects of cannabidiol (CBD) in generalized social anxiety disorder: A preliminary report. *J. Psychopharmacol.* **2011**, *25*, 121–130. [CrossRef] [PubMed]
45. Sales, A.J.; Fogaça, M.V.; Sartim, A.G.; Pereira, V.S.; Wegener, G.; Guimarães, F.S.; Joca, S.R.L. Cannabidiol Induces Rapid and Sustained Antidepressant-Like Effects Through Increased BDNF Signaling and Synaptogenesis in the Prefrontal Cortex. *Mol. Neurobiol.* **2019**, *56*, 1070–1081. [CrossRef]
46. Shoval, G.; Shbiro, L.; Hershkovitz, L.; Hazut, N.; Zalsman, G.; Mechoulam, R.; Weller, A. Prohedonic effect of cannabidiol in a rat model of depression. *Neuropsychobiology* **2016**, *73*, 123–129. [CrossRef] [PubMed]
47. Sales, A.J.; Crestani, C.C.; Guimarães, F.S.; Joca, S.R.L. Antidepressant-like effect induced by Cannabidiol is dependent on brain serotonin levels. *Prog. Neuro Psychopharmacol. Biol. Psychiatry* **2018**, *86*, 255–261. [CrossRef]
48. Kolcsar, M.; Gáll, Z.; Dogaru, M.T. Dose dependent effects of serotonergic agents on anxiety. *Acta Physiol. Hung.* **2014**, *101*, 479–487. [CrossRef]
49. Schrantee, A.; Solleveld, M.M.; Schwantje, H.; Bruin, W.B.; Mutsaerts, H.-J.M.; Adriaanse, S.M.; Lucassen, P.; Booij, J.; Reneman, L. Dose-dependent effects of the selective serotonin reuptake inhibitor citalopram: A combined SPECT and phMRI study. *J. Psychopharmacol.* **2019**, *33*, 660–669. [CrossRef]
50. Millar, S.A.; Maguire, R.F.; Yates, A.S.; O'Sullivan, S.E. Towards Better Delivery of Cannabidiol (CBD). *Pharmaceuticals* **2020**, *13*, 219. [CrossRef] [PubMed]
51. Izgelov, D.; Davidson, E.; Barasch, D.; Regev, A.; Domb, A.J.; Hoffman, A. Pharmacokinetic investigation of synthetic cannabidiol oral formulations in healthy volunteers. *Eur. J. Pharm. Biopharm.* **2020**, *154*, 108–115. [CrossRef] [PubMed]
52. Xu, C.; Chang, T.; Du, Y.; Yu, C.; Tan, X.; Li, X. Pharmacokinetics of oral and intravenous cannabidiol and its antidepressant-like effects in chronic mild stress mouse model. *Environ. Toxicol. Pharmacol.* **2019**, *70*, 103202. [CrossRef] [PubMed]
53. Gray, R.A.; Stott, C.G.; Jones, N.A.; Di Marzo, V.; Whalley, B.J. Anticonvulsive Properties of Cannabidiol in a Model of Generalized Seizure Are Transient Receptor Potential Vanilloid 1 Dependent. *Cannabis Cannabinoid Res.* **2020**, *5*, 145–149. [CrossRef] [PubMed]
54. Castillo, A.; Tolón, M.R.; Fernández-Ruiz, J.; Romero, J.; Martinez-Orgado, J. The neuroprotective effect of cannabidiol in an in vitro model of newborn hypoxic–ischemic brain damage in mice is mediated by CB2 and adenosine receptors. *Neurobiol. Dis.* **2010**, *37*, 434–440. [CrossRef] [PubMed]
55. Leo, A.; Russo, E.; Elia, M. Cannabidiol and epilepsy: Rationale and therapeutic potential. *Pharmacol. Res.* **2016**, *107*, 85–92. [CrossRef]
56. Coles, M.; Watt, G.; Kreilaus, F.; Karl, T. Medium-Dose Chronic Cannabidiol Treatment Reverses Object Recognition Memory Deficits of APP Swe /PS1ΔE9 Transgenic Female Mice. *Front. Pharmacol.* **2020**, *11*, 587604. [CrossRef]
57. Antunes, M.; Biala, G. The novel object recognition memory: Neurobiology, test procedure, and its modifications. *Cogn. Process.* **2012**, *13*, 93–110. [CrossRef]
58. Baj, G.; D'alessandro, V.; Musazzi, L.; Mallei, A.; Sartori, C.R.; Sciancalepore, M.; Tardito, D.; Langone, F.; Popoli, M.; Tongiorgi, E. Physical Exercise and Antidepressants Enhance BDNF Targeting in Hippocampal CA3 Dendrites: Further Evidence of a Spatial Code for BDNF Splice Variants. *Neuropsychopharmacology* **2012**, *37*, 1600–1611. [CrossRef]
59. Mahmoud, F.; El-Hakim, A.A.; El Deen Amer, A.; Fidal, M. Effect of exposure to cadmium on the hippocampus in adult albino rat and the possible role of L-carnitine. *J. Curr. Med. Res. Pract.* **2019**, *4*, 240. [CrossRef]
60. Lin, N.; Xiong, L.-L.; Zhang, R.; Zheng, H.; Wang, L.; Qian, Z.-Y.; Zhang, P.; Chen, Z.; Gao, F.-B.; Wang, T.-H. Injection of Aβ1-40 into hippocampus induced cognitive lesion associated with neuronal apoptosis and multiple gene expressions in the tree shrew. *Apoptosis* **2016**, *21*, 621–640. [CrossRef]
61. Stringer, J.L. Repeated seizures increase GFAP and vimentin in the hippocampus. *Brain Res.* **1996**, *717*, 147–153. [CrossRef]
62. Verhoog, Q.P.; Holtman, L.; Aronica, E.; van Vliet, E.A. Astrocytes as Guardians of Neuronal Excitability: Mechanisms Underlying Epileptogenesis. *Front. Neurol.* **2020**, *11*, 591690. [CrossRef]
63. van Vliet, E.A.; Aronica, E.; Vezzani, A.; Ravizza, T. Review: Neuroinflammatory pathways as treatment targets and biomarker candidates in epilepsy: Emerging evidence from preclinical and clinical studies. *Neuropathol. Appl. Neurobiol.* **2018**, *44*, 91–111. [CrossRef] [PubMed]
64. Rana, A.; Musto, A.E. The role of inflammation in the development of epilepsy. *J. Neuroinflamm.* **2018**, *15*, 144. [CrossRef] [PubMed]
65. Cerbai, F.; Lana, D.; Nosi, D.; Petkova-Kirova, P.; Zecchi, S. The Neuron-Astrocyte-Microglia Triad in Normal Brain Ageing and in a Model of Neuroinflammation in the Rat Hippocampus. *PLoS ONE* **2012**, *7*, 45250. [CrossRef] [PubMed]

66. Lana, D.; Iovino, L.; Nosi, D.; Wenk, G.L.; Giovannini, M.G. The neuron-astrocyte-microglia triad involvement in neuroinflammaging mechanisms in the CA3 hippocampus of memory-impaired aged rats. *Exp. Gerontol.* **2016**, *83*, 71–88. [CrossRef] [PubMed]
67. Lana, D.; Ugolini, F.; Giovannini, M.G. Space-dependent glia–neuron interplay in the hippocampus of transgenic models of β-amyloid deposition. *Int. J. Mol. Sci.* **2020**, *21*, 9441. [CrossRef] [PubMed]

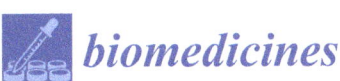

Article

Differential Effects of D9 Tetrahydrocannabinol (THC)- and Cannabidiol (CBD)-Based Cannabinoid Treatments on Macrophage Immune Function In Vitro and on Gastrointestinal Inflammation in a Murine Model

Zhanna Yekhtin [1], Iman Khuja [1], David Meiri [2], Reuven Or [1,†] and Osnat Almogi-Hazan [1,*,†]

[1] Laboratory of Immunotherapy and Bone Marrow Transplantation, Hadassah Medical Center, The Faculty of Medicine, Hebrew University of Jerusalem, Jerusalem 91120, Israel; zhannay@hadassah.org.il (Z.Y.); iman.khuja@mail.huji.ac.il (I.K.); reuvenor@hadassah.org.il (R.O.)

[2] The Laboratory of Cancer Biology and Cannabinoid Research, Department of Biology, Technion—Israel Institute of Technology, Haifa 320003, Israel; dmeiri@technion.ac.il

[*] Correspondence: osnath@hadassah.org.il; Tel.: +972-26778247; Fax: +972-25344081

[†] These authors contributed equally to this work.

Abstract: Phytocannabinoids possess a wide range of immune regulatory properties, mediated by the endocannabinoid system. Monocyte/macrophage innate immune cells express endocannabinoid receptors. Dysregulation of macrophage function is involved in the pathogenesis of different inflammatory diseases, including inflammatory bowel disease. In our research, we aimed to evaluate the effects of the phytocannabinoids D9 tetrahydrocannabinol (THC) and cannabidiol (CBD) on macrophage activation. Macrophages from young and aged C57BL/6 mice were activated in vitro in the presence of pure cannabinoids or cannabis extracts. The phenotype of the cells, nitric oxide (NO•) secretion, and cytokine secretion were examined. In addition, these treatments were administered to murine colitis model. The clinical statuses of mice, levels of colon infiltrating macrophages, and inflammatory cytokines in the blood, were evaluated. We demonstrated inhibition of macrophage NO• and cytokine secretion and significant effects on expression of cell surface molecules. In the murine model, clinical scores were improved and macrophage colon infiltration reduced following treatment. We identified higher activity of cannabis extracts as compared with pure cannabinoids. Each treatment had a unique effect on cytokine composition. Overall, our results establish that the effects of cannabinoid treatments differ. A better understanding of the reciprocal relationship between cannabinoids and immunity is essential to design targeted treatment strategies.

Keywords: cannabinoid; cannabis; immune; macrophage; elderly; inflammatory bowel disease; cannabidiol; D9 tetrahydrocannabinol; nitric oxide

Citation: Yekhtin, Z.; Khuja, I.; Meiri, D.; Or, R.; Almogi-Hazan, O. Differential Effects of D9 Tetrahydrocannabinol (THC)- and Cannabidiol (CBD)-Based Cannabinoid Treatments on Macrophage Immune Function In Vitro and on Gastrointestinal Inflammation in a Murine Model. *Biomedicines* 2022, 10, 1793. https://doi.org/10.3390/biomedicines10081793

Academic Editors: Wesley M. Raup-Konsavage and Raffaele Capasso

Received: 7 June 2022
Accepted: 22 July 2022
Published: 26 July 2022

Publisher's Note: MDPI stays neutral with regard to jurisdictional claims in published maps and institutional affiliations.

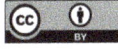

Copyright: © 2022 by the authors. Licensee MDPI, Basel, Switzerland. This article is an open access article distributed under the terms and conditions of the Creative Commons Attribution (CC BY) license (https://creativecommons.org/licenses/by/4.0/).

1. Introduction

Macrophages are specialized innate immune cells that orchestrate homeostatic, inflammatory, and reparative activities. Murine macrophages are located in the brain, skin, liver, kidney, lungs, and heart and originate from the yolk sac or fetal liver; their maintenance in adulthood in the absence of stressors is independent of circulating monocytic precursors. In other tissues, such as the gastrointestinal tract, monocytic precursors contribute to tissue macrophages [1]. In the steady state, tissue macrophages have intrinsic anti-inflammatory functions. Tissue stress, including infection, drives the production of monocytes and neutrophils. Bone marrow-derived monocytes are recruited to the damaged site, differentiate into macrophages and dendritic cells, and begin the inflammatory processes [2]. These events must be tightly regulated. Dysregulation of macrophage differentiation and function is involved in the pathogenesis of different diseases, including inflammatory bowel disease (IBD).

Immunological dysregulation in IBD is characterized by epithelial damage, expansion of inflammation driven by intestinal flora, a large number of cells infiltrating into the lamina propria, and a failure of immune regulation to control the inflammatory response [3]. In IBD patients, the number of macrophages increase in the inflamed mucosa [3].

The endocannabinoid system (ECS) regulates various aspects of physiological, behavioral, immunological, and metabolic functions. It is now clear that many of the components of the endocannabinoid system function as key regulators of the immune system and the immune response [4]. Endocannabinoid ligands and receptors are involved in the regulation of both innate and adaptive immune cells. Murine and human monocytes/macrophages and microglial cells express the endocannabinoid receptors CB1 and CB2. CB2 receptors in macrophages have anti-inflammatory properties [5–8], while CB1 receptors have proinflammatory properties and are involved in phagocytosis [9–12]. Importantly, the expression levels of cannabinoid receptors in leukocytes are influenced by different inflammatory factors [13].

Phytocannabinoids, the biologically active constituents of cannabis, possess a wide range of immune regulatory properties, mediated by the endocannabinoid system. Two cannabinoids have been the focus of most of the studies that have examined medical uses, i.e., D9 tetrahydrocannabinol (THC) and cannabidiol (CBD). THC and some of the other phytocannabinoids mediate their biological effects primarily through the classical cannabinoid receptors CB1 and CB2. In addition, THC can act as an agonist of the receptors/channels GPR55, GPR18, PPARγ, transient TRPA1, TRPV2, TRPV3, and TRPV4, and as an antagonist of the receptors/channels TRPM8 and 5-HT3A. Interestingly, although CBD affects the immune function, it has a very weak affinity to CB2 or CB1, where it can act as a negative allosteric modulator. Several reports have demonstrated that CBD acts as an agonist of other receptors/channels, such as TRPA1, TRPV1, TRPV2, TRPV3, PPARγ, and 5-HT1A, and as an antagonist of the receptors GPR55, GPR18, and 5-HT3A. CBD is also an inverse agonist of the receptors GPR3, GPR6, and GPR12 [4].

Previously, we compared the influence of cannabinoid-based treatments on lymphocyte function [14]. The aim of the current research was to examine the consequences of treatment with THC and CBD on macrophage activation and in macrophage-related inflammation. Since THC and CBD mediate their actions on mammal cells though different receptors, we hypothesized that each cannabinoid has selective effects on macrophage phenotype and function, and hence, a different impact on activation and inflammation. Therefore, the aim of our research was to elucidate the differential effects of THC- and CBD-based treatments on macrophage immune function. Our previous results suggested that the combination of cannabinoids with other active molecules in the plant may achieve better clinical results than pure cannabinoids, therefore, we also examined the differences between the effects of high THC and high CBD cannabis extracts (Table 1).

Table 1. Chemical analysis of the main phytocannabinoids and terpenoids in the cannabis extracts.

		THCE	CBDE
Phytocannabinoids (%) HPLC-UV	Total THC	24.58	1.3488
	Total CBD	9.62	36.0906
	Total CBG	0.3	0.4412
Terpenoids (ppm) SHS-GC/MS/MS	Linalool	346.1	1087.0
	Fenchyl alcohol	850.9	924.1
	α-Terpineol	825.8	992.0
	β-Caryophyllene	1548.7	695.3
	α-Humulene	406.9	265.2

While Cannabis is not yet registered as a drug, the potential of cannabinoid-based medicines for the treatment of various conditions has led many countries to authorize their clinical use. As a result, in recent years, there has been a rapid increase in the medical use of cannabis and a wide range of cannabinoid-based treatments are offered to patients. THC and CBD are considered to be the two essential elements in these treatments. Therefore, it is crucial to explore the various biological effects of these molecules. A better understanding of the effects of THC, CBD, and other active molecules on the immune response will assist physicians in providing the best possible individually targeted treatment for their patients and will allow the design of new treatments.

2. Materials and Methods

2.1. Cannabis Extracts and Cannabinoids

This research was performed under the approval of The Medical Cannabis Unit in the Israeli Ministry of Health (REQ46). Pure THC was generously provided by the laboratory of Prof. Raphael Mechoulam. Synthetic CBD was purchased from STI Pharmaceuticals Ltd., Newtown, UK. Cannabis Sativa and Indica extract with high content in THC or CBD (i.e., THCE/CBDE, respectively) were supplied by Cannabliss (Cannabliss Ltd., Tel Aviv, Israel). Extraction was obtained using ethanol, and evaporated. Identification and quantification of phytocannabinoids in the cannabis extracts were done by ultrahigh performance liquid chromatography with an ultraviolet detector (UHPLC/UV) system (Thermo Scientific, Bremen, Germany). The terpenoid analysis was performed by static headspace gas chromatography tandem mass spectrometry (SHS-GC/MS/MS) using full evaporation technique with external calibrations, as previously described [15,16]. The main molecules are listed in Table 1.

2.2. Mice

Female and male 8- to 11-week-old and 8-month-old C57BL/6 female mice were purchased from Envigo, Jerusalem, Israel and were acclimated for at least 7 days before the experiment in the specific pathogen-free (SPF) facility of the Authority of Biological and Biomedical Models at the Hebrew University of Jerusalem. The aged mice were up to 18 months old in the SPF animal facility. The study was approved by the Institutional Animal Care and Use Committee of the Hebrew University of Jerusalem in accordance with national laws and regulations for the protection of animals (MD-22-16868-4, MD-20-16432-4, and MD-18-15565-5). The mice were housed under specific SPF conditions in the animal facility under the AAALAC accreditation, throughout the experiments.

2.3. Peritoneal Macrophages

Peritoneal exudate cells were induced in mice by an intraperitoneal injection of 0.5 mL of 3% thioglycollate (BD DIFCO, Franklin Lakes, NJ, USA). After 4 days, mice were anesthetized with ketamine and xylazine, and then killed by cervical dislocation. Peritoneal exudate cells were washed from the peritoneal cavity of mice by lavage with 5 mL of ice-cold, sterile phosphate buffered saline (PBS). Cells were washed with PBS and re-suspended in Dulbecco's modified Eagle medium (DMEM) (Sartorius, Israel) supplemented with 10% fetal calf serum (FCS), 1% penicillin/streptomycin, and 1% L-glutamine (Biological industries/Sartorius, Beit Haemek, Israel). Cell viability was determined by MTT colorimetric assay in which a yellow tetrazole, is reduced to purple formazan in living cells (MP Biomedicals, LLC, Solon, OH, USA). The resultant color was measured at 450 nm using a Biotek PowerWave XS Microplate Reader.

2.4. Nitric Oxide (NO•) Determination

Peritoneal macrophages were seeded at a density of 2.5×10^5 cells/well in 96-well plates and incubated overnight at 37 °C and 5% CO_2. On the following day, the medium was changed to fresh DMEM containing 5 μg/mL CBD, THC, or cannabis extracts. The cells were then stimulated for 24 h by the addition of lipopolysaccharide (LPS) to a concentration of 1 μg/mL. After 24 h, cell supernatants (SNs) were harvested for nitric oxide radical (NO•) assay by addition of 100 μL SN to an equal volume of Griess reagent (1% sulfanilamide, 0.1% naphthalene diamine, and 2% H_3PO_4). After 10 min of incubation, the resultant color was measured at 550 nm. The amount of NO• produced, and any inhibition by the tested materials, was calculated from a standard curve prepared with $NaNO_2$. Controls: non-activated cells, activated cells + vehicle, activated cells + 1400W dihydrochloride (NOS2 inhibitor, Enzo Life Sciences Inc., Lausen, Switzerland).

2.5. Flow Cytometry

5×10^5 cells/sample were washed once in ice-cold staining buffer (PBS containing 1% FBS, pH 7.2). Then, cells were stained in the dark at 4 °C for 30 min with fluorochrome-labeled anti-mouse mAb (Biolegend, San Diego, CA, USA), specific for cell surface antigens: F4/80, I-Ad (MHC class II), and CD16/32. Cells were subsequently washed, re-suspended in staining buffer, and analyzed by flow cytometry.

2.6. RNA Extraction and Real-Time PCR Analysis

Total cellular RNA was extracted using RNeasy Mini Kit columns (Geneaid, New Taipei City, Taiwan), according to the manufacturer's protocol. One microgram of total RNA was used to synthesize cDNA using a high-capacity cDNA kit (Applied Biosystems, Waltham, MA, USA), following the supplier's instructions. Detection of transcript levels of CB1 and CB2 was performed using a TaqMan Gene Expression Assay Kit (Applied Biosystems, Waltham, MA, USA), with HPRT-1 as a reference. All primers were purchased from Applied Biosystems (Waltham, MA, USA). Real-Time PCR reactions were conducted using a QuantStudio 5 instrument (Applied Biosystems, Waltham, MA, USA). Data were analyzed using the QuantStudio design and analysis Software (Applied Biosystems, Waltham, MA, USA).

2.7. Induction of Colitis in Mice

Colitis was induced in C57BL/6 mice with 2% DSS dissolved in drinking water given ad libitum (Days 1–7), and then replaced with plain drinking water for 3 days. Then, 5 mg/kg cannabis/cannabinoids were prepared in 5% Cremophor EL (Sigma, St. Louis, MO, USA), 5% ethanol (Gadot, Haifa, Israel) in PBS, and 0.1 mL were administered IP every other day, starting from Day 1. Body weight and stool were monitored once a day. Changes of body weight are indicated as loss of baseline body weight (% of initial weight). Clinical score (0–9) included: stool score (0–3), rectal score (0–3), and general clinical parameters (fur texture, behavior, and posture, 0–3). On the tenth day of colitis induction, blood was collected from the mouse tails into ethylenediaminetetraacetic acid (EDTA)-coated capillary tubes, and then the mice were anesthetized using ketamine and xylazine, and then killed by cervical dislocation. The intestines were excised, measured, and carefully rinsed with saline. Blood tubes were centrifuged at 1500 rpm, room temperature, for 5 min; plasma was collected and kept at −80 °C for cytokine and chemokine analysis.

2.8. Histopathology and Immunohistochemistry

Colon tissue was fixed in 4% buffered formaldehyde (Bio-Lab, Jerusalem, Israel) and embedded in paraffin. For histology, the sections were stained with H&E according to standard protocols. Histological scoring (0–9) was based on 3 parameters: Crypt damage (0–3), percent involvement (0–3), and damage to bowel wall structure (0–3).

For immunostaining, paraffin embedded sections were heated to 60 °C, deparaffinized using xylene, dehydrated using ethanol, and washed with H_2O. Sections were treated with 3% H_2O_2 and antigens retrieved by incubation with 1 mg/mL pronase. Then, the samples were washed in PBS and blocked in CAS blocking reagent (Rhenium, Modi'in, Israel). The slides were stained with anti-F480 (Bio-Rad, Hercules, CA, USA). Anti-rat IgG universal immune peroxidase polymer (Nichirei Biosciences Inc., Tokyo, Japan) was used as secondary antibody. Sections were incubated with Stable Peroxidase Substrate Buffer (Thermo Scientific, Waltham, MA, USA), washed with H_2O, and analyzed on a BX41 microscope (Olympus Corporation, Tokyo, Japan).

2.9. Proinflammatory Chemokine and Cytokine Analysis

Peritoneal macrophages were activated for 24 h with LPS, in the presence of 5 µg/mL CBD, THC, or cannabis extracts. The supernatant was collected and analyzed using a LEGENDplex™ MU Macrophage/Microglia Panel cytokine array assay (Biolegend, San Diego, CA, USA), according to the manufacturer's instructions.

Plasma samples from DSS model mice were analyzed using a LEGENDplex™ Mouse Inflammation Panel cytokine array (Biolegend, San Diego, CA, USA), according to the manufacturer's instructions.

2.10. Statistical Analysis

Data from in vitro studies are represented as mean ± SE. The mean was calculated from the indicated number of experiments. The mean of triplicates from each experiment was used for this calculation. For statistical analysis of the macrophage NO• secretion experiments in female and male mice, we used Friedman test. For statistical analysis of the macrophage NO• secretion and cannabinoid receptors expression, macrophage cytokine secretion, and flow cytometry experiments in young and aged mice, we used the Mann–Whitney test. For statistical analysis of colon length, colon histopathology, macrophage infiltration to the colon, and blood cytokines in the DSS model experiments, we used the Kruskal–Wallis test. For statistical analysis of weight loss and clinical score in the DSS model experiments, we used the Kruskal–Wallis test of area under the curve (AUC). In all experiments, p value < 0.05 were considered statistically significant.

3. Results

3.1. Cannabinoid Treatments Reduce Nitric Oxide and Cytokine Production of LPS-Activated Peritoneal Macrophages

Upon activation, macrophages produce large amounts of nitric oxide (NO•). To test the effect of cannabinoid treatments on macrophage activation, NO• secretion was determined. Macrophages from previously thioglycollate (tg)-injected C57BL/6 mice were collected by peritoneal lavage, and then activated for 24 h with lipopolysaccharide (LPS), in the presence of cannabinoid treatments; 1400W dihydrochloride, a specific iNOS inhibitor, served as control. All treatments show dose dependent effect on NO• secretion (Figure S1). For our further experiments, we used 5 µg/mL of each treatment (THC, CBD, or cannabis extracts). Our results demonstrate 42–72% inhibition of activation-induced NO• secretion from peritoneal macrophages from female (Figure 1a) and male (Figure 1b) mice in the presence of cannabinoid treatments. The reduced NO• secretion was not caused by decreasing cell number, since the treatments showed no toxic effect on the cells in MTT viability assay (Figure S2). The differences between THC and CBD treatments were significant only in the female mice. Importantly, both extracts were significantly more efficient ($p < 0.0001$) than the pure cannabinoids in female and male mice. A treatment with the combination of THC and CBD (2.5 µg/mL of each) was less effective than the pure cannabinoids (Figure S3).

Next, we examined the influence of aging on the responsiveness of macrophages to cannabinoid treatments. For this aim, we obtained peritoneal macrophages from aged (18 months old) mice and compared their NO• secretion with macrophages from young (2 months old) mice. Figure 1c (left) shows elevated secretion of NO• from non-activated cells and reduced secretion upon activation of old peritoneal macrophages. The effect of cannabinoid treatments on NO• secretion was significantly reduced as compared with cells from young mice (Figure 1c, right). In addition, peritoneal macrophages from aged mice demonstrate alleviated expression of the cannabinoid receptors (Figure 1d).

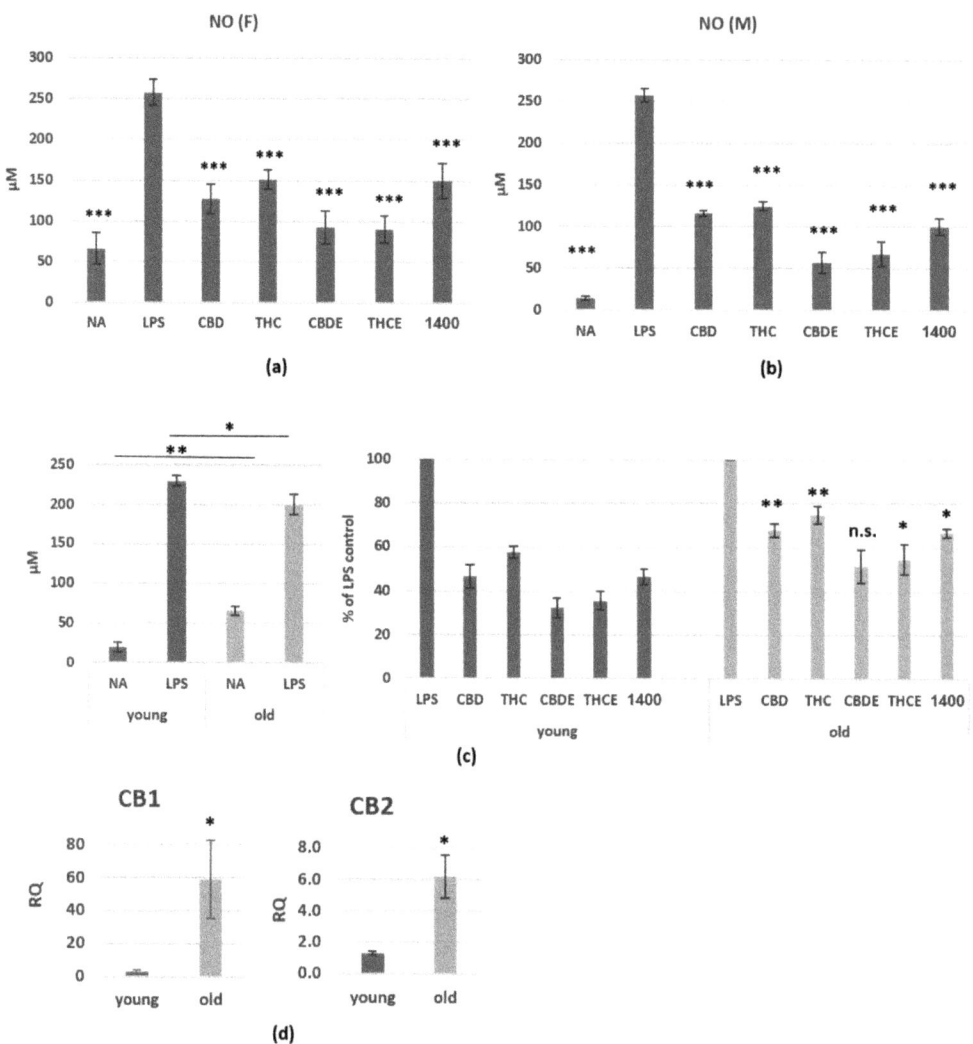

Figure 1. The influence of pure CBD/THC and cannabis extracts on nitric oxide production of LPS-activated peritoneal macrophages. Peritoneal macrophages from C57BL/6 female (**a**) and male (**b**) mice were activated for 24 h with LPS, in the presence of cannabinoid treatments (5 µg/mL). 1400W (1400), a specific iNOS inhibitor, served as control. NO• levels in the supernatant were analyzed. (**a**)—n = 10 mice, from 3 independent experiments; (**b**)—n = 7 mice, from 3 independent experiments. The differences of all treatments as compare with LPS-activated control (indicated on the graphs) are highly significant. The differences of THCE and THC between CBDE and CBD are significant in (**a**,**b**); (**c**) NO• levels in the supernatant of activated peritoneal macrophages from young (2 months old) and aged (18 months old) C57BL/6 female and male mice. n = 7 mice per group, from 3 independent experiments. The differences between aged and young mice in each treatment, are indicated on the graph; (**d**) the expression levels of CB1 and CB2 in peritoneal macrophages from young and aged C57BL/6 female mice (n = 3/group) were assessed by real-time PCR analysis. The results are expressed as mean + SEM. p-value *, <0.05; **, <0.01; ***, <0.001. NA—non-activated; LPS—lipopolysaccharide-activated macrophages; THC—D9 tetrahydrocannabino; CBD—cannabidiol; THCE—high THC cannabis extract; CBDE—high CBD cannabis extract; n.s.—not significant.

To examine the effect of the treatments on inflammatory cytokine/chemokine secretion from peritoneal macrophages, we collected the supernatant of 24 h LPS-activated cells and analyzed the levels of different cytokines using a LEGENDplex™ MU Macrophage/Microglia Panel cytokine array assay. IL6, TNF-alpha, CXCL2, and G-CSF levels in the culture media increased upon activation (Figure 2a–d). Our results demonstrate 40–74% inhibition of activation-induced IL6 secretion from peritoneal macrophages (Figure 2a), 22–66% inhibition of TNF-alpha secretion (Figure 2b), 4–44% inhibition of CXCL2 secretion (Figure 2c), and 0–58% inhibition of GM-CSF secretion (Figure 2d). CBD and CBDE had more significant inhibitory effect on cytokine/chemokine secretion as compared with THC and THCE. The differences between CBD and THC are significant in TNF-alpha, CXCL2, and G-CSF. IL12p40, CCL22, and IL18 were also elevated following activation, however, the cannabinoid-based treatments did not have clear effects on their levels (Figure S4).

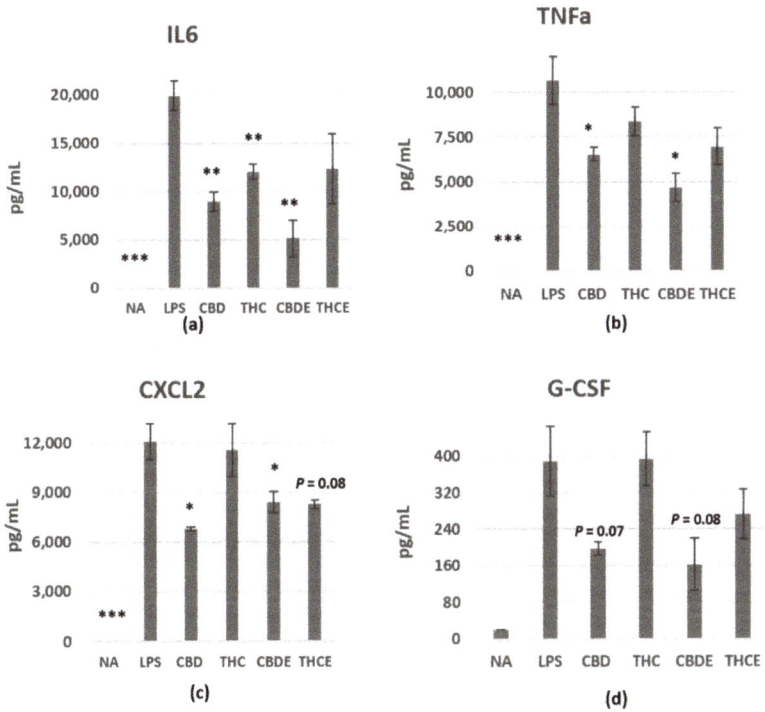

Figure 2. The influence of pure CBD/THC and cannabis extracts on cytokine/chemokine production of LPS-activated peritoneal macrophages. Peritoneal macrophages were activated for 24 h with LPS, in the presence of cannabinoid treatments (5 µg/mL), as in Figure 1. $n = 3$ mice. IL6 (**a**), TNF-alpha (**b**), CXCL2 (**c**), and G-CSF (**d**) levels in the culture supernatant were detected. The results are expressed as mean + SEM. p-value as compare with LPS-activated control cells *, <0.05; **, <0.01; ***, <0.001. NA—non-activated; LPS—lipopolysaccharide-activated macrophages; THC—D9 tetrahydrocannabinol; CBD—cannabidiol; THCE—high THC cannabis extract; CBDE—high CBD cannabis extract.

3.2. Cannabinoid Treatments Affect the Phenotype of Activated Peritoneal Macrophages

To learn more about CBD and THC molecular effects in macrophages, we tested cell surface expression of several molecules in the activated macrophages. Class II molecules of the major histocompatibility complex (MHCII) is upregulated on some polarized macrophage populations upon activation. We found that both THC and CBD treatments induce small, but significant, further elevation in MHCII expression (Figure 3a). R. A. Ezekowitz and S. Gordon have demonstrated that expression levels of the F4/80 glycoprotein and the Fc receptor CD16/32 on peritoneal macrophages are dependent on the activator [17]. In our study, in tg-induced macrophages activated with LPS, F4/80 was elevated by THC (15%), but reduced by CBD treatment (32%) (Figure 3b). CD16/32 cell surface expression was elevated on LPS-activated cells, but the cannabinoid treatments had no significant effect on its expression (Figure 3c).

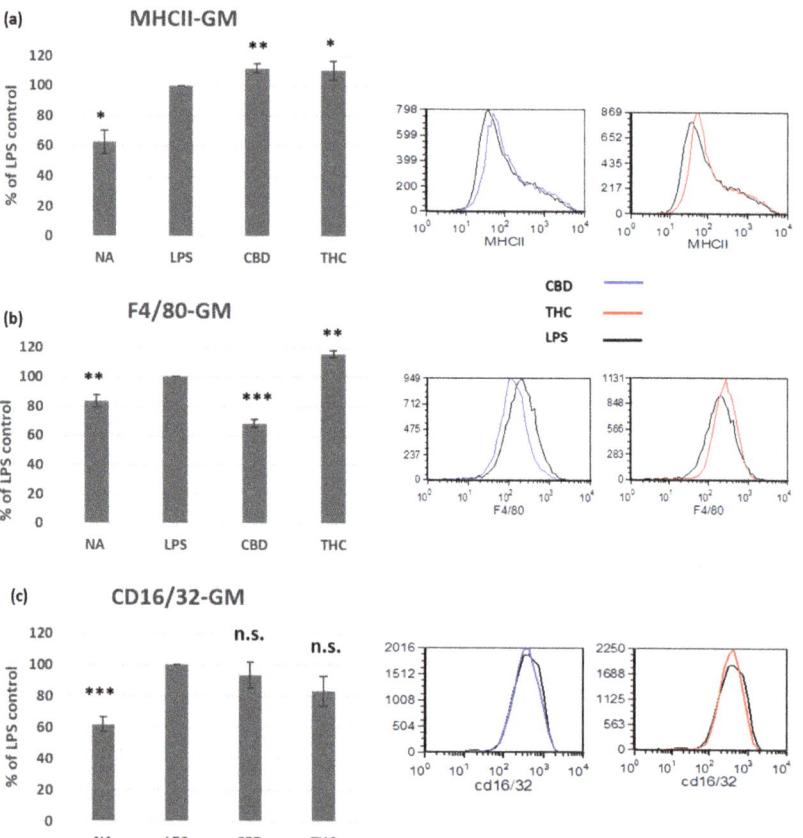

Figure 3. The effect of CBD and THC on the phenotype of LPS-activated peritoneal macrophages. Peritoneal macrophages from C57BL/6 female mice were activated for 24 h with LPS, in the presence of cannabinoid treatments (5 µg/mL). Cell surface expression levels of MHCII ((**a**), $n = 5$), F4/80 ((**b**), $n = 6$), and CD16/32 ((**c**), $n = 7$) were determined by flow cytometry. The results are expressed as mean + SEM. *p*-value as compare with LPS-activated control cells *, <0.05; **, <0.01; ***, <0.001. NA—non-activated; LPS—lipopolysaccharide-activated macrophages; THC—D9 tetrahydrocannabinol; CBD—cannabidiol; n.s.—not significant.

3.3. Cannabis Extracts Have Improved Effect in Murine Colitis DSS Model Mice as Compared with Pure Cannabinoids

We chose the murine colitis dextran sodium sulfate (DSS) model to compare the efficacy of the different cannabinoid treatments in macrophage-related inflammation in vivo. DSS is a chemical colitogen with anticoagulant properties. In the acute intestinal inflammation model, DSS causes disruption of the intestinal epithelial monolayer lining, leading to the entry of luminal bacteria and associated antigens into the mucosa and activation of the innate immunity [18].

Acute colitis was induced by adding DSS to the mice drinking water at 2% (w/v) ad libitum for 7 days, and then replaced with plain water. Cannabinoid treatments, 5 mg/kg, were administered intraperitoneal, every other day, from Day 1 to Day 10 (Figure 4a). All treatments, but particularly the CBD extract (CBDE), significantly inhibited weight loss in the DSS mice (Figure 4b). THC and CBD extracts both had better effect on the disease clinical score as compared with the pure cannabinoids (Figure 4c). This improved effect was also evident in the measurement of colon length (Figure 4d); the average length of the colon in the CBDE-treated mice was 4.8 cm, significantly higher than the average length of the colon in the CBD-treated mice 3.9 cm ($p < 0.0001$). In THCE-treated mice, the average length of the colon was 4.8 cm vs. 4.1 cm in the THC-treated mice ($p < 0.0001$). All treatment significantly improved the clinical condition of the mice as compared with the vehicle DSS group. The difference between the CBD and THC groups was not significant.

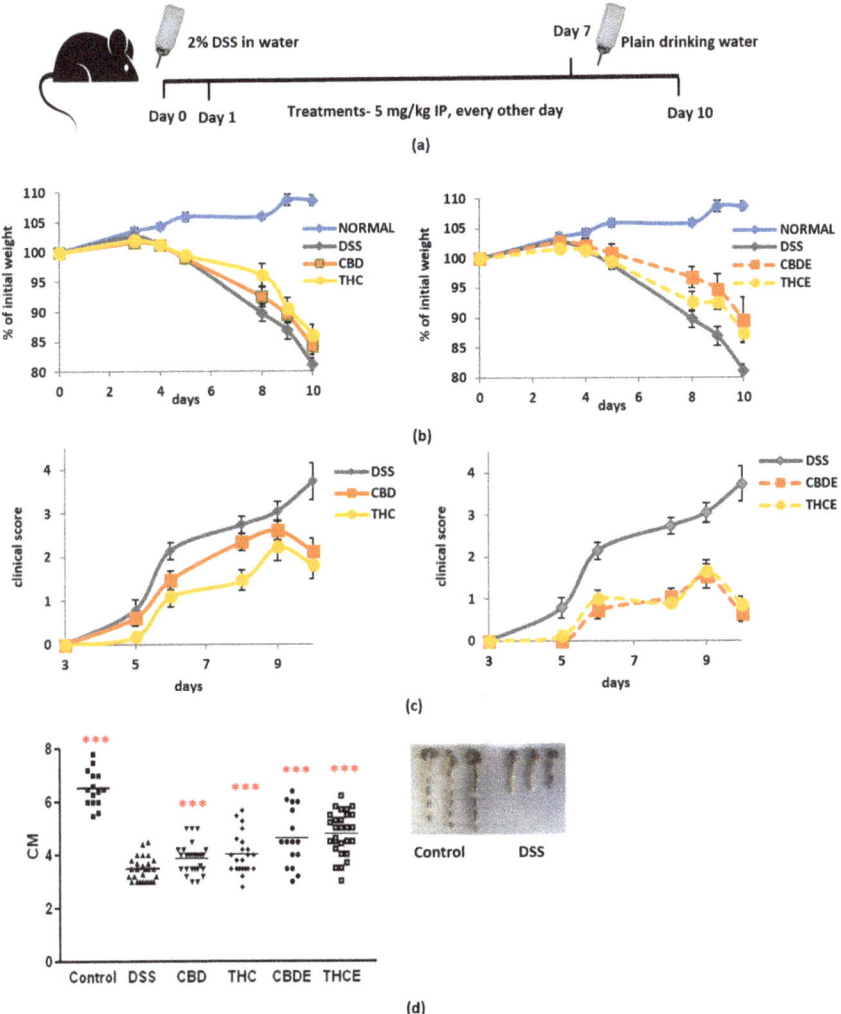

Figure 4. Cannabis/cannabinoids administration for treatment of murine colitis in DSS model mice: (a) Acute colitis was induced by adding DSS to the mice drinking water at 2% (w/v) ad libitum for 7 days,

and then replaced with plain water. 5 mg/kg cannabis/cannabinoids were administered IP every other day, starting from Day 1; (**b**) the effect of pure cannabinoids (left) and cannabis extracts (right) on weight loss. Differences between DSS group and THCE- as well as CBDE-treated groups are significant. The difference between the CBD- and CBDE-treated groups is significant $p < 0.05$; (**c**) the effect of pure cannabinoids (left) and cannabis extracts (right) on clinical score. Differences between the DSS group and all cannabinoid-treated groups are significant $p < 0.005$. Differences between cannabis extracts and pure cannabinoids are significant $p < 0.008$. The difference between the CBD- and THC-treated groups is significant $p < 0.05$; (**d**) the effect of pure cannabinoids and cannabis extracts on colon length, at the end of the experiment (Day 10). *p*-value as compare with the DSS control group ***, <0.001. The differences between THCE and THC and between CBDE and CBD are significant. Data are summarized from 5 independent experiments, 5–7 mice/group in each experiment. DSS—dextran sodium sulfate; THC—D9 tetrahydrocannabinol; CBD—cannabidiol; THCE—high THC cannabis extract; CBDE—high CBD cannabis extract.

The improved clinical outcome of all cannabinoid-based treatments is also demonstrated in the histopathology of the colon (Figure 5a,b). Colon sections were stained with haematoxylin/eosin and scored for the infiltration with inflammatory cells, damage in crypt architecture, and thickening of the bowel wall. In this assay, no significant differences between the four cannabinoid-based treatments were found.

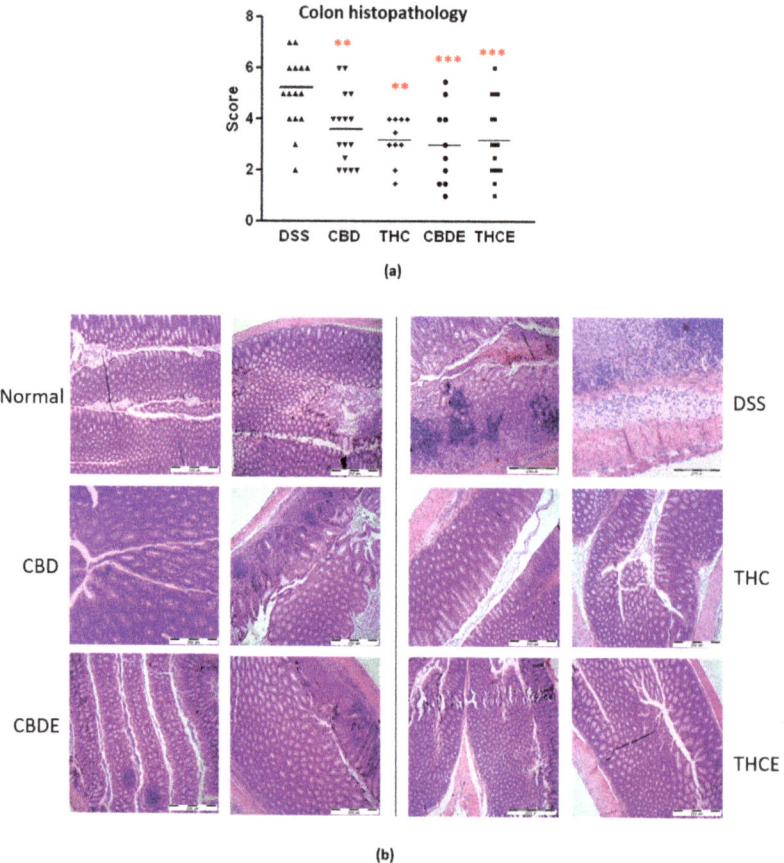

Figure 5. Histopathology of the colons of DSS model mice. Paraffin sections were stained with H&E and scored for inflammation and tissue damage; (**a**) Summary of average scores. *p*-value as compare

with the DSS control group **, <0.01; ***, <0.001; (**b**) representative pictures of H&E stained sections. DSS—dextran sodium sulfate; THC—D9 tetrahydrocannabinol; CBD—cannabidiol; THCE—high THC cannabis extract; CBDE—high CBD cannabis extract.

3.4. Cannabinoid Treatments Reduce Intestinal Macrophage Infiltration and the Levels of Inflammatory Cytokines in the Plasma of DSS Mice

Next, we examined the effects of the treatments on macrophages and inflammation in the DSS model. In IBD patients, an increased number of macrophages in the inflamed mucosa initiate a rapid response to luminal microbial antigens [3]. Immunohistochemistry with F4/80 antibody was performed to detect macrophages in the colon. As demonstrated in Figure 6a,b, the number of macrophages in the colon tissue is highly elevated in the DSS mice. All the cannabinoid-based treatments significantly inhibited colon infiltration of macrophages in the DSS mice (40–60% inhibition). CBDE treatment inhibition of macrophage infiltration was significantly more effective than pure CBD treatment ($p = 0.03$). The THCE and THC treatments were not significantly different.

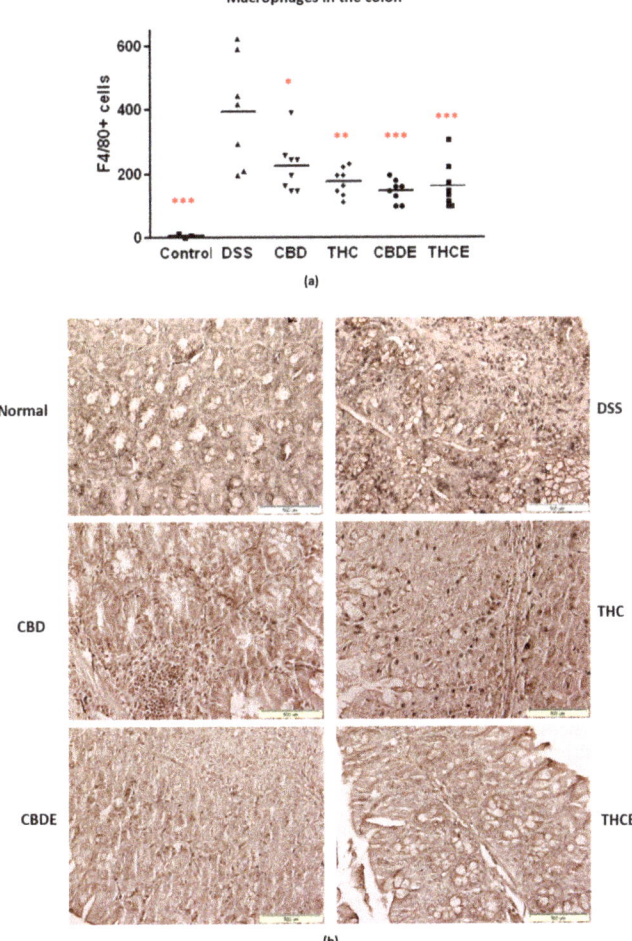

Figure 6. Immunostaining for macrophages in the colons of DSS model mice. Paraffin sections were stained with anti-F4/80 antibodies: (**a**) Average number of positive cells. *p*-value as compare with the

DSS control group *, <0.05; **, <0.01; ***, <0.001. The difference between the CBDE and CBD groups is significant; (**b**) representative pictures of F4/80 immunostained sections. DSS—dextran sodium sulfate; THC—D9 tetrahydrocannabinol; CBD—cannabidiol; THCE—high THC cannabis extract; CBDE—high CBD cannabis extract.

Cytokine levels in the blood reflect the inflammatory status in the body. It was also demonstrated that inflammatory cytokines have a crucial role in the pathogenesis of IBD, where they control multiple aspects of the inflammatory response [19]. We, therefore, tested the plasma levels of inflammatory cytokines of treated DSS mice using a mouse inflammation cytokine array assay. Interestingly, we found that the different treatments have unique effects on plasma cytokines (Figure 7). IL6 levels were reduced by all treatments, but particularly by CBDE. The levels of TNF-alpha were significantly reduced only by the cannabis extracts; but pure cannabinoids had stronger effect on IFN-beta levels. The levels of other tested cytokines were not significantly changed in the plasma of DSS mice as compared with healthy controls.

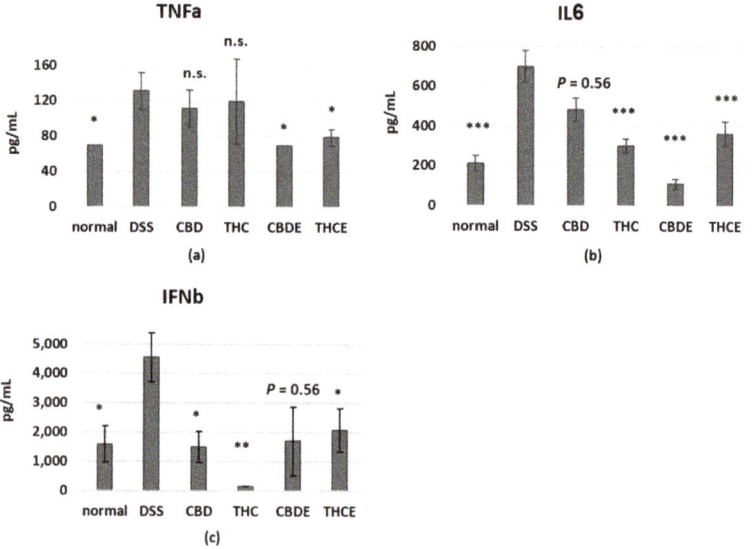

Figure 7. The influence of pure CBD/THC and cannabis extracts on inflammatory cytokines in the blood of DSS model mice. Blood samples for cytokine analysis were obtained at Day 10. The levels of TNFa (**a**), IL6 (**b**), and IFNb (**c**) in the plasma were determined using a LEGENDplex™ Mouse Inflammation Panel cytokine array; n = 5–10 mice/group. The results are expressed as mean + SEM. p-value as compare with the DSS group *, <0.05; **, <0.01; ***, <0.001. DSS—dextran sodium sulfate; THC—D9 tetrahydrocannabinol; CBD—cannabidiol; THCE—high THC cannabis extract; CBDE—high CBD cannabis extract; n.s.—not significant.

4. Discussion

Macrophages play key roles in innate immunity. They are specialized cells involved in the detection and destruction of bacteria and other harmful pathogens. In addition, they can present antigens to T cells and initiate inflammation. Macrophages and microglial cells express the Gi protein-coupled seven transmembrane cannabinoid receptors, CB1 and CB2 [12,20–24]. On the one hand, CB2 receptors in macrophages have anti-inflammatory properties, can affect macrophage polarization, and are involved in promoting autophagy [3,5,6,8]. CB1 receptors in macrophages, on the other hand, have proinflammatory properties and are involved in phagocytosis [9–12].

Phytocannabinoids possess a wide range of immune regulatory properties, mediated by the endocannabinoid system [4]. Two cannabinoids have been the focus of most of the studies examining medical uses: THC and CBD. These two phyto-cannabinoids utilize different endocannabinoid receptors to mediate their effects. A few studies have demonstrated anti-inflammatory effect for phytocannabinoid treatments on macrophage function, however, these studies have generally focused on a single cannabinoid [25–29].

Previously, we compared the influence of THC, CBD, and cannabis extracts on lymphocyte activation in vitro and in a murine graft versus host disease (GvHD) model [14]. In the current research, we aimed to compare the consequences of treatment with THC or CBD on macrophage activation and in DSS murine model for gastrointestinal inflammation. We use this model as a model for acute inflammation with involvement of macrophages in the pathophysiology of the disease [19].

First, we examined the effect of cannabinoid treatments on NO• secretion from peritoneal macrophages, ex vivo. Macrophages produce large amounts of NO• as a defense mechanism. However, in pathological conditions, such as autoimmune diseases, there is excessive simultaneous production of NO• and O_2•− by macrophages and other cells. NO• and O_2•− generate large quantities of the toxic molecule peroxynitrite (ONOO−), an oxidant and nitrating agent which can damage a wide array of molecules in cells, including DNA and proteins [30]. Elevated NO• bioavailability has been implicated in the etiology of a number of pathological events including IBD. It is now clear that the ECS plays a key role in regulating NO• formation via CB1R, CB2R, and/or alternative molecular targets [31]. We found that both THC and CBD, as well as cannabis extracts treatments, inhibit activation-induced NO• secretion from both female and male peritoneal macrophages. These results were in agreement with the results of Romano et al. who demonstrated a similar effect with the cannabinoid THCV [32]. Cannabis extracts and pure cannabinoids were used in a concentration of 5 µg/mL; the extracts had stronger effect than the pure cannabinoids, although cannabinoids constituted only 35–38% of their content. This could result either from inhibitory signaling of other molecules in the plant (not THC/CBD) or from a synergistic function of THC/CBD with other molecules. Interestingly, CBD signaling has been associated with inhibition of cytokine/chemokine secretion, since both pure CBD and CBDE had greater effect on the levels of peritoneal macrophage's secreted cytokines as compared with THC and THCE. It should be noted that the cannabis extracts had no significant advantage over the pure cannabinoids in inhibition of cytokine/chemokine secretion from peritoneal macrophages. The inhibitory effect of CBD, on the one hand, IL6 and TNF-alpha, and on the other hand, CXCL2 and G-CSF may suggest its ability to regulate both local inflammation and periphery bone marrow interactions.

Aging is concurrent with a slow and constant functional deterioration of the immune system, known as immunosenescence, which is accompanied by an increase in chronic inflammatory processes, a phenomenon known as "inflammaging". The devastating consequences of an aged immune system include impairment of the ability to cope with infections and an increased risk of developing chronic diseases such as cancer and heart disease—the two leading causes of death in old age [33]. Indeed, our results demonstrate elevated NO• secretion from non-activated peritoneal macrophages from aged mice, which indicated pre-existing inflammatory process. In addition, the reduced secretion upon LPS activation of aged mice peritoneal macrophages, may indicate immunosenescence. The old cells also showed decreased responsiveness to cannabinoid treatments and alleviated expression of CB1 and CB2 receptors. These results corresponds with earlier studies which demonstrated age-related alterations in the endocannabinoid system [34,35], and may be accompanied with other age-related changes in the endocannabinoid receptors and enzymes in the cells.

The effect of THC and CBD treatments on the expression of cell surface molecules on activated peritoneal macrophages was examined. Stimulation with LPS, a major component of the outer membrane of Gram-negative bacteria, leads to an effective classical, proinflammatory, macrophage activation. MHC-II molecules, expressed by antigen presenting cells, are central in the initiation of cellular and humoral immune responses. Upon LPS activation, MHCII is upregulated in macrophages [36], and hence increased antigen presentation. MHCII levels can also be affected by different soluble factors, such as cytokines [37]. In a previous study by Paul W. Wacnik et al. THC reduced MHCII expression in LPS-activated dendritic cells [38]. Since cannabinoid treatments reduced nitric oxid secretion, we expected similar reduced expression of MHCII. Surprisingly, we found that both treatments did not reduce, but induced, a small elevation of MHCII expression in the activated macrophages. The combination of these results may indicate that treatment of cannabinoids together with LPS may lead to M2b polarization of the peritoneal macrophages. M2b macrophages are a population of regulatory macrophages, classically induced by LPS and immune complexes, G-protein coupled receptor ligands, or prostaglandins [39,40].

F4/80 is widely used as a mouse macrophage antigen marker. Although the ligands for F4/80 have not been defined, evidence shows that this molecule is required for peripheral tolerance [41]. In addition, it has been demonstrated that F4/80 and Fc receptor CD16/32 expression levels in peritoneal macrophages are dependent on the activator [17]. In our experiments, the expression of F4/80 was elevated by THC, but reduced by CBD treatment as compared with the activated control cells. This result demonstrates the different consequences of the treatment with different cannabinoids. However, the functional relevance of this result is yet to be determined. CD16 and CD32 are low affinity IgG Fc receptors. Immune complexes signaling through the Fc receptors can lead to M2B polarization [39]. In our experiments, CD16/32 cell surface expression was elevated in LPS-activated cells, however, the cannabinoid treatments had no significant effect on their expression. Therefore, it is possible that the cannabinoids bypass CD16/32 signaling, for example, by binding to PPARγ, which may provide the second signal for M2B polarization.

IBD is comprised of well-known gastrointestinal autoimmune inflammatory disorders such as ULcerative colitis (UC) and Crohn's (CD). Cannabinoid receptor stimulation attenuates murine colitis, while cannabinoid receptor antagonism and cannabinoid receptor deficient models reverse these anti-inflammatory effects [4]. Phytocannabinoids have been used in preclinical models of gastrointestinal inflammation [42,43] and several clinical trial have tested the efficacy of cannabinoid-based treatments in IBD patients [42,44]. Indeed, in our DSS murine colitis model, cannabinoid treatments improved the clinical condition of the mice. Similar to the in vitro nitric oxide secretion assay and to our previous results in the murine GvHD model [14], the results of treatment with cannabis extracts were superior to pure-cannabinoid treatments. This unique effect could be a result of either a synergistic function of THC/CBD with other components or from independent anti-inflammatory properties of other molecules in the plant.

Dysregulated macrophages have a key role in the pathogenesis of IBD. In IBD patients, the number of macrophages increases in the inflamed mucosa. The phenotype and functions of the macrophages in the inflamed sites differ from those in physical conditions. For instance, they express high levels of costimulatory molecules and produce high levels of IL-12 and IL-23 in vitro under the microbial stimulation [3]. Our results demonstrate that cannabinoid-based treatments inhibit colon infiltration of macrophages in DSS mice. The average number of colon infiltrating macrophages in each treatment group correlated with the severity of the disease.

Inflammatory cytokines are produced by macrophages, but also by other cells such as dendritic cells, fibroblasts, and lymphocytes. The cannabinoid treatments all affected the levels of inflammatory cytokines in the mice blood. However, each treatment had a unique effect on the composition of cytokines: CBD treatment reduced the levels of IL6 and the more regulatory cytokine, interferon-beta; THC treatment reduced the levels of IL6 and interferon-beta better than CBD; CBDE treatment reduced the levels of TNF-alpha and had the strongest effect on the level of IL6; and THCE treatment reduced the levels of IL6, interferon-beta; and TNF-alpha. These results demonstrate, once again, the different consequences of treatment with different cannabinoid-based treatments. Interestingly, IL6, a key cytokine in IBD [19] was reduced by all the cannabinoid treatments, but TNF-alpha, another cytokine involved in the pathogenesis of IBD, was significantly affected, in the murine model, only by the cannabis extracts. Therefore it is possible that the reduced levels of TNF-alpha are responsible for the improved clinical effect. Importantly, anti-TNF agents are often used for IBD treatment in the clinic, due to the central role of this cytokine in the pathogenesis of the disease in human subjects too. CBDE was the most effective treatment in IL6 and TNF-alpha inhibition, both in activated peritoneal macrophages and in the murine model. This result was in agreement with the recently published results of Aswad et al., who demonstrated similar effects for a different high-CBD cannabis extract in human PBMCs and neutrophils and in murine models for systemic and lung inflammation [45].

5. Conclusions

Overall, our results indicate both similarities and differences between the impact of CBD- and THC-based drugs. Although all the tested treatments had an anti-inflammatory effect, their specific effects (for example, on phenotype of the cells and on cytokine production) differed. These differences may influence the clinical outcome of the treatment. We were surprised to find very similar anti-inflammatory results for the two cannabis extracts, which had diverse content of THC and CBD. This could suggest that THC/CBD content may not be the best indicator for anti-inflammatory properties of a cannabis-based drug. These results highlight the need to expand the research on the interplay between cannabinoids and other phytochemicals in the cannabis extracts. A better understanding of the effects of each molecule and the synergism between these molecules on the immune response will assist physicians to provide the best possible individually targeted treatment for their patients and will allow the design of new treatments.

Supplementary Materials: The following supporting information can be downloaded at: https://www.mdpi.com/article/10.3390/biomedicines10081793/s1, Figure S1: Dose dependent inhibition of nitric oxide production by peritoneal macrophages treated with pure CBD/THC or cannabis extracts. Figure S2: MTT viability assay. Figure S3: Combination of THC and CBD (2.5 µg/mL of each) is less effective than the pure cannabinoids. Figure S4: IL12p40, CCL22, and IL18 secretion from activated peritoneal macrophages.

Author Contributions: Conceptualization, O.A.-H. and R.O.; methodology, Z.Y. and I.K.; validation, O.A.-H., D.M. and R.O.; formal analysis, O.A.-H., Z.Y., D.M. and I.K.; investigation, O.A.-H. and R.O.; resources, R.O.; data curation, O.A.-H.; writing—original draft preparation, O.A.-H.; writing—review and editing, R.O.; supervision, O.A.-H.; funding acquisition, R.O. All authors have read and agreed to the published version of the manuscript.

Funding: This study was supported (in part) by the Gassner Fund for Medical Research. The sponsors of this study are public or nonprofit organizations that support science in general. They had no role in gathering, analyzing, or interpreting the data.

Institutional Review Board Statement: The animal study protocol was approved by the Institutional Animal Care and Use Committee of the Hebrew University of Jerusalem in accordance with national laws and regulations for the protection of animals (MD-22-16868-4, MD-20-16432-4, and MD-18-15565-5).

Informed Consent Statement: Not applicable.

Data Availability Statement: Not applicable.

Acknowledgments: We thank Raphael Mechoulam and Aviva Brener for the THC and for their helpful advice. We thank Cannabliss Ltd. for providing cannabis extracts. Cannabliss Ltd. had no role in study design, the collection, analysis and interpretation of results. We thank Zichron Menachem nonprofit organization for their support. We thank Norman Grover for his help with statistical analysis. We thank Tamara Silberberg for her help in editing the manuscript.

Conflicts of Interest: The authors declare no conflict of interest.

Abbreviations

D9 tetrahydrocannabinol (THC); cannabidiol (CBD); high THC extract (THCE); high CBD extract (CBDE); nitric oxide (NO•); inflammatory bowel disease (IBD); endocannabinoid system (ECS); specific pathogen-free (SPF); phosphate buffered saline (PBS); Dulbecco's modified Eagle medium (DMEM); fetal calf serum (FCS); lipopolysaccharide (LPS); supernatant (SN); thioglycollate (tg); area under the curve (AUC); non-activated (NA); dextran sodium sulfate (DSS); graft versus host disease (GvHD).

References

1. Locati, M.; Curtale, G.; Mantovani, A. Diversity, Mechanisms, and Significance of Macrophage Plasticity. *Annu. Rev. Pathol.* **2020**, *15*, 123–147. [CrossRef] [PubMed]
2. Murray, P.J.; Wynn, T.A. Protective and pathogenic functions of macrophage subsets. *Nat. Rev. Immunol.* **2011**, *11*, 723–737. [CrossRef]
3. Guan, Q. A Comprehensive Review and Update on the Pathogenesis of Inflammatory Bowel Disease. *J. Immunol. Res.* **2019**, *2019*, 7247238. [CrossRef]
4. Almogi-Hazan, O.; Or, R. Cannabis, the Endocannabinoid System and Immunity-the Journey from the Bedside to the Bench and Back. *Int. J. Mol. Sci.* **2020**, *21*, 4448. [CrossRef]
5. Tomar, S.; Zumbrun, E.E.; Nagarkatti, M.; Nagarkatti, P.S. Protective role of cannabinoid receptor 2 activation in galactosamine/lipopolysaccharide-induced acute liver failure through regulation of macrophage polarization and microRNAs. *J. Pharmacol. Exp. Ther.* **2015**, *353*, 369–379. [CrossRef] [PubMed]
6. Liu, A.P.; Yuan, Q.H.; Zhang, B.; Yang, L.; He, Q.W.; Chen, K.; Liu, Q.S.; Li, Z.; Zhan, J. Cannabinoid receptor 2 activation alleviates septic lung injury by promoting autophagy via inhibition of inflammatory mediator release. *Cell. Signal.* **2020**, *69*, 109556. [CrossRef] [PubMed]
7. Jiang, L.; Chen, Y.; Huang, X.; Yuan, A.; Shao, Q.; Pu, J.; He, B. Selective activation of CB2 receptor improves efferocytosis in cultured macrophages. *Life Sci.* **2016**, *161*, 10–18. [CrossRef]
8. Denaes, T.; Lodder, J.; Chobert, M.N.; Ruiz, I.; Pawlotsky, J.M.; Lotersztajn, S.; Teixeira-Clerc, F. The Cannabinoid Receptor 2 Protects Against Alcoholic Liver Disease Via a Macrophage Autophagy-Dependent Pathway. *Sci. Rep.* **2016**, *6*, 28806. [CrossRef]
9. Duncan, M.; Galic, M.A.; Wang, A.; Chambers, A.P.; McCafferty, D.M.; McKay, D.M.; Sharkey, K.A.; Pittman, Q.J. Cannabinoid 1 receptors are critical for the innate immune response to TLR4 stimulation. *Am. J. Physiol. Regul. Integr. Comp. Physiol.* **2013**, *305*, R224–R231. [CrossRef]
10. Mai, P.; Yang, L.; Tian, L.; Wang, L.; Jia, S.; Zhang, Y.; Liu, X.; Yang, L.; Li, L. Endocannabinoid System Contributes to Liver Injury and Inflammation by Activation of Bone Marrow-Derived Monocytes/Macrophages in a CB1-Dependent Manner. *J. Immunol.* **2015**, *195*, 3390–3401. [CrossRef]
11. Mai, P.; Tian, L.; Yang, L.; Wang, L.; Yang, L.; Li, L. Cannabinoid receptor 1 but not 2 mediates macrophage phagocytosis by G(alpha)i/o/RhoA/ROCK signaling pathway. *J. Cell. Physiol.* **2015**, *230*, 1640–1650. [CrossRef] [PubMed]
12. Miranda, K.; Mehrpouya-Bahrami, P.; Nagarkatti, P.S.; Nagarkatti, M. Cannabinoid Receptor 1 Blockade Attenuates Obesity and Adipose Tissue Type 1 Inflammation Through miR-30e-5p Regulation of Delta-Like-4 in Macrophages and Consequently Downregulation of Th1 Cells. *Front. Immunol.* **2019**, *10*, 1049. [CrossRef] [PubMed]
13. Simard, M.; Rakotoarivelo, V.; Di Marzo, V.; Flamand, N. Expression and Functions of the CB2 Receptor in Human Leukocytes. *Front Pharmacol.* **2022**, *13*, 826400. [CrossRef] [PubMed]
14. Khuja, I.; Yekhtin, Z.; Or, R.; Almogi-Hazan, O. Cannabinoids Reduce Inflammation but Inhibit Lymphocyte Recovery in Murine Models of Bone Marrow Transplantation. *Int. J. Mol. Sci.* **2019**, *20*, 668. [CrossRef]
15. Berman, P.; Futoran, K.; Lewitus, G.M.; Mukha, D.; Benami, M.; Shlomi, T.; Meiri, D. A new ESI-LC/MS approach for comprehensive metabolic profiling of phytocannabinoids in Cannabis. *Sci. Rep.* **2018**, *8*, 14280. [CrossRef]
16. Shapira, A.; Berman, P.; Futoran, K.; Guberman, O.; Meiri, D. Tandem Mass Spectrometric Quantification of 93 Terpenoids in Cannabis Using Static Headspace Injections. *Anal. Chem.* **2019**, *91*, 11425–11432. [CrossRef]
17. Ezekowitz, R.A.; Gordon, S. Surface properties of activated macrophages: Sensitized lymphocytes, specific antigen and lymphokines reduce expression of antigen F4/80 and FC and mannose/fucosyl receptors, but induce Ia. *Adv. Exp. Med. Biol.* **1982**, *155*, 401–407. [CrossRef]
18. Eichele, D.D.; Kharbanda, K.K. Dextran sodium sulfate colitis murine model: An indispensable tool for advancing our understanding of inflammatory bowel diseases pathogenesis. *World J. Gastroenterol.* **2017**, *23*, 6016–6029. [CrossRef]
19. Neurath, M.F. Cytokines in inflammatory bowel disease. *Nat. Rev. Immunol.* **2014**, *14*, 329–342. [CrossRef]
20. Chiurchiu, V.; Lanuti, M.; Catanzaro, G.; Fezza, F.; Rapino, C.; Maccarrone, M. Detailed characterization of the endocannabinoid system in human macrophages and foam cells, and anti-inflammatory role of type-2 cannabinoid receptor. *Atherosclerosis* **2014**, *233*, 55–63. [CrossRef]

21. Galiegue, S.; Mary, S.; Marchand, J.; Dussossoy, D.; Carriere, D.; Carayon, P.; Bouaboula, M.; Shire, D.; Le Fur, G.; Casellas, P. Expression of central and peripheral cannabinoid receptors in human immune tissues and leukocyte subpopulations. *Eur. J. Biochem.* **1995**, *232*, 54–61. [CrossRef] [PubMed]
22. Lee, S.F.; Newton, C.; Widen, R.; Friedman, H.; Klein, T.W. Differential expression of cannabinoid CB(2) receptor mRNA in mouse immune cell subpopulations and following B cell stimulation. *Eur. J. Pharmacol.* **2001**, *423*, 235–241. [CrossRef]
23. Staiano, R.I.; Loffredo, S.; Borriello, F.; Iannotti, F.A.; Piscitelli, F.; Orlando, P.; Secondo, A.; Granata, F.; Lepore, M.T.; Fiorelli, A.; et al. Human lung-resident macrophages express CB1 and CB2 receptors whose activation inhibits the release of angiogenic and lymphangiogenic factors. *J. Leukoc. Biol.* **2016**, *99*, 531–540. [CrossRef] [PubMed]
24. Sugamura, K.; Sugiyama, S.; Nozaki, T.; Matsuzawa, Y.; Izumiya, Y.; Miyata, K.; Nakayama, M.; Kaikita, K.; Obata, T.; Takeya, M.; et al. Activated endocannabinoid system in coronary artery disease and antiinflammatory effects of cannabinoid 1 receptor blockade on macrophages. *Circulation* **2009**, *119*, 28–36. [CrossRef] [PubMed]
25. Rajan, T.S.; Scionti, D.; Diomede, F.; Grassi, G.; Pollastro, F.; Piattelli, A.; Cocco, L.; Bramanti, P.; Mazzon, E.; Trubiani, O. Gingival Stromal Cells as an In Vitro Model: Cannabidiol Modulates Genes Linked With Amyotrophic Lateral Sclerosis. *J. Cell. Biochem.* **2017**, *118*, 819–828. [CrossRef] [PubMed]
26. Yeisley, D.J.; Arabiyat, A.S.; Hahn, M.S. Cannabidiol-Driven Alterations to Inflammatory Protein Landscape of Lipopolysaccharide-Activated Macrophages In Vitro May Be Mediated by Autophagy and Oxidative Stress. *Cannabis Cannabinoid Res.* **2021**, *6*, 253–263. [CrossRef]
27. Fitzpatrick, J.M.; Minogue, E.; Curham, L.; Tyrrell, H.; Gavigan, P.; Hind, W.; Downer, E.J. MyD88-dependent and -independent signalling via TLR3 and TLR4 are differentially modulated by Delta(9)-tetrahydrocannabinol and cannabidiol in human macrophages. *J. Neuroimmunol.* **2020**, *343*, 577217. [CrossRef]
28. Muthumalage, T.; Rahman, I. Cannabidiol differentially regulates basal and LPS-induced inflammatory responses in macrophages, lung epithelial cells, and fibroblasts. *Toxicol. Appl. Pharmacol.* **2019**, *382*, 114713. [CrossRef]
29. Dopkins, N.; Miranda, K.; Wilson, K.; Holloman, B.; Nagarkatti, P.; Nagarkatti, M. Effects of Orally Administered Cannabidiol on Neuroinflammation and Intestinal Inflammation in the Attenuation of Experimental Autoimmune Encephalomyelitis. *J. Neuroimmune Pharmacol.* **2021**, 1–18. [CrossRef]
30. Pacher, P.; Beckman, J.S.; Liaudet, L. Nitric oxide and peroxynitrite in health and disease. *Physiol. Rev.* **2007**, *87*, 315–424. [CrossRef]
31. Lipina, C.; Hundal, H.S. The endocannabinoid system: 'NO' longer anonymous in the control of nitrergic signalling? *J. Mol. Cell Biol.* **2017**, *9*, 91–103. [CrossRef] [PubMed]
32. Romano, B.; Pagano, E.; Orlando, P.; Capasso, R.; Cascio, M.G.; Pertwee, R.; Marzo, V.D.; Izzo, A.A.; Borrelli, F. Pure Delta(9)-tetrahydrocannabivarin and a Cannabis sativa extract with high content in Delta(9)-tetrahydrocannabivarin inhibit nitrite production in murine peritoneal macrophages. *Pharmacol. Res.* **2016**, *113*, 199–208. [CrossRef] [PubMed]
33. Muller, L.; Di Benedetto, S.; Pawelec, G. The Immune System and Its Dysregulation with Aging. *Subcell. Biochem.* **2019**, *91*, 21–43. [CrossRef] [PubMed]
34. Pascual, A.C.; Gaveglio, V.L.; Giusto, N.M.; Pasquare, S.J. Aging modifies the enzymatic activities involved in 2-arachidonoylglycerol metabolism. *Biofactors* **2013**, *39*, 209–220. [CrossRef]
35. Paradisi, A.; Oddi, S.; Maccarrone, M. The endocannabinoid system in ageing: A new target for drug development. *Curr. Drug Targets* **2006**, *7*, 1539–1552. [CrossRef]
36. Mosser, D.M. The many faces of macrophage activation. *J. Leukoc. Biol.* **2003**, *73*, 209–212. [CrossRef]
37. Samadi, N.; Polak, D.; Kitzmuller, C.; Steinberger, P.; Zlabinger, G.J.; Jahn-Schmid, B.; Bohle, B. T-cell-derived cytokines enhance the antigen-presenting capacity of human neutrophils. *Eur. J. Immunol.* **2019**, *49*, 1441–1443. [CrossRef]
38. Wacnik, P.W.; Luhr, K.M.; Hill, R.H.; Ljunggren, H.G.; Kristensson, K.; Svensson, M. Cannabinoids affect dendritic cell (DC) potassium channel function and modulate DC T cell stimulatory capacity. *J. Immunol.* **2008**, *181*, 3057–3066. [CrossRef]
39. Palma, A.; Jarrah, A.S.; Tieri, P.; Cesareni, G.; Castiglione, F. Gene Regulatory Network Modeling of Macrophage Differentiation Corroborates the Continuum Hypothesis of Polarization States. *Front. Physiol.* **2018**, *9*, 1659. [CrossRef]
40. Wang, L.X.; Zhang, S.X.; Wu, H.J.; Rong, X.L.; Guo, J. M2b macrophage polarization and its roles in diseases. *J. Leukoc. Biol.* **2019**, *106*, 345–358. [CrossRef]
41. Lin, H.H.; Faunce, D.E.; Stacey, M.; Terajewicz, A.; Nakamura, T.; Zhang-Hoover, J.; Kerley, M.; Mucenski, M.L.; Gordon, S.; Stein-Streilein, J. The macrophage F4/80 receptor is required for the induction of antigen-specific efferent regulatory T cells in peripheral tolerance. *J. Exp. Med.* **2005**, *201*, 1615–1625. [CrossRef] [PubMed]
42. Ambrose, T.; Simmons, A. Cannabis, Cannabinoids, and the Endocannabinoid System-Is there Therapeutic Potential for Inflammatory Bowel Disease? *J. Crohns Colitis* **2019**, *13*, 525–535. [CrossRef] [PubMed]
43. Scheau, C.; Caruntu, C.; Badarau, I.A.; Scheau, A.E.; Docea, A.O.; Calina, D.; Caruntu, A. Cannabinoids and Inflammations of the Gut-Lung-Skin Barrier. *J. Pers. Med.* **2021**, *11*, 494. [CrossRef] [PubMed]
44. Nso, N.; Nyabera, A.; Nassar, M.; Alshamam, M.S.; Sumbly, V.; Vest, M.; Patel, N.; Ojong, G.; Rizzo, V. Cannabis and Its Potential Protective Role Against Inflammatory Bowel Disease: A Scoping Review. *Cureus* **2021**, *13*, e18841. [CrossRef] [PubMed]
45. Aswad, M.; Hamza, H.; Pechkovsky, A.; Zikrach, A.; Popov, T.; Zohar, Y.; Shahar, E.; Louria-Hayon, I. High-CBD extract (CBD-X) downregulates cytokine storm systemically and locally in inflamed lungs. *Front. Immunol.* **2022**, *13*, 875546. [CrossRef] [PubMed]

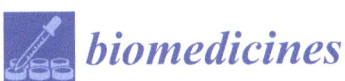

Article

Enhancing Endocannabinoid Signaling via β-Catenin in the Nucleus Accumbens Attenuates PTSD- and Depression-like Behavior of Male Rats

Tomer Mizrachi Zer-Aviv [1], Larglinda Islami [1], Peter J. Hamilton [2], Eric M. Parise [2], Eric J. Nestler [2], Brenda Sbarski [1] and Irit Akirav [1,*]

[1] Department of Psychology, School of Psychological Sciences, and the Integrated Brain and Behavior Research Center, University of Haifa, Haifa 3498838, Israel; tomer.mizrachi6@gmail.com (T.M.Z.-A.); laislami@uni-mainz.de (L.I.); bsbarski@gmail.com (B.S.)

[2] Nash Family Department of Neuroscience and Friedman Brain Institute, Icahn School of Medicine at Mount Sinai, New York, NY 10029, USA; peter.hamilton@vcuhealth.org (P.J.H.); eric.parise@mssm.edu (E.M.P.); eric.nestler@mssm.edu (E.J.N.)

* Correspondence: iakirav@psy.haifa.ac.il

Abstract: Inhibition of fatty acid amide hydrolase (FAAH), which increases anandamide levels, has been suggested as a potential treatment for stress-related conditions. We examined whether the stress-preventing effects of the FAAH inhibitor URB597 on behavior are mediated via β-catenin in the nucleus accumbens (NAc). Male rats were exposed to the shock and reminders model of PTSD and then treated with URB597 (0.4 mg/kg; i.p.). They were tested for anxiety- (freezing, startle response), depression-like behaviors (despair, social preference, anhedonia), and memory function (T-maze, social recognition). We also tested the involvement of the CB1 receptor (CB1r), β-catenin, and metabotropic glutamate receptor subtype 5 (mGluR5) proteins. URB597 prevented the shock- and reminders-induced increase in anxiety- and depressive-like behaviors, as well as the impaired memory via the CB1r-dependent mechanism. In the NAc, viral-mediated β-catenin overexpression restored the behavior of rats exposed to stress and normalized the alterations in protein levels in the NAc and the prefrontal cortex. Importantly, when NAc β-catenin levels were downregulated by viral-mediated gene transfer, the therapeutic-like effects of URB597 were blocked. We suggest a potentially novel mechanism for the therapeutic-like effects of FAAH inhibition that is dependent on β-catenin activation in the NAc in a PTSD rat model.

Keywords: rat; post-traumatic stress disorder (PTSD); cannabinoids; URB597; mGluR5; CB1 receptor; fatty acid amide hydrolase (FAAH); β-catenin

1. Introduction

Stressful life events can substantially impact the brain and induce psychiatric disorders such as post-traumatic stress disorder (PTSD) and depression [1].

A large body of evidence, including our own findings, points to the endocannabinoid (ECB) system as a possible therapeutic target to help treat PTSD [2–15]. The ECB system contains the cannabinoid receptors CB1 (CB1r) and CB2 (CB2r); endogenous ligands: N-arachidonyl ethanolamine (anandamide; AEA) and 2-arachidonoyl glycerol (2-AG); and their degrading enzymes: 2 monoacylglycerol lipase (MAGL) for 2-AG and fatty acid amide hydrolase (FAAH) for AEA.

Using a rat model for PTSD in an inhibitory avoidance apparatus, wherein rats are exposed to a single severe foot shock followed by exposure to contextual reminders, we found that acute administration of the FAAH inhibitor URB597 or the CB1/CB2 receptor agonist WIN55,212-2 after shock exposure prevented anxiety- and depression-like behaviors [3,15–17]. Unlike direct cannabinoid agonists, URB597 does not cause classical

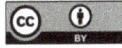

cannabinoid side effects such as catalepsy, hypothermia, hyperphagia, and abuse potential [18,19]. However, the mechanism for the therapeutic-like effects of URB597 requires further investigation.

The Wnt/β-catenin pathway was found to play a significant role in anxiety and depressive symptoms [20,21] and to regulate pro-resilient and anxiolytic-like effects in the nucleus accumbens (NAc) by activating a network that includes Dicer1 and downstream microRNAs [22]. Moreover, overexpressing GSK-3β (i.e., the kinase which phosphorylates β-catenin) in the NAc induced depressive-like behavior, whereas GSK-3β inhibition promoted resilience [23]. Similarly, contextual and cued fear memory increased GSK-3β phosphorylation in the hippocampus and amygdala [21,24,25]. We have previously demonstrated that enhanced extinction kinetics in rats exposed to shock and reminders was significantly associated with increased expression of β-catenin in the NAc; hence, suggesting that the expression of β-catenin in the NAc is linked with a resilient response to the stressor [26]. When β-catenin levels in the NAc were inhibited using the non-selective β-catenin antagonist sulindac, it blocked the therapeutic-like effects of WIN55,212-2 on extinction [26]. The involvement of the Wnt/β-catenin pathway in antidepressant and pro-cognitive effects also has been observed in the medial prefrontal cortex (mPFC) [27,28].

In vivo and in vitro evidence suggests that Wnt/β-catenin signaling is downstream of metabotropic glutamate receptor subtype 5 (mGluR5); hence, mGluR5 signaling plays a key role in controlling neuronal gene expression by regulating the assembly of the N-cadherin/β-catenin complex and consequently the expression of REST/NRSF (Repressor element 1-silencing transcription factor/neuron-restrictive silencer factor) in primary corticostriatal neurons [29]. Importantly, mGluR5 is implicated in the pathophysiology of several psychiatric disorders [30]. The direction of mGluR5 modulation that elicits antidepressant/anxiolytic-like effects has been inconsistent across studies [31–33]. However, the PFC of postmortem brains of major depressive disorder patients shows reduced mGluR5 protein expression [34]; in rodents, an essential role for mGluR5 in the NAc was found in promoting stress resilience, suggesting that a deficit in mGluR5-mediated signaling in this region may represent an endophenotype for stress-induced depression [35]. In a recent study, NAc mGluR5 activation ameliorated the effects of stress on depression-like behavior and pain, through ECB mediation, suggesting an association between ECB signaling and the expression of mGluR5 in stressed rats [36].

The aim of the current study is to examine the role of β-catenin in the stress-attenuating effects of FAAH inhibition and to assess its function in anxiety- (freezing, startle response), and depression-like behaviors (forced swim test, social preference, saccharin preference), as well as memory function (water T-maze, social recognition). To that end, we overexpressed and downregulated β-catenin in the NAc by viral-mediated gene transfer and assessed the effects of URB597 in these relevant stress-related behaviors and several proteins of interest (i.e., β-catenin, mGluR5 and CB1r) in the NAc, PFC, hippocampus and amygdala. We hypothesized that URB597 would prevent the shock- and reminders-induced alterations in behavior, and that these therapeutic-like effects of URB597 would be mediated via β-catenin in the NAc.

2. Materials and Methods

2.1. Subjects

Male Sprague Dawley rats (60 days old, ~225 g; Envigo, Jerusalem, Israel) were caged together according to their treatment group (4 per cage; 59 × 28 × 20 cm) at 22 ± 2 °C under 12 h light/dark cycles. Plastic hoses were placed in each cage to enrich the animals' environment. For the saccharin preference test, each rat was placed in a separate cage. Rats were allowed water and laboratory rodent food ad libitum.

2.2. Drug Treatment

The FAAH inhibitor URB597 (0.4 mg/kg, i.p.) and the CB1r antagonist AM251 (0.3 mg/kg, i.p.) (Cayman Chemicals, Ann Arbor, MI, USA) were dissolved in dimethylsulfoxide 5%, Tween-80 and saline 90% (Sigma-Aldrich, Rehovot, Israel). Drug doses are based on previous findings [3,4,16,37].

2.3. Shock and Situational Reminders

Rats were exposed to a single shock in a passive avoidance apparatus divided into two equal-size compartments (one light and one dark), which were separated by a guillotine door [15,17]. On shock day, rats were placed in the light compartment; once the rat entered the dark compartment, a single foot shock (1.5 mA, 10 s) was delivered (Coulbourn Instruments, Whitehall, PA, USA). The no-shock groups received the same treatment, but with the shock mechanism inactivated.

For situational reminders (SRs), a rat was placed in the lighted start chamber for 60 s, with the guillotine door closed to prevent the rat from entering the shock compartment (to avoid extinction). No further shocks were administered. We used a video camera to monitor the duration of freezing behavior during the 60 s SR in the lighted chamber. Freezing was measured before shock administration (baseline) and during the five days of SRs (SR1-SR5). The percentage of changed pixels between two adjacent 1 s images was calculated, and if the percentage of change in images was <0.05%, the rat was scored as "freezing" [38]. Freezing was defined as the absence of all movement except for respiration [39].

2.4. Behavioral Testing

All rats were tested in all behavioral procedures in the same order. The most aversive test (forced swim test—FST) was last. Tests were separated by a 24 h period. All behavioral tests were conducted under dim lighting (15–20 lx) and took place between 12:00 and 16:00. Behavioral testing was taken after SR5 in order to examine the long-term effects of the traumatic event. In a previous study, we found that shocked rats exposed to SRs persistently avoided the dark chamber, whereas, shocked rats not exposed to SRs demonstrated increased avoidance on the first extinction trial, but their extinction kinetic was intact [7].

2.5. Acoustic Startle Response (ASR)

A soundproof chamber (25 × 25 × 25 cm) containing an acrylic animal holder (8 × 8 × 16 cm; Coulbourn Instruments, Whitehall, PA, USA) that is connected to a piezoelectric accelerometer. For consistency between chambers and experiments, calibration of sensitivity to the movement and sound levels was applied. A single rat was placed in the holder for a 5 min acclimatization period; 30 acoustic startle trials (98 or 120 dB; 50 ms duration, 20–40 s intertrial interval) were presented over the 68 dB white noise background. We analyzed the mean startle amplitude which indicates the averaged response to the 98 and 120 dB in mV [40].

2.6. Social Preference and Social Recognition

This task assesses sociability and short-term social memory. Habituation for 1 h to the transparent corrals in the home cages of the juvenile and experimental rats preceded the training. The object and the juvenile rat were confined to the corrals that were placed 10 cm from the two opposite corners of the arena. The corrals (9 cm in diameter) allowed physical contact with the experimental rat [3]. The objects were children's Lego blocks.

For the preference and recognition phases, the experimental rat was given 5 min exploration with an intertrial interval of 30 min in a holding cage. For preference, the rat explored the novel object and the unfamiliar juvenile. The ratio was calculated as the time spent exploring the juvenile rat divided by the total exploration time (juvenile rat + novel object). For recognition, the rat explored a novel juvenile and the familiarized juvenile. The ratio was calculated as the time spent exploring the novel juvenile divided by total exploration time (familiar + novel juveniles). The trials were videotaped (Logiteck, C922 Pro Stream, Newark, CA, USA) and recorded (NCH Software, Greenwood Village, CO, USA) and the time spent in corral exploration was analyzed using EthoVision XT9 software.

2.7. Water T-Maze (WTM)

The WTM is a black Plexiglas maze (length of stem, 64 cm; length of arms, 43 cm; width, 13 cm; height of walls, 42 cm). A transparent plastic escape platform (12 × 12 cm) is hidden at the end of one of the two arms that are filled with water ($23 \pm 1\ °C$). The test has two phases: acquisition and reversal.

For the first acquisition phase, a rat needs to choose the right arm out of two. If it chooses the right arm, it remains on the platform for 10 more seconds. If it chooses the wrong arm, the rat is confined to the arm for 20 s.

In the second reversal phase (performed 24 h after the acquisition phase), each rat was first tested in a probe trial without the platform. Once the rat entered an arm, it was removed from the maze. If the non-reinforced arm was chosen, the rat was retrained on the discrimination of the previous day and tested again 24 h later. If the reinforced arm was chosen, the rat was trained on the reversal of that discrimination, i.e., the platform was moved to the opposite arm [41]. In both phases, the number of correct trials was recorded until the rat reached five consecutive correct trials.

2.8. Forced Swim Test (FST)

This test is based on the assumption that when a rat is placed in a container filled with water, it will at first make efforts to escape but eventually will exhibit immobility that may reflect despair [42]. An acrylic cylindrical container (62 cm diameter, 40 cm height) was filled with water at a temperature of 24 °C. The water level (34 cm) was such that a rat could not touch the bottom with its hind paws. A rat was forced to swim for 15 min inside the container. Then, after 24 h in the home cage, the rat was put back in the container and forced to swim for 5 min. The time spent immobile was recorded. Immobility was defined as the lack of motion, except for movements necessary to keep the rat's head above water [43,44].

2.9. Saccharin Preference Test

Water bottles were removed before the dark part of the cycle and replaced with two bottles, one filled with water and the other with saccharin (0.01 mg/L, dissolved in water, Sigma-Aldrich, Rehovot, Israel). Saccharin consumption was measured during the 12 dark hours of the cycle. Following one night of habituation to saccharin, the saccharin preference ratio was calculated as the saccharin consumption divided by the total consumption (consumption of saccharin/water + saccharin).

2.10. Western Blotting (WB)

Rats were euthanized and brain tissues of the mPFC (prelimbic and infralimbic punched together), NAc shell, basolateral amygdala (BLA), and CA1 area of the hippocampus were removed by cryostat using a 0.5 mm puncher (coordinates relative to Bregma in mm: mPFC: anteroposterior (AP), +3.72; medial–lateral (ML), ±0.4; ventral (V), −4.8; NAc shell: AP, +1.6; ML, ±1; V, −5.5; BLA: AP, −1.596; ML, ±4.2; V, 8.45; CA1: AP, −4.2; ML, ±2.5; V: −2.5). Protein levels were determined by the bicinchoninic acid protein assay kit (Thermo Fisher Scientific, Waltham, MA, USA). The samples were then diluted in an SDS sample buffer, boiled for 5 min at 100 °C, and then stored at −80 °C. On running day, wells were loaded with 30 µL of samples. Each gel contained at least one sample from each group. Aliquots were subjected to SDS–PAGE (7.5% polyacrylamide; Sigma-Aldrich, Rehovot, Israel) and immunoblot analysis.

Blots were incubated with CB1r (1:1000; abcam, Cambridge, UK; ab25932 [ERP23934-20]), β–catenin (1:5000; abcam, Cambridge, UK; ab32572 [E247]), or mGluR5 (1:5000; abcam, Cambridge, UK; ab76316 [ERP2425Y]) antibodies overnight at 4 °C. This was followed by a 1 h incubation with an HRP-linked secondary antibody at room temperature (1:10,000; goat anti-rabbit IgG; Jackson ImmunoResearch Laboratories, West Grove, PA, USA; 111-035-144). Blots were visualized with ECL (Bio-Lab, Jerusalem, Israel) and an XRS charge-coupled device camera (BioRad Laboratories, Hercules, CA, USA). We used the Quantity One software (BioRad Laboratories, Hercules, CA, USA) to assess blot density. All protein samples were standardized with β-actin (1:1000; Cell Signaling, Danvers, MA, USA; #5125 [13E5]). For antibody specificity, see the Supplementary File, Figure S1.

2.11. Viral-Mediated Gene Transfer

The replication-deficient *herpes simplex virus* (HSV) p1005 vector is a "short-term" vector, derived from herpes simplex virus-1 with a high titer range ($3-5 \times 10^8$ transduction unit, TU/mL; an illustration of a modified HSV amplicon plasmid is presented in the Supplementary File, Figure S2). Stereotactic surgery was performed on rats under anesthesia of Domitor (2%, 10 mg/kg, i.p.) and ketamine (10%, 100 mg/kg, s.c.) (Vetmarket, Modiin, Israel). A total of 1 µL of the HSV viral vector or green fluorescent protein (GFP) was infused bilaterally into the NAc (Stoelting, Wood Dale, IL, USA) at a rate of 0.1 µL/min (coordinates relative to Bregma: AP, +1.6 mm; LM, ±1 mm; V, −5.5 mm). Vectors were used to overexpress (OE) or downregulate (DR) the expression of β-catenin compared to a GFP control five days before shock day; the vector is expressed in vivo within 2–3 h, with maximal expression from 3–5 days post-injection that lasts only 8 days in vivo [23,45–47]. The viral dose was determined by rendering the >90% cell infection rate in brain tissue, diluted in 60% PBS.

The needle was held in place for 5 additional minutes before being slowly withdrawn. Animals were allowed 5 days of recovery before behavioral experiments began.

2.12. Perfusion and Immunohistochemistry (IHC)

Perfusion:

In anesthetized rats (Domitor and ketamine), brains were perfused with 4% paraformaldehyde solution (Santa Cruz Biochemicals, Dallas, TX, USA). Post-fixation brains were kept at −80 °C [48].

GFP detection:

Brains were sectioned in 35-µm-thick slices using cryostat microtome (Leica Biosystems, Deer Park, IL, USA) and stored at 4 °C in PBS. Then, slices were washed three times for 15 min each in 1 × PBS (Sigma-Aldrich, St. Louis, MO, USA). After the washing procedure, the brain slices were mounted on super frost glass slides using PBS as a mounting solution and left to dry for 24 h. Glass slides were then stored at 4 °C in a dark chamber. Staining was documented using a confocal microscope at 5×, 10×, and 40× zoom (ZEISS, Jena, Germany).

2.13. Experimental Design

a. Study design for experiments 1 and 2: on day 0, male rats were exposed to a single, severe foot shock (1.5 mA, 10 s) in an inhibitory avoidance apparatus, followed by exposure to contextual 1 min situational reminders (SRs) of the shock on days 5, 10, 15, 20, and 25 (Scheme 1a). Freezing was measured during exposure to SR. Drugs (Vehicle, URB597, AM251, AM251 + URB597) were administered i.p. 1 h after shock exposure. Following habituation to saccharin on day −3 (sacc' hab; pre-shock), preference was tested on day −2 pre-shock and on days 2, 7, and 14 post-shock. Acoustic startle response (ASR) testing was administered twice: one day before the shock (−1; ASR1) and one day after the last reminder (day 26; ASR2). On day 27, rats were exposed to the social preference and recognition tests, on days 28–29 to the water T-maze (WTM), and on days 30–31 to the forced swim test (FST). In experiment 1, four groups (n = 10 for all groups) were administered with vehicle or URB597, and brains were removed on day 32 for western blotting (WB). In experiment 2, six groups (n = 8 for all groups) were administered with vehicle, AM251, or AM 251 + URB597. No rats were excluded from the experiments.

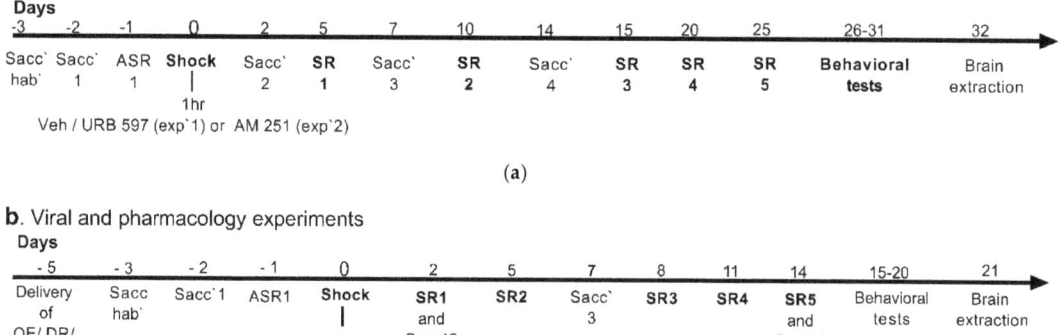

Scheme 1. (a) Study design for experiments 1 and 2. Rats were exposed to a severe foot shock (1.5 mA, 10 s) followed by exposure to contextual 1 min situational reminders (SRs). Drugs were administered i.p. 1 h after shock exposure followed by a battery of behavioral tests and brain extraction. (b) Study design for experiments 3 and 4. On day −5, the herpes simplex virus (HSV) vector was injected bilaterally into the nucleus accumbens (NAc) to overexpress (OE) or downregulate (DR) β-catenin. On day 0, rats were exposed to a single severe foot shock (1.5 mA, 10 s) followed by exposure to contextual 1 min situational reminders (SRs). In experiment 4, drugs (Vehicle, URB59751) were administered i.p. 1 h after shock exposure. All rats were exposed to a battery of behavioral tests. For experiment 3, the brains were removed following the tests.

b. Study design for experiments 3 and 4: on day −5, the herpes simplex virus (HSV) vector was injected bilaterally into the nucleus accumbens (NAc) to overexpress (OE) or downregulate (DR) β-catenin (Scheme 1b). On day 0, male rats were exposed to a single severe foot shock (1.5 mA, 10 s) in an inhibitory avoidance apparatus followed by exposure to contextual 1 min situational reminders (SRs) of the shock on days: 2, 5, 8, 11, and 14. Following habituation to saccharin on day −3 (sacc' hab; pre-shock), preference was tested on days −2 pre-shock and on days 2, 7, and 14 post-shock. Acoustic startle response (ASR) testing was administered before the shock (day 1; ASR1) and one day after the last reminder (day 15; ASR2). In experiment 4, drugs (Vehicle, URB59751) were administered i.p. 1 h after shock exposure. On day 16 rats were exposed to the social preference and recognition tests, on days 17–18 to the water T-maze (WTM), and on days 19–20 to the forced swim test (FST). For experiment 3, the brains were removed on day 21, and β-catenin, mGluR5, and CB1r expression were measured using western blotting (WB). In experiment 3, GFP or OE was delivered to four groups (n = 7–10 for all groups). In experiment 4, GFP or DR was delivered to eight groups (n = 8 for all groups). No rats were excluded from the experiments.

2.14. Statistical Analysis

The results are expressed as means ± SEM. For statistical analysis, we used one-way ANOVAs, two-way ANOVAs, repeated measures ANOVAs, t-tests, and Pearson bivariate correlation tests, as indicated. All post hoc comparisons were made using Tukey's range test. Significance was chosen at $p \leq 0.05$. Data were analyzed using SPSS 27 (IBM, Chicago, IL, USA). Normality assumption was examined using the Kolmogorov–Smirnov and Shapiro–Wilk tests.

3. Results

3.1. Experiment 1: The Effects of URB597 on Behavior and the Expression of β-Catenin in Rats Exposed to Shock and Reminders

Rats were exposed to a single severe foot shock followed by situational reminders. Drugs were administered i.p. 1 h after shock exposure, and then the rats performed a battery of behavioral tests; brains were removed after 24 h and β-catenin expression was measured (for detailed study design, see Section 2.13 Experimental Design).

3.1.1. Freezing

Freezing behavior was monitored during the 1 min exposure to the SR conditions (baseline and SR1–SR5) (Figure 1a). Repeated measures ANOVA (shock × drug × SR; 2 × 2 × 6) revealed significant main effects of drug [$F(1,36) = 37.737$, $p < 0.001$], shock [$F(1,36) = 78.650$, $p < 0.001$], SR day [$F(5,180) = 11.773$, $p < 0.001$]. We also detected the following interactions: shock × drug [$F(1,36) = 36.301$, $p < 0.001$], shock × SR [$F(5,180) = 10.960$, $p < 0.001$], drug × SR [$F(5,180) = 4.910$, $p < 0.001$], and shock × drug × SR [$F(5,180) = 4.823$, $p < 0.001$]. Post hoc analysis revealed that on SR1 to SR5 the Shock/Veh group demonstrated a significant increase in freezing levels compared with the NoShock/Veh group ($p < 0.001$) and the Shock/URB group (SR1; SR2; SR4; SR5: $p < 0.01$; SR3: $p < 0.001$). This suggests that URB597 prevented the shock-induced increase in freezing behavior. In addition, the Shock/URB group showed increased freezing levels compared with the NoShock/URB group (SR1: $p < 0.001$; SR2; SR3: $p < 0.01$; SR4: $p < 0.05$).

3.1.2. Saccharin Preference

Saccharin preference was tested on day 2 pre-shock and on days 2, 7, and 14 post-shock (Figure 1b). Repeated measures ANOVA (shock × drug × day; 2 × 2 × 4) revealed significant effects of drug [$F(1,36) = 16.109$, $p < 0.001$] and day [$F(3,108) = 5.633$, $p < 0.01$]; with the following interactions: shock × drug [$F(1,36) = 8.970$, $p < 0.01$], shock × day [$F(3,108) = 2.896$, $p < 0.05$], drug × day [$F(3,108) = 5.723$, $p < 0.01$], shock × drug × day [$F(3,108) = 6.052$, $p < 0.01$]. Post hoc analysis revealed that on days 2 and 7, the Shock/Veh group demonstrated decreased saccharin preference compared with the NoShock/Veh (day 2: $p < 0.001$; day 7: $p < 0.01$) and Shock/URB ($p < 0.001$) groups. Hence, URB597 prevented the shock and reminders induced a decrease in saccharin preference (i.e., anhedonia).

3.1.3. Acoustic Startle Response

The ASR test was performed on days 1 (pre-shock) and 26 (Figure 1c). We performed a repeated measures ANOVA (shock × drug × time; 2 × 2 × 2) on mean amplitude, and identified significant effects of shock [$F(1,36) = 4.060$, $p < 0.05$] and time [$F(1,36) = 7.799$, $p < 0.01$], with the following significant interactions: shock × time [$F(1,36) = 5.3$, $p < 0.05$], drug × time [$F(1,36) = 6.779$, $p < 0.05$], and shock × drug × time [$F(1,36) = 8.646$, $p < 0.01$]. Post hoc analysis on ASR2 revealed a significant increase in amplitude in Shock/Veh compared with Shock/URB and NoShock/Veh ($p < 0.05$ in both cases). This suggests that URB597 restored the shock/reminders-induced increase in startle response.

3.1.4. Social Tests

We performed the social tests on day 27 (Figure 1d). We ran a two-way ANOVA (shock × drug; 2 × 2) and found significant effects of shock [preference: $F(1,36) = 4.537$, $p < 0.05$; recognition: $F(1,36) = 23.199$, $p < 0.001$] and drug [preference: $F(1,36) = 22.928$, $p < 0.001$; recognition: $F(1,36) = 6.619$, $p < 0.05$], with a significant drug × shock interaction [preference: $F(1,36) = 6.259$, $p < 0.05$; recognition: $F(1,36) = 5.905$, $p < 0.05$]. Post hoc analysis revealed a significant decrease in the exploration ratio in both tasks in the Shock/Veh group compared with the NoShock/Veh group (preference: $p < 0.01$; recognition: $p < 0.001$) and Shock/URB597 group ($p < 0.001$ for both preference and recognition). Hence, URB597 restored the impairing effects of shock and reminders on social behavior. For total exploration time, see the Supplementary File, Figure S3.

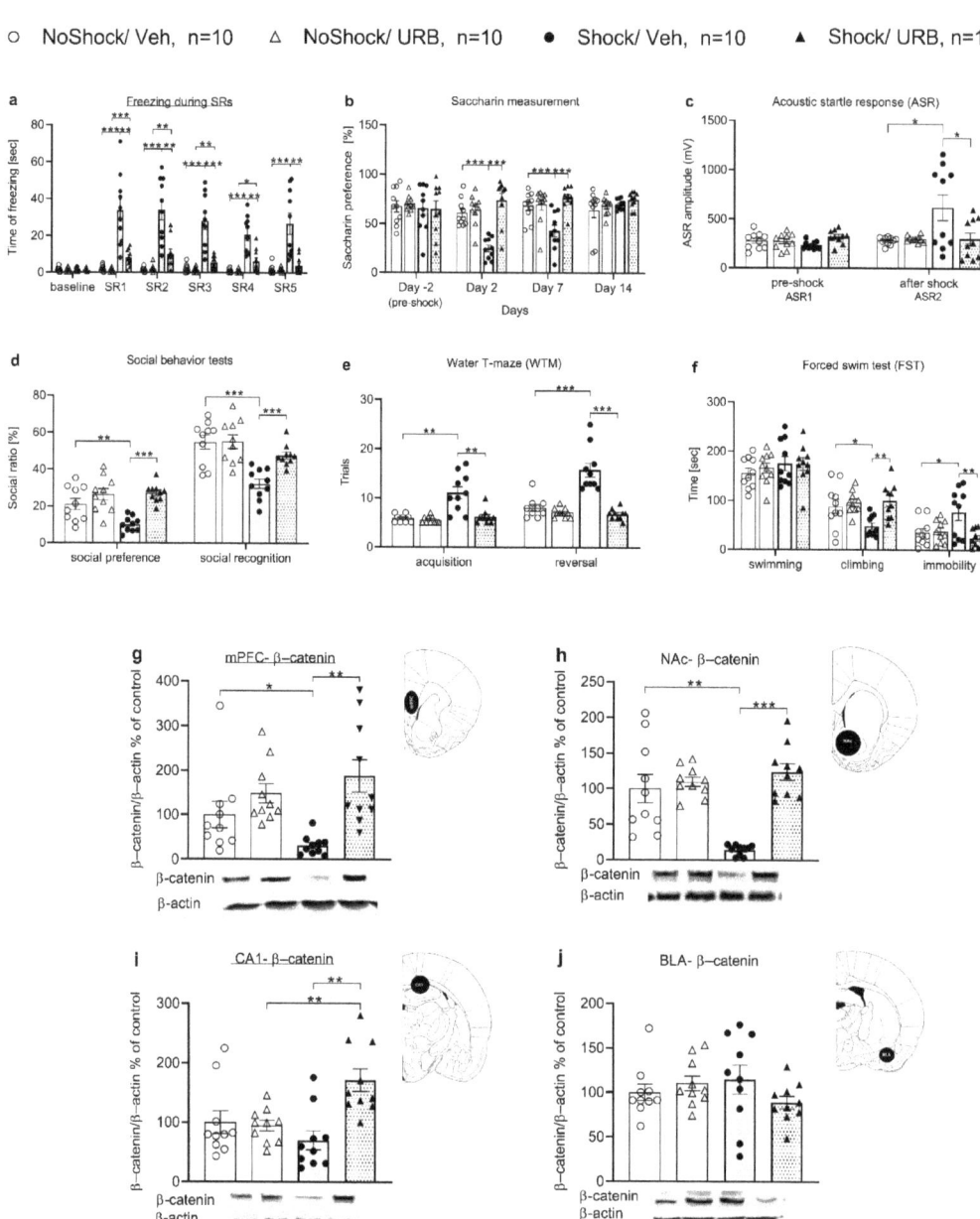

Figure 1. The effects of URB597 on behavior and β-catenin expression in rats exposed to shock and reminders. Compared with non-shocked rats treated with vehicle (NoShock/Veh) and shocked rats treated with URB597 (Shock/URB597), rats that were exposed to shock and treated with vehicle (Shock/Veh) demonstrated the following: increased freezing on SR1 to SR5 (SR—situational reminder) (**a**), decreased saccharin preference on days 2 and 7 (**b**), increased acoustic startle amplitude (ASR) on ASR2 (**c**); decreased social preference and social recognition (**d**); impaired performance in the acquisition and reversal phases in the water T-maze (WTM) (**e**), increased immobility in the forced swim test (FST) (**f**); downregulation in β-catenin protein levels in the medial prefrontal cortex (mPFC) (**g**),

and in the nucleus accumbens (NAc) (h); in the CA1, the Shock/Veh group and the NoShock/URB597 group demonstrated downregulation in β-catenin levels compared with the Shock/URB597 group (i); in the basolateral amygdala (BLA), no significant differences between the groups were observed (j) rat brain atlas illustration indicating punch location are also shown (data is shown as mean ± sem; *, $p < 0.05$; **, $p < 0.01$; ***, $p < 0.001$).

3.1.5. Water T-Maze

For the WTM, tested on days 28–29 (Figure 1e), a repeated measures ANOVA (shock × drug × test; 2 × 2 × 2) revealed significant effects of shock [$F(1,35) = 60.717$, $p < 0.001$], drug [$F(1,35) = 77.881$, $p < 0.001$] and test [$F(1,35) = 13.271$, $p < 0.01$], with a significant shock × drug interaction [$F(1,36) = 53.689$, $p < 0.01$]. Post hoc analysis revealed that the Shock/Veh group showed a significant increase in the number of trials required to reach the criterion in both phases compared with the NoShock/Veh and Shock/URB groups (for both groups: acquisition, $p < 0.01$; reversal, $p < 0.001$). This suggests that URB597 prevented the shock and reminders-induced impairment in performance in the WTM task.

3.1.6. Forced Swim Test

For the FST, performed on days 30–31 (Figure 1f), a two-way ANOVA [shock × drug; 2 × 2] on immobility revealed significant effects of drug [$F(1,36) = 6.047$, $p < 0.05$], and drug × shock interaction [$F(1,36) = 7.389$, $p < 0.05$]. Post hoc analysis revealed an increase in immobility in the Shock/Veh group compared with the NoShock/Veh group ($p < 0.05$) and the Shock/URB597 group ($p < 0.01$), suggesting that URB597 restored the shock- and reminders-induced despair-like behavior.

3.1.7. β-Catenin

Punches were extracted from the rat mPFC, NAc, CA1, and BLA (Figure 1g–j, respectively; also shown are brain sites from where the tissue samples were extracted).

For β-catenin levels, a two-way ANOVA [shock × drug; 2 × 2] revealed significant effects of shock [NAc: $F(1,36) = 8.52$, $p < 0.01$], drug [mPFC: $F(1,36) = 15.324$, $p < 0.001$; NAc: $F(1,36) = 24.099$, $p < 0.001$; CA1: $F(1,36) = 8.749$, $p < 0.01$], and shock × drug interaction [mPFC: $F(1,36) = 4.320$, $p < 0.05$; NAc: $F(1,36) = 16.888$, $p < 0.001$; CA1: $F(1,36) = 10.863$, $p < 0.01$]. Post hoc comparisons revealed a significant decrease in β-catenin levels in the mPFC and NAc in the Shock/Veh group compared with the NoShock/Veh group (mPFC: $p < 0.05$; NAc: $p < 0.01$) and the Shock/URB597 group (mPFC: $p < 0.01$; NAc $p < 0.001$). In CA1, the Shock/URB597 group demonstrated increased β-catenin levels compared with the NoShock/URB597 group and the Shock/Veh group (both $p < 0.01$). No significant effects were observed in the BLA. Hence, exposure to shock and reminders downregulated β-catenin levels in the mPFC and NAc, and URB597 normalized these effects.

The same blots were rehybridized with antibodies specific for β-actin in order to confirm equal protein loading. As there were no differences between the groups in the levels of β-actin in the brain regions we examined, we concluded that the treatment had no effect on the levels of β-actin.

3.1.8. Correlation between β-Catenin Levels and Behavior

We conducted Pearson bivariate correlation tests (Supplementary File; Table S1) between the expression of β-catenin and behavior to explore the association between the β-catenin levels and the anxiety- and depressive-like phenotype of the rats. The most robust correlations were found between β-catenin levels in the NAc and the following behaviors: freezing (SR1: $r = -0.560$; SR2: $r = -0.550$; SR3: $r = -0.610$; SR4: $r = -0.572$; SR1: $r = -0.541$; all $p < 0.01$); ASR ($r = -0.461$, $p < 0.01$); WTM acquisition ($r = -0.437$, $p < 0.01$) and reversal ($r = -0.694$, $p < 0.01$), and saccharin preference (Day 2: $r = 0.618$, $p < 0.01$; Day 7: $r = 0.597$, $p < 0.01$). This suggests that decreased β-catenin levels in the NAc are associated with enhanced freezing and startle response, anhedonia, and impaired performance in the WTM. A robust correlation was also found between mPFC β-catenin levels and climbing in the FST (r = 0.419, $p < 0.01$).

3.2. Experiment 2: The Preventing Effects of URB597 on Behavior of Rats Exposed to Shock and Reminders Are Mediated by CB1 Receptors

As URB597 is a FAAH inhibitor, we aimed to examine whether its effects on stress behavior are mediated through CB1r-dependent mechanisms. We used a low dose of the CB1r antagonist AM251 (am; 0.3 mg/kg) to block CB1r, as previous results have demonstrated that a low dose of this antagonist had no effect on behavior by itself but prevented the therapeutic effects of the cannabinoid agonists (Segev et al., 2018). Therefore, AM251 and URB597 were administered concurrently in order to examine the involvement of CB1rs in the effects of the FAAH inhibitor on behavior (for a detailed study design, see Section 2.13 Experimental Design).

3.2.1. Freezing

Freezing behavior was monitored during the 1 min exposure to the SRs. A repeated measures ANOVA (shock × drug × SR; 2 × 3 × 6) revealed significant main effects of shock [$F(1,42) = 551.682, p < 0.001$] and SR [$F(5,210) = 33.124, p < 0.001$]; with a shock × SR interaction [$F(5,210) = 32.356, p < 0.001$] (Figure 2a). Post hoc analysis revealed that on SR1 to SR5, the shock groups (Veh; am; am + URB) demonstrated a significant increase in freezing levels compared with the NoShock groups (Veh; am; am + URB; $p < 0.001$). Hence, the preventive effect of URB597 on freezing behavior was blocked by AM251.

3.2.2. Saccharin Preference

Saccharin preference was tested on day 2 pre-shock and on days 2, 7, and 14 post-shock. A repeated measures ANOVA (2 × 2 × 4) revealed a significant effect of shock [$F(1,54) = 99.552, p < 0.001$] and drug [$F(2,54) = 6.626, p < 0.01$], with a shock × drug interaction [$F(1,54) = 4.021, p < 0.05$] (Figure 2b). Post hoc analysis revealed that the shock groups (Veh, am, am + URB) demonstrated a decrease in saccharin preference compared with their corresponding NoShock groups: NoShock/Veh (days 2, 7, and 14: all $p < 0.001$), NoShock/am (day 2: $p < 0.05$; day 7: $p < 0.01$), NoShock/am + URB (day 2: $p < 0.01$; day 7: $p < 0.001$; days 14 and 21: $p< 0.05$). Moreover, compared with the NoShock/Veh group, we found that the NoShock/am group (days 2 and 14: $p < 0.01$; day 7: $p < 0.001$), and the NoShock/am + URB group (days 2 and 14: $p < 0.05$; day 7: $p < 0.01$) demonstrated decreased saccharin preference. Hence, co-administration of URB597 + AM251 shows that the restoring effect of URB597 on saccharin preference was blocked by AM251 treatment.

The shock-induced decrease in saccharin preference was short-termed (observed only one or two weeks after shock exposure). We have previously shown that in rats exposed to severe shock and to SRs 7, 14, and 21 days after shock exposure, the shock-induced decrease lasted till day 14 post-shock but not till day 28 post-shock (Burstein et al., 2018). In a previous study, we found that the chronic stress-induced decrease in sucrose consumption only lasted 1 week after the stress ended (Segev et al., 2014). Hence, there are fluctuations in saccharin preference at different times after stress exposure.

3.2.3. Acoustic Startle Response

We tested ASR on days 1 and 26, and a repeated measures ANOVA on startle amplitude indicated significant main effects of shock [$F(1,54) = 4.060, p < 0.001$] and time [$F(1,54) = 17.854, p < 0.001$], as well as a shock × time interaction [$F(1,54) = 17.854, p < 0.001$] (Figure 2c). Post hoc analysis revealed that on ASR2, a significant increase in amplitude was found in the shocked groups treated with vehicle (Shock/Veh), AM251 alone (Shock/am), and AM251 and URB597 (Shock/am + URB597) compared with the non-shocked groups (NoShock/Veh: $p < 0.01$, NoShock/am: $p < 0.01$, NoShock/am + URB597: $p < 0.001$). Hence, AM251 had no effect on ASR by itself; the co-administration of URB597 and AM251 in rats exposed to shock and reminders increased their startle response amplitude, suggesting that the effects of URB597 on startle response were blocked by AM251 treatment.

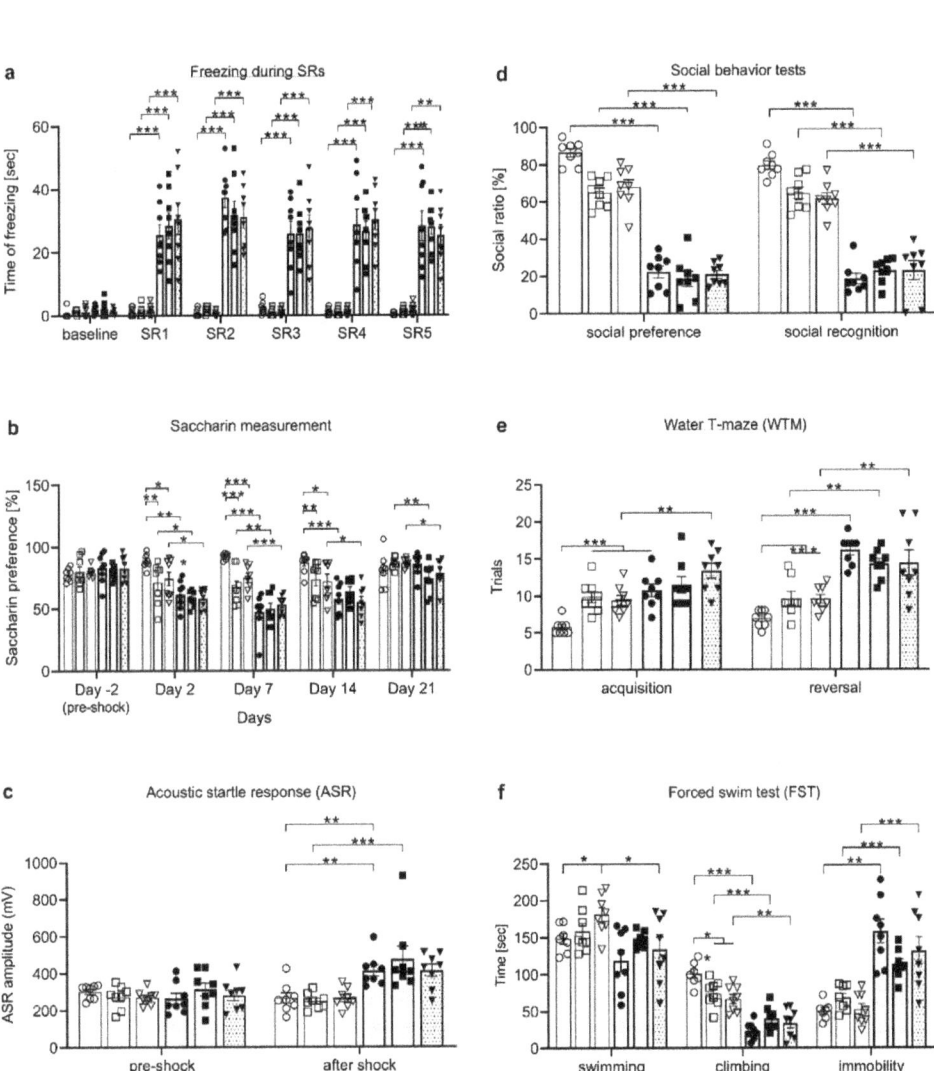

Figure 2. The effects of URB597 on behavior in rats exposed to shock and reminders are mediated by CB1 receptors. The shocked groups (Shock/Veh, Shock/am, Shock/am + URB597) compared with the non-shocked groups (NoShock/Veh, NoShock/am, NoShock/am + URB597), demonstrated the following: increased freezing levels (**a**); a decrease in saccharin preference on days 2, 7, 14, and 21 (**b**); increased acoustic startle response (ASR) amplitude on ASR2 (**c**); decreased social preference and social recognition (**d**); impaired performance in the acquisition and reversal phases in the water T-maze (WTM) (**e**); and increased immobility (**f**) (data is shown as mean ± sem; *, $p < 0.05$; **, $p < 0.01$; ***, $p < 0.001$).

3.2.4. Social Tests

For the social tests performed on day 27, a two-way ANOVA revealed significant main effects of shock [preference: $F(1,42) = 419.047$, $p < 0.001$; recognition: $F(1,42) = 315.307$, $p < 0.001$] and drug [preference: $F(2,42) = 9.021$, $p < 0.01$], with a shock × drug interaction [preference: $F(2,42) = 5.161$, $p < 0.05$; recognition: $F(2,42) = 6.969$, $p < 0.01$] (Figure 2d). Post hoc analysis revealed a significant decrease in the exploration ratio in both tasks in the shocked groups (Shock/Veh, Shock/am, Shock/am + URB597) compared to the non-shocked groups (NoShock/Veh, NoShock/am, NoShock/am + URB597; all $p < 0.001$). Hence, AM251 had no effect on social behavior by itself; shocked rats co-administrated with URB597 and AM251 behaved similarly to shocked rats treated with vehicle, suggesting that the effects of URB597 on social behavior were blocked by AM251 treatment. For total exploration time, see Supplementary File, Figure S4.

3.2.5. Water T-Maze

Rats were tested in the WTM on days 28–29. Repeated measures ANOVA (2 × 2 × 2) revealed significant main effects of shock [$F(1,54) = 85.307$, $p < 0.001$], drug [$F(2,54) = 5.788$, $p < 0.01$], and time [$F(1,54) = 9.179$, $p < 0.01$]. We also detected two interactions: shock × drug [$F(2,54) = 5.840$, $p < 0.01$] and time × shock [$F(1,54) = 6.950$, $p < 0.01$] (Figure 2e). Post hoc analysis revealed that fewer trials were needed to reach the criterion in the NoShock groups (Veh, am, am + URB) compared with their corresponding shock groups: Shock/Veh (acquisition and reversal, both $p < 0.001$), Shock/am (reversal, $p < 0.01$), and Shock/am + URB (acquisition and reversal, both $p < 0.01$). In addition, the NoShock/Veh group needed fewer trials to reach criterion compared with the NoShock/am group (acquisition, $p < 0.001$; reversal, $p < 0.01$) and the NoShock/am + URB group (acquisition, $p < 0.001$; reversal, $p = 0.05$) groups. Hence, the co-administration of URB597 + AM251 shows that the restoring effect of URB597 on performance in this task was blocked by AM251 treatment.

3.2.6. Forced Swim Test

For FST performed on days 30–31, a two-way ANOVA on immobility revealed a significant main effect of shock [$F(1,42) = 70.807$, $p < 0.001$] as well as a shock × drug interaction [$F(1,42) = 3.660$, $p < 0.05$] (Figure 2f). Post hoc analysis revealed that, compared to the non-shocked groups, the shocked groups demonstrated a significant increase in immobility (Shock/Veh, $p < 0.01$; Shock/am, Shock/am + URB597, $p < 0.001$). Hence, the effects of URB597 on immobility were blocked by AM251 treatment.

No significant differences were observed between the Shock/Veh and Shock/am groups in any of the tests, suggesting that this low dose of AM251 had no effect on behavior by itself. We did detect differences between the Noshock/Veh and Noshock/am groups in the saccharin and WTM tests, suggesting an effect of AM251 in these tests in control rats. The fact that AM251 had an effect by itself in these two tests in non-stressed rats could suggest that under these conditions, the co-administration of URB with AM251 has additive effects (i.e., the combining effects of the two drugs equal the sum of the effects of the two drugs acting independently); hence, the effects of URB597 in WTM performance and social preference are not necessarily mediated by CB1r.

3.3. Experiment 3: The Effects of NAc β-Catenin Overexpression on Behavior in Rats Exposed to Shock and Reminders

We found that exposure to shock and reminders induced a behavioral phenotype that includes anxiety- and depressive-like behaviors, impaired memory performance, and decreased expression of β-catenin in the NAc and mPFC compared to non-shocked rats. Pearson correlations indicated that the behavioral phenotype was highly associated with decreased levels of β-catenin in the NAc. Hence, we next examined whether the overexpression (OE) of β-catenin in the NAc would prevent the effects of exposure to shock and reminders on behavior.

3.3.1. Verifying β-Catenin Overexpression and Accuracy of Injection

In a preliminary experiment, we delivered overexpression (OE) vectors into the NAc (Figure 3a). In one set of rats (n = 12) we measured β-catenin expression in the NAc using WB (Figure 3b). An independent sample t-test revealed that overexpressing β-catenin in the NAc resulted in significant upregulation of β-catenin levels in the NAc 5 days after viral delivery [t(10) = 3.230, $p < 0.05$] compared to the GFP group. In the second set of rats (n = 12) we verified the accuracy of injection in the NAc using GFP detection (Figure 3c).

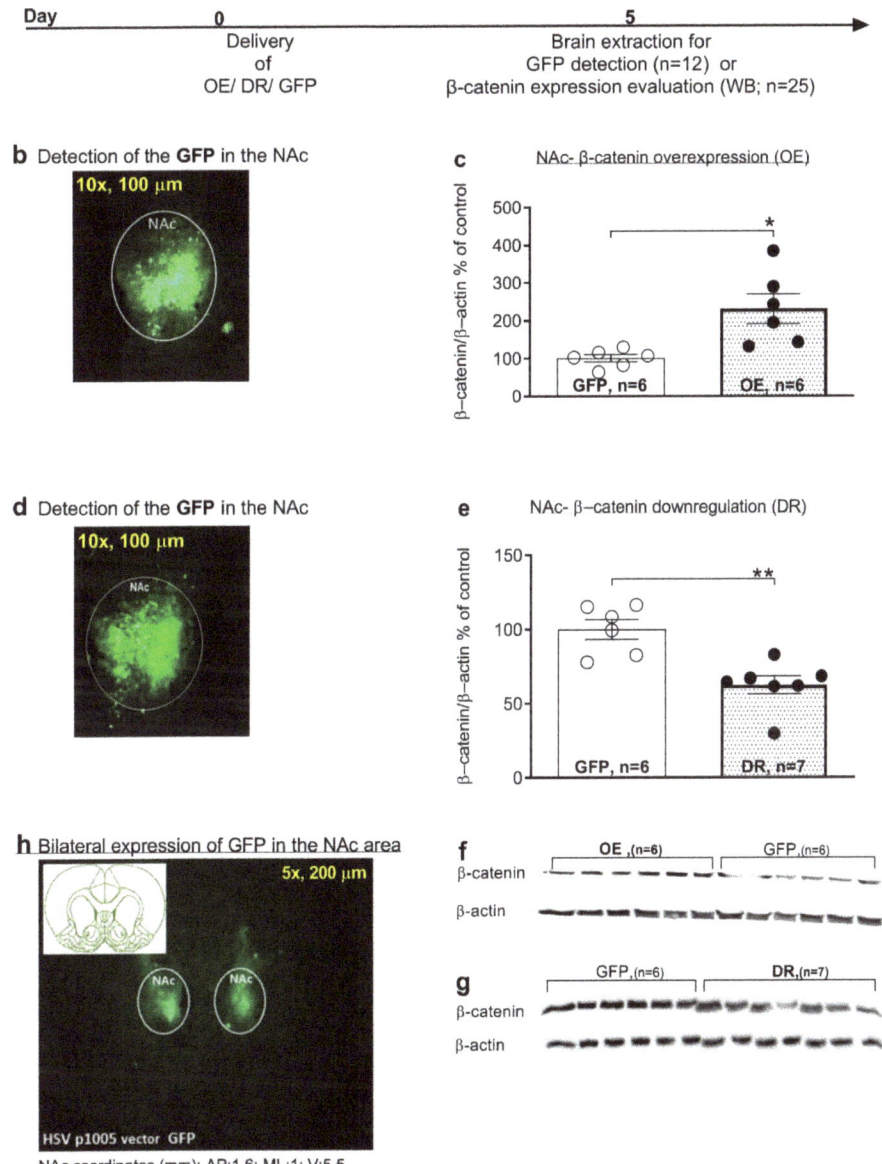

Figure 3. The delivery of the viral overexpression (OE) or downregulation (DR) vectors affects β-catenin levels in the nucleus accumbens (NAc). On day 0, overexpression (OE), downregulation (DR),

or green fluorescent protein (GFP) vectors were injected bilaterally into the rat nucleus accumbens (NAc). After five days of recovery, brains were removed and taken for GFP detection and β-catenin expression evaluation (**a**); the overexpression (OE) group demonstrated increased β-catenin levels compared to the green fluorescent protein (GFP) group (**b**); GFP detection revealed successful delivery of the OE vector to NAc (**b**); the OE group demonstrated increased β-catenin levels compared to the GFP group (**c**); GFP detection revealed successful delivery of the DR vector to the NAc (**d**); the DR group demonstrated decreased β-catenin levels compared to the GFP group (**e**); the expression of β-catenin in the NAc, after the delivery of viral vectors (OE/DR) were quantified by western blotting (**f**,**g**); bilateral expression of GFP in the NAc area (**h**); (data is shown as mean ± sem (*, $p < 0.05$; **, $p < 0.01$). (NA coordinates are relative to Bregma; AP: anterior–posterior; ML: medial–lateral; NAc: nucleus accumbens; OE: overexpression; DR: downregulation; V: ventral; WB: western blotting).

We examined whether viral-mediated OE of β-catenin in the NAc can restore the effects of shock and reminders on behavior, compared to rats injected with GFP (see Section 2.13 Experimental Design).

3.3.2. Freezing

A repeated measures ANOVA (shock × virus × SR; 2 × 2 × 6) on freezing behavior during SRs (Figure 4a) indicated significant main effects of drug [$F(1,30) = 27.535$, $p < 0.001$], shock [$F(1,30) = 56.779$, $p < 0.001$], and SR [$F(5,150) = 14.616$, $p < 0.001$]. We also detected the following significant interactions: shock × virus [$F(1,30) = 23.092$, $p < 0.001$], shock × SR [$F(5,150) = 7.636$, $p < 0.05$], virus × SR [$F(5,150) = 20.135$, $p < 0.001$], and shock × virus × SR [$F(5,150) = 12.028$, $p < 0.01$]. Post hoc analysis revealed that on SR1–SR5, the Shock/GFP group demonstrated a significant increase in freezing levels compared with the NoShock/GFP group (SR1, $p < 0.01$; SR2–SR5, $p < 0.001$) and Shock/OE group (SR1, $p < 0.05$; SR2, $p < 0.01$, SR3–SR5: $p < 0.001$). Moreover, the Shock/OE group showed increased freezing levels compared with the NoShock/OE group (SR1, $p < 0.01$; SR2, SR3, SR5: $p < 0.05$). Taken together, the findings suggest that β-catenin OE ameliorated the shock- and reminders-induced increase in freezing behavior.

Next, we examined whether viral–mediated OE of β-catenin in the NAc can restore the effects of shock and reminders on behavior, compared to rats injected with GFP (see Section 2.13 Experimental Design). In this experiment, the brains were taken for analysis 26 days after virus delivery and following behavioral testing.

3.3.3. Saccharin Preference

A mixed design three-way ANOVA on saccharin preference (shock × virus × days; 2 × 2 × 4) indicated significant main effects of shock [$F(1,30) = 8.739$, $p < 0.01$] and days [$F(3,30) = 35.374$, $p < 0.001$], with the following significant interactions: shock × virus [$F(1,30) = 7.196$, $p < 0.05$]; shock × days [$F(1,30) = 7.90$, $p < 0.001$]; and shock × virus × days [$F(1,30) = 2.577$, $p = 0.05$] (Figure 4b). Post hoc comparisons revealed that the Shock/GFP group demonstrated decreased saccharin preference compared with the NoShock/GFP group (day 2: $p < 0.001$) and the Shock/OE group (day 2: $p < 0.001$; day 14: $p < 0.05$). This suggests that NAc β-catenin overexpression prevented the shock- and reminders-induced decrease in saccharin preference.

3.3.4. Acoustic Startle Response

A repeated measures ANOVA [shock × virus × time] on startle amplitude in the ASR indicated a significant main effect of virus [$F(1,30) = 12.943$, $p < 0.01$], and a significant shock × virus interaction [$F(1,30) = 6.737$, $p < 0.05$] (Figure 4c). Post hoc analysis revealed that the Shock/GFP group demonstrated a significant increase in startle amplitude compared with the Shock/OE and NoShock/GFP groups (both $p < 0.001$). Hence, upregulation of β-catenin in the NAc restored startle amplitude in rats exposed to shock and reminders.

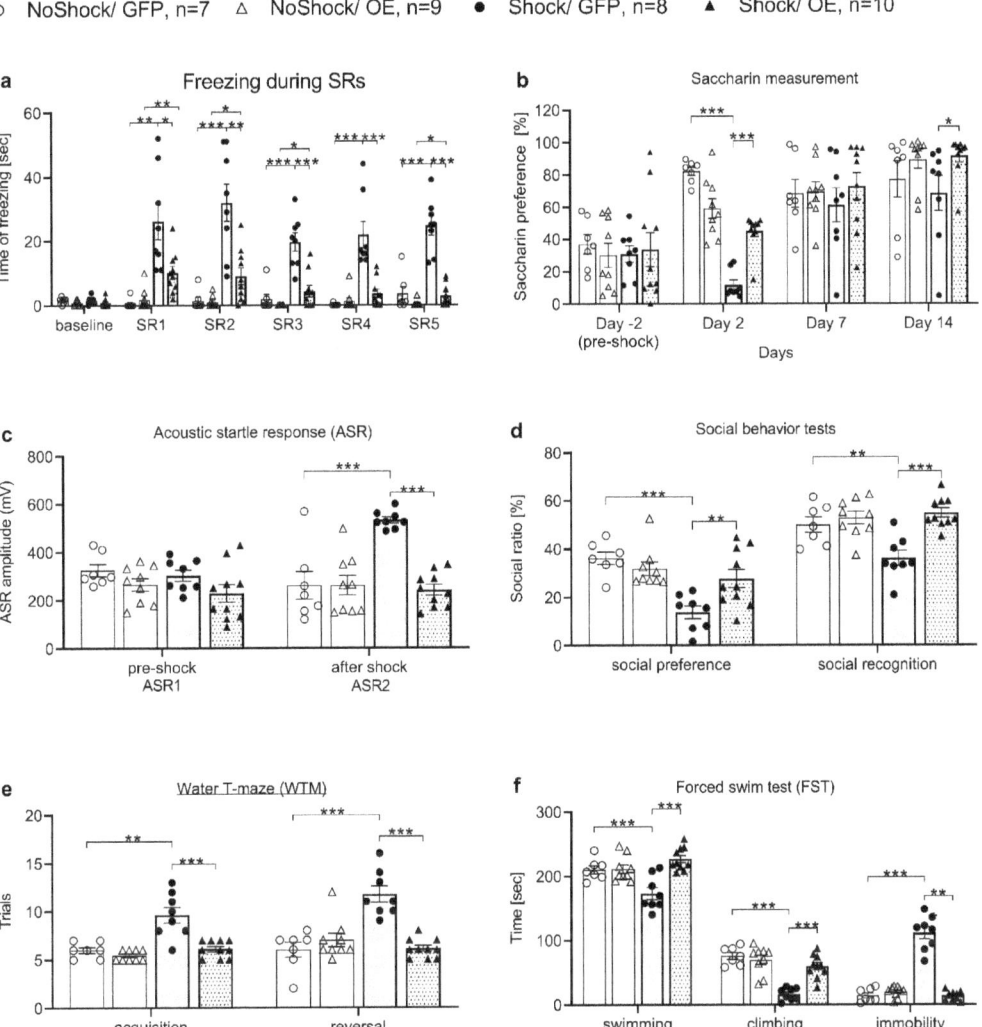

Figure 4. The effects of nucleus accumbens (NAc) β-catenin overexpression on behavior in rats exposed to shock and reminders. Compared with shocked rats with β-catenin overexpression in the nucleus accumbens (NAc) (Shock/OE) and non-shocked rats treated with green fluorescent protein (GFP) (NoShock/GFP), shocked rats treated with GFP (Shock/GFP) demonstrated the following: increased freezing on SR1 to SR5 (SR—situational reminder) (**a**); decreased saccharin preference on days 2 and 7 (only the NoShock/GFP group) (**b**); increased acoustic startle amplitude (ASR) on ASR2 (**c**); decreased social preference and social recognition (**d**); impaired performance in the acquisition and reversal phases in the water T-maze (WTM) (**e**); and increased immobility in the forced swim test (FST) (**f**) (data is shown as mean ± sem; *, $p < 0.05$; **, $p < 0.01$; ***, $p < 0.001$).

3.3.5. Social Tests

A two-way ANOVA for the social tests revealed significant main effects of shock [preference: $F(1,30) = 17.652$, $p < 0.001$; recognition: $F(1,30) = 4.751$, $p < 0.05$] and virus [preference: $F(1,30) = 16.185$, $p < 0.001$], with a significant shock × virus interaction [preference: $F(1,30) = 8.402$; recognition: $F(1,30) = 8.727$, both $p < 0.01$] (Figure 4d). Post hoc analysis revealed a lower exploration ratio in both tasks in the Shock/GFP group compared with the Shock/OE group (preference, $p < 0.01$; recognition, $p < 0.001$) and the NoShock/GFP group (preference, $p < 0.001$; recognition, $p < 0.01$). This suggests that NAc β-catenin overexpression prevented the effects of shock and reminders on social behaviors. For total exploration time, see Supplementary File, Figure S5.

3.3.6. Water T-Maze

A mixed design three-way ANOVA (shock × virus × test; 2 × 2 × 2) on the WTM experiment revealed significant main effects of shock [$F(1,30) = 25.88, p < 0.001$] and virus [$F(1,30) = 23.67, p < 0.001$]; with two significant interactions: shock × virus [$F(1,30) = 28.735, p < 0.001$] and test × shock × virus [$F(1,30) = 7.50, p = 0.01$] (Figure 4e). Post hoc comparisons revealed that the Shock/GFP group showed a significant increase in the number of trials required to reach the criterion in the acquisition and reversal phases compared with the NoShock/GFP group (acquisition, $p < 0.01$; reversal, $p < 0.001$) and Shock/OE group (acquisition and reversal, both $p < 0.001$). Hence, overexpression of β-catenin in the NAc prevented the shock- and reminders-induced impairment in performance in the WTM task.

3.3.7. Forced Swim Test

Two-way ANOVA for the FST experiment revealed significant main effects on immobility of shock [$F(1,30) = 78.646, p < 0.001$] and virus [$F(1,30) = 78.695, p < 0.001$], with a significant shock × virus interaction [$F(1,30) = 98.321, p < 0.01$] (Figure 4f). Post hoc analysis revealed an increase in immobility in the Shock/GFP group compared with the NoShock/GFP and Shock/OE (both $p < 0.001$) groups, suggesting that overexpression of β-catenin in the NAc prevented the shock- and reminders-induced impairment in the FST.

No significant differences were observed between the NoShock/GFP and NoShock/OE groups in any of the behavioral measures, suggesting that the virus had no effect in non-shocked control rats.

3.4. β-Catenin, mGluR5, and CB1 Receptors Regulation by Overexpressing NAc β-Catenin in Rats Exposed to Shock and Reminders

3.4.1. β-Catenin

Following the behavioral battery (Figure 4a) and the sacrifice of the rats, the expression of β-catenin was measured in the mPFC (Figure 5a), NAc (Figure 5b), CA1 (Figure 5c), and BLA (Figure 5d). A two-way ANOVA on β-catenin levels revealed significant main effects of shock [mPFC: $F(1,30) = 13.278, p < 0.01$; NAc: $F(1,31) = 11.402, p < 0.01$] and virus [BLA: $F(1,31) = 11.593$; CA1: $F(1,31) = 9.944$, all $p < 0.01$], as well as a shock × virus interaction [mPFC: $F(1,30) = 13.781, p < 0.01$; NAc: $F(1,31) = 9.515, p < 0.01$; CA1: $F(1,31) = 19.697, p < 0.001$]. Post hoc analysis revealed decreased β-catenin levels in the mPFC, NAc, and CA1 in the Shock/GFP group compared with the NoShock/GFP group (mPFC, $p < 0.001$; NAc and CA1, both $p < 0.01$) and the Shock/OE group (mPFC, $p < 0.05$; Nac and CA1, both $p < 0.001$). Additionally, in the CA1 the Shock/OE group demonstrated increased expression compared to the NoShock/OE group ($p < 0.05$), and in the BLA, the Shock/OE group demonstrated increased expression compared to the Shock/GFP group ($p < 0.01$). Hence, exposure to shock and reminders downregulated β-catenin levels in the mPFC, Nac, and CA1, and overexpressing β-catenin in the NAc normalized these effects.

For β-actin levels, no significant between-group differences were observed in any of these brain areas, suggesting that β-actin levels were not affected by the treatment.

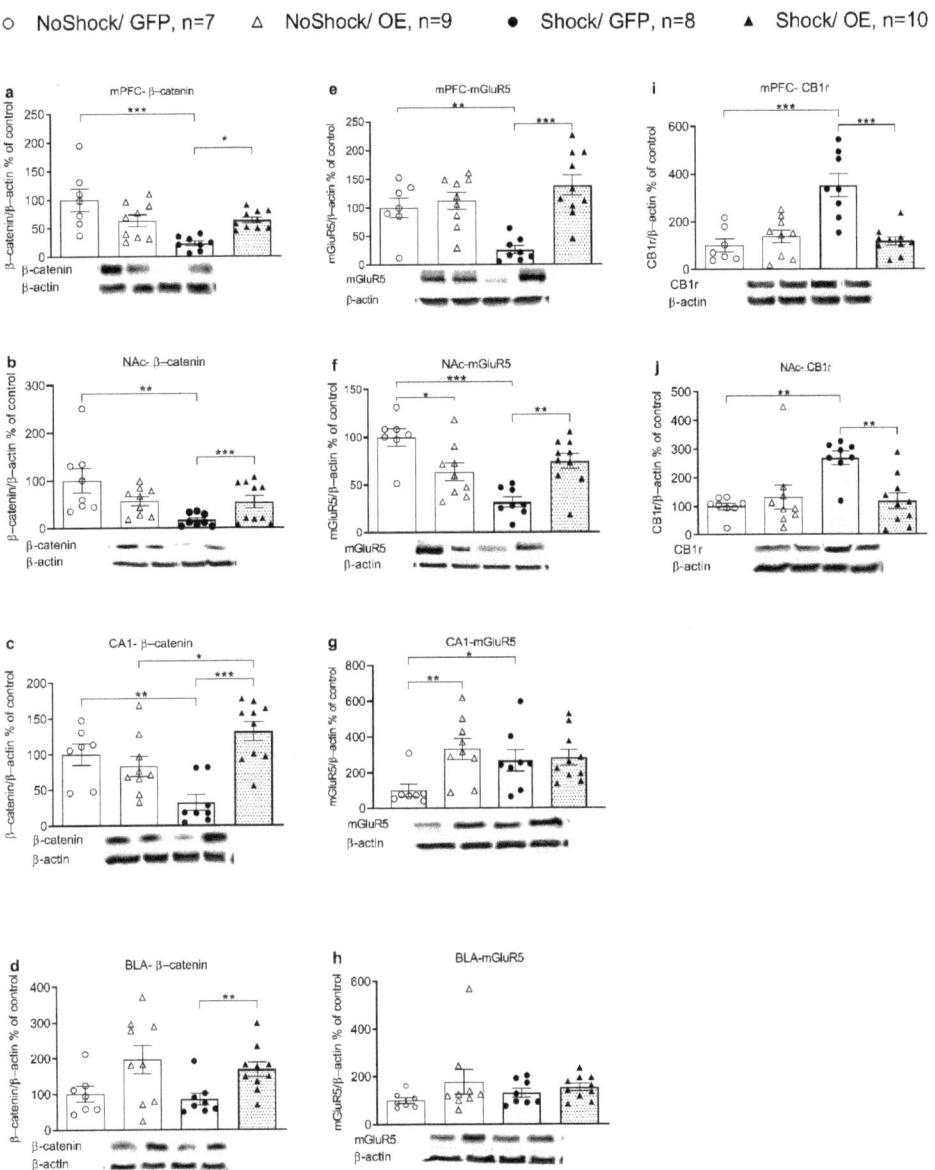

Figure 5. β-catenin, mGluR5, and CB1 receptors regulation by overexpressing nucleus accumbens (NAc) β-catenin in rats exposed to shock and reminders. β-catenin expression (**a–d**): The Shock/GFP (green fluorescent protein) group demonstrated a significant decrease in β-catenin levels compared with NoShock/GFP and Shock/OE (overexpression) groups in the medial prefrontal cortex (mPFC) (**a**), nucleus accumbens (NAc) (**b**), and CA1. Additionally, in the CA1, the Shock/OE group demonstrated increased expression compared to the NoShock/OE group (**c**); in the basolateral amygdala (BLA), the Shock/OE group demonstrated increased expression compared to the Shock/GFP group (**d**). Metabotropic glutamate receptor subtype 5 (mGluR5) expression (**e–h**): The Shock/GFP group

demonstrated a significant decrease in mGluR5 levels compared with the NoShock/GFP and Shock/OE groups in the mPFC (**e**) and NAc. Additionally, in the NAc, the NoShock/GFP group demonstrated increased expression compared with the NoShock/OE group (**f**); in the CA1, the NoShock/GFP group demonstrated decreased expression of mGluR5 compared to the NoShock/OE and Shock/GFP groups (**g**); in the BLA, no significant differences in mGluR5 levels were observed (**h**). Cannabinoid receptor type 1 (CB1r) expression (**i,j**): the Shock/GFP group demonstrated increased levels of CB1r compared with the NoShock/GFP and Shock/OE groups in the mPFC (**i**); and NAc (**j**) (data is shown as mean ± sem; *, $p < 0.05$; **, $p < 0.01$; ***, $p < 0.001$).

3.4.2. mGluR5

The expression of mGluR5 was measured in the mPFC (Figure 5e), NAc (Figure 5f), CA1 (Figure 5g), and BLA (Figure 5h). A two-way ANOVA on mGluR5 protein levels revealed significant main effects of shock [NAc: $F(1,31) = 13.209, p < 0.01$] and virus [CA1: $F(1,31) = 6.252, p < 0.05$; mPFC: $F(1,31) = 17.391, p < 0.001$], as well as a shock × virus interaction [mPFC: $F(1,31) = 11.468, p < 0.01$; NAc: $F(1,31) = 24.915, p < 0.001$; CA1: $F(1,31) = 4.682, p < 0.05$]. Post hoc analysis revealed a decrease in mGluR5 levels in the mPFC and NAc in the Shock/GFP group compared with the NoShock/GFP group (mPFC: $p < 0.01$; NAc: $p < 0.001$) and the Shock/OE group (mPFC: $p < 0.001$; NAc: $p < 0.01$). Additionally, in the NAc the NoShock/GFP group demonstrated increased expression compared with the NoShock/OE group ($p < 0.05$), and in the CA1 the NoShock/GFP group demonstrated decreased expression compared with the NoShock/OE group ($p < 0.01$) and the Shock/GFP group ($p < 0.05$). No effects were observed in the BLA. Hence, exposure to shock and reminders downregulated mGluR5 levels in the mPFC and NAc, and overexpressed β-catenin in the NAc normalized these effects. OE decreased mGluR5 levels compared to the GFP group in the non-shocked groups. Nevertheless, OE restored the shock- and reminders-induced decrease in mGluR5 levels compared to GFP-shocked rats.

3.4.3. CB1

Our findings regarding the involvement of β-catenin in the effects of shock and reminders on the amygdala-hippocampal-cortico-striatal circuit suggest a key role for the mPFC and the NAc in mediating the effects on behavior. Hence, we also examined the expression of CB1r in the mPFC and NAc. A two-way ANOVA on CB1r protein levels revealed significant main effects of shock [mPFC: $F(1,31) = 14.405, p < 0.01$; NAc: $F(1,31) = 6.839, p < 0.05$] and virus [mPFC: $F(1,31) = 10.727, p < 0.01$; NAc: $F(1,31) = 4.030, p = 0.05$], as well as a shock × virus interaction [mPFC: $F(1,31) = 20.238, p < 0.001$; NAc: $F(1,31) = 24.915, p < 0.001$]. Post hoc analysis revealed increased CB1r levels in the mPFC (Figure 5i) and NAc (Figure 5j) in the Shock/GFP group compared with the NoShock/GFP and Shock/OE groups (mPFC: both $p < 0.001$; NAc: both $p < 0.01$). Hence, exposure to shock and reminders upregulated CB1r levels in the mPFC and NAc, and overexpressing β-catenin in the NAc normalized these effects.

3.5. Experiment 4: The Effects of NAc β-Catenin Downregulation on Behavior of Rats Exposed to Shock and Reminders and Treated with URB597

3.5.1. Verifying β-Catenin Downregulation

In a preliminary experiment, we delivered an HSV P1005 vector, which expresses a mutant of β-catenin, into the NAc (Figure 3a). In one set of rats (n = 13) we measured β-catenin expression in the NAc using WB (Figure 3d). An independent sample t-test revealed that β-catenin protein levels in the NAc were downregulated ($t(11) = 4.179$, $p < 0.01$) compared to the HSV-GFP group. In another set of rats (n = 12), we verified the accuracy of injection in the NAc using GFP detection (Figure 3e).

Next, we examined whether the effects of URB597 on behavior in rats exposed to shock and reminders are mediated by β-catenin. To do so, we used a viral approach to downregulate (DR) β-catenin in the NAc (see Section 2.13 Experimental Design).

3.5.2. Freezing

For freezing during the SRs (Figure 6a), a repeated measures ANOVA (shock × virus × drug × SRs; 2 × 2 × 2 × 6) indicated significant main effects of drug [$F(1,56) = 57.964$, $p < 0.001$], shock [$F(1,56) = 628.020$, $p < 0.001$], virus [$F(1,56) = 50.831$, $p < 0.001$], and SR [$F(5,280) = 21.893$, $p < 0.001$]. The results also indicated the following interactions: shock × virus [$F(1,56) = 52.261$, $p < 0.001$], shock × drug [$F(1,56) = 51.441$, $p < 0.001$]; virus × drug [$F(1,56) = 32.402$, $p < 0.001$]; shock × virus × drug [$F(1,56) = 41.557$, $p < 0.001$]; shock × SR [$F(5,280) = 20.870$, $p < 0.001$], drug × SR [$F(5,280) = 2.851$, $p < 0.05$], shock × virus × SR [$F(5,280) = 2.886$, $p < 0.05$], and shock × virus × drug × SR [$F(5,280) = 2.233$, $p = 0.05$]. Post hoc analysis revealed that the Shock/GFP + Veh, Shock/DR + URB, and Shock/DR + Veh groups demonstrated a significant increase in freezing levels compared with their corresponding control groups (SR1–SR5: all $p < 0.001$). Moreover, the Shock/DR + URB group showed decreased freezing levels compared with the Shock/GFP + Veh group and the Shock/DR + URB group (SR1–SR5: all $p < 0.001$), and increased freezing levels compared with the NoShock/GFP + URB group (SR1, SR2, SR4, and SR5: all $p < 0.05$). Hence, downregulation of β-catenin in the NAc had no effect on freezing behavior by itself, but it blocked the preventive effects of URB597 in shocked rats.

3.5.3. Saccharin Preference

For saccharin preference (Figure 6b), a repeated measures ANOVA (shock × virus × drug × time; 2 × 2 × 2 × 4) revealed significant main effects of shock [$F(1,56) = 36.663$, $p < 0.001$] and time [$F(3,168) = 15.689$, $p < 0.001$]. We also identified the following interactions: shock × virus [$F(1,56) = 4.108$, $p < 0.05$], shock × time [$F(3,168) = 17.943$, $p < 0.001$], and drug × time [$F(3,168) = 3.263$, $p < 0.05$]. Post hoc analysis revealed that on post-shock days 2 and 7, a significant decrease in saccharin preference was observed in the Shock/GFP + Veh group compared with the Shock/GFP + URB group (day 2: $p < 0.05$; day 7: $p < 0.01$) and the NoShock/GFP + Veh group (days 2 and 7: both $p < 0.01$). Additionally, a significant decrease was observed in the Shock groups (GFP + URB, DR + Veh, and DR + URB) compared their corresponding NoShock groups: Shock/GFP + URB (day 2: $p < 0.01$), Shock/DR + Veh (day 2: $p < 0.01$; day 7: $p < 0.001$), and Shock/DR + URB (day 2: $p < 0.05$; day 7: $p < 0.01$). Hence, downregulating β-catenin in the NAc had no effect on saccharin preference-shocked rats by itself; however, it blocked the restoring effects of URB597.

3.5.4. Acoustic Startle Response

For ASR (Figure 6c), a repeated measures ANOVA revealed significant main effects of shock [$F(1,56) = 108.120$, $p < 0.001$], virus [$F(1,56) = 19.008$, $p < 0.001$], and drug [$F(1,56) = 24.204$, $p < 0.001$], as well as the following interactions: shock × virus [$F(1,56) = 5.597$, $p < 0.05$], shock × drug [$F(1,56) = 34.653$, $p < 0.001$], and shock × virus × drug [$F(1,56) = 11.692$, $p < 0.01$]. Post hoc analysis on ASR2 revealed decreased amplitude in shocked rats treated with URB597 (Shock/GFP + URB597) compared to the Shock/GFP + Veh and Shock/DR + URB597 groups (both $p < 0.001$). In addition, the shocked groups (Shock/GFP + Veh, Shock/DR + URB597, and Shock/DR + Veh) demonstrated increased startle compared to the non-shocked groups (NoShock/GFP + Veh, NoShock/DR + URB597, and NoShock/DR + Veh; all $p < 0.001$). The Shock/DR + URB597 group showed decreased amplitude compared to the Shock/DR + Veh group ($p < 0.05$). Hence, downregulating β-catenin in the NAc prevented the URB597 normalization of the startle response in shocked rats.

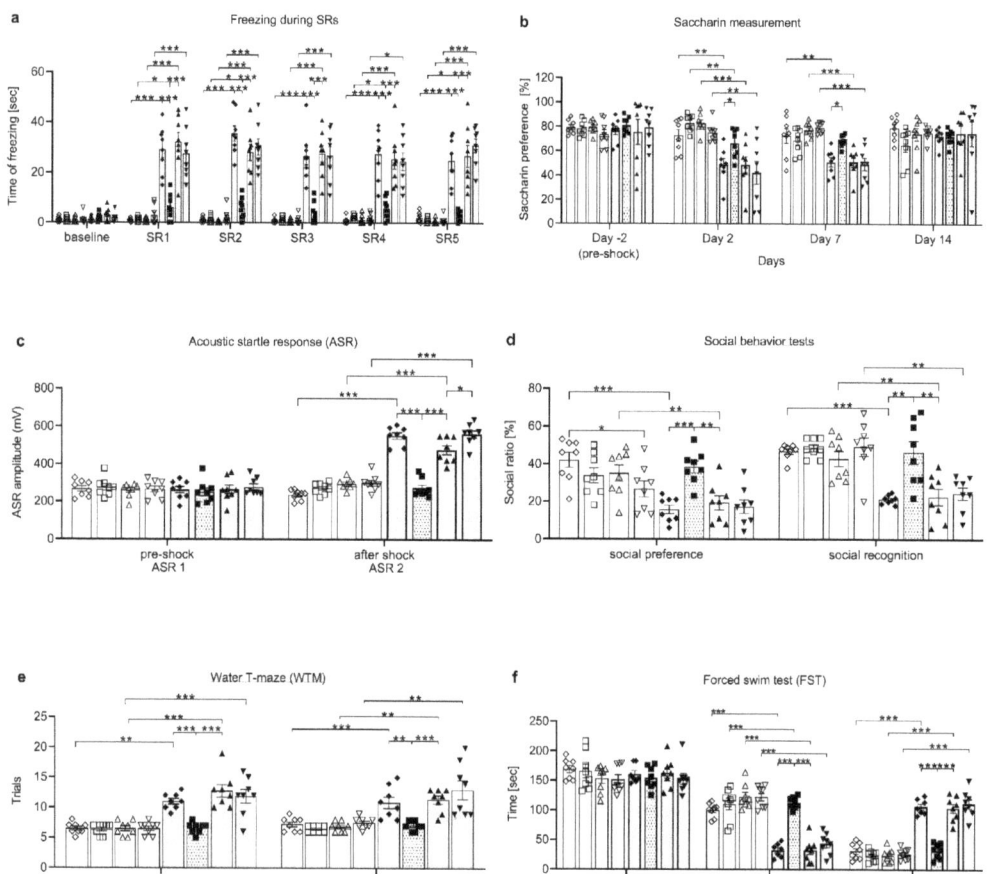

Figure 6. Nucleus accumbens (NAc) β-catenin downregulation (DR) blocked the preventive effects of URB597 on behavior in rats exposed to shock and reminders. Compared to shocked rats injected with vehicle (Shock/GFP + Veh) or shocked rats with β-catenin downregulation (DR) and URB597 injection (Shock/DR + URB597), shocked rats treated with URB597 (Shock/GFP + URB597) demonstrated the following: decreased freezing on SR1 to SR5 (SR: situational reminder; GFP: green fluorescent protein) (**a**); higher saccharin preference (only compared with the Shock/DR + URB group) (**b**); decreased acoustic startle response (ASR) on ASR2 (**c**); increased social preference and social recognition (**d**); intact performance in the acquisition and reversal phases in the water T-maze (WTM) (**e**); and decreased immobility in the forced swim test (FST) (**f**) (data is shown as mean ± sem; *, $p < 0.05$; **, $p < 0.01$; ***, $p < 0.001$).

3.5.5. Social Tests

For the social tests (Figure 6d), a three-way ANOVA revealed significant main effects of shock [preference: $F(1,56) = 19.525$; recognition: $F(1,56) = 46.854$; both $p < 0.001$], virus [preference: $F(1,56) = 8.982$, $p < 0.01$; recognition: $F(1,56) = 4.958$, $p < 0.05$], and drug [preference:

$F(1,56) = 4.008$; recognition: $F(1,56) = 4.447$; both $p < 0.05$]. We also identified the following interactions: shock × drug [recognition: $F(1,56) = 8.885, p < 0.01$]; virus × drug [recognition: $F(1,56) = 8.744, p < 0.01$]; and shock × virus × drug [preference: $F(1,56) = 15.375, p < 0.001$]. Post hoc analysis revealed a significant increase in the exploration ratio in both tasks in the Shock/GFP + URB597 group compared to the Shock/GFP + Veh group (preference: $p < 0.001$; recognition: $p < 0.01$) and the Shock/DR + URB597 group ($p < 0.01$). This suggests that downregulation blocked the effects of URB597 on social behavior.

In addition, we observed a decrease in the shocked groups (Shock/GFP + Veh, Shock/DR + URB597, Shock/DR + Veh) compared to the non-shocked groups (NoShock/GFP + Veh: preference, $p < 0.05$, recognition: $p < 0.001$; NoShock/DR + URB597: preference and recognition, $p < 0.01$; NoShock/DR + Veh: recognition, $p < 0.01$). In the preference task, an increase was observed in the NoShock/GFP + Veh group compared with NoShock/DR + Veh group ($p < 0.05$). Hence, NAc β-catenin downregulation blocked the preventive effects of URB597 on social behavior in rats exposed to shock and reminders. For total exploration time, see the Supplementary File, Figure S6.

3.5.6. Water T-Maze

For the WTM (Figure 6e), a repeated measures ANOVA (shock × virus × drug × time; 2 × 2 × 2 × 2) revealed significant main effects of shock [$F(1,56) = 117.663, p < 0.001$], virus [$F(1,56) = 25.030, p < 0.001$], and drug [$F(1,56) = 13.504, p < 0.01$]. We also identified the following significant interactions: shock × virus [$F(1,56) = 19.996, p < 0.001$], shock × drug [$F(1,56) = 6.823, p < 0.05$], virus × drug [$F(1,56) = 7.294, p < 0.01$], and shock × virus × drug [$F(1,56) = 6.368, p < 0.05$]. Post hoc analysis revealed that in the acquisition and the reversal phases, fewer trials were needed to reach the criterion in the non-shocked groups (GFP + Veh, DR + Veh, DR + URB) compared with the shocked groups: Shock/GFP + Veh (acquisition, $p < 0.01$; reversal, $p < 0.001$), Shock/DR + Veh (acquisition, $p < 0.001$; reversal: $p < 0.01$) and Shock/DR + URB (acquisition, $p < 0.001$; reversal, $p < 0.01$). The Shock/GFP + URB group also demonstrated a decreased number of trials compared with the Shock/GFP + Veh group (acquisition, $p < 0.001$; reversal, $p < 0.01$) and the Shock/DR + URB group (acquisition: $p < 0.001$; reversal: $p < 0.01$). Hence, downregulating β-catenin in the NAc had no effect on WTM performance, but it did block the preventative effects of URB597 in shocked rats.

3.5.7. Forced Swim Test

For the FST (Figure 6f), a three-way ANOVA on immobility revealed significant main effects of shock [$F(1,56) = 283.367, p < 0.001$], virus [$F(1,56) = 23.916, p < 0.001$], and drug [$F(1,56) = 23.916, p < 0.001$], as well as the following significant interactions: shock × virus [$F(1,56) = 30.606, p < 0.001$], shock × drug [$F(1,56) = 23.423, p < 0.001$], virus × drug [$F(1,56) = 24.432, p < 0.001$], and shock × virus × drug [$F(1,56) = 17.059, p < 0.001$]. Post hoc analysis revealed that the Shock/GFP + URB597 group demonstrated decreased immobility compared with the Shock/GFP + Veh and Shock/DR + URB597 (both $p < 0.001$) groups. In addition, an increase in immobility was observed in the other shocked groups (Shock/GFP + Veh, Shock/DR + URB597, and Shock/DR + Veh) compared to the non-shocked counterparts (NoShock/GFP + Veh, NoShock/DR + URB597, and NoShock/DR + Veh; all $p < 0.001$). Hence, downregulating β-catenin in the NAc blocked the preventive effects of URB597 on despair-like behavior in the FST in rats exposed to shock and reminders.

No significant differences were observed between the Shock/GFP + Veh and Shock/DR + Veh groups, suggesting that downregulation had no effect on behavior by itself in shocked rats. In the non-shocked groups, we observed a difference between the NoShock/GFP + Veh and NoShock/DR + Veh groups in the social preference test, suggesting that downregulation decreased social preference.

4. Discussion

Our findings suggest a potentially novel mechanism for the stress-protective effects of URB597 through β-catenin activation in the NAc in a rat model for PTSD and depression.

We found that exposing rats to shock and reminders induced anxiety-like behavior (i.e., increased freezing and startle response) and depressive-like behavior (i.e., decreased social behavior, induced anhedonia, and despair-like behavior), and also impaired memory function in the social recognition and water maze tasks. Administering the FAAH inhibitor URB597 1 h after shock exposure prevented these effects, as had been previously demonstrated [3,17]. Most of the effects of URB597 on behavior were found to be CB1r-dependent, as co-administration of the CB1r antagonist AM251 with URB597 prevented the ameliorating effects of URB597.

Importantly, exposure to shock and reminders decreased β-catenin levels in the NAc and mPFC. Decreased β-catenin levels in the NAc were associated with the behavioral phenotype, including enhanced freezing and startle response, anhedonia, and impaired performance in the WTM. This association led us to focus on upregulating and downregulating β-catenin levels in the NAc. Overexpression of NAc β-catenin in rats exposed to shock and reminders resulted in intact behavior (restores freezing and startle response, no indication of depressive-like behavior, intact memory function) and restored expression of β-catenin, mGluR5, and CB1r in the NAc. It is interesting that overexpressing β-catenin in the NAc also restored these same normal levels in the mPFC. Future studies might test the overexpression of β-catenin in the mPFC. Another future study is to examine the potential therapeutic effects of URB597 and the involvement of β-catenin in female rats.

Increased β-catenin levels were reported to promote resilient responses to stress in the NAc [26]. Mice with stabilized β-catenin in the hippocampus showed resilience to some anxious/depressive manifestations when subjected to the corticosterone model of depression [49]. NAc β-catenin upregulation in mice exposed to social defeat stress resulted in a pro-resilient phenotype, demonstrating less social avoidance and better performance in the FST and elevated plus maze (Dias et al., 2014). Similarly, intra-NAc LiCl (2 μg/side), which upregulates β-catenin activity via inhibition of GSK-3β, facilitated inhibitory extinction [26].

In rats exposed to shock and reminders, we found that β-catenin overexpression restored the decrease in mGluR5 and the increase in CB1r expression in the NAc and mPFC. Decreased mGluR5 levels were observed in animal models of depression and the mPFC of depressed individuals [34,35], and blocking mGluR5 has therapeutic effects in PTSD patients and animal models [34,50]. Increased CB1r in the BLA and CA1 were observed in animal models for PTSD [4,15,17], and increased CB1r availability in the amygdala-hippocampal-cortico-striatal circuit in human subjects with PTSD [10].

Other studies have shown a stress-induced decrease in β-catenin levels in the mPFC and NAc that was accompanied by highly susceptible behavioral responses [22,51–53]. Mice with dysfunctional NAc Wnt signaling demonstrated increased depression-like behavior and susceptibility to social defeat stress [23], and β-catenin inactivation in the astrocyte-specific glutamate transporter (GLAST)-expressing cells enhanced anxious/depressive-like responses [49]. In depressed patients, lowered β-catenin protein levels, but not mRNA levels were found in the NAc, suggesting that depression may be associated with reduced activity of β-catenin, and perhaps not a defect at the transcriptional level [49,54].

Importantly, URB597 did not prevent the effects of exposure to shock and reminders on behavior in rats with viral-mediated NAc downregulation of β-catenin. This indicates that β-catenin is crucial for URB597 to exert its ameliorating effects on behavior. In a previous study, we showed that downregulating β-catenin using sulindac prevented the facilitating effect of the CB1/2 agonist WIN55,212-2 on extinction [26]. Taken together, these findings suggest a strong functional interaction between CB1r and β-catenin. Indeed, cannabinoids regulate neuronal precursor proliferation via β-catenin; the activation of CB1r enhances the activity of PI3K/AKT; this results in AKT-mediated phosphorylation of GSK-3β, followed by the stabilization of β-catenin that translocates into the nucleus; in the nucleus, β-catenin regulates transcription and gene expression such as cyclin D1 that is involved in cell proliferation regulation [55]. β-catenin may activate TCF/Lef transcription factors [56] and microRNAs [57], which promote anti-stress responses. This could be a possible explanation for the therapeutic-like effects of URB597, acting through CB1r to modulate β-catenin and produce pro-resilient responses.

There are other relevant pathways that might play a critical role in explaining our results. For example, AEA affects CB1r but also has other targets that might be involved in the effects of URB597 [i.e., AEA is a full agonist of TRPV1, which probably participates in ECB signaling [58]]. Garro-Martinez et al. (2020) suggested a link between β-catenin levels and 5-HT1A receptor functionality underlying the vulnerability or resilience to stress-related disorders [59].

5. Conclusions

In many cases, drugs are used in clinical settings without a full understanding of the molecular mechanisms through which they function. Understanding the mechanism of action for a given drug in greater detail has the potential to support further pharmacological development efforts and mitigate the risk of failed clinical trials by stratifying patients to focus on subpopulations most likely to respond to such treatment. We suggest a potentially novel mechanism for the stress-ameliorating effects of URB597 that involves activation of CB1 and the Wnt/β-catenin pathway in the NAc. Overall our findings suggest that FAAH inhibitors may be a viable approach for the treatment of stress-related neuropsychiatric disorders and PTSD in particular and that these therapeutic effects are mediated via a β-catenin-dependent mechanism.

Supplementary Materials: The following supporting information can be downloaded at: https://www.mdpi.com/article/10.3390/biomedicines10081789/s1, Figure S1: Antibody specificity; Figure S2: An illustration of a modified herpes simplex virus (HSV) amplicon plasmid; Figure S3: The effects of URB597 on exploration time during the social preference and the social recognition tests; Figure S4: The effects of URB597 and AM251 on exploration time during the social preference and the social recognition tests; Figure S5: The effects of nucleus accumbens (NAc) β-catenin overexpression on exploration time during the social preference and the social recognition tests; Figure S6: The effects of nucleus accumbens (NAc) β-catenin downregulation on exploration time during the social preference and the social recognition tests; Table S1: Pearson bivariate correlation between the expression of β-catenin and behavior.

Author Contributions: Conceptualization, I.A. and T.M.Z.-A.; Formal analysis, T.M.Z.-A.; Funding acquisition, I.A.; Investigation, T.M.Z.-A., L.I. and B.S.; Methodology, I.A., T.M.Z.-A., P.J.H., E.M.P. and E.J.N.; Project administration, I.A.; Resources, I.A., P.J.H., E.M.P. and E.J.N.; Supervision, I.A.; Validation, I.A.; Writing—original draft, I.A. and T.M.Z.-A.; Writing—review and editing, I.A. and T.M.Z.-A. All authors have read and agreed to the published version of the manuscript.

Funding: This research was funded by the Israel Science Foundation (ISF), grant number 993/20 to IA.

Institutional Review Board Statement: The animal study protocol was approved by the Institutional Ethics Committee of the University of Haifa (protocol codes 403/2016, 535/2017).

Informed Consent Statement: Not applicable.

Data Availability Statement: Not applicable.

Conflicts of Interest: The authors declare no conflict of interest. The funders had no role in the design of the study; in the collection, analyses, or interpretation of data; in the writing of the manuscript, or in the decision to publish the results.

References

1. Kessler, R.C.; Sonnega, A.; Bromet, E.; Hughes, M.; Nelson, C.B. Posttraumatic Stress Disorder in the National Comorbidity Survey. *Arch. Gen. Psychiatry* **1995**, *52*, 1048–1060. [CrossRef] [PubMed]
2. Berardi, A.; Trezza, V.; Campolongo, P. Modeling specific phobias and posttraumatic stress disorder in rodents: The chal-lenge to convey both cognitive and emotional features. *Rev. Neurosci.* **2012**, *23*, 645–657. [CrossRef] [PubMed]

3. Burstein, O.; Shoshan, N.; Doron, R.; Akirav, I. Cannabinoids prevent depressive-like symptoms and alterations in BDNF expression in a rat model of PTSD. *Prog. Neuro-Psychopharmacol. Biol. Psychiatry* **2018**, *84*, 129–139. [CrossRef] [PubMed]
4. Fidelman, S.; Zer-Aviv, T.M.; Lange, R.; Hillard, C.J.; Akirav, I. Chronic treatment with URB597 ameliorates post-stress symptoms in a rat model of PTSD. *Eur. Neuropsychopharmacol.* **2018**, *28*, 630–642. [CrossRef] [PubMed]
5. Fraser, G.A. The Use of a Synthetic Cannabinoid in the Management of Treatment-Resistant Nightmares in Posttraumatic Stress Disorder (PTSD). *CNS Neurosci. Ther.* **2009**, *15*, 84–88. [CrossRef] [PubMed]
6. Hill, M.N.; Campolongo, P.; Yehuda, R.; Patel, S. Integrating Endocannabinoid Signaling and Cannabinoids into the Biology and Treatment of Posttraumatic Stress Disorder. *Neuropsychopharmacology* **2017**, *43*, 80–102. [CrossRef]
7. Korem, N.; Akirav, I. Cannabinoids Prevent the Effects of a Footshock Followed by Situational Reminders on Emotional Processing. *Neuropsychopharmacology* **2014**, *39*, 2709–2722. [CrossRef]
8. Lutz, B. The Endocannabinoid System and Extinction Learning. *Mol. Neurobiol.* **2007**, *36*, 92–101. [CrossRef]
9. Morena, M.; Patel, S.; Bains, J.; Hill, M.N. Neurobiological Interactions between Stress and the Endocannabinoid System. *Neuropsychopharmacology* **2015**, *41*, 80–102. [CrossRef]
10. Neumeister, A. The endocannabinoid system provides an avenue for evidence-based treatment development for ptsd. *Depress Anxiety* **2013**, *30*, 93–96. [CrossRef]
11. Patel, S.; Hill, M.N.; Cheer, J.; Wotjak, C.T.; Holmes, A. The endocannabinoid system as a target for novel anxiolytic drugs. *Neurosci. Biobehav. Rev.* **2017**, *76*, 56–66. [CrossRef]
12. Roitman, P.; Mechoulam, R.; Cooper-Kazaz, R.; Shalev, A. Preliminary, open-label, pilot study of add-on oral Δ9-tetrahydrocannabinol in chronic post-traumatic stress disorder. *Clin. Drug Investig.* **2014**, *34*, 587–591. [CrossRef]
13. Sbarski, B.; Akirav, I. Cannabinoids as therapeutics for PTSD. *Pharmacol. Ther.* **2020**, *211*, 107551. [CrossRef]
14. Shoshan, N.; Segev, A.; Abush, H.; Zer-Aviv, T.M.; Akirav, I. Cannabinoids prevent the differential long-term effects of exposure to severe stress on hippocampal- and amygdala-dependent memory and plasticity. *Hippocampus* **2017**, *27*, 1093–1109. [CrossRef]
15. Trezza, V.; Campolongo, P. The endocannabinoid system as a possible target to treat both the cognitive and emotional features of post-traumatic stress disorder (PTSD). *Front. Behav. Neurosci.* **2013**, *7*, 100. [CrossRef]
16. Segev, A.; Korem, N.; Zer-Aviv, T.M.; Abush, H.; Lange, R.; Sauber, G.; Hillard, C.J.; Akirav, I. Role of endocannabinoids in the hippocampus and amygdala in emotional memory and plasticity. *Neuropsychopharmacology* **2018**, *43*, 2017–2027. [CrossRef]
17. Shoshan, N.; Akirav, I. The effects of cannabinoid receptors activation and glucocorticoid receptors deactivation in the amygdala and hippocampus on the consolidation of a traumatic event. *Neurobiol. Learn. Mem.* **2017**, *144*, 248–258. [CrossRef]
18. Piomelli, D.; Tarzia, G.; Duranti, A.; Tontini, A.; Mor, M.; Compton, T.R.; Dasse, O.; Monaghan, E.P.; Parrott, J.A.; Putman, D. Pharmacological Profile of the Selective FAAH Inhibitor KDS-4103 (URB597). *CNS Drug Rev.* **2006**, *12*, 21–38. [CrossRef]
19. Van Esbroeck, A.C.; Janssen, A.P.; Cognetta, A.B.; Ogasawara, D.; Shpak, G.; Van Der Kroeg, M.; Kantae, V.; Baggelaar, M.P.; De Vrij, F.M.; Deng, H. Activity-based protein profiling reveals off-target proteins of the FAAH inhibitor BIA 10-2474. *Science* **2017**, *356*, 1084–1087. [CrossRef]
20. Gould, T.D.; O'Donnell, K.C.; Picchini, A.M.; Dow, E.R.; Chen, G.; Manji, H.K. Generation and behavioral characterization of β-catenin forebrain-specific conditional knock-out mice. *Behav. Brain Res.* **2008**, *189*, 117–125. [CrossRef]
21. Maguschak, K.A.; Ressler, K.J. β-catenin is required for memory consolidation. *Nat. Neurosci.* **2008**, *11*, 1319–1326. [CrossRef] [PubMed]
22. Dias, C.; Feng, J.; Sun, H.; Mazei-Robison, M.S.; Damez-Werno, D.; Scobie, K.; Bagot, R.; LaBonté, B.; Ribeiro, E.; Liu, X.; et al. β-catenin mediates stress resilience through Dicer1/microRNA regulation. *Nature* **2014**, *516*, 51. [CrossRef] [PubMed]
23. Wilkinson, M.B.; Dias, C.; Magida, J.; Mazei-Robison, M.; Lobo, M.; Kennedy, P.; Dietz, D.; Covington, H.; Russo, S.; Neve, R. A novel role of the WNT-dishevelled-GSK3β signaling cascade in the mouse nucleus accumbens in a social defeat model of de-pression. *J. Neurosci.* **2011**, *31*, 9084–9092. [CrossRef] [PubMed]
24. Dahlhoff, M.; Siegmund, A.; Golub, Y.; Wolf, E.; Holsboer, F.; Wotjak, C.T. AKT/GSK-3β/β-catenin signalling within hippocampus and amygdala reflects genetically determined differences in posttraumatic stress disorder like symptoms. *Neuroscience* **2010**, *169*, 1216–1226. [CrossRef]
25. Fujio, J.; Hosono, H.; Ishiguro, K.; Ikegami, S.; Fujita, S.C. Tau phosphorylation in the mouse brain during aversive conditioning. *Neurochem. Int.* **2007**, *51*, 200–208. [CrossRef]
26. Korem, N.; Lange, R.; Hillard, C.J.; Akirav, I. Role of beta-catenin and endocannabinoids in the nucleus accumbens in extinction in rats exposed to shock and reminders. *Neuroscience* **2017**, *357*, 285–294. [CrossRef]
27. Cuesta, S.; Funes, A.; Pacchioni, A.M. Social Isolation in Male Rats During Adolescence Inhibits the Wnt/β-Catenin Pathway in the Prefrontal Cortex and Enhances Anxiety and Cocaine-Induced Plasticity in Adulthood. *Neurosci. Bull.* **2020**, *36*, 611–624. [CrossRef]
28. Mohamed, A.M.; Habib, M.Z.; Ebeid, M.A.; Abdelraouf, S.M.; el Faramawy, Y.; Aboul-Fotouh, S.; Magdy, Y. Amisulpride alleviates chronic mild stress-induced cognitive deficits: Role of prefrontal cortex microglia and Wnt/β-catenin pathway. *Eur. J. Pharmacol.* **2020**, *885*, 173411. [CrossRef]
29. de Souza, J.M.; Abd-Elrahman, K.S.; Ribeiro, F.M.; Ferguson, S.S. mGluR5 regulates REST/NRSF signaling through N-cadherin/β-catenin complex in Huntington's disease. *Mol. Brain* **2020**, *13*, 118. [CrossRef]
30. Nicoletti, F.; Bockaert, J.; Collingridge, G.L.; Conn, P.J.; Ferraguti, F.; Schoepp, D.D.; Wroblewski, J.T.; Pin, J.P. Metabotropic glu-tamate receptors: From the workbench to the bedside. *Neuropharmacology* **2011**, *60*, 1017–1041. [CrossRef]

31. Li, Z.; Zhou, Q.; Li, L.; Mao, R.; Wang, M.; Peng, W.; Dong, Z.; Xu, L.; Cao, J. Effects of unconditioned and conditioned aversive stimuli in an intense fear conditioning paradigm on synaptic plasticity in the hippocampal CA1 area in vivo. *Hippocampus* **2005**, *15*, 815–824. [CrossRef]
32. Tatarczyńska, E.; Kłodzińska, A.; Chojnacka-Wójcik, E.; Pałucha, A.; Gasparini, F.; Kuhn, R.; Pilc, A. Potential anxiolyt-ic-and antidepressant-like effects of MPEP, a potent, selective and systemically active mGlu5 receptor antagonist. *Br. J. Pharmacol.* **2001**, *132*, 1423–1430. [CrossRef]
33. Xu, J.; Zhu, Y.; Contractor, A.; Heinemann, S.F. mGluR5 Has a Critical Role in Inhibitory Learning. *J. Neurosci.* **2009**, *29*, 3676–3684. [CrossRef]
34. Deschwanden, A.; Karolewicz, B.; Feyissa, A.M.; Treyer, V.; Ametamey, S.M.; Johayem, A.; Burger, C.; Auberson, Y.P.; Sovago, J.; Stockmeier, C.A.; et al. Reduced Metabotropic Glutamate Receptor 5 Density in Major Depression Determined by [^{11}C]ABP688 PET and Postmortem Study. *Am. J. Psychiatry* **2011**, *168*, 727–734. [CrossRef]
35. Shin, S.; Kwon, O.; Kang, J.I.; Kwon, S.; Oh, S.; Choi, J.; Kim, C.H.; Kim, D.G. mGluR5 in the nucleus accumbens is critical for promoting resilience to chronic stress. *Nat. Neurosci.* **2015**, *18*, 1017–1024. [CrossRef]
36. Xu, X.; Wu, K.; Ma, X.; Wang, W.; Wang, H.; Huang, M.; Luo, L.; Su, C.; Yuan, T.; Shi, H.; et al. mGluR5-Mediated eCB Signaling in the Nucleus Accumbens Controls Vulnerability to Depressive-Like Behaviors and Pain after Chronic Social Defeat Stress. *Mol. Neurobiol.* **2021**, *58*, 4944–4958. [CrossRef]
37. Alteba, S.; Portugalov, A.; Hillard, C.J.; Akirav, I. Inhibition of Fatty Acid Amide Hydrolase (FAAH) during Adolescence and Exposure to Early Life Stress may Exacerbate Depression-like Behaviors in Male and Female Rats. *Neuroscience* **2021**, *455*, 89–106. [CrossRef]
38. Akirav, I.; Segev, A.; Motanis, H.; Maroun, M. D-Cycloserine into the BLA Reverses the Impairing Effects of Exposure to Stress on the Extinction of Contextual Fear, but Not Conditioned Taste Aversion. *Learn. Mem.* **2009**, *16*, 682–686.
39. Fanselow, M.S. Conditional and unconditional components of post-shock freezing. *Pavlov. J. Biol. Sci.* **1980**, *15*, 177–182. [CrossRef]
40. Maymon, N.; Zer-Aviv, T.M.; Sabban, E.L.; Akirav, I. Neuropeptide Y and cannabinoids interaction in the amygdala after exposure to shock and reminders model of PTSD. *Neuropharmacology* **2019**, *162*, 107804. [CrossRef]
41. Bauminger, H.; Zaidan, H.; Akirav, I.; Gaisler-Salomon, I. Anandamide Hydrolysis Inhibition Reverses the Long-Term Behavioral and Gene Expression Alterations Induced by MK-801 in Male Rats: Differential CB1 and CB2 Receptor-Mediated Effects. *Schizophr. Bull.* **2022**; Online ahead of print.
42. Yankelevitch-Yahav, R.; Franko, M.; Huly, A.; Doron, R. The Forced Swim Test as a Model of Depressive-like Behavior. *J. Vis. Exp.* **2015**, *2*, e52587. [CrossRef]
43. Abush, H.; Akirav, I. Cannabinoids Ameliorate Impairments Induced by Chronic Stress to Synaptic Plasticity and Short-Term Memory. *Neuropsychopharmacology* **2013**, *38*, 1521–1534. [CrossRef]
44. Segev, A.; Rubin, A.S.; Abush, H.; Richter-Levin, G.; Akirav, I. Cannabinoid Receptor Activation Prevents the Effects of Chronic Mild Stress on Emotional Learning and LTP in a Rat Model of Depression. *Neuropsychopharmacology* **2013**, *39*, 919–933. [CrossRef]
45. Kim, H.-D.; Hesterman, J.; Call, T.; Magazu, S.; Keeley, E.; Armenta, K.; Kronman, H.; Neve, R.L.; Nestler, E.J.; Ferguson, D. SIRT1 Mediates Depression-Like Behaviors in the Nucleus Accumbens. *J. Neurosci.* **2016**, *36*, 8441–8452. [CrossRef]
46. Neve, R.L.; Neve, K.A.; Nestler, E.J.; Carlezon, W.A., Jr. Use of herpes virus amplicon vectors to study brain disorders. *Biotechniques* **2005**, *39*, 381–391. [CrossRef]
47. Wang, Z.-J.; Martin, J.A.; Mueller, L.E.; Caccamise, A.; Werner, C.T.; Neve, R.L.; Gancarz, A.M.; Li, J.-X.; Dietz, D.M. BRG1 in the Nucleus Accumbens Regulates Cocaine-Seeking Behavior. *Biol. Psychiatry* **2016**, *80*, 652–660. [CrossRef]
48. Gage, G.J.; Kipke, D.R.; Shain, W. Whole Animal Perfusion Fixation for Rodents. *J. Vis. Exp.* **2012**, e3564. [CrossRef]
49. Vidal, R.; Garro-Martínez, E.; Díaz, Á.; Castro, E.; Florensa-Zanuy, E.; Taketo, M.M.; Pazos, Á.; Pilar-Cuéllar, F. Targeting β-catenin in GLAST-expressing cells: Impact on anxiety and depression-related behavior and hippocampal proliferation. *Mol. Neurobiol.* **2019**, *56*, 553–566. [CrossRef]
50. Holmes, S.E.; Girgenti, M.J.; Davis, M.T.; Pietrzak, R.H.; DellaGioia, N.; Nabulsi, N.; Matuskey, D.; Southwick, S.; Duman, R.S.; Carson, R.E.; et al. Altered metabotropic glutamate receptor 5 markers in PTSD: In vivo and postmortem evidence. *Proc. Natl. Acad. Sci. USA* **2017**, *114*, 8390–8395. [CrossRef]
51. Chen, Y.; Tan, Q.; Dang, W.; Wang, H.; Zhang, R.; Li, Z.; Lin, H.; Liu, R. The effect of citalopram on chronic stress-induced depressive-like behavior in rats through GSK3β/β-catenin activation in the medial prefrontal cortex. *Brain Res. Bull.* **2012**, *88*, 338–344. [CrossRef] [PubMed]
52. Gould, T.D.; Einat, H.; Bhat, R.; Manji, H.K. AR-A014418, a Selective GSK-3 Inhibitor, Produces Antidepressant-like Effects in the Forced Swim Test. *Int. J. Neuropsychopharmacol.* **2004**, *7*, 387–390. [CrossRef] [PubMed]
53. Teo, C.H.; Soga, T.; Parhar, I.S. Brain Beta-Catenin Signalling during Stress and Depression. *Neurosignals* **2018**, *26*, 31–42. [CrossRef] [PubMed]
54. Karege, F.; Perroud, N.; Burkhardt, S.; Fernandez, R.; Ballmann, E.; La Harpe, R.; Malafosse, A. Protein levels of β-catenin and activation state of glycogen synthase kinase-3β in major depression. A study with postmortem prefrontal cortex. *J. Affect. Dis-Ord.* **2012**, *136*, 185–188. [CrossRef]
55. Trazzi, S.; Steger, M.; Mitrugno, V.M.; Bartesaghi, R.; Ciani, E. CB1 cannabinoid receptors increase neuronal precursor pro-liferation through AKT/glycogen synthase kinase-3β/β-catenin signaling. *J. Biol. Chem.* **2010**, *285*, 10098–10109. [CrossRef]

56. Vidal, R.; Pilar-Cuellar, F.; Dos Anjos, S.; Linge, R.; Treceno, B.; Vargas, V.I.; Rodriguez-Gaztelumendi, A.; Mostany, R.; Castro, E.; Diaz, A.; et al. New Strategies in the Development of Antidepressants: Towards the Modulation of Neuroplasticity Pathways. *Curr. Pharm. Des.* **2011**, *17*, 521–533. [CrossRef]
57. Nestler, E.J. Role of the brain's reward circuitry in depression: Transcriptional mechanisms. *Int. Rev. Neu-Robiol.* **2015**, *124*, 151–170.
58. Di Marzo, V.; De Petrocellis, L. Why do cannabinoid receptors have more than one endogenous ligand? *Philos. Trans. R. Soc. B Biol. Sci.* **2012**, *367*, 3216–3228. [CrossRef]
59. Garro-Martínez, E.; Vidal, R.; Adell, A.; Díaz, Á.; Castro, E.; Amigó, J.; Gutiérrez-Lanza, R.; Florensa-Zanuy, E.; Gómez-Acero, L.; Taketo, M.M. β-Catenin Role in the Vulnerability/Resilience to Stress-Related Disorders Is Associated to Changes in the Serotonergic System. *Mol. Neurobiol.* **2020**, *57*, 1704–1715. [CrossRef]

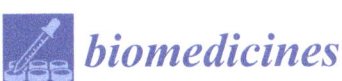

Article

A Placebo-Controlled Trial of Cannabinoid Treatment for Disruptive Behavior in Children and Adolescents with Autism Spectrum Disorder: Effects on Sleep Parameters as Measured by the CSHQ

Aviad Schnapp [1], Moria Harel [2], Dalit Cayam-Rand [2], Hanoch Cassuto [3], Lola Polyansky [2] and Adi Aran [2,4,*]

[1] Department of Pediatrics, Hadassah Medical Center, Jerusalem 91120, Israel; aviad.schnapp@gmail.com
[2] Neuropediatric Unit, Shaare Zedek Medical Center, Jerusalem 9103102, Israel; moriaharel@gmail.com (M.H.); dalitc@szmc.org.il (D.C.-R.); lolapol@szmc.org.il (L.P.)
[3] Child Development Centers, Leumit Health Services, Jerusalem 9439121, Israel; han.cass@gmail.com
[4] Faculty of Medicine, Hebrew University of Jerusalem, Jerusalem 9112102, Israel
* Correspondence: aaran@szmc.org.il

Citation: Schnapp, A.; Harel, M.; Cayam-Rand, D.; Cassuto, H.; Polyansky, L.; Aran, A. A Placebo-Controlled Trial of Cannabinoid Treatment for Disruptive Behavior in Children and Adolescents with Autism Spectrum Disorder: Effects on Sleep Parameters as Measured by the CSHQ. *Biomedicines* **2022**, *10*, 1685. https://doi.org/10.3390/biomedicines10071685

Academic Editor: Wesley M. Raup-Konsavage

Received: 7 June 2022
Accepted: 12 July 2022
Published: 13 July 2022

Publisher's Note: MDPI stays neutral with regard to jurisdictional claims in published maps and institutional affiliations.

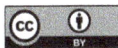

Copyright: © 2022 by the authors. Licensee MDPI, Basel, Switzerland. This article is an open access article distributed under the terms and conditions of the Creative Commons Attribution (CC BY) license (https://creativecommons.org/licenses/by/4.0/).

Abstract: Autism spectrum disorder (ASD) is often associated with debilitating sleep disturbances. While anecdotal evidence suggests the positive effect of cannabinoids, randomized studies are lacking. Here, we report the effects of cannabinoid treatment on the sleep of 150 children and adolescents with ASD, as part of a double-blind, placebo-controlled study that assessed the impact of cannabinoid treatment on behavior (NCT02956226). Participants were randomly assigned to one of the following three treatments: (1) whole-plant cannabis extract, containing cannabidiol (CBD) and Δ9-Tetrahydrocannabinol (THC) in a 20:1 ratio, (2) purified CBD and THC extract in the same ratio, and (3) an oral placebo. After 12 weeks of treatment (Period 1) and a 4-week washout period, participants crossed over to a predetermined, second 12-week treatment (Period 2). Sleep disturbances were assessed using the Children's Sleep-Habit Questionnaire (CSHQ). We found that the CBD-rich cannabinoid treatment was not superior to the placebo treatment in all aspects of sleep measured by the CSHQ, including bedtime resistance, sleep-onset delay, and sleep duration. Notably, regardless of the treatment (cannabinoids or placebo), improvements in the CSHQ total score were associated with improvements in the autistic core symptoms, as indicated by the Social Responsiveness Scale total scores (Period 1: r = 0.266, p = 0.008; Period 2: r = 0.309, p = 0.004). While this study failed to demonstrate that sleep improvements were higher with cannabinoids than they were with the placebo treatment, further studies are required.

Keywords: autism spectrum disorder; cannabinoids; cannabidiol; tetrahydrocannabinol; clinical trials; randomized controlled; sleep; child psychiatry; developmental disorders

1. Introduction

Autism spectrum disorder (ASD) is a heterogeneous neurodevelopmental disorder that is characterized by persistent deficits in social interaction and communication, restricted interests, and repetitive behaviors [1]. Phenotypes among individuals with ASD are highly diverse in terms of cognition, language abilities, irritability, sensory perception, anxiety, motor skills, executive functions, epilepsy, gastrointestinal problems, and more [1,2]. Up to 80% of children with ASD also have sleep disorders, including prolonged sleep onset latency, extended night awakenings, and early morning awakenings [3,4].

The etiology of sleep disorders in ASD is presumed to include multiple neuropsychological factors [5], among which alterations in the circadian sleep–wake cycle are the most well established [6,7]. Accordingly, the most common pharmacological treatment for sleep disorders in individuals with ASD is exogenous melatonin, given as an add on to behavioral interventions, and parental education [8].

One of the main regulators of the sleep–wake cycle is the endocannabinoid system [9]. The primary components of this cell-signaling system are the cannabinoid receptors and their endogenous ligands (endocannabinoids) [10]. The cannabis plant contains unique compounds (phytocannabinoids) that can interact with the endocannabinoid system either directly, using ∆9-tetrahydrocannabinol (THC), or indirectly, using cannabidiol (CBD). THC is the major psychoactive component of the cannabis plant. It activates the type 1 cannabinoid receptor (CB_1R) in the brain and might lead to anxiety and psychosis [11]. CBD is the major non-psychoactive phytocannabinoid. While it is an allosteric modulator of the CB_1R, which may decrease the effects of CB_1R agonists, it concomitantly increases the levels of the endocannabinoids that activate the CB_1R (Figure 1) [11]. As opposed to THC, CBD has a relatively high toxicity threshold and it also appears to have anxiolytic, antipsychotic, antiepileptic, and neuroprotective properties that may be mediated through receptors, such as serotonin $5\text{-}HT_{1A}$, TRPV1, GPR55, $GABA_A$, and PPARγ, and through the inhibition of adenosine reuptake (Figure 1) [12–16].

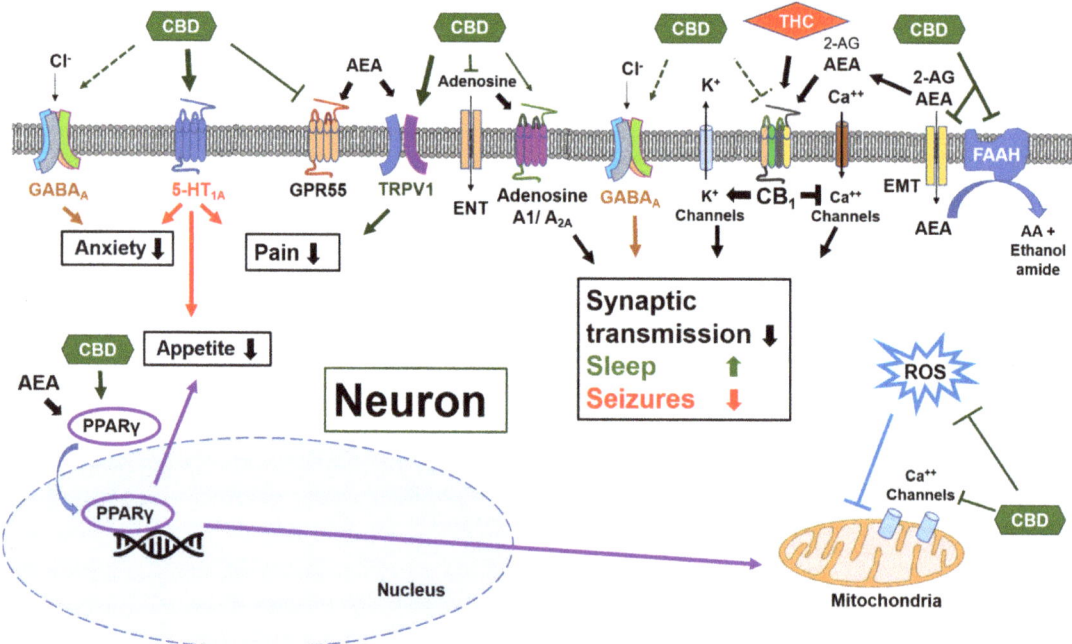

Figure 1. Multiple molecular targets for cannabidiol (CBD) in neurons.

Alterations in the endocannabinoid system have been found in several animal models of ASD [17,18]. Recent human studies have demonstrated lower circulating endocannabinoid levels in children with ASD [19–21] and evidence of successful CBD-rich cannabinoid treatment for the core symptoms and comorbidities in children with ASD is accumulating [22–25]. However, the effect of phytocannabinoids on the sleep of ASD children is still unclear.

In general, cannabinoid therapy with various THC to CBD ratios is being increasingly used to alleviate sleep disorders, regardless of the cause. Among patients with chronic pain, treatment with medical cannabis seems to result in a small improvement in sleep quality [26]. Preliminary evidence of successful treatment is also available for sleep apnea, and post-traumatic stress disorder-related nightmares [27]. However, currently there is insufficient evidence to support this line of treatment for any individual sleep disorder [27–29].

In the current study, we aimed to evaluate the impact of a CBD-rich cannabinoid treatment on sleep, as part of a placebo-controlled trial, which assessed the effects of cannabinoids on the behavior of children and adolescents with ASD. We used two CBD-rich preparations. The first contained only purified CBD and purified THC isolates (pure cannabinoids) and the second contained a full-spectrum (whole-plant) extract, which, in addition to the same amounts of CBD and THC, also contained minor cannabinoids, terpenes, and flavonoids that might enhance the efficacy and tolerability.

We found that an improvement in sleep (after receiving either cannabinoids or the placebo) was associated with an improvement in the autistic core symptoms and disruptive behavior. However, CBD-rich cannabinoid treatment did not improve sleep disturbances more than the placebo treatment.

The main cannabinoid receptor in neurons is cannabinoid receptor type 1 (CB_1R). The primary neuronal effect of the CB_1R is a decrease in the synaptic transmission during increased synaptic activity, which can also promote sleep and reduce seizures and excitotoxicity. CBD is a negative allosteric modulator of the CB_1R. However, CBD can activate the endocannabinoid system through the CB_1R by inhibiting the endocannabinoid membrane transporter (EMT) and the degradation of anandamide (AEA) through fatty acid amide hydrolase (FAAH). This, in turn, increases the levels of the endocannabinoids AEA (main agonist of CB_1R) and 2-Arachidonoylglycerol (2-AG). Other neuronal effects of CBD are mediated through agonism at the $5-HT_{1A}$ serotonin receptors and at the TRPV1 channel, reducing anxiety and pain, and through agonism of the nuclear PPARγ receptors, increasing the expression of the cytoprotective enzymes. CBD also has direct antioxidative effects.

ENT—equilibrative nucleotide transporter; $5-HT_{1A}$—5-hydroxytryptamine 1A receptor; GPR55—G protein coupled receptor 55; PPARγ—peroxisome proliferator-activated receptor gamma; ROS—reactive oxygen species; TRPV1—transient receptor potential vanilloid 1.

2. Materials and Methods

2.1. Study Design

NCT02956226 was a proof-of-concept, randomized, double-blind, placebo-controlled trial, and methods were previously described [23]. The primary objective of this trial was to assess the impact of cannabinoid treatment on ASD-associated disruptive behavior. We previously reported the effects of the cannabinoid treatment on disruptive behavior and the ASD core symptoms, as well as adverse effects of the treatment [23]. We report here the effect of the cannabinoid treatment on sleep parameters.

2.2. Standard Protocol Approvals and Patient Consent

The study was conducted in a single referral center for ASD diagnosis and treatment: Shaare Zedek Medical Center, Jerusalem, Israel. It was approved by the Institutional Review Board at Shaare Zedek Medical Center and the Israeli Ministry of Health prior to participant enrollment. Participants' parents provided written informed consent and written consent was also obtained from participants, when appropriate.

2.3. Study Population

Eligible participants were children and adolescents between 5 and 21 years old, with an ASD diagnosis, as per the Diagnostic and Statistical Manual of Mental Disorders, fifth edition (DSM-5), criteria, and as confirmed by the Autism Diagnostic Observation Schedule (ADOS-2), and moderate or greater behavioral problems rating (rating ≥ 4) on the Clinical Global Impression's (CGI) severity scale. The full list of inclusion and exclusion criteria appears in Table S1.

2.4. Treatment Scheme

Participants were randomly allocated for treatment with two out of three oral preparations, each given in a distinct 12-week treatment period. Treatment options were as follows: (1) BOL-DP-O-01-W (BOL Pharma, Revadim Israel), a whole-plant (full spectrum) cannabis extract, containing CBD and THC at a 20:1 ratio; (2) BOL-DP-O-01 (BOL Pharma, Revadim, Israel), purified CBD and THC at the same ratio; and (3) placebo (BOL Pharma, Revadim, Israel). In each treatment period, starting dose was 1 mg/kg/d CBD (and 0.05 mg/kg/d THC) or an equivalent placebo. The dose was increased by 1 mg/kg/d CBD (and 0.05 mg/kg/d THC) every other day, up to 10 mg/kg body weight per day CBD (and 0.5 mg/kg/d THC), for children weighing 20–40 kg or 7.5 mg/kg/d CBD (and 0.375 mg/kg/d THC) for weight >40 kg (maximum 420 mg CBD and 21 mg THC per day), divided into 3 daily doses. Treatments were given orally (sublingual whenever possible), as an add-on to any ongoing stable medication (Table 1). At the end of the first treatment period, the study treatment was gradually decreased over 2 weeks, followed by 2 weeks of no study treatment to enable full elimination of the cannabinoids given in the first period [30].

Table 1. Participants' baseline characteristics.

	All (n = 150)	Group A (n = 50)	Group B (n = 50)	Group C (n = 50)	Sig.
Treatment 1st period		Placebo	Pure cannabinoids	Whole plant	
Treatment 2nd period		Whole plant	Placebo	Pure cannabinoids	
Sex					
Males n (%)	120 (80%)	42 (84%)	42 (84%)	36 (72%)	0.22 *
Age					
Mean ± SD	11.8 ± 4.1	11.7 ± 3.8	11.6 ± 4.3	12.1 ± 4.3	0.79 #
[median, range]	[11.3, 5.1–20.8]	[10.7, 5.8–20.0]	[10.3, 5.1–20.4]	[12.6, 5.1–20.8]	
BMI					
Mean ± SD	20.8 ± 5.7	20.5 ± 5.2	20.5 ± 6.0	21.3 ± 6.1	0.72 #
[median, range]	[19.0, 12.3–39.6]	[19.1, 12.8–34.0]	[19.1, 12.3–39.6]	[19.0, 13.9–39.5]	
ADOS comparison score					
Mean ± SD	8.8 ± 1.5	8.6 ± 1.6	9.2 ± 1.3	8.6 ± 1.6	0.07 #
[median, range]	[10.0, 4.0–10.0]	[9.0, 4.0–10.0]	[10.0, 6.0–10.0]	[9.0, 4.0–10.0]	
VABS composite score					
Mean ± SD	52.3 ± 14.5	52.0 ± 15.0	52.4 ± 15.2	52.3 ± 13.6	0.99 #
[median, range]	[51.0, 20.0–102.0]	[49.0, 26.0–102.0]	[54.0, 25.0–89.0]	[52.0, 20.0–78.0]	
CARS total score					
Mean ± SD	45.4 ± 8.4	46.0 ± 8.5	45.5 ± 8.9	44.6 ± 7.8	0.68 #
[median, range]	[47.5, 29.5–59.0]	[47.3, 30.5–59.0]	[48.5, 29.5–57.5]	[46.5, 31.0–56.5]	
SRS					
Mean ± SD	119 ± 27	122 ± 23	118 ± 31	117 ± 27	0.37 #
[median, range]	[121, 53–180]	[124, 53–159]	[118, 64–178]	[117, 66–180]	
Concomitant medications					
Atypical antipsychotics n (%)	76 (50.7%)	28 (56.0%)	20 (40.0%)	28 (56.0%)	0.18 *
Typical antipsychotics n (%)	13 (8.7%)	5 (10.0%)	3 (6.0%)	5 (10.0%)	0.82 *
Anticonvulsants n (%)	18 (8.7%)	6 (12.0%)	4 (8.0%)	8 (16.0%)	0.47 *
Stimulants n (%)	20 (13.3%)	5 (8.0%)	11 (22.0%)	5 (10.0%)	0.08 *
Benzodiazepines n (%)	5 (3.3%)	1 (2.0%)	2 (4.0%)	2 (4.0%)	1.00 *
Melatonin n (%)	12 (8.0%)	6 (12.0%)	4 (8.0%)	2 (4.0%)	0.39 *
SSRIs n (%)	21 (14.0%)	6 (12.0%)	8 (16.0%)	7 (4.0%)	0.84 *
Total CSHQ score					
Mean ± SD	49.9 ± 9.2	49.7 ± 8.7	50.1 ± 9.4	49.7 ± 9.6	0.97 #
[median, range]	[48.5, 34.0–73.5]	[49.0, 34.0–69.2]	[47.5, 36.0–72.0]	[35.0, 34.0–73.5]	
Bedtime Resistance					
Mean ± SD	9.4 ± 3.3	9.7 ± 3.2	9.4 ± 3.4	9.1 ± 3.3	0.63 #
[median, range]	[8.0, 6.0–17.0]	[9.0, 6.0–17.0]	[6.0–16.0]	[8.0, 6.0–17.0]	

Table 1. Cont.

	All (n = 150)	Group A (n = 50)	Group B (n = 50)	Group C (n = 50)	Sig.
Sleep Onset Delay Mean ± SD [median, range]	1.9 ± 0.8 [2.0, 1.0–3.0]	1.9 ± 0.8 [2.0, 1.0–3.0]	1.9 ± 0.9 [2.0, 1.0–3.0]	2.0 ± 0.8 [2.0, 1.0–3.0]	0.99 #
Sleep Duration Mean ± SD [median, range]	4.6 ± 1.8 [4.0, 3.0–9.0]	4.6 ± 1.8 [4.0, 3.0–9.0]	4.6 ± 1.8 [4.0, 3.0–9.0]	4.5 ± 1.8 [4.0, 3.0–9.0]	0.96 #
Sleep Anxiety Mean ± SD [median, range]	6.3 ± 2.3 [6.0, 4.0–12.0]	6.4 ± 2.1 [6.0, 4.0–11.0]	6.5 ± 2.4 [6.0, 4.0–12.0]	6.1 ± 2.3 [5.0, 4.0–12.0]	0.64 #
Night Wakings Mean ± SD [median, range]	4.9 ± 1.9 [4.0, 3.0–9.0]	4.8 ± 1.7 [4.5, 3.0–9.0]	5.13 ± 2.0 [5.0, 3.0–9.0]	4.7 ± 2.0 [4.0, 3.0–9.0]	0.52 #
Parasomnias Mean ± SD [median, range]	9.2 ± 2.0 [9.0, 7.0–18.2]	8.6 ± 1.7 [9.0, 7.0–12.0]	9.5 ± 2.0 [9.0, 7.0–14.0]	9.3 ± 2.3 [8.8, 7.0–18.2]	0.44 #
Sleep Disordered Breathing Mean ± SD [median, range]	3.9 ± 1.4 [3.0, 3.0–9.0]	3.9 ± 1.2 [3.5, 3.0–7.0]	3.7 ± 1.3 [3.0, 3.0–9.0]	4.1 ± 1.6 [3.0, 3.0–7.0]	0.40 #
Daytime Sleepiness Mean ± SD [median, range]	14.4 ± 3.6 [14.0, 9.0–24.0]	14.2 ± 3.7 [14.0, 9.0–23.0]	14.3 ± 3.7 [13.1, 9.0–24.0]	14.7 ± 3.5 [15.0, 9.0–24.0]	0.79 #

Baseline characteristics of participants stratified to treatment arms. ADOS-2—Autism Diagnostic Observation Schedule, comparison score of 8–10 indicated severe autistic symptoms; BMI—body mass index; CARS—Childhood Autism Rating Scale, scores above 36.5 are indicative of severe ASD; CSHQ—Children's Sleep Habits Questionnaire; SRS—Social Responsiveness Scale, total score ≥ 75 indicates severe autistic symptoms; VABS—Vineland Adaptive Behavior Scale, composite score ≤ 70 indicates low adaptive level. * Categorical parameters (sex and medications) were compared using Pearson chi-square tests. # Continuous parameters were compared using one-way analysis of variance (ANOVA).

The CBD:THC ratio and daily dose were chosen based on our clinical experience and previous open-label studies on the effect of medical cannabis on ASD core symptoms and comorbidities, including sleep problems [22,24,25]. Further details regarding the cannabinoids' preparations and randomization process appear in the Supplemental Information.

2.5. Baseline Evaluations

Baseline assessments at study onset (day 1) included the following: ADOS-2 [31], a systematic and standardized assessment of communication, social interaction, play, and imaginary use of materials, which was administered by a developmental psychologist (MH), with research reliability; Vineland Adaptive Behavior Scales (VABS) [32], a caregiver interview assessing communication, socialization, and daily living skills, which was administered by the same psychologist; and Childhood Autism Rating Scale, second edition (CARS2-ST) [33]—A quantitative measure of direct behavior observation–which was administered by a trained pediatric neurologist (AA).

2.6. Outcomes

Children's Sleep Habits Questionnaire (CSHQ) [34]. This parent-rated questionnaire has been used and validated in multiple studies of ASD [35–39]. It comprises 33 scored questions, and additional items intended to provide other relevant information on sleep behavior. Each scored question is rated on a 3-point scale, as occurring 'usually' (i.e., 5–7 times within the past week), 'sometimes' (i.e., 2–4 times within the past week), or 'rarely (i.e., never or 1 time within the past week). A higher score reflects more significant sleep disturbances. Items are combined to form the following 8 subscales: bedtime resistance, sleep onset delay, sleep duration, sleep anxiety, night waking, parasomnias, sleep disordered breathing, and daytime sleepiness. A total score is calculated as the sum of all CSHQ scored items and can range from 33 to 99. A total score of 41 and above indicates a pediatric sleep disorder, as this cutoff has been shown to accurately identify 80% of children with a clinically diagnosed sleep disorder [34]. Parents were instructed to answer questions regarding their child's sleep during a typical recent week. The questionnaire was completed at the onset and end of each treatment period. The completed CSHQ questionnaires were excluded from analysis if more than 20% of the data were missing.

Clinical Global Impression–Improvement scale (CGI-I) [40] was used to measure the improvement in disruptive behaviors from the baseline. Scores range from 1 (very much improved), to 4 (unchanged), to 7 (very much worse). Scores of 1 or 2 (much improved) were defined as a positive response and all others indicated a negative response [40]. CGI-I was assessed at the end of each treatment period. Anchoring instructions were used to rate improvement in behavioral difficulties on the CGI-I, rather than improvement in overall ASD symptoms. The same clinician (AA) assessed and rated the CGI-S and CGI-I of all participants. Notably, while the CGI-S and CGI-I were developed to assess 'overall function', we used anchor points that were 'domain-specific' for disruptive behavior.

Social Responsiveness Scale (SRS-2): [41] this 65-item, caregiver questionnaire quantifies autism symptom severity (total scores range from 0 to 195, with higher scores indicating worsening severity). The questionnaire was completed at the onset and end of each treatment period.

2.7. Statistical Analyses

The impact of treatment on sleep was assessed using the change in CSHQ scores in each treatment period. Difference in the CSHQ total score was assessed both as a continuous and a dichotomous variable, using the cutoff score of 41. We adjusted for the following variables: sex, age at enrollment, and maternal education.

Continuous variables were assessed by two-tailed paired t-tests or ANOVA (after confirmation for normal/near normal distribution). Categorical variables were assessed by Pearson χ^2 test. Treatment efficacy was compared between groups during the first and second treatment period and within treatment groups for participants who completed both treatment periods (per protocol [PP] analysis). Analyses were performed using IBM SPSS® version 25 (2017). All p values were two-sided. p-value < 0.05 was considered significant.

3. Results

3.1. Participants

Between 11 January 2017 and 12 April 2018, 150 children and adolescents (mean age 11.8 ± 4.1 years, median 11.25, range 5.1–20.8; 80% boys) entered the trial. The ASD symptoms were 'severe' in 78.7% per ADOS-2 (comparison score = 8–10) [31] and the adaptive levels were 'low' (composite score ≤ 70) in 88%, as per the Vineland Behavior Scales [32].

The participant's characteristics are provided in Table 1. Fifty participants were randomly assigned to each of the three treatments in Period 1 and 44 participants per group completed the study (Figure 2).

Among the 150 participants who underwent randomization, 131 (87%) submitted valid questionnaires at the onset and end of the first treatment period (Figure 2), enabling a between-subject analysis in this period (i.e., to compare the change in sleep parameters between the participants who received cannabinoids and the participants who received the placebo). In total, 107 participants (71%) submitted valid questionnaires at the onset and the end of both the first and second treatment period, enabling a within-subject analysis (i.e., to compare the change in sleep parameters while receiving cannabinoids, while receiving the placebo, and in participants who received both treatments).

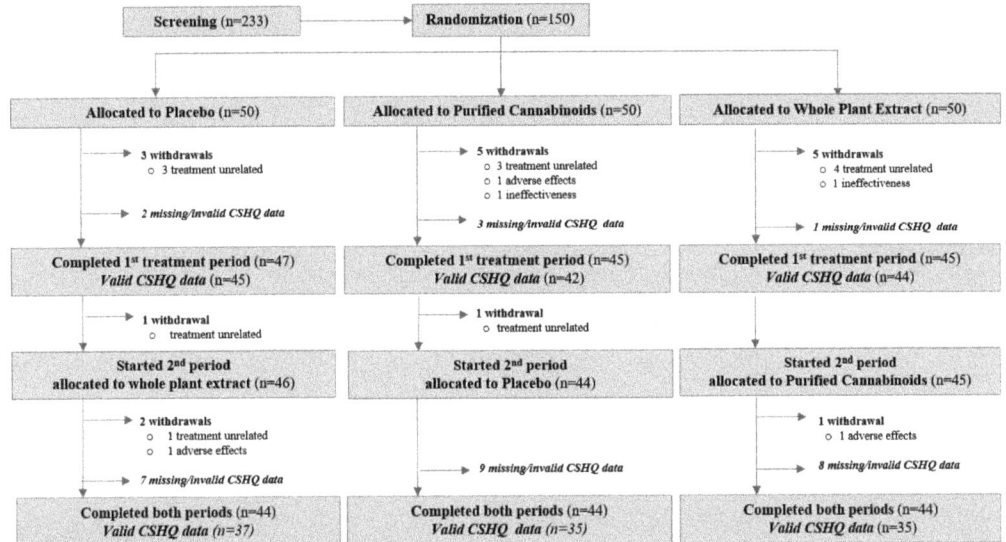

Figure 2. Participants' allocation and adherence.

The participants' baseline characteristics, including sleep disturbances, as indicated by the CSHQ total and sub scores, were similar in the three treatment arms (Table 1).

Overall, 18 participants (12%) withdrew from the trial for the following reasons: 13 for reasons unrelated to treatment, three due to adverse events, and two due to ineffectiveness. In total, 131 participants (87%) had valid CSHQ scores before and after the treatment in the first treatment period. In total, 107 participants (71%) had valid pre-and post-treatment scores in both treatment periods, allowing a within-subject comparison.

3.2. Baseline Sleep Disturbances

Among the 146 participants who had valid CSHQ scores at the baseline, 125 (86%) had a CSHQ total score ≥ 41, indicating a sleep disorder. Higher CSHQ scores (indicating more prominent sleep disorder symptoms) at the baseline were correlated with a younger age (Pearson correlation r = -0.288, $p < 0.001$) and with higher SRS total scores, indicating more severe core autistic traits (r = 0.175, $p = 0.036$). The CSHQ scores were not associated with sex or adaptive behavior, as indicated by the VABS composite scores.

Notably, the baseline characteristics were not different between the participants included in the per-protocol analysis and the participants who were excluded due to withdrawal or missing data, including age ($p = 0.83$); sex ($p = 0.86$); the severity of sleep disorders, as reflected by the CSHQ total score ($p = 0.63$); adaptive behavior, as evaluated by the VABS Composite scores ($p = 0.57$); and the severity of the core autistic symptoms, as assessed by the ADOS-2 ($p = 0.58$), CARS ($p = 0.75$), and the SRS ($p = 0.25$).

3.3. Impact of Cannabinoid Treatment on Sleep

The impact of the cannabinoid treatment on sleep disturbances was assessed using the CSHQ. In total, 131 participants had valid CSHQ scores, both pre-treatment and post-treatment, in the first 12-week treatment period. Among these 131 participants, 44 received a whole-plant extract (BOL-DP-O-01-W, CBD:THC ratio = 20:1), 42 received pure cannabinoids (BOL-DP-O-01, CBD, and THC at a 20:1 ratio), and 45 received a placebo. The CSHQ total scores and the subscale scores did not differ significantly between the participants who received cannabinoids and the participants who received the placebo

(Table 2). None of these measures differed significantly between the participants who received the whole-plant extract versus the pure cannabinoids (Table 2).

Table 2. Impact of cannabinoid treatment on sleep. Comparison of treatment effects in the 1st 12-week period.

	Placebo n = 45 [Change in Points]	Pure Cannabinoids n = 42 [Change in Points]	Whole Plant n = 44 [Change in Points]	Total n = 131 [Change in Points]	Sig ^
Total CSHQ score					
Mean ± SD	−1.4 ± 6.6	−2.9 ± 9.2	−2.3 ± 5.6	−2.2 ± 7.2	0.63
[median, range]	[−1.9, −20.3–13.0]	[−1.5, −27.9–18.0]	[−1.5, −18.0–7.3]	[−1.9, −27.9–18.0]	
Bedtime Resistance					
Mean ± SD	−0.6 ± 1.6	−0.5 ± 2.7	−0.3 ± 1.6	−0.4 ± 2.0	0.79
[median, range]	[0.0, −4.0–3.0]	[0.0, −9.0–5.7]	[0.0, −6.0–3.0]	[0.0, −9.0–5.7]	
Sleep Onset Delay					
Mean ± SD	−0.1 ± 0.6	−0.1 ± 0.8	−0.2 ± 0.8	−0.2 ± 0.7	0.98
[median, range]	[0.0, −1.0–2.0]	[0.0, −2.0–2.0]	[0.0, −2.0–1.0]	[0.0, −2.0–2.0]	
Sleep Duration					
Mean ± SD	−0.1 ± 1.6	0.0 ± 2.0	−0.5 ± 1.9	−0.2 ± 1.8	0.38
[median, range]	[0.0, −4.0–4.0]	[0.0, −5.0–4.0]	[0.0, −5.0–4.0]	[0.0, −5.0–4.0]	
Sleep Anxiety					
Mean ± SD	−0.4 ± 1.2	−0.6 ± 1.3	−0.2 ± 1.5	−0.4 ± 1.3	0.59
[median, range]	[0.0, −4.0–2.0]	[0.0, −4.0–1.7]	[0.0, −4.0–2.0]	[0.0, −4.0–2.0]	
Night Wakings					
Mean ± SD	−0.2 ± 1.3	−0.8 ± 1.5	−0.6 ± 1.2	−0.5 ± 1.4	0.11
[median, range]	[0.0, −3.0–3.0]	[−0.5, −4.0–1.0]	[0.0, −4.0–1.0]	[0.0, −4.0–3.0]	
Parasomnias					
Mean ± SD	−0.2 ± 1.6	−0.6 ± 1.9	−0.5 ± 1.4	−0.5 ± 1.6	0.53
[median, range]	[0.0, −4.0–4.0]	[−0.9, −7.0–4.0]	[0.0, −4.5–2.3]	[0.0, −7.0–4.0]	
Sleep Disordered Breathing					
Mean ± SD	−0.0 ± 0.9	−0.3 ± 1.0	−0.1 ± 0.8	−0.2 ± 0.9	0.36
[median, range]	[0.0, −2.0–3.0]	[−0.0, −4.0–1.0]	[0.0, −2.0–1.0]	[0.0, −4.0–3.0]	
Daytime Sleepiness					
Mean ± SD	0.1 ± 3.0	0.2 ± 3.5	0.0 ± 2.7	0.1 ± 3.1	0.96
[median, range]	[0.0, −9.0–7.8]	[0.0, −7.0–7.0]	[0.0, −5.0–5.0]	[0.0, −9.0–7.8]	

Between-subject analyses of the change in the CSHQ scores following treatment in the first treatment period. CSHQ—Children's Sleep Habits Questionnaire. Positive change (increment of CSHQ scores) indicates worsening of the sleep disorder. Change in the CSHQ scores from baseline following treatment is compared between the 3 treatment arms. ^ One-way ANOVA for influence of treatments between study groups. Notably, the difference between cannabinoid treatment and placebo was not statistically significant, even when combining the two cannabinoid treatments into one group, compared to placebo (data not shown).

Similar negative results were found in the second treatment period (Table S2) and when comparing the two treatments that each participant received, using a within-participant analysis (Table S3).

3.4. Longitudinal Associations between Sleep, Behavior, and Autistic Core Symptoms

Regardless of the treatment, improvements in the sleep disturbances, as indicated by a decline in the CSHQ total score, were associated with improvements in the autistic core symptoms, as well as the associated disruptive behaviors in both treatment periods.

The autistic core symptoms were assessed using the SRS total score (higher scores indicate higher severity of symptoms). Changes in the SRS total score correlated with changes in the CSHQ total score in Period 1 (Pearson correlation: r = 0.266, p = 0.008) and Period 2 (r = 0.309, p = 0.004).

Improvements in the ASD-associated disruptive behaviors were evaluated by the Clinical Global Impression–Improvement rate (CGI-I: lower rates indicate improvement). The CGI-I rate was associated with a change in the CSHQ total score in Period 1 (one-way ANOVA: f = 4.5, p = 0.013) and Period 2 (f = 3.36, p = 0.038).

4. Discussion

Interest in cannabis preparations as therapeutic agents in neuropsychiatric disorders is growing in both the scientific and lay communities [42,43]. This interest is particularly strong in disorders with substantial unmet needs, such as refractory epilepsy and pediatric ASD, which lacks medications that target its core symptoms [44]. Currently, robust evidence exists only for Epidiolex, a plant-derived pure CBD isolate, to treat the following specific types of refractory epilepsy: Dravet syndrome [45], Lennox–Gastaut syndrome [46], and tuberous sclerosis complex [47]. Nevertheless, full-spectrum extracts of various cannabis strains and synthetic cannabinoids are being widely used to treat adults living with chronic pain [48–50], chemotherapy-induced nausea and vomiting [51,52], sleep disorders [26], depression, anxiety, psychosis [53], PTSD [54], and to treat children with various types of refractory epilepsy [55], and irritability associated with autism spectrum disorder (ASD) [22,24,25,56].

The endocannabinoid system is involved in the pathophysiology of both sleep disorders [9] and ASD [19], which might contribute to the high incidence of sleep disturbances in people with ASD. These associations make the endocannabinoid system an attractive target for the treatment of sleep disturbances in ASD.

There is much anecdotal evidence, as well as several reports of uncontrolled case series, suggesting an improvement in sleep disturbances following treatment with various strains of medical cannabis [24,25,57,58]. However, placebo-controlled studies have not been published so far.

In this randomized, placebo-controlled trial we used the following two CBD-rich preparations: a full-spectrum (whole-plant) extract, and purified CBD and THC isolates (pure cannabinoids). This is particularly relevant for sleep disturbances as it is commonly believed that, in addition to the main cannabinoids, other components of the cannabis plant, such as terpenes and flavonoids, also assist in alleviating sleep disturbances (an entourage effect) [59–61].

In our cohort, the effect of these two cannabinoid preparations at a dose of ~5.5 mg CBD and ~0.3 mg THC per kg, per day, was not superior to the placebo in all aspects of sleep measured by the CSHQ.

These findings are in line with a recent report on the negative acute effect of CBD on the sleep–wake cycle of healthy adults in a placebo-controlled study [62]. Of note, while a recent meta-analysis of randomized clinical trials demonstrated that cannabinoids provided a small benefit for impaired sleep, the studies that were analyzed were mainly in adults living with chronic pain, who used THC-rich preparations [26].

Accordingly, future studies of cannabinoid treatment for sleep disorders should consider using a more balanced CBD to THC ratio. Indeed, recreational cannabis strains that contain high THC and low CBD concentrations were associated with serious adverse events when used during youth, including decreased motivation [63–65], addiction [66], mild cognitive decline [64,67–69], and schizophrenia [64,70–72]. However, all of these risks are higher in cannabis strains with a high ratio of THC to CBD [73], than in the more balanced strains.

Consistent with previous studies [39,74], we also found that the severity of sleep disturbances, as indicated by the CSHQ total score at the baseline, correlated with a younger age and with the severity of the autistic core symptoms. Most of the participants in our cohort had severe autistic symptoms (78.7% had a comparison score of 8–10 in the ADOS-2). This might explain the higher rate of participants (86%) who screened positive for sleep disturbances, compared to a rate of approximately 70% that was reported in a US registry study [74] and in a Chinese multicenter survey [39].

Notably, we found a longitudinal association between changes in the CSHQ total score (in participants who received either cannabinoids or the placebo) and changes in the disruptive behavior and the severity of the core symptoms, suggesting the possibility of a cause-and-effect relationship (better sleep leads to lower symptoms). These findings are congruent with associations between sleep quality, behavior, and the severity of autistic core symptoms that have been reported in cross-sectional studies [39,75]. This finding also underscores the importance of sleep quality in children with ASD, the impact of which may exceed that of their typically developing peers.

Our study had several limitations: The study was designed as a cross-over study, which allows within-participant analyses, comparing the two treatments that each participant received. However, a treatment order effect (all treatments were more effective in the first period, probably due to a greater initial placebo effect) made this analysis less accurate. Therefore, we reported the more accurate between-subject analyses of the first treatment period (Table 2). We also present, in the Supplemental Information, the within-participant analyses (Table S3) and the between-participant analyses of Period 2 (Table S3), which yielded similar negative results. Another limitation of this study was the use of a caregiver's report for assessing sleep quality, without more objective measures of sleep such as actigraphy and sleep logs. Additionally, our study was not powered to detect the effects of age, the level of function, and other baseline characteristics on the treatment response.

5. Conclusions

Sleep disturbances are very common in children with ASD, and they have a substantial impact on the quality of life of the child and the family. Preliminary clinical evidence and preclinical studies, which implicate the endocannabinoid system in the pathophysiology of both ASD and sleep disorders, suggest that cannabinoid treatment might improve sleep in children with ASD. In a controlled study of 150 participants, we found that a whole-plant extract and a pure cannabinoid preparation, which contained CBD and THC in a 20:1 ratio did not improve the sleep parameters, as reflected in the CSHQ scores. Future studies should consider using actigraphy and sleep logs and recruiting participants within narrower ranges of age and functional levels, this might enable the identification of target populations within the autism spectrum that might benefit from this line of treatment.

Supplementary Materials: The following supporting information can be downloaded at https://www.mdpi.com/article/10.3390/biomedicines10071685/s1, Supplementary Methods: interventions, randomization, and blinding; Table S1: inclusion and exclusion criteria for study participation; Table S2: impact of cannabinoid treatment on sleep; comparison of treatment effects in 2nd period; Table S3: comparison of changes in CSHQ scores (Mean ± SE), following the 1st and 2nd treatment that each participant received.

Author Contributions: Conceptualization, A.A. and H.C.; methodology, A.A.; software, A.S. and L.P.; validation, A.A., L.P, D.C.-R. and M.H.; formal analysis, A.A. and A.S.; resources, A.A.; data curation, A.A., A.S. and M.H.; writing—original draft preparation, A.S. and A.A.; writing—review and editing, A.A. and D.C.-R.; supervision, A.A. and H.C.; project administration, L.P.; funding acquisition, A.A. All authors have read and agreed to the published version of the manuscript.

Funding: This research was funded by the National Institute for Psychobiology in Israel, grant number 203-17-18, and BOL Pharma, Revadim, Israel. The funding bodies were not involved in any way in the study design, the collection, analysis, and interpretation of data, or in the writing of the manuscript.

Institutional Review Board Statement: The study was conducted in accordance with the Declaration of Helsinki and approved by the Institutional Review Board of Shaare Zedek Medical center (protocol code 0175-16, date of approval 15 September 2016) and the Israeli Ministry of Health (application number: 20162153, date of approval 27 September 2016).

Informed Consent Statement: Informed consent was obtained from all subjects involved in the study. Participants' parents provided written informed consent and written consent was also obtained from participants when appropriate.

Data Availability Statement: The authors declare that the data supporting the findings of this study are available within the paper and its Supplemental Information. The remainder of the data are available from the corresponding author upon reasonable request.

Conflicts of Interest: Adi Aran reports receiving personal fees and stock options for advisory roles at BOL Pharma between 2018 and 2020. The remaining authors declare no conflict of interest. The funders had no role in the design of the study; in the collection, analyses, or interpretation of the data; in the writing of the manuscript; or in the decision to publish the results.

References

1. Lord, C.; Elsabbagh, M.; Baird, G.; Veenstra-Vanderweele, J. Autism spectrum disorder. *Lancet* **2018**, *392*, 508–520. [CrossRef]
2. Masi, A.; DeMayo, M.M.; Glozier, N.; Guastella, A.J. An Overview of Autism Spectrum Disorder, Heterogeneity and Treatment Options. *Neurosci. Bull.* **2017**, *33*, 183–193. [CrossRef] [PubMed]
3. Tesfaye, R.; Wright, N.; Zaidman-Zait, A.; Bedford, R.; Zwaigenbaum, L.; Kerns, C.M.; Duku, E.; Mirenda, P.; Bennett, T.; Georgiades, S.; et al. Investigating longitudinal associations between parent reported sleep in early childhood and teacher reported executive functioning in school-aged children with autism. *Sleep* **2021**, *44*, zsab122. [CrossRef] [PubMed]
4. Reynolds, A.M.; Soke, G.N.; Sabourin, K.R.; Hepburn, S.; Katz, T.; Wiggins, L.D.; Schieve, L.A.; Levy, S.E. Sleep Problems in 2- to 5-Year-Olds with Autism Spectrum Disorder and Other Developmental Delays. *Pediatrics* **2019**, *143*, e20180492. [CrossRef]
5. Johnson, K.P.; Zarrinnegar, P. Autism Spectrum Disorder and Sleep. *Child Adolesc. Psychiatr. Clin. N. Am.* **2021**, *30*, 195–208. [CrossRef]
6. Lorsung, E.; Karthikeyan, R.; Cao, R. Biological Timing and Neurodevelopmental Disorders: A Role for Circadian Dysfunction in Autism Spectrum Disorders. *Front. Neurosci.* **2021**, *15*, 642745. [CrossRef]
7. Pinato, L.; Galina Spilla, C.S.; Markus, R.P.; da Silveira Cruz-Machado, S. Dysregulation of Circadian Rhythms in Autism Spectrum Disorders. *Curr. Pharm Des.* **2019**, *25*, 4379–4393. [CrossRef]
8. Williams Buckley, A.; Hirtz, D.; Oskoui, M.; Armstrong, M.J.; Batra, A.; Bridgemohan, C.; Coury, D.; Dawson, G.; Donley, D.; Findling, R.L.; et al. Practice guideline: Treatment for insomnia and disrupted sleep behavior in children and adolescents with autism spectrum disorder: Report of the Guideline Development, Dissemination, and Implementation Subcommittee of the American Academy of Neurology. *Neurology* **2020**, *94*, 392–404. [CrossRef]
9. Kesner, A.J.; Lovinger, D.M. Cannabinoids, Endocannabinoids and Sleep. *Front. Mol. Neurosci.* **2020**, *13*, 125. [CrossRef]
10. Guerrero-Alba, R.; Barragan-Iglesias, P.; Gonzalez-Hernandez, A.; Valdez-Morales, E.E.; Granados-Soto, V.; Condes-Lara, M.; Rodriguez, M.G.; Marichal-Cancino, B.A. Some Prospective Alternatives for Treating Pain: The Endocannabinoid System and Its Putative Receptors GPR18 and GPR55. *Front. Pharmacol.* **2018**, *9*, 1496. [CrossRef]
11. Szkudlarek, H.J.; Desai, S.J.; Renard, J.; Pereira, B.; Norris, C.; Jobson, C.E.L.; Rajakumar, N.; Allman, B.L.; Laviolette, S.R. Delta-9-Tetrahydrocannabinol and Cannabidiol produce dissociable effects on prefrontal cortical executive function and regulation of affective behaviors. *Neuropsychopharmacology* **2019**, *44*, 817–825. [CrossRef] [PubMed]
12. Campos, A.C.; Fogaca, M.V.; Scarante, F.F.; Joca, S.R.L.; Sales, A.J.; Gomes, F.V.; Sonego, A.B.; Rodrigues, N.S.; Galve-Roperh, I.; Guimaraes, F.S. Plastic and Neuroprotective Mechanisms Involved in the Therapeutic Effects of Cannabidiol in Psychiatric Disorders. *Front. Pharmacol.* **2017**, *8*, 269. [CrossRef] [PubMed]
13. McGuire, P.; Robson, P.; Cubala, W.J.; Vasile, D.; Morrison, P.D.; Barron, R.; Taylor, A.; Wright, S. Cannabidiol (CBD) as an Adjunctive Therapy in Schizophrenia: A Multicenter Randomized Controlled Trial. *Am. J. Psychiatry* **2018**, *175*, 225–231. [CrossRef] [PubMed]
14. Devinsky, O.; Cilio, M.R.; Cross, H.; Fernandez-Ruiz, J.; French, J.; Hill, C.; Katz, R.; Di Marzo, V.; Jutras-Aswad, D.; Notcutt, W.G.; et al. Cannabidiol: Pharmacology and potential therapeutic role in epilepsy and other neuropsychiatric disorders. *Epilepsia* **2014**, *55*, 791–802. [CrossRef]
15. Iannotti, F.A.; Hill, C.L.; Leo, A.; Alhusaini, A.; Soubrane, C.; Mazzarella, E.; Russo, E.; Whalley, B.J.; Di Marzo, V.; Stephens, G.J. Nonpsychotropic plant cannabinoids, cannabidivarin (CBDV) and cannabidiol (CBD), activate and desensitize transient receptor potential vanilloid 1 (TRPV1) channels in vitro: Potential for the treatment of neuronal hyperexcitability. *ACS Chem. Neurosci.* **2014**, *5*, 1131–1141. [CrossRef]
16. Cifelli, P.; Ruffolo, G.; De Felice, E.; Alfano, V.; van Vliet, E.A.; Aronica, E.; Palma, E. Phytocannabinoids in Neurological Diseases: Could They Restore a Physiological GABAergic Transmission? *Int. J. Mol. Sci.* **2020**, *21*, 723. [CrossRef]
17. Zamberletti, E.; Gabaglio, M.; Parolaro, D. The Endocannabinoid System and Autism Spectrum Disorders: Insights from Animal Models. *Int. J. Mol. Sci.* **2017**, *18*, 1916. [CrossRef]
18. Pietropaolo, S.; Bellocchio, L.; Bouzón-Arnáiz, I.; Yee, B.K. The role of the endocannabinoid system in autism spectrum disorders: Evidence from mouse studies. *Prog. Mol. Biol. Transl. Sci.* **2020**, *173*, 183–208. [CrossRef]
19. Zou, M.; Liu, Y.; Xie, S.; Wang, L.; Li, D.; Li, L.; Wang, F.; Zhang, Y.; Xia, W.; Sun, C.; et al. Alterations of the endocannabinoid system and its therapeutic potential in autism spectrum disorder. *Open Biol.* **2021**, *11*, 200306. [CrossRef]
20. Karhson, D.S.; Krasinska, K.M.; Dallaire, J.A.; Libove, R.A.; Phillips, J.M.; Chien, A.S.; Garner, J.P.; Hardan, A.Y.; Parker, K.J. Plasma anandamide concentrations are lower in children with autism spectrum disorder. *Mol. Autism.* **2018**, *9*, 18. [CrossRef]
21. Aran, A.; Eylon, M.; Harel, M.; Polianski, L.; Nemirovski, A.; Tepper, S.; Schnapp, A.; Cassuto, H.; Wattad, N.; Tam, J. Lower circulating endocannabinoid levels in children with autism spectrum disorder. *Mol. Autism.* **2019**, *10*, 2. [CrossRef] [PubMed]

22. Aran, A.; Cassuto, H.; Lubotzky, A.; Wattad, N.; Hazan, E. Brief Report: Cannabidiol-Rich Cannabis in Children with Autism Spectrum Disorder and Severe Behavioral Problems-A Retrospective Feasibility Study. *J. Autism. Dev. Disord.* **2019**, *49*, 1284–1288. [CrossRef] [PubMed]
23. Aran, A.; Harel, M.; Cassuto, H.; Polyansky, L.; Schnapp, A.; Wattad, N.; Shmueli, D.; Golan, D.; Castellanos, F.X. Cannabinoid treatment for autism: A proof-of-concept randomized trial. *Mol. Autism.* **2021**, *12*, 6. [CrossRef] [PubMed]
24. Bar-Lev Schleider, L.; Mechoulam, R.; Saban, N.; Meiri, G.; Novack, V. Real life Experience of Medical Cannabis Treatment in Autism: Analysis of Safety and Efficacy. *Sci. Rep.* **2019**, *9*, 200. [CrossRef] [PubMed]
25. Barchel, D.; Stolar, O.; De-Haan, T.; Ziv-Baran, T.; Saban, N.; Fuchs, D.O.; Koren, G.; Berkovitch, M. Oral Cannabidiol Use in Children With Autism Spectrum Disorder to Treat Related Symptoms and Co-morbidities. *Front. Pharmacol.* **2018**, *9*, 1521. [CrossRef]
26. AminiLari, M.; Wang, L.; Neumark, S.; Adli, T.; Couban, R.J.; Giangregorio, A.; Carney, C.E.; Busse, J.W. Medical Cannabis and Cannabinoids for Impaired Sleep: A Systematic Review and Meta-Analysis of Randomized Clinical Trials. *Sleep* **2021**, *45*, zsab234. [CrossRef]
27. Suraev, A.S.; Marshall, N.S.; Vandrey, R.; McCartney, D.; Benson, M.J.; McGregor, I.S.; Grunstein, R.R.; Hoyos, C.M. Cannabinoid therapies in the management of sleep disorders: A systematic review of preclinical and clinical studies. *Sleep Med. Rev.* **2020**, *53*, 101339. [CrossRef]
28. Kaul, M.; Zee, P.C.; Sahni, A.S. Effects of Cannabinoids on Sleep and their Therapeutic Potential for Sleep Disorders. *Neurotherapeutics* **2021**, *18*, 217–227. [CrossRef]
29. Spanagel, R.; Bilbao, A. Approved cannabinoids for medical purposes—Comparative systematic review and meta-analysis for sleep and appetite. *Neuropharmacology* **2021**, *196*, 108680. [CrossRef]
30. Lucas, C.J.; Galettis, P.; Schneider, J. The pharmacokinetics and the pharmacodynamics of cannabinoids. *Br. J. Clin. Pharmacol.* **2018**, *84*, 2477–2482. [CrossRef]
31. Lord, C.; Risi, S.; Lambrecht, L.; Cook, E.H., Jr.; Leventhal, B.L.; DiLavore, P.C.; Pickles, A.; Rutter, M. The autism diagnostic observation schedule-generic: A standard measure of social and communication deficits associated with the spectrum of autism. *J. Autism. Dev. Disord.* **2000**, *30*, 205–223. [CrossRef] [PubMed]
32. Sparrow, S.S.; Balla, D.A.; Cicchetti, D.V. *Vineland Adaptive Behavior Scales: Survey Form Manual*; American Guidance Service: Circle Pines, MN, USA, 1984.
33. Schopler, E.; Reichler, R.J.; DeVellis, R.F.; Daly, K. Toward objective classification of childhood autism: Childhood Autism Rating Scale (CARS). *J. Autism. Dev. Disord.* **1980**, *10*, 91–103. [CrossRef] [PubMed]
34. Owens, J.A.; Spirito, A.; McGuinn, M. The Children's Sleep Habits Questionnaire (CSHQ): Psychometric properties of a survey instrument for school-aged children. *Sleep* **2000**, *23*, 1043–1051. [CrossRef] [PubMed]
35. Johnson, C.R.; DeMand, A.; Lecavalier, L.; Smith, T.; Aman, M.; Foldes, E.; Scahill, L. Psychometric properties of the children's sleep habits questionnaire in children with autism spectrum disorder. *Sleep Med.* **2016**, *20*, 5–11. [CrossRef]
36. Hatch, B.; Nordahl, C.W.; Schwichtenberg, A.J.; Ozonoff, S.; Miller, M. Factor Structure of the Children's Sleep Habits Questionnaire in Young Children with and Without Autism. *J. Autism. Dev. Disord.* **2021**, *51*, 3126–3137. [CrossRef] [PubMed]
37. Zaidman-Zait, A.; Zwaigenbaum, L.; Duku, E.; Bennett, T.; Szatmari, P.; Mirenda, P.; Smith, I.; Vaillancourt, T.; Volden, J.; Waddell, C.; et al. Factor analysis of the children's sleep habits questionnaire among preschool children with autism spectrum disorder. *Res. Dev. Disabil.* **2020**, *97*, 103548. [CrossRef] [PubMed]
38. Petruzzelli, M.G.; Matera, E.; Giambersio, D.; Marzulli, L.; Gabellone, A.; Legrottaglie, A.R.; Margari, A.; Margari, L. Subjective and Electroencephalographic Sleep Parameters in Children and Adolescents with Autism Spectrum Disorder: A Systematic Review. *J. Clin. Med.* **2021**, *10*, 3893. [CrossRef] [PubMed]
39. Chen, H.; Yang, T.; Chen, J.; Chen, L.; Dai, Y.; Zhang, J.; Li, L.; Jia, F.; Wu, L.; Hao, Y.; et al. Sleep problems in children with autism spectrum disorder: A multicenter survey. *BMC Psychiatry* **2021**, *21*, 406. [CrossRef] [PubMed]
40. McCracken, J.T.; McGough, J.; Shah, B.; Cronin, P.; Hong, D.; Aman, M.G.; Arnold, L.E.; Lindsay, R.; Nash, P.; Hollway, J.; et al. Risperidone in children with autism and serious behavioral problems. *N. Engl. J. Med.* **2002**, *347*, 314–321. [CrossRef]
41. Constantino, J.N.; Gruber, C.P. *The Social Responsiveness Scale (SRS) (Manual)*; Western Psychological Services: Los Angeles, CA, USA, 2005.
42. Friedman, D.; French, J.A.; Maccarrone, M. Safety, efficacy, and mechanisms of action of cannabinoids in neurological disorders. *Lancet Neurol.* **2019**, *18*, 504–512. [CrossRef]
43. Kirkland, A.E.; Fadus, M.C.; Gruber, S.A.; Gray, K.M.; Wilens, T.E.; Squeglia, L.M. A scoping review of the use of cannabidiol in psychiatric disorders. *Psychiatry Res.* **2022**, *308*, 114347. [CrossRef] [PubMed]
44. Agarwal, R.; Burke, S.L.; Maddux, M. Current state of evidence of cannabis utilization for treatment of autism spectrum disorders. *BMC Psychiatry* **2019**, *19*, 328. [CrossRef] [PubMed]
45. Devinsky, O.; Cross, J.H.; Laux, L.; Marsh, E.; Miller, I.; Nabbout, R.; Scheffer, I.E.; Thiele, E.A.; Wright, S. Trial of Cannabidiol for Drug-Resistant Seizures in the Dravet Syndrome. *N. Engl. J. Med.* **2017**, *376*, 2011–2020. [CrossRef]
46. Devinsky, O.; Patel, A.D.; Cross, J.H.; Villanueva, V.; Wirrell, E.C.; Privitera, M.; Greenwood, S.M.; Roberts, C.; Checketts, D.; VanLandingham, K.E.; et al. Effect of Cannabidiol on Drop Seizures in the Lennox-Gastaut Syndrome. *N. Engl. J. Med.* **2018**, *378*, 1888–1897. [CrossRef] [PubMed]

47. Thiele, E.A.; Bebin, E.M.; Bhathal, H.; Jansen, F.E.; Kotulska, K.; Lawson, J.A.; O'Callaghan, F.J.; Wong, M.; Sahebkar, F.; Checketts, D.; et al. Add-on Cannabidiol Treatment for Drug-Resistant Seizures in Tuberous Sclerosis Complex: A Placebo-Controlled Randomized Clinical Trial. *JAMA Neurol.* **2021**, *78*, 285–292. [CrossRef] [PubMed]
48. Stockings, E.; Campbell, G.; Hall, W.D.; Nielsen, S.; Zagic, D.; Rahman, R.; Murnion, B.; Farrell, M.; Weier, M.; Degenhardt, L. Cannabis and cannabinoids for the treatment of people with chronic noncancer pain conditions: A systematic review and meta-analysis of controlled and observational studies. *Pain* **2018**, *159*, 1932–1954. [CrossRef] [PubMed]
49. Wang, L.; Hong, P.J.; May, C.; Rehman, Y.; Oparin, Y.; Hong, C.J.; Hong, B.Y.; AminiLari, M.; Gallo, L.; Kaushal, A.; et al. Medical cannabis or cannabinoids for chronic non-cancer and cancer related pain: A systematic review and meta-analysis of randomised clinical trials. *BMJ* **2021**, *374*, n1034. [CrossRef]
50. Häuser, W.; Welsch, P.; Klose, P.; Radbruch, L.; Fitzcharles, M.A. Efficacy, tolerability and safety of cannabis-based medicines for cancer pain: A systematic review with meta-analysis of randomised controlled trials. *Schmerz* **2019**, *33*, 424–436. [CrossRef]
51. Grimison, P.; Mersiades, A.; Kirby, A.; Lintzeris, N.; Morton, R.; Haber, P.; Olver, I.; Walsh, A.; McGregor, I.; Cheung, Y.; et al. Oral THC:CBD cannabis extract for refractory chemotherapy-induced nausea and vomiting: A randomised, placebo-controlled, phase II crossover trial. *Ann. Oncol.* **2020**, *31*, 1553–1560. [CrossRef]
52. Chow, R.; Valdez, C.; Chow, N.; Zhang, D.; Im, J.; Sodhi, E.; Lock, M. Oral cannabinoid for the prophylaxis of chemotherapy-induced nausea and vomiting-a systematic review and meta-analysis. *Support Care Cancer* **2020**, *28*, 2095–2103. [CrossRef]
53. Black, N.; Stockings, E.; Campbell, G.; Tran, L.T.; Zagic, D.; Hall, W.D.; Farrell, M.; Degenhardt, L. Cannabinoids for the treatment of mental disorders and symptoms of mental disorders: A systematic review and meta-analysis. *Lancet Psychiatry* **2019**, *6*, 995–1010. [CrossRef]
54. Bonn-Miller, M.O.; Sisley, S.; Riggs, P.; Yazar-Klosinski, B.; Wang, J.B.; Loflin, M.J.E.; Shechet, B.; Hennigan, C.; Matthews, R.; Emerson, A.; et al. The short-term impact of 3 smoked cannabis preparations versus placebo on PTSD symptoms: A randomized cross-over clinical trial. *PLoS ONE* **2021**, *16*, e0246990. [CrossRef] [PubMed]
55. de Carvalho Reis, R.; Almeida, K.J.; da Silva Lopes, L.; de Melo Mendes, C.M.; Bor-Seng-Shu, E. Efficacy and adverse event profile of cannabidiol and medicinal cannabis for treatment-resistant epilepsy: Systematic review and meta-analysis. *Epilepsy Behav.* **2019**, *102*, 106635. [CrossRef] [PubMed]
56. Fleury-Teixeira, P.; Caixeta, F.V.; Ramires da Silva, L.C.; Brasil-Neto, J.P.; Malcher-Lopes, R. Effects of CBD-Enriched Cannabis sativa Extract on Autism Spectrum Disorder Symptoms: An Observational Study of 18 Participants Undergoing Compassionate Use. *Front. Neurol.* **2019**, *10*, 1145. [CrossRef] [PubMed]
57. Holdman, R.; Vigil, D.; Robinson, K.; Shah, P.; Contreras, A.E. Safety and Efficacy of Medical Cannabis in Autism Spectrum Disorder Compared with Commonly Used Medications. *Cannabis Cannabinoid Res.* **2021**, *ahead of print*. [CrossRef]
58. McVige, J.; Headd, V.; Alwahaidy, M.; Lis, D.; Kaur, D.; Albert, B.; Mechtler, L. *Medical Cannabis in the Treatment of Patients with Autism Spectrum Disorder (1648)*; AAN Enterprises: Apex, NC, USA, 2020.
59. Yau, J.C.; Yu, S.M.; Panenka, W.J.; Pearce, H.; Gicas, K.M.; Procyshyn, R.M.; MacCallum, C.; Honer, W.G.; Barr, A.M. Characterization of mental health in cannabis dispensary users, using structured clinical interviews and standardized assessment instruments. *BMC Psychiatry* **2019**, *19*, 335. [CrossRef]
60. Ferber, S.G.; Namdar, D.; Hen-Shoval, D.; Eger, G.; Koltai, H.; Shoval, G.; Shbiro, L.; Weller, A. "The Entourage Effect": Terpenes Coupled with Cannabinoids for the Treatment of Mood Disorders and Anxiety Disorders. *Curr. Neuropharmacol.* **2020**, *18*, 87–96. [CrossRef]
61. Russo, E.B. The Case for the Entourage Effect and Conventional Breeding of Clinical Cannabis: No "Strain", No Gain. *Front. Plant Sci.* **2018**, *9*, 1969. [CrossRef]
62. Linares, I.M.P.; Guimaraes, F.S.; Eckeli, A.; Crippa, A.C.S.; Zuardi, A.W.; Souza, J.D.S.; Hallak, J.E.; Crippa, J.A.S. No Acute Effects of Cannabidiol on the Sleep-Wake Cycle of Healthy Subjects: A Randomized, Double-Blind, Placebo-Controlled, Crossover Study. *Front. Pharmacol.* **2018**, *9*, 315. [CrossRef]
63. Morgan, C.J.; Freeman, T.P.; Schafer, G.L.; Curran, H.V. Cannabidiol attenuates the appetitive effects of Delta 9-tetrahydrocannabinol in humans smoking their chosen cannabis. *Neuropsychopharmacol. Off. Publ. Am. Coll. Neuropsychopharmacol.* **2010**, *35*, 1879–1885. [CrossRef]
64. Morgan, C.J.; Gardener, C.; Schafer, G.; Swan, S.; Demarchi, C.; Freeman, T.P.; Warrington, P.; Rupasinghe, I.; Ramoutar, A.; Tan, N.; et al. Sub-chronic impact of cannabinoids in street cannabis on cognition, psychotic-like symptoms and psychological well-being. *Psychol. Med.* **2012**, *42*, 391–400. [CrossRef]
65. Zlebnik, N.E.; Cheer, J.F. Beyond the CB1 Receptor: Is Cannabidiol the Answer for Disorders of Motivation? *Annu. Rev. Neurosci.* **2016**, *39*, 1–17. [CrossRef] [PubMed]
66. Hurd, Y.L.; Yoon, M.; Manini, A.F.; Hernandez, S.; Olmedo, R.; Ostman, M.; Jutras-Aswad, D. Early Phase in the Development of Cannabidiol as a Treatment for Addiction: Opioid Relapse Takes Initial Center Stage. *Neurother. J. Am. Soc. Exp. NeuroTherapeutics* **2015**, *12*, 807–815. [CrossRef]
67. Morgan, C.J.; Schafer, G.; Freeman, T.P.; Curran, H.V. Impact of cannabidiol on the acute memory and psychotomimetic effects of smoked cannabis: Naturalistic study. *Br. J. Psychiatry J. Ment. Sci.* **2010**, *197*, 285–290. [CrossRef] [PubMed]
68. Lorenzetti, V.; Solowij, N.; Yucel, M. The Role of Cannabinoids in Neuroanatomic Alterations in Cannabis Users. *Biol. Psychiatry* **2016**, *79*, e17–e31. [CrossRef] [PubMed]
69. Krebs, M.O.; Kebir, O.; Jay, T.M. Exposure to cannabinoids can lead to persistent cognitive and psychiatric disorders. *Eur. J. Pain* **2019**, *23*, 1225–1233. [CrossRef] [PubMed]

70. Iseger, T.A.; Bossong, M.G. A systematic review of the antipsychotic properties of cannabidiol in humans. *Schizophr. Res.* **2015**, *162*, 153–161. [CrossRef] [PubMed]
71. Silva, T.B.; Balbino, C.Q.; Weiber, A.F. The relationship between cannabidiol and psychosis: A review. *Ann. Clin. Psychiatry Off. J. Am. Acad. Clin. Psychiatr.* **2015**, *27*, 134–141.
72. Ortiz-Medina, M.B.; Perea, M.; Torales, J.; Ventriglio, A.; Vitrani, G.; Aguilar, L.; Roncero, C. Cannabis consumption and psychosis or schizophrenia development. *Int. J. Soc. Psychiatry* **2018**, *64*, 690–704. [CrossRef]
73. Volkow, N.D.; Baler, R.D.; Compton, W.M.; Weiss, S.R. Adverse health effects of marijuana use. *N. Engl. J. Med.* **2014**, *370*, 2219–2227. [CrossRef]
74. Malow, B.A.; Katz, T.; Reynolds, A.M.; Shui, A.; Carno, M.; Connolly, H.V.; Coury, D.; Bennett, A.E. Sleep Difficulties and Medications in Children With Autism Spectrum Disorders: A Registry Study. *Pediatrics* **2016**, *137* (Suppl. S2), S98–S104. [CrossRef]
75. Bangerter, A.; Chatterjee, M.; Manyakov, N.V.; Ness, S.; Lewin, D.; Skalkin, A.; Boice, M.; Goodwin, M.S.; Dawson, G.; Hendren, R.; et al. Relationship Between Sleep and Behavior in Autism Spectrum Disorder: Exploring the Impact of Sleep Variability. *Front. Neurosci.* **2020**, *14*, 211. [CrossRef] [PubMed]

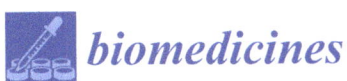

Article

Serum Concentrations of the Endocannabinoid, 2-Arachidonoylglycerol, in the Peri-Trauma Period Are Positively Associated with Chronic Pain Months Later

Colleen M. Trevino [1,*], Cecilia J. Hillard [2], Aniko Szabo [3] and Terri A. deRoon-Cassini [1,4]

[1] Division of Trauma and Acute Care Surgery, Department of Surgery, Medical College of Wisconsin, Milwaukee, WI 53226, USA; tcassini@mcw.edu
[2] Department of Pharmacology and Toxicology, Neuroscience Research Center, Medical College of Wisconsin, Milwaukee, WI 53226, USA; chillard@mcw.edu
[3] Department of Biostatistics, Medical College of Wisconsin, Milwaukee, WI 53226, USA; aszabo@mcw.edu
[4] Comprehensive Injury Center, Medical College of Wisconsin, Milwaukee, WI 53226, USA
* Correspondence: ctrevino@mcw.edu; Tel.: +1-414-955-1726; Fax: +1-414-955-0072

Abstract: Endocannabinoid signaling and the hypothalamic-pituitary-adrenal axis are activated by trauma and both stress systems regulate the transition from acute to chronic pain. This study aimed to develop a model of relationships among circulating concentrations of cortisol and endocannabinoids (eCBs) immediately after traumatic injury and the presence of chronic pain months later. Pain scores and serum concentrations of eCBs and cortisol were measured during hospitalization and 5–10 months later in 147 traumatically injured individuals. Exploratory correlational analyses and path analysis were completed. The study sample was 50% Black and Latino and primarily male (69%); 34% percent endorsed a pain score of 4 or greater at follow-up and were considered to have chronic pain. Path analysis was used to model relationships among eCB, 2-arachidonoylglycerol (2-AG), cortisol, and pain, adjusting for sex and injury severity (ISS). Serum 2-AG concentrations at the time of injury were associated with chronic pain in 3 ways: a highly significant, independent positive predictor; a mediator of the effect of ISS, and through a positive relationship with cortisol concentrations. These data indicate that 2-AG concentrations at the time of an injury are positively associated with chronic pain and suggest excessive activation of endocannabinoid signaling contributes to risk for chronic pain.

Keywords: N-arachidonoylethanolamine; cortisol; chronic pain; injury

1. Introduction

Acute pain is inevitable and important following injury as it protects the individual against further tissue damage. However, pain that persists after tissue injury has healed, so-called "chronic pain," is not protective and has a significant, negative effect on the quality of life [1]. Chronic pain is defined as pain persisting after surgery or trauma for greater than three months [2]. Previous studies from our group and others have found that the incidence of chronic pain in traumatically injured patients can be as high as 70% and there is a strong correlation between pain severity and life interference [3–5]. Unlike acute pain, chronic pain is not primarily related to tissue injury [6] and traditional therapies for pain, including opioids, have poor efficacy in their treatment [7,8]. Not all injured individuals develop chronic pain, and few reliable or clinically significant biomarkers have been identified that predict the progression of acute to chronic pain in the traumatically injured population. Thus, this research could contribute to an improvement in our ability to predict who will develop chronic pain through the validation of biomarkers. A secondary long-term goal of this research project is to better understand the biological factors that contribute to the development of chronic pain, which could improve our ability to treat or prevent this transition.

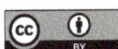

Preclinical research suggests a role for the endocannabinoid signaling system (ECSS) in pain [9,10]. The endogenous ligands for cannabinoid (CB) receptors, called endocannabinoids (eCBs), are N-arachidonoylethanolamine (AEA or anandamide) and 2-arachidonoylglycerol (2-AG). Noxious stimuli and tissue injury increase eCB mobilization [11,12] and chronic pain can up-regulate the expression of CB1 [13] and CB2 [14] receptors. Although preclinical studies largely support the hypothesis that endogenous activation of CB receptors reduces acute pain [9,10], eCBs produced by intense nociceptive stimuli render nociceptive neurons in the spinal cord excitable by non-painful stimuli, suggesting that eCB/CB signaling can also promote pain sensitization and thus contribute to the development of chronic pain [15].

Multiple studies have examined the relationships between the concentrations of circulating eCBs and related lipids with the presence of chronic pain in humans. Circulating concentrations of 2-AG are higher compared to pain-free control groups in several types of chronic pain, including fibromyalgia, irritable bowel syndrome, and neuropathic pain [16–18]. Similarly, circulating AEA concentrations in individuals with fibromyalgia are three times higher than in matched controls [19]. Patients with complex regional pain syndrome (CRPS), a neuropathic pain syndrome precipitated by extremity injury, have significantly higher plasma concentrations of AEA than controls [20]. Women with endometriosis-associated pain, compared to those without endometriosis, exhibited elevated concentrations of both AEA and 2-AG [21]. Thus, while preclinical data indicate that eCB-mediated signaling reduces pain sensation at multiple sites within the neuronal pain circuit, the peripheral pool of eCBs is positively associated with chronic pain in humans. However, the presence of an association is not indicative of a causal relationship; it is possible that the high circulating eCBs are a physiological response to the stress of the pain experience.

Human studies also support the role of cortisol in developing chronic pain [22–24]. The imposition of acute pain (such as the cold pressor test) in healthy individuals elicits cortisol secretion, which is in accord with pain as a stressor [25]. On the other hand, inappropriate activation of the hypothalamic-pituitary-adrenal (HPA) axis is associated with the presence or development of chronic pain [26,27]. In particular, inappropriately low concentrations of cortisol have been associated with a diagnosis of chronic pain from fibromyalgia and low back pain [28,29].

Both the HPA axis [30] and the ECSS [31] are activated by exposure to physical and psychological stress, and these systems have diverging and converging effects on the stress response. HPA axis activation via actions of cortisol and the ECSS reduce pain and inflammation. In the brain, there are considerable data that cortisol increases the 2-AG synthesis and that CB1 receptor activation links brain cortisol to changes in synaptic activity. On the other hand, ECSS activation in the brain reduces HPA axis activation by stress and enhances recovery to baseline following stress. Importantly, both the ECSS and HPA axis are downregulated in situations of chronic stimulation, so excessive activation of either system can lead to loss of critical homeostatic processes.

This study aimed to develop a model of the relationships between circulating cortisol and eCBs, and the development of chronic pain after a traumatic injury. Our working hypothesis is that both the HPA axis and the ECSS are mobilized by the severe stress that accompanies traumatic injury and both contribute to reduced pain at that time point. However, we hypothesize that excessive concentrations of both at the time of injury will increase the risk for chronic pain development. The specific hypotheses for this study were: (1) circulating concentrations of the eCBs positively correlate with circulating cortisol concentrations at the time of injury, both reflecting the physical and psychological stress of the injury; (2) at the time of injury, pain measures negatively correlate with circulating eCB and cortisol concentrations due to the ability of both mediators to reduce pain; and (3) circulating eCBs concentrations at the time of hospitalization positively correlate with measures of pain months after the injury, possibly due to down-regulation of the ECSS.

2. Materials and Methods

2.1. Participants

The Institutional Review Board (IRB) at the Medical College of Wisconsin approved all study procedures (PRO00022827, approved on 3 May 2019) and participants were monetarily compensated for their time. Participants in this study were subjects of a prospective, exploratory, longitudinal cohort study entitled "Study on Trauma and Resilience (STAR)". We have previously reported some demographic and clinical data and the relationship between endocannabinoids and depression [32] and risk for post-traumatic stress disorder (PTSD) [33] in the same cohort. Two hundred eighty participants were recruited and consented at the time of injury in the parent study; 147 completed the follow-up pain assessments and blood draw and are included in these analyses.

2.2. Study Design

Individuals with any type of traumatic injury who were admitted to the inpatient trauma service at Froedtert Hospital, a level 1 American College of Surgery verified trauma center, were eligible for recruitment. Recruitment occurred over a 19-month period by daily review of the trauma division inpatient census for those who experienced a traumatic event; were at least 18 years of age, English speaking, and able to provide written informed consent within seven days of admission. Excluded were those who did not have appropriate cognitive capacity defined as Glasgow Coma Scale of 13 or less (e.g., moderate or severe TBI; obtained from chart review) and greater than 30 min of peritraumatic amnesia; were in police custody, or were having active psychotic or self-harm symptoms. Participants returned to the campus translational research unit 5–10 months (average 192 days, range 156–286) after their injury for a follow-up visit.

2.3. Measures

After providing informed consent and during hospitalization, study participants completed a series of questionnaires as a part of the parent study of trauma and resilience. Participant demographics, injury-related data, and a blood sample were obtained. The mean time of blood sampling was 1156 h, SD 1.6 h (approximately noon). The pain was assessed at the time of hospitalization via the numeric pain score (NPS), using a Likert scale with anchors at 0 (no pain) and 10 (worst pain imaginable) [34]. We utilized the injury severity score (ISS) as an anatomical measure of the severity of multiple physical traumatic injuries based upon the worst injury of six body systems [35]. Each system is scored from 1–6 depending on the level of severity and the sum of squares is taken from the three most injured systems. The highest score is 75 and denotes a non-survivable injury. The ISS for mild injury is 1–8, moderate injury is 9–15, severe injury is 16–24, and very severe is 25 and higher. The ISS was measured once at the time of hospitalization.

At the follow-up visit, blood was collected, and questionnaires were administered. The mean time of blood collection at follow-up was 1217 h, SD = 2.39 h. The Brief Pain Inventory (BPI) [36] was collected at the follow-up visit. The BPI measures both the intensity of the pain (sensory dimension) and interference of pain in the patient's life (reactive dimension), with higher scores indicating greater pain intensity and interference, respectively [36]. Pain measures were asked within the context of the patient's initial traumatic injuries. In our exploratory analyses, we used NPS of equal to or greater than 4 out of 10 to determine chronic pain since moderate and severe pain are associated with compromised physical functioning [37].

2.4. Study Procedures

Whole blood samples were drawn at hospitalization and the follow-up visit using serum collecting tubes (red-top tubes). After incubation at room temperature for 30–60 min, serum was harvested by centrifugation. Serum concentrations of the eCBs (2-AG and AEA) were measured in lipid extracts using isotope dilution and liquid chromatography-mass spectrometry to quantify daughter ions of AEA and 2-AG as described previously [38]. Concentrations of cortisol were measured in the same serum samples using radioimmunoassay (Cort-Cote 06B256440; MP Biomedical, San Diego, CA, USA). The sensitivity for cortisol assay was 57.5 pg/mL and no data lower than the minimum detection level were found. Based on the manufacturer's reporting, intra-assay precision varies from 7.3–10.5, and inter-assay precision varies from 8.6–13.4 for high-to-low cortisol levels.

2.5. Analyses

For descriptive statistics and summary tables, chronic pain (CP) was defined as pain severity (NPS) of greater than or equal to 4 at the second time point. The continuous underlying indices of NPS and pain interference were used in other analyses.

Demographic and clinical characteristics were summarized using counts with percentages for categorical variables and mean with standard deviation and range for continuous variables. These were compared between groups using the chi-squared test and Mann-Whitney test, respectively. The comparisons of CP between individual injury mechanisms used Fisher's exact tests with permutation-based adjustment over the possible mechanisms to control the overall type I error rate.

Based on initial bivariate exploratory analyses, the biomarkers (2-AG, AEA, cortisol) were log-transformed to improve the linearity of the relationships and reduce skewness. Pearson's correlation coefficient was used to quantify the strength of association between different biomarkers and between biomarkers and pain indices as continuous variables. The p-values were adjusted for multiple comparisons using the Benjamini–Hochberg method that controls the false discovery rate. For these exploratory analyses, FDR < 0.1 was considered a significant correlation.

A path model was developed to analyze the relationships among the circulating eCB and cortisol concentrations and pain measures at both time points, adjusting for covariates. The initial model structure was constructed based on biological plausibility, measurement timing, and the results of our exploratory correlational data. Specifically, the following variable groups were considered: sex and injury severity score (ISS); hospital and follow-up 2-AG and cortisol concentrations; self-reported pain score at hospitalization; and pain severity and interference scores obtained from the BPI at follow-up. In the initial model, sex and ISS were allowed to influence both hospitalization and follow-up pain measures. In addition, concentrations of 2-AG and cortisol were assumed to be correlated and could affect pain and biomarker measures at either time point. No direct effect of pain on 2-AG or cortisol was included. Hospitalization pain scores were included as a predictor of the follow-up pain measures. The effects of sex, cortisol, and 2-AG on pain were constrained to have equal strength at both hospitalization and follow-up, and the correlation between 2-AG and cortisol was also constrained to be the same at both time points. The model was fitted using the full information maximum likelihood method, which is a maximum-likelihood-based method that can incorporate missing-at-random observations [39].

The initial model was then simplified to find a more parsimonious description. Paths with non-significant effects with standardized coefficients under 0.1 in absolute value were removed, monitoring that goodness of fit indices continue to fall in their acceptable ranges and prioritizing models with lower Bayesian Information Criterion (BIC). Table 1 shows the goodness of fit indices of the initial and reduced models, indicating an excellent fit for both.

All analyses were performed using SAS 9.4 (SAS Institute, Cary, NC, USA) using the CALIS procedure for the path analysis. Unless otherwise noted, a two-sided 5% significance level was used.

Table 1. Goodness of fit indices of the initial and reduced models.

Goodness-of-Fit Measure	Guideline for Acceptable Fit	Initial Model	Reduced Model
X^2/df	<3	14.9/11 = 1.3	20.9/23 = 0.91
Standardized root mean square residual (SRMR)	<0.080	0.041	0.049
Root mean square error of approximation (RMSEA) with 90% confidence interval	<0.06, upper limit < 0.08	0.05 (0.0–0.11)	0.0 (0.0–0.06)
Comparative fit index (CFI)	>0.95	0.98	1.0
Bayesian information criterion (BIC)	Lower value implies more parsimonious fit	228.6	175.9

3. Results

3.1. Demographic Results

Demographic information, pain data, and biospecimens were collected from hospitalized participants an average of 2.5 days following injury (range 1–10 days; hospitalization time point). Pain data and blood samples were also obtained 5–10 months post-injury (average 192 days; range 156–286; follow-up time point). The demographic and clinical information related to the injury for the total population of participants are shown in the second column of Table 2. The sample was predominately male (69.4%) and spanned the entire adult age range. Forty-five percent of the sample self-identified as Black or African American and 7.5% as Hispanic or Latino.

Table 2. Demographic and clinical data of the study participants.

Parameter	Total Sample	NCP (NPS Score < 4)	CP (NPS Score ≥ 4)	p-Value (NCP Compared to CP)
N	147	97	50 (34%)	
Mean Age (SD, range)	42.5 (16.4, 18–89)	42.2 (17.5, 18–89)	42.9 (14.0, 20–74)	$p > 0.1$
Sex				$p > 0.1$
Female (percent)	45 (30.6)	28 (28.9)	17 (34.0)	
Male (percent)	102 (69.4)	69 (71.1)	33 (66.0)	
Race/Ethnicity				0.09
Non-Hispanic White	68 (46.3)	52 (53.6)	16 (32.0)	
Black or African American	66 (44.9)	37 (38.1)	29 (58.0)	
Hispanic or Latino	11 (7.5)	7 (7.2)	4 (8.0)	
Native American/Alaskan Native	2 (1.4)	1 (1)	1 (2)	
Highest Educational Level Completed				0.09
Advanced degree (master's or higher)	10 (6.8)	10 (10.3)	0 (0.0)	
College graduate	24 (16.3)	15 (15.5)	9 (18.0)	
Graduated high school, some college	52 (35.4)	37 (38.1)	15 (30.0)	
High school graduate, no college	36 (24.4)	20 (20.6)	16 (32.0)	
Less than high school	25 (17.0)	15 (15.5)	10 (20.0)	
In a committed relationship				0.056
No	57 (39.3)	32 (33.7)	25 (50.0)	
Yes	88 (60.7)	63 (66.3)	25 (50.0)	
Time between injury and follow-up assessment for chronic pain and blood draw (SD, range)	192 days (22, 156–286)	191 (19, 156–240)	194 (26, 160–286)	$p > 0.1$
Injury severity score (ISS; SD, range)	10.1 (5.9, 0–29)	9.1 (5.2, 0–24)	12.2 (6.6, 0–29)	0.002
Numerical pain score at hospitalization (SD, range)	5.8 (2.4, 0–10)	5.2 (2.3, 0–10)	6.9 (2.3, 1–10)	<0.001

NCP: no chronic pain and CP: chronic pain subgroups determined at follow-up. Age, time between injury and follow-up, severity scores (ISS), and acute pain scores were compared between the NCP and CP groups using Mann–Whitney non-parametric t-tests; other comparisons were made using the Chi-squared test.

The presence of pain was assessed at the follow-up visit and chronic pain (CP) was defined as an NPS of 4 or greater and was endorsed by 50 individuals (34%). The demographic and clinical characteristics of the no chronic pain (NCP; NPS < 4) and CP subgroups of the sample were determined and compared (Table 2). There were no significant differences between the NCP and CP subgroups with regard to age or sex. There was no difference in the time that elapsed between the injury and follow-up visit between the NCP and CP subgroups. The ISS and NPS scores at the time of hospitalization were both significantly higher in the CP group than in the NCP group. Those not in a committed relationship were more likely to have chronic pain. One hundred forty-five of the 147 subjects in the study were treated with opiate analgesics at the time of injury, so the impact of opiates on chronic pain could not be studied in this cohort. Individuals were asked about cannabis use at both the time of hospitalization and at the follow-up assessment; there was no difference in reported use between the NCP and CP subgroups (data not shown).

3.2. Mechanisms of Injury

The mechanisms of traumatic injury were examined in the entire sample and compared between the NCP and CP subgroups. The three most prevalent mechanisms of injury were motor vehicle crashes (32%), falls (17%), and gunshot wounds (16%). A significantly greater proportion of those in the CP than the NCP subgroup was injured by gunshot wounds (28%, $p = 0.023$).

3.3. Correlational Analyses of Biomarkers and Pain

Correlational analyses were used to test our initial hypotheses that circulating concentrations of the eCBs and cortisol are correlated with acute and chronic pain (Table 2). For these exploratory analyses, False Discovery Rate (FDR) <0.1 was considered a significant correlation. At the time of hospitalization, cortisol concentrations were significantly, negatively correlated with acute pain; neither 2-AG nor AEA concentrations were correlated with acute pain. There was a modest, positive correlation between cortisol and 2-AG at hospitalization.

At follow-up, none of the biomarkers were correlated with pain measures. However, a significant, positive relationship between 2-AG and cortisol occurred while the concentrations of AEA and cortisol were negatively correlated.

To test the predictive value of the biomarkers, correlational analyses were carried out between biomarker concentrations at the time of hospitalization and indices of chronic pain 5–10 months after injury. 2-AG concentrations at the time of hospitalization were positively correlated with the degree of pain interference with activities of daily living 5–10 months after the injury.

3.4. Model Incorporating Biomarkers, Demographics, and Pain Measures

A path model was developed to analyze the relationships among the biomarkers, pain measures, and covariates (Figure 1). Table 1 shows the goodness of fit indices of the initial and reduced models, indicating an excellent fit for both.

The strongest relationships identified using this model were: (1) a positive relationship between serum concentrations of 2-AG at hospitalization and pain severity at follow-up; and (2) a negative relationship between cortisol and pain severity at both time points. Both 2-AG and cortisol concentrations at hospitalization were positively correlated with 2-AG concentrations at follow-up, and cortisol concentrations at hospitalization and follow-up were positively correlated with each other. ISS influenced pain severity at follow-up directly and indirectly through a relationship with 2-AG concentrations at hospitalization. The female sex exerted a significant, positive effect on pain severity at both time points, independent of other factors in the model. Cortisol at hospitalization affected cortisol at follow-up, and pain severity affected interference with activities of daily living at follow-up.

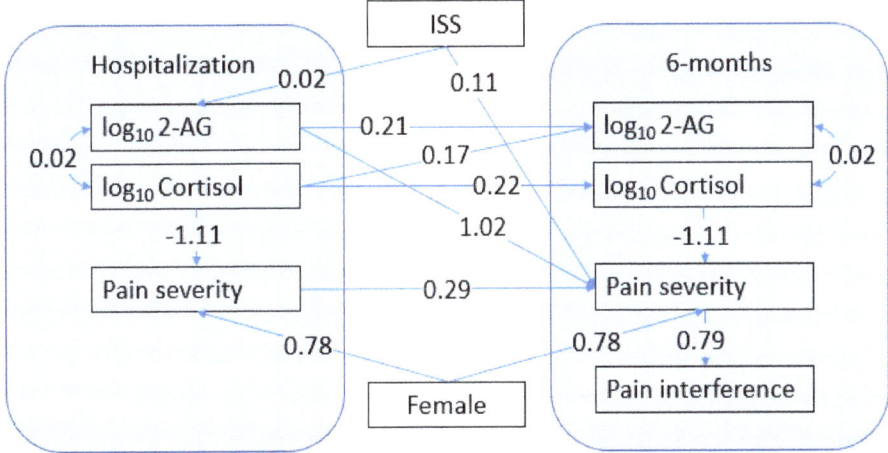

Figure 1. Model of the Relationship of Traumatic Pain, Cortisol, and Endocannabinoid Levels. The numbers on the arrows are regression coefficients, representing the effect of a 1-unit increase in the predictor on the outcome. For the log-transformed biomarkers, a 1 unit increase on the log scale corresponds to a 10-fold increase in the original value. All coefficients shown are significant with $p < 0.05$.

4. Discussion

While pain after injury is an expected outcome, continued, unresolved pain is a troubling consequence of traumatic injury. This study explored relationships among biomarkers of stress and pain severity measured at two-time points (hospitalization and five to ten months post-injury) in a sample of 147 traumatically injured subjects to explore biological relationships underlying the transition from acute to chronic pain. Biomarkers, clinical measures, and pain scores were determined within days of the traumatic injury and again five to ten months later-a time period when physical injuries are healed. Moderate to severe chronic pain was present in 34% of subjects 5–10 months after injury, which is a lower percentage than found in a previous study of an injured patient population in a community-based sample [3]. In that study, which was carried out four months after the injury, 43% of patients had moderate to severe pain, 50% had moderate to severe life interference associated with the development of chronic pain, and 50% continued to use opioids to treat their chronic pain four months after a traumatic injury [3].

In the current study, those without a committed relationship were significantly more likely to have chronic pain. This is aligned with the results of a recently published large study (>900 participants) which found that those with limited social support were significantly more likely to exhibit chronic pain, functional limitations, and poor mental health outcomes following moderate-severe traumatic injury [40].

In our study, those injured due to a gunshot wound were more likely to develop chronic pain. Given that civilian gunshot injuries are associated with interpersonal violence, these data support the role of distress as a risk factor for developing chronic pain [41].

As has been reported previously [42], the path analysis demonstrated a significant, positive effect of the female sex on both acute and chronic pain. Likely because our sample was only about one-third women, this difference did not reach significance in univariate analyses, but it did go in the same direction as the path analysis. This difference was most likely because the path analysis had more power with pain scores as a continuous variable and the path model explained some of the variability in the pain scores reducing the unexplained variability and making it easier to detect other effects.

Numerical pain scores at the time of injury were positively associated with the severity of chronic pain. This is in accord with the well-accepted notion that acute pain causes changes in the sensory pathway and pain-related brain circuits resulting in sensitization and chronic pain [43]. Both univariate and path analyses also identified a significant positive correlation between the severity of the physical injury (measured using the ISS) and acute pain at the time of injury and path analysis revealed a moderate but significant positive association between ISS and chronic pain. This result differed from findings in a previous study by our group that did not find ISS to correlate with the development of chronic pain [44], which suggests that ISS has a weak influence on chronic pain. Interestingly, the path model did not identify a significant association between ISS and acute pain, suggesting that ISS contributes to the risk for chronic pain beyond solely an enhancement of acute pain.

Cortisol concentrations were significantly negatively correlated with contemporaneous pain measures both in the univariate analyses and in the path analysis. For the path analysis, we made the assumption that the relationship between pain and cortisol would be independent of sampling time, reasoning that the biological relationship between them would not be altered by time since injury. A rerun of the model without this assumption did not appreciably change the relationships between cortisol and pain at either time, suggesting that this is a valid assumption.

While acute pain tends to increase concentrations of cortisol in healthy individuals, we found a significant, negative relationship between contemporaneous measures of circulating cortisol and pain both in the days after the traumatic injury and at 5–10 months follow-up. The expectation of high cortisol during acute pain was not seen in this sample. There are several possible explanations; the first is the timing of the cortisol measurements, which were several days on average after the injury. It is possible that cortisol was depleted at this stage due to the significant stress of the injury itself. Interestingly, previous studies have found that Blacks and Whites differ in cortisol responses to pain and stress, with Blacks exhibiting a lower response than Whites [45]. Given that our study population was enriched in individuals from racial and ethnic minorities, it is possible that the demographics of our sample contributed to this relationship. On the other hand, hypocortisolism has been linked to chronic pain disorders, including fibromyalgia, chronic fatigue syndrome, chronic pelvic pain, and temporomandibular disorder [46,47]. As suggested by Hannibal and Bishop, hypocortisolemia can potentiate and prolong chronic pain due to increased inflammation, which can increase pain and increase the risk for depressed mood, an additional risk factor for chronic pain [48].

The lack of association between levels of eCBs at hospitalization and acute pain refutes our hypothesis that pain measures correlate with eCBs at baseline. However, the positive correlation between cortisol and 2-AG at the time of hospitalization supports our hypothesis and is in accord with preclinical data demonstrating that glucocorticoid receptor (GR) activation increases 2-AG synthesis in the brain [49] and periphery [50], although the possibility that cortisol and 2-AG are elevated independently cannot be ruled out. In this regard, ISS and 2-AG were positively associated, suggesting that the severity of the traumatic injury may contribute to 2-AG concentrations independently from cortisol.

Our primary goal in this study was to test the predictive value of the biomarkers measured at the time of injury for the development of chronic pain. Bivariate analyses indicated that 2-AG concentrations at the time of hospitalization were positively associated with the degree of pain interference with activities of daily living measured using the Brief Pain Inventory at follow-up. The path analysis also identified a significant and positive association between circulating 2-AG concentrations at the time of injury and pain severity at the follow-up visit and a nearly one-to-one correspondence between pain severity and pain interference. These data support our hypothesis that circulating concentrations of 2-AG have value as a biomarker for the risk of developing chronic pain.

On the other hand, neither analysis demonstrated significant associations between measures of pain severity or interference at follow-up and circulating concentrations of 2-AG measured at the same time. This finding contrasts with studies in which circulating 2-AG was found to be higher compared to pain-free control groups in individuals with several types of chronic pain, including fibromyalgia, irritable bowel syndrome, and neuropathic pain [17,18,51]. Differences in the duration and type of chronic pain could underlie the difference in findings.

It is yet unknown if elevated 2-AG concentrations during the time of injury *per se* are mechanistically involved in the severity of pain months later. Given the preclinical data that CB1R activation is associated with reduced pain in many models and that highly elevated 2-AG concentrations result in reduced CB1R density [52], it is possible that CB1R signaling is down-regulated by the high 2-AG concentrations that occur following injury. This could result in increased pain perception at the time of injury, a known risk factor for the development of persistent pain [53]. Our finding of a significant relationship between pain severity at hospitalization and follow-up supports this notion, as do the extremely high concentrations of 2-AG during the peritraumatic period. However, pain severity was not related to circulating 2-AG concentrations at hospitalization, which would be expected if this were the mechanism. An alternative hypothesis, based upon the findings that chronic pain is accompanied by widespread changes in brain circuits [43] and 2-AG/CB1 signaling affects synaptic activity throughout the brain [54], is that excessive 2-AG-mediated signaling at the time of injury contributes to lasting changes in circuits that subserve chronic pain. Further studies are needed to explore these and other possible mechanisms.

There were no interactions between circulating concentrations of the second endocannabinoid, AEA, and the other measures in this study. While 2-AG and AEA are both endogenous ligands of the cannabinoid receptors, there are differences in the triggers for their mobilization and their reported associations with psychological indicators in humans [55]. Previous studies in humans have found that AEA concentrations are more likely to be associated with anxiety while 2-AG is more likely to be associated with depression [56,57]. Interestingly, 2-AG concentrations at hospitalization were also associated with increased risk for depression at follow-up [32], while AEA concentrations at hospitalization were associated with risk for the development of chronic PTSD [33] in the participants of this study.

This study was not without limitations. First, we measured the endocannabinoids at only two time points (hospitalization and at least 5 months later), which provided partial longitudinal data over a period of time when the participants were recovering from their injury and were undergoing important changes in symptoms. However, we do not know the trajectory, and importantly, we do not know when the elevated 2-AG concentrations returned to normal values. Our hypothesis that excessive elevation of eCB signaling suggests that individuals with a prolonged increase in 2-AG would be at greater risk for chronic pain. Measuring the eCBs over multiple time points would allow us to test this hypothesis. In addition, the follow-up visits occurred over a broad range of times (5.2 months to nearly 10 months), which could add significant variability to the results. The blood collection times were dictated by the situation of the participant, which resulted in a fairly wide range of elapsed time since injury and did not differ between the NCP and CP groups. Similarly, the time of day for the blood collections was not controlled for, which is a limitation because of the circulating concentrations of both cortisol and 2-AG exhibit strong circadian rhythms [58]. Moreover, the literature has noted that the microbiota can affect the ECSS [59–61]. However, this was not evaluated within our study. Finally, we did not screen participants for pre-existing chronic pain, which could be a possible confound for assessing chronic pain associated with the current traumatic injury. However, the participants were asked at the follow-up to evaluate the severity of their pain related to the injury a few months earlier.

5. Conclusions

In conclusion, the results of this preliminary study suggest that both 2-AG and cortisol concentrations are associated with the risk for development of chronic pain following injury and add the endocannabinoid system to the list of stress-responsive systems that are associated with long-term consequences of an injury. We have previously published that 2-AG concentrations at the time of injury are also positively associated with risk for the development of major depression 6–9 months later [32]. Together, these studies indicate that 2-AG concentrations, which are roughly six times higher following trauma than under normal conditions, could serve as a general biomarker for risk for negative psychological states following traumatic injury. Future studies will probe the more interesting possibility that strong engagement of endocannabinoid signaling in the periphery and brain occurs in the aftermath of significant physiological stress and while this response may be beneficial at the time of injury, it could result in long-term negative effects in certain individuals.

Author Contributions: All four authors; C.M.T., C.J.H., A.S. and T.A.d.-C. contributed to all aspects of conceptualization, methodology, validation, and formal analysis, writing—original draft preparation, review and editing, and T.A.d.-C. and C.J.H. completed funding acquisition. All authors have read and agreed to the published version of the manuscript.

Funding: Funding for this study was provided by a grant from the National Institute on Mental Health (5R21MH102838 TA deRoon-Cassini and CJ Hillard, MPI).

Institutional Review Board: The study was conducted in accordance with the Declaration of Helsinki and approved by the Institutional Review Board of Medical College of Wisconsin IRB# PRO00022827 approved on 3 May 2019 for studies involving humans.

Informed Consent Statement: Informed consent was obtained from all subjects involved in the study.

Data Availability Statement: Not applicable.

Conflicts of Interest: Cecilia Hillard is a member of the Scientific Advisory Boards of Phytecs, Inc. and Formulate Biosciences; and has equity in Formulate Biosciences.

References

1. Hadi, M.A.; McHugh, G.A.; Closs, S.J. Impact of Chronic Pain on Patients' Quality of Life: A Comparative Mixed-Methods Study. *J. Patient Exp.* **2019**, *6*, 133–141. [CrossRef] [PubMed]
2. Treede, R.-D.; Rief, W.; Barke, A.; Aziz, Q.; Bennett, M.I.; Benoliel, R.; Cohen, M.; Evers, S.; Finnerup, N.B.; First, M.B.; et al. A classification of chronic pain for ICD-11. *Pain* **2015**, *156*, 1003–1007. [CrossRef] [PubMed]
3. Trevino, C.M.; Essig, B.; deRoon-Cassini, T.A.; Brasel, K. Chronic pain at 4 months in hospitalized trauma patients: Incidence and life interference. *J. Trauma Nurs.* **2012**, *19*, 154–159. [CrossRef] [PubMed]
4. Kolstadbraaten, K.M.; Spreng, U.J.; Wisloeff-Aase, K.; Gaarder, C.; Naess, P.A.; Raeder, J. Incidence of chronic pain 6 y after major trauma. *Acta Anaesthesiol. Scand.* **2019**, *63*, 1074–1078. [CrossRef] [PubMed]
5. Rivara, F.P.; MacKenzie, E.J.; Jurkovich, G.J.; Nathens, A.B.; Wang, J.; Scharfstein, D.O. Prevalence of Pain in Patients 1 Year After Major Trauma. *Arch. Surg.* **2008**, *143*, 282–287. [CrossRef]
6. Cohen, S.P.; Vase, L.; Hooten, W.M. Chronic pain: An update on burden, best practices, and new advances. *Lancet* **2021**, *397*, 2082–2097. [CrossRef]
7. Ballantyne, J.C.; Shin, N.S. Efficacy of opioids for chronic pain: A review of the evidence. *Clin. J. Pain* **2008**, *24*, 469–478. [CrossRef]
8. Rosenblum, A.; Marsch, L.A.; Joseph, H.; Portenoy, R.K. Opioids and the treatment of chronic pain: Controversies, current status, and future directions. *Exp. Clin. Psychopharmacol.* **2008**, *16*, 405–416. [CrossRef]
9. Piomelli, D.; Sasso, O. Peripheral gating of pain signals by endogenous lipid mediators. *Nat. Neurosci.* **2014**, *17*, 164–174. [CrossRef]
10. Woodhams, S.G.; Chapman, V.; Finn, D.P.; Hohmann, A.G.; Neugebauer, V. The cannabinoid system and pain. *Neuropharmacology* **2017**, *124*, 105–120. [CrossRef]
11. Walker, J.M.; Huang, S.M.; Strangman, N.M.; Tsou, K.; Sañudo-Peña, M.C. Pain modulation by release of the endogenous cannabinoid anandamide. *Proc. Natl. Acad. Sci. USA* **1999**, *96*, 12198–12203. [CrossRef] [PubMed]
12. Arevalo-Martin, A.; Garcia-Ovejero, D.; Sierra-Palomares, Y.; Paniagua-Torija, B.; González-Gil, I.; Ortega-Gutiérrez, S.; Molina-Holgado, E. Early Endogenous Activation of CB1 and CB2 Receptors after Spinal Cord Injury Is a Protective Response Involved in Spontaneous Recovery. *PLoS ONE* **2012**, *7*, e49057. [CrossRef] [PubMed]
13. Siegling, A.; Hofmann, H.A.; Denzer, D.; Mauler, F.; De Vry, J. Cannabinoid CB1 receptor upregulation in a rat model of chronic neuropathic pain. *Eur. J. Pharmacol.* **2001**, *415*, R5–R7. [CrossRef]
14. Zhang, J.; Hoffert, C.; Vu, H.K.; Groblewski, T.; Ahmad, S.; O'Donnell, D. Induction of CB2 receptor expression in the rat spinal cord of neuropathic but not inflammatory chronic pain models. *Eur. J. Neurosci.* **2003**, *17*, 2750–2754. [CrossRef] [PubMed]
15. Pernía-Andrade, A.J.; Kato, A.; Witschi, R.; Nyilas, R.; Katona, I.; Freund, T.F.; Watanabe, M.; Filitz, J.; Koppert, W.; Schüttler, J.; et al. Spinal endocannabinoids and CB1 receptors mediate C-fiber-induced heterosynaptic pain sensitization. *Science* **2009**, *325*, 760–764. [CrossRef]
16. Stensson, N.; Ghafouri, N.; Ernberg, M.; Mannerkorpi, K.; Kosek, E.; Gerdle, B.; Ghafouri, B. The Relationship of Endocannabinoidome Lipid Mediators with Pain and Psychological Stress in Women with Fibromyalgia: A Case-Control Study. *J. Pain* **2018**, *19*, 1318–1328. [CrossRef]

17. Fichna, J.; Wood, J.T.; Papanastasiou, M.; Vadivel, S.K.; Oprocha, P.; Sałaga, M.; Sobczak, M.; Mokrowiecka, A.; Cygankiewicz, A.I.; Zakrzewski, P.K.; et al. Endocannabinoid and Cannabinoid-like Fatty Acid Amide Levels Correlate with Pain-Related Symptoms in Patients with IBS-D and IBS-C: A Pilot Study. *PLoS ONE* **2013**, *8*, e85073. [CrossRef]
18. Pellkofer, H.L.; Havla, J.; Hauer, D.; Schelling, G.; Azad, S.C.; Kuempfel, T.; Magerl, W.; Huge, V. The Major Brain Endocannabinoid 2-AG Controls Neuropathic Pain and Mechanical Hyperalgesia in Patients with Neuromyelitis Optica. *PLoS ONE* **2013**, *8*, e71500. [CrossRef]
19. Kaufmann, I.; Schelling, G.; Eisner, C.; Richter, H.P.; Krauseneck, T.; Vogeser, M.; Hauer, D.; Campolongo, P.; Chouker, A.; Beyer, A.; et al. Anandamide and neutrophil function in patients with fibromyalgia. *Psychoneuroendocrinology* **2008**, *33*, 676–685. [CrossRef]
20. Kaufmann, I.; Hauer, D.; Huge, V.; Vogeser, M.; Campolongo, P.; Chouker, A.; Thiel, M.; Schelling, G. Enhanced Anandamide Plasma Levels in Patients with Complex Regional Pain Syndrome following Traumatic Injury: A Preliminary Report. *Eur. Surg. Res.* **2009**, *43*, 325–329. [CrossRef]
21. Sanchez, A.M.; Cioffi, R.; Viganò, P.; Candiani, M.; Verde, R.; Piscitelli, F.; Di Marzo, V.; Garavaglia, E.; Panina-Bordignon, P. Elevated Systemic Levels of Endocannabinoids and Related Mediators Across the Menstrual Cycle in Women with Endometriosis. *Reprod. Sci.* **2016**, *23*, 1071–1079. [CrossRef] [PubMed]
22. Ehlert, U.; Gaab, J.; Heinrichs, M. Psychoneuroendocrinological contributions to the etiology of depression, posttraumatic stress disorder, and stress-related bodily disorders: The role of the hypothalamus–pituitary–adrenal axis. *Biol. Psychol.* **2001**, *57*, 141–152. [CrossRef]
23. Tsigos, C.; Chrousos, G.P. Hypothalamic–pituitary–adrenal axis, neuroendocrine factors and stress. *J. Psychosom. Res.* **2002**, *53*, 865–871. [CrossRef]
24. Fries, E.; Hesse, J.; Hellhammer, J.; Hellhammer, D.H. A new view on hypocortisolism. *Psychoneuroendocrinology* **2005**, *30*, 1010–1016. [CrossRef]
25. Bali, A.; Jaggi, A.S. Clinical experimental stress studies: Methods and assessment. *Rev. Neurosci.* **2015**, *26*, 555–579. [CrossRef]
26. McBeth, J.; Silman, A.J.; Gupta, A.; Chiu, Y.H.; Ray, D.; Morriss, R.; Dickens, C.; King, Y.; Macfarlane, G. Moderation of psychosocial risk factors through dysfunction of the hypothalamic–pituitary–adrenal stress axis in the onset of chronic widespread musculoskeletal pain: Findings of a population-based prospective cohort study. *Arthritis Care Res.* **2007**, *56*, 360–371. [CrossRef] [PubMed]
27. Paananen, M.; O'Sullivan, P.; Straker, L.; Beales, D.; Coenen, P.; Karppinen, J.; Pennell, C.; Smith, A. A low cortisol response to stress is associated with musculoskeletal pain combined with increased pain sensitivity in young adults: A longitudinal cohort study. *Arthritis Res. Ther.* **2015**, *17*, 355. [CrossRef]
28. Riva, R.; Mork, P.J.; Westgaard, R.H.; Lundberg, U. Comparison of the cortisol awakening response in women with shoulder and neck pain and women with fibromyalgia. *Psychoneuroendocrinology* **2012**, *37*, 299–306. [CrossRef]
29. Muhtz, C.; Rodriguez-Raecke, R.; Hinkelmann, K.; Moeller-Bertram, T.; Kiefer, F.; Wiedemann, K.; May, A.; Otte, C. Cortisol Response to Experimental Pain in Patients with Chronic Low Back Pain and Patients with Major Depression. *Pain Med.* **2013**, *14*, 498–503. [CrossRef]
30. McEwen, B.S.; Stellar, E. Stress and the individual. Mechanisms leading to disease. *Arch. Intern. Med.* **1993**, *153*, 2093–2101. [CrossRef]
31. Hillard, C.J.; Beatka, M.; Sarvaideo, J. Endocannabinoid signaling and the hypothalamic-pituitary-adrenal axis. *Compr. Physiol.* **2016**, *7*, 1. [PubMed]
32. Fitzgerald, J.M.; Chesney, S.A.; Lee, T.S.; Brasel, K.; Larson, C.L.; Hillard, C.J.; Deroon-Cassini, T.A. Circulating endocannabinoids and prospective risk for depression in trauma-injury survivors. *Neurobiol. Stress* **2021**, *14*, 100304. [CrossRef] [PubMed]
33. Deroon-Cassini, T.A.; Bergner, C.L.; Chesney, S.A.; Schumann, N.R.; Lee, T.S.; Brasel, K.J.; Hillard, C.J. Circulating endocannabinoids and genetic polymorphisms as predictors of posttraumatic stress disorder symptom severity: Heterogeneity in a community-based cohort. *Transl. Psychiatry* **2022**, *12*, 48. [CrossRef] [PubMed]
34. Dworkin, R.H.; Turk, D.C.; Farrar, J.T.; Haythornthwaite, J.A.; Jensen, M.P.; Katz, N.P.; Kerns, R.D.; Stucki, G.; Allen, R.R.; Bellamy, N.; et al. Core outcome measures for chronic pain clinical trials: IMMPACT recommendations. *Pain* **2005**, *113*, 9–19. [CrossRef]
35. Baker, S.P.; O'Neill, B.; Haddon, W., Jr.; Long, W.B. The injury severity score: A method for describing patients with multiple injuries and evaluating emergency care. *J. Trauma Acute Care* **1974**, *14*, 187–196. [CrossRef]
36. Cleeland, C.S.; Ryan, K.M. Pain assessment: Global use of the Brief Pain Inventory. *Ann. Acad. Med. Singap.* **1994**, *23*, 129–138.
37. Boonstra, A.M.; Stewart, R.E.; Köke, A.J.A.; Oosterwijk, R.F.A.; Swaan, J.L.; Schreurs, K.M.G.; Preuper, H.R.S. Cut-Off Points for Mild, Moderate, and Severe Pain on the Numeric Rating Scale for Pain in Patients with Chronic Musculoskeletal Pain: Variability and Influence of Sex and Catastrophizing. *Front. Psychol.* **2016**, *7*, 1466. [CrossRef]
38. Crombie, K.; Brellenthin, A.G.; Hillard, C.J.; Koltyn, K.F. Psychobiological Responses to Aerobic Exercise in Individuals with Posttraumatic Stress Disorder. *J. Trauma Stress* **2018**, *31*, 134–145. [CrossRef]
39. Yung, Y.F.; Zhang, W. Making Use of Incomplete Observations in the Analysis of Structural Equation Models: The CALIS Procedure's Full Information Maximum Likelihood Method in SAS/STAT 9.3. In *Proceedings of the SAS Global Forum 2011 Conference*; SAS Institute Inc.: Cary, NC, USA, 2011. Available online: http://support.sas.com/resources/papers/proceedings11/333-2011.pdf (accessed on 1 January 2019).
40. Orlas, C.P.; Herrera-Escobar, J.P.; Hau, K.M.; Velmahos, G.; Patel, N.; Sanchez, S.; Kaafarani, H.M.; Salim, A.; Nehra, D. Perceived social support is strongly associated with recovery after injury. *J. Trauma Acute Care Surg.* **2021**, *91*, 552–558. [CrossRef]
41. Mills, S.E.; Nicolson, K.P.; Smith, B.H. Chronic pain: A review of its epidemiology and associated factors in population-based studies. *Br. J. Anaesth.* **2019**, *123*, e273–e283. [CrossRef]

42. Mogil, J.S. Qualitative sex differences in pain processing: Emerging evidence of a biased literature. *Nat. Rev. Neurosci.* **2020**, *21*, 353–365. [CrossRef] [PubMed]
43. Kuner, R.; Kuner, T. Cellular Circuits in the Brain and Their Modulation in Acute and Chronic Pain. *Physiol. Rev.* **2021**, *101*, 213–258. [CrossRef] [PubMed]
44. Trevino, C.M.; deRoon-Cassini, T.A.; Brasel, K. Does opiate use in traumatically injured individuals worsen pain and psychological outcomes? *J. Pain* **2013**, *14*, 424–430. [CrossRef] [PubMed]
45. Herbert, M.S.; Goodin, B.R.; Bulls, H.; Sotolongo, A.; Petrov, M.; Edberg, J.C.; Bradley, L.A.; Fillingim, R. Ethnicity, Cortisol, and Experimental Pain Responses Among Persons with Symptomatic Knee Osteoarthritis. *Clin. J. Pain* **2017**, *33*, 820–826. [CrossRef]
46. Tak, L.M.; Rosmalen, J. Dysfunction of stress responsive systems as a risk factor for functional somatic syndromes. *J. Psychosom. Res.* **2010**, *68*, 461–468. [CrossRef]
47. Quartana, P.J.; Buenaver, L.F.; Edwards, R.R.; Klick, B.; Haythornthwaite, J.A.; Smith, M.T. Pain catastrophizing and salivary cortisol responses to laboratory pain testing in temporoman-dibular disorder and healthy participants. *J. Pain* **2010**, *11*, 186–194. [CrossRef]
48. Hannibal, K.E.; Bishop, M. Chronic Stress, Cortisol Dysfunction, and Pain: A Psychoneuroendocrine Rationale for Stress Management in Pain Rehabilitation. *Phys. Ther.* **2014**, *94*, 1816–1825. [CrossRef]
49. Hill, M.N.; McLaughlin, R.; Pan, B.; Fitzgerald, M.L.; Roberts, C.; Lee, T.T.-Y.; Karatsoreos, I.N.; Mackie, K.; Viau, V.; Pickel, V.M.; et al. Recruitment of Prefrontal Cortical Endocannabinoid Signaling by Glucocorticoids Contributes to Termination of the Stress Response. *J. Neurosci.* **2011**, *31*, 10506–10515. [CrossRef]
50. Bowles, N.P.; Karatsoreos, I.N.; Li, X.; Vemuri, V.K.; Wood, J.-A.; Li, Z.; Tamashiro, K.L.K.; Schwartz, G.J.; Makriyannis, A.M.; Kunos, G.; et al. A peripheral endocannabinoid mechanism contributes to glucocorticoid-mediated metabolic syndrome. *Proc. Natl. Acad. Sci. USA* **2015**, *112*, 285–290. [CrossRef]
51. Stensson, N.; Ghafouri, B.; Gerdle, B.; Ghafouri, N. Alterations of anti-inflammatory lipids in plasma from women with chronic widespread pain—A case control study. *Lipids Health Dis.* **2017**, *16*, 112. [CrossRef]
52. Schlosburg, J.E.; Blankman, J.L.; Long, J.Z.; Nomura, D.K.; Pan, B.; Kinsey, S.G.; Nguyen, P.T.; Ramesh, D.; Booker, L.; Burston, J.J.; et al. Chronic monoacylglycerol lipase blockade causes functional antagonism of the endocannabinoid system. *Nat. Neurosci.* **2010**, *13*, 1113–1119. [CrossRef] [PubMed]
53. Trevino, C.; Harl, F.; Deroon-Cassini, T.; Brasel, K.; Litwack, K. Predictors of Chronic Pain in Traumatically Injured Hospitalized Adult Patients. *J. Trauma Nurs.* **2014**, *21*, 50–56. [CrossRef] [PubMed]
54. Hillard, C.J. The endocannabinoid signaling system in the CNS: A primer. *Int. Rev. Neurobiol.* **2015**, *125*, 1–47. [PubMed]
55. Deroon-Cassini, T.A.; Stollenwerk, T.M.; Beatka, M.; Hillard, C.J. Meet Your Stress Management Professionals: The Endocannabinoids. *Trends Mol. Med.* **2020**, *26*, 953–968. [CrossRef]
56. Hill, M.; Miller, G.; Ho, W.-S.; Gorzalka, B.; Hillard, C. Serum Endocannabinoid Content is Altered in Females with Depressive Disorders: A Preliminary Report. *Pharmacopsychiatry* **2008**, *41*, 48–53. [CrossRef]
57. Dlugos, A.; Childs, E.; Stuhr, K.L.; Hillard, C.J.; de Wit, H. Acute Stress Increases Circulating Anandamide and Other N-Acylethanolamines in Healthy Humans. *Neuropsychopharmacology* **2012**, *37*, 2416–2427. [CrossRef]
58. Hanlon, E.C.; Tasali, E.; Leproult, R.; Stuhr, K.L.; Doncheck, E.; De Wit, H.; Hillard, C.J.; Van Cauter, E. Circadian Rhythm of Circulating Levels of the Endocannabinoid 2-Arachidonoylglycerol. *J. Clin. Endocrinol. Metab.* **2015**, *100*, 220–226. [CrossRef]
59. Freitas, M.; Vasconcelos, A.; Gonçalves, E.; Ferrarini, E.; Vieira, G.; Cicia, D.; Cola, M.; Capasso, R.; Dutra, R. Involvement of Opioid System and TRPM8/TRPA1 Channels in the Antinociceptive Effect of *Spirulina platensis*. *Biomolecules* **2021**, *11*, 592. [CrossRef]
60. Vieira, G.; Cavalli, J.; Gonçalves, E.C.D.; Braga, S.F.P.; Ferreira, R.S.; Santos, A.R.S.; Cola, M.; Raposo, N.R.B.; Capasso, R.; Dutra, R.C. Antidepressant-Like Effect of Terpineol in an Inflammatory Model of Depression: Involvement of the Cannabinoid System and D2 Dopamine Receptor. *Biomolecules* **2020**, *10*, 792. [CrossRef]
61. Gonçalves, E.C.D.; Baldasso, G.M.; Bicca, M.A.; Paes, R.S.; Capasso, R.; Dutra, R.C. Terpenoids, Cannabimimetic Ligands, beyond the *Cannabis* Plant. *Molecules* **2020**, *25*, 1567. [CrossRef]

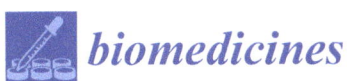

Article

Anti-Tumorigenic Effect of a Novel Derivative of 2-Hydroxyoleic Acid and the Endocannabinoid Anandamide on Neuroblastoma Cells

Hana Golan [1,2,3], Raphael Mechoulam [4], Reem Smoum [4], Efrat Cohen-Zada [1], Sara Pri-Chen [1], Sapir Wiener [1], Igor Grinberg [1], Dekel D. Bar-Lev [1], Christeeneh G. Haj [4], Tamar Fisher [1,†] and Amos Toren [1,2,3,*,†]

- [1] Pediatric Hematology Oncology Research Laboratory, Cancer Research Center, The Chaim Sheba Medical Center, Tel-Hashomer, Ramat Gan 52621, Israel; hana.golan@sheba.health.gov.il (H.G.); efratco1@gmail.com (E.C.-Z.); sara.prichen@sheba.health.gov.il (S.P.-C.); sapirneeman24@gmail.com (S.W.); igor.grinberg@sheba.health.gov.il (I.G.); dekeldov.barlev@sheba.health.gov.il (D.D.B.-L.); tamar.fisher@sheba.health.gov.il (T.F.)
- [2] Department of Pediatric Hematology Oncology, The Edmond and Lily Safra Children's Hospital, The Chaim Sheba Medical Center, Tel-Hashomer, Ramat Gan 52621, Israel
- [3] Sackler Faculty of Medicine, Tel-Aviv University, Tel-Aviv 6997801, Israel
- [4] Medicinal Chemistry Laboratory, The Institute for Drug Research, School of Pharmacy, Faculty of Medicine, The Hebrew University of Jerusalem, Jerusalem 9112001, Israel; raphaelm@ekmd.huji.ac.il (R.M.); reems@ekmd.huji.ac.il (R.S.); christeeneh@ekmd.huji.ac.il (C.G.H.)
- * Correspondence: amost@post.tau.ac.il
- † These authors contributed equally to this work.

Abstract: Modulation of the endogenous cannabinoid system has been suggested as a potential anticancer strategy. In the search for novel and less toxic therapeutic options, structural modifications of the endocannabinoid anandamide and the synthetic derivative of oleic acid, Minerval (HU-600), were done to obtain 2-hydroxy oleic acid ethanolamide (HU-585), which is an HU-600 derivative with the anandamide side chain. We showed that treatment of SK-N-SH neuroblastoma cells with HU-585 induced a better anti-tumorigenic effect in comparison to HU-600 as evidenced by 3-[4,5-dimethylthiazole-2-yl]-2,5-diphenyltetrazolium bromide assay, colony-forming assay, and migration assay. Moreover, HU-585 demonstrated pro-apoptotic properties shown by increased levels of activated caspase-3 following treatment and a better senescence induction effect in comparison to HU-600, as demonstrated by increased activity of lysosomal β-galactosidase. Finally, we observed that combined treatment of HU-585 with the senolytic drugs ABT-263 in vitro, and ABT-737 in vivo resulted in enhanced anti-proliferative effects and reduced neuroblastoma xenograft growth in comparison to treatment with HU-585 alone. Based on these results, we suggest that HU-585 is a pro-apoptotic and senescence-inducing compound, better than HU-600. Hence, it may be a beneficial option for the treatment of resistant neuroblastoma especially when combined with senolytic drugs that enhance its anti-tumorigenic effects.

Keywords: 2-hydroxy oleic acid; anandamide; anti Bcl2; endocannabinoid system; membrane lipid therapy; neuroblastoma

Citation: Golan, H.; Mechoulam, R.; Smoum, R.; Cohen-Zada, E.; Pri-Chen, S.; Wiener, S.; Grinberg, I.; Bar-Lev, D.D.; Haj, C.G.; Fisher, T.; et al. Anti-Tumorigenic Effect of a Novel Derivative of 2-Hydroxyoleic Acid and the Endocannabinoid Anandamide on Neuroblastoma Cells. *Biomedicines* **2022**, *10*, 1552. https://doi.org/10.3390/biomedicines10071552

Academic Editor: Wesley M. Raup-Konsavage

Received: 18 May 2022
Accepted: 22 June 2022
Published: 29 June 2022

Publisher's Note: MDPI stays neutral with regard to jurisdictional claims in published maps and institutional affiliations.

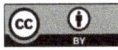

Copyright: © 2022 by the authors. Licensee MDPI, Basel, Switzerland. This article is an open access article distributed under the terms and conditions of the Creative Commons Attribution (CC BY) license (https:// creativecommons.org/licenses/by/ 4.0/).

1. Introduction

Neuroblastoma (NBL) is the most common extracranial solid tumor of childhood. Children with high-risk neuroblastoma currently have long-term survival rates under 50% despite intensive, multimodal treatment regimens that include chemotherapy, surgical tumor resection, autologous stem cell transplantation, radiation therapy, and maintenance immunotherapy combined with 13-*cis*-retinoic acid [1,2]. In addition, the aggressive chemo-radiotherapy used for the treatment of these children is associated with severe side effects and multi-organ damage [3]. Therefore, new, less toxic therapeutic combinations directed at relevant targets are needed for these children to reduce relapse rates and improve survival.

The cannabinoids are a group of more than 100 chemically related compounds found in the marijuana plant *Cannabis sativa*, that have been found to possess diverse pharmacological activities in cancer, including cytostatic, apoptotic, and antiangiogenic effects [4]. Tetrahydrocannabinol (THC), the main psychoactive constituent in *Cannabis sativa*, acts mainly through the activation of specific cannabinoid receptors CB1 and CB2 and thus mimics the binding of the animal endogenous cannabinoids (named endocannabinoids) [5–7]. Endocannabinoids are known to participate in many biological processes in the immune, respiratory, circulatory, and reproductive systems. On a cellular level, they have been shown to modulate cell proliferation, viability, and differentiation [8]. The cytotoxicity of endocannabinoids on tumoral cells has been frequently reported, hence, their potential use in the treatment of malignant diseases [9]. Several different mechanisms have been implicated in the anti-tumorigenic actions of endocannabinoids and include cytotoxic or cytostatic effects, apoptosis induction, and anti-metastatic effects, such as inhibition of neo-angiogenesis and tumor cell migration [10]. One of the best-known endocannabinoids with anti-tumorigenic effects is anandamide (AEA). AEA has been shown to inhibit cholangiocarcinoma growth [11], to exert cytotoxic and antiproliferative effects on colorectal carcinoma cells [12], and to cause apoptosis of osteosarcoma cells [13] and glioma cells [14].

AEA is the ethanolamide of the fatty acid arachidonic acid. The anti-cancer drug Minerval is a 2-hydroxy derivative of another fatty acid, oleic acid. Minerval (HU-600) is one of the most studied synthetic lipid compounds that was shown to be safe and effective in patients with glioma and other advanced solid tumors [15]. In contrast to most anticancer drugs, HU-600 targets the plasma membrane and mediates its anti-tumor effect by affecting the biophysical properties of membranes [16–18].

Based on the anti-cancer effects of HU-600 and AEA, we assumed that a molecule that is a derivative of both compounds may be a novel anti-cancer drug with a promising anticancer therapeutic profile. Hence, structural modification of HU-600 was done to obtain 2-hydroxy-oleic acid (2-OHOA) ethanolamide (HU-585), a novel compound, which is an HU-600 derivative with the AEA side chain.

To further our research on this subject [19], we explored and compared the anti-tumorigenic effects of HU-600 and its novel derivate HU-585 on the NBL cell line. The results obtained in our study indicate that of the two compounds tested, HU-585 was indeed more effective on the NBL cell line in comparison to HU-600. Furthermore, HU-585 demonstrated pro-apoptotic and senescence-inducing properties, and combined treatment with senolytic drugs further enhanced its anti-tumorigenic effect. Our findings add contemporary information, attractive strategy, and an effective and less toxic therapeutic option for the treatment of refractory NBL.

2. Materials and Methods

2.1. Preparation of 2-Hydroxyoleoyl Ethanolamide (HU-585)

The 2-hydroxy oleic acid (HU-600) was synthesized according to Lazarus et al. [20]. The ethanolamide derivative (HU-585) of HU-600 was prepared according to the following procedure: To a solution of 2-hydroxyoleic acid sodium salt (100 mg, 0.3125 mmol) and N,N-dimethylformamide (23.65 µL, 0.3125 mmol) in dry methylene chloride (4.7 mL) was added dropwise oxalyl chloride (2.0 M solution in methylene chloride, 0.312 mL, 0.62 mmol) under nitrogen atmosphere at 0–5 °C. The reaction mixture was stirred for 10 min, and then the solvent was evaporated under nitrogen flow. The crude material in methylene chloride (4.7 mL) was added to an ice-cold solution of ethanolamide (0.214 mL, 3.55 mmol) in methylene chloride (4.7 mL). The reaction mixture was stirred for 10 min, then it was washed with water (3 × 20 mL) and dried ($MgSO_4$), and the solvent was evaporated under reduced pressure. The residue was chromatographed on silica gel. White solid, melting point: 63 °C, NMR ($CDCl_3$, ppm): 5.37 [m, 2H]; 4.15 [dd, 1H]; 3.75 [m, 2H]; 3.52–3.45 [m, 2H]; 2.04 [m, 4H]; 1.85–1.66 [m, 2H]; 1.44–1.29 [m, 20H]; 0.92 [t, 3H]. LC-MS (+p) = 342.2.

2.2. Cell Culture

Human neuroblastoma cell line SK-N-SH was obtained from ATCC (Manassas, VA, USA). SK-N-SH cells were cultured in Eagle minimum essential medium (ATCC), supplemented with 10% fetal bovine serum (FBS) and 100 U/mL penicillin—streptomycin (Gibco, Paisley, UK). Fibroblasts were obtained from dermal human fibroblasts, per protocol #7044 (approved by the Institutional Review Board at Sheba Medical Center, Tel Hashomer, Ramat Gan, Israel). Fibroblasts cells were cultured in high glucose DMEM supplemented with 20% FBS, penicillin-streptomycin, 1% non-essential amino acids and 0.2% β-mercaptoethanol (Invitrogen, Life Technologies, Grand Island, NY, USA). Normal human astrocytes (HA) obtained from Science Cell Research Laboratories (Carlsbad, CA, USA). HA cells were cultured in HA medium (Catalog #1801) with supplement from Science Cell Research Laboratories (Carlsbad, CA, USA). All cells were routinely tested for the presence of mycoplasma. The cell lines were cultured at 37 °C in a humidified atmosphere containing 5% CO_2. As they approached confluence, the cells were sub-cultured following treatment with 6% trypsin-EDTA.

2.3. MTT Test

The effect of HU-600 and HU-585 on the SK-N-SH NBL cell line was studied using the 3-(4, 5-dimethylthiazol-2-yl)-2,5diphenyltetrazolium bromide (MTT) assay (Sigma-Aldrich Co., St. Louis, MO, USA). SK-N-SH cells (4×10^3 cells/well) were plated (200 µL) in triplicates in flat bottom 96-well plates in appropriate medium as mentioned above. The cells were allowed to adhere to the plate surface overnight and then cultured with increasing doses of HU-600 or HU-585 (0–200 µM) for 72 h. Cell viability was then determined using MTT assay, which measures reduction of MTT to formazan by mitochondria of viable cells. Formazan was measured spectrophotometrically by absorption at 560 nm in a PowerWaveX™ (BioTek, Santa Clara, CA, USA) plate reader. All experiments were repeated at least 3 times. Cell morphologies were assessed daily by light microscopy.

2.4. Colony-Forming Assay (CFA)

CFA was used to determine the effect of HU-600 and HU-585 treatment on the ability of a single cell to grow into a colony. SK-N-SH cells (500 cells/well) were plated in triplicates in 6-well plates (3 mL) and were treated according to treatment regimen mentioned below with 12.5, 37.5, and 75 µM of HU-600 or HU-585 for 14 days. Subsequently, colonies were fixed with ethanol 70%, stained with crystal violet solution (0.5% w/v), rinsed extensively by tap water, dried, and counted using EPSON scan software. Colonies were counted using ImageJ software.

2.5. Cell Migration Assay

Wound healing assay was performed to compare the effect of HU-600 and HU-585 on cell migration ability. SK-N-SH cells (1×10^6 cells/well) were plated in duplicates in 6-well plates (3 mL) and were allowed to adhere overnight, then treated with 75 µM of HU-600 or HU-585, and were allowed to grow into a confluent cell monolayer. Cells then were starved using starvation medium (FBS free) overnight. A single scratch along each well was made by micropipette, fresh medium was supplemented, and cells were incubated for 24 h. Cell migration was quantified by taking pictures with a regular inverted microscope at two time points: right after scratching and 24 h later. Gap intervals were measured using ImageJ software, and the percentage of migration and gap closure was calculated using the formula:

$$\% \; migration = \frac{average \; wound \; width \; 0h - average \; wound \; width \; 24h}{average \; wound \; width \; 0h} \times 100$$

2.6. Western Blot Assay

To assess apoptotic activity following treatment with HU-585, caspase-3 and Bcl-2 protein levels were evaluated by western blot assay. One day before HU-585 treatment (100 μM for 24 h and 48 h), cells were plated (1 × 10^6 cells per 9-cm plate). Cells were harvested and proteins were extracted with RIPA buffer supplemented with phosphatase and protease inhibitors (Sigma–Aldrich). Protein concentrations were calibrated using the BCA Protein Assay Reagent Kit (Pierce, Rockford, IL, USA). Equal amounts of protein (30 μg) were loaded onto 12.5% SDS-PAGE gels and transferred onto nitrocellulose membranes (Bio-Rad, Rishon Le Zion, Israel). The blots were reacted using caspase-3 (9662S) or Bcl-2 (D55G8, 4223S) rabbit monoclonal antibody (Cell Signaling Technology, Danvers, MA, USA) as the primary antibody. The secondary antibody, horseradish peroxidase conjugated goat anti-rabbit antibody (Jackson ImmunoResearch Laboratories, Farmington, CT, USA), was detected by chemiluminescence. Signals were detected using an ECL Kit (CYANAGEN, Bologna, Italy) and visualized using the ChemiDocTM MP Imaging System. Quantification of caspase-3 and Bcl-2 was done by Image Lab software.

2.7. Senescence-Associated β-Galactosidase Activity Assay

Senescence-associated β-galactosidase (SA-β-gal) activity was measured with a β-galactosidase staining kit (Senescence B-Galactosidase Staining KIT, Cell Signaling Technology, #9860) according to the manufacturer's instructions. Briefly, SK-N-SH cells (5 × 10^4 cells\well) were plated in 6-well plates (3 mL) and treated according to the previously described treatment regimen [19] with 50, 75 and 100 μM of HU-600 or HU-585 for 48 h and then fixed and incubated overnight at 37 °C in CO_2 free environment. Accumulation of a distinctive blue color in senescent cells was then observed by microscope (Olympus Scientific Solutions, Waltham, MA, USA). Pictures of three representative fields of each well were taken, blue colored cells were counted by ImageJ software, and the percentage of β-galactosidase positive cells was determined and normalizing to the control.

2.8. In Vitro Senolytic Studies

In vitro senolytic studies were performed using Navitoclax (ABT-263) dissolved in DMSO (Sigma-Aldrich, Rehovot, Israel). SK-N-SH cells (2 × 10^4 cells/well) were plated in triplicates in 96-well plates (200 μL) and were cultured according to the previously described regimen, with increasing concentrations of HU-600 or HU-585 (0–200 μM) for 48 h. Subsequently, cells were cultured with ABT-263 (2.5 μM) for 24 h, then an MTT test was performed according to the MTT assay mentioned above. ABT-263 concentration was chosen following several dose response MTT assays. The maximal dose with no effect on survival was 2.5 μM (data not shown).

2.9. Murine Xenograft Therapeutic Studies

In vivo experiments were carried out according to protocols approved by the Ethical Committee of the Chaim Sheba Medical Center. Female athymic nude mice (Foxn1nu) 6–8 weeks of age (ENVIGO RMS, Jerusalem, Israel) were used for the tumor xenograft (Xn) model. In total, 5 × 10^6 SK-N-SH mCherry expressing cells were subcutaneously inoculated in the right flank of each mouse. Following cell injection, tumor burden was determined once a week by a Spectrum Animals in vivo imaging system (IVIS®), and the mice were allocated into four homogeneous groups according to the intensity of the average total radiant efficiency signal measured by IVIS: Control vehicle; HU-585 (120 mg/kg); ABT-737 (75 mg/kg); combined treatment with HU-585 (120 mg/kg) and ABT-737 (75 mg/kg), (n = 8 per group). ABT-737 (S1002, Selleckchem, Houston, TX, USA) was formulated in a mixture of 30% propylene glycol, 5% Tween 80, and 65% DsW (5% dextrose in DDW). Treatment started 4 weeks following cell injection and was administered intraperitoneally (IP) once daily for a total of 21 days. Tumor burden was determined once a week by the IVIS system and by external electronic caliper measurements throughout treatments. Tumor volumes were calculated by the following formula: $A \times B^2/2$, where A is the greatest diameter, and B is the diameter perpendicular to A. At the end of treatment, the animals were then euthanized, and tumor Xns were immediately removed, weighed, stored, and fixed.

2.10. Statistical Analysis

An estimating equations (GEE) test was used to evaluate significant differences in all in vitro experiments except for apoptosis assay in which Two-way ANOVA was used. The Kruskal-Wallis test was performed with the post hoc Dunn's multiple comparisons to evaluate significant differences in the growth rate of xenografts between treatment groups. All analyses were performed using the IBM SPSS Statistics software application (version 24: IBM, Armonk, NY, USA). Excluding MTT analysis, all results are shown as means ± SE. $p < 0.05$ was considered to indicate statistical significance.

3. Results

3.1. Structural Modification of HU-600

The syntheses 2-OHOA ethanolamide (HU-585) was done by the addition of anandamide side chain to 2-OHOA (HU-600) (Figure 1).

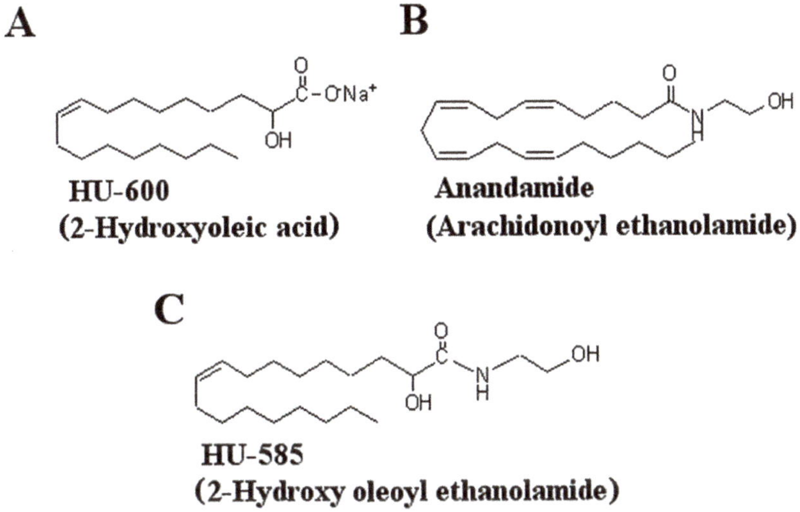

Figure 1. Structures of the synthetic compounds tested for anticancer activity. Structures of (**A**) HU−600 (Minerval, 2−hydroxyoleic acid), (**B**) anandamide (AEA) and (**C**) HU−585 that was obtained by structural modification and the addition of AEA side chain to HU−600.

3.2. HU-585 Induces Cell Growth Inhibition, Reduced Colony Formation, and Reduced Migration in the Neuroblastoma Cell Line SK-N-SH In Vitro

In order to evaluate the antitumorigenic effects of HU-600 and its derivative, HU-585, on SK-N-SH cells, we used MTT, CFU, and migration assays (Figure 2). The choice of concentrations used in these assays (12.5–200 µM) is based on previous data showing that the IC_{50} of HU600 for most cancer cells studied is in the range of 30–250 µM [16,21,22]. A similar and significant dose-dependent decrease in cell viability was demonstrated by both compounds at a concentration of 12.5 µM (16.7%, $p < 0.05$). The effect on cell viability reduction was significantly better for HU-585 treatment in comparison to HU-600 treatment at concentration of 75 µM and above: 33.5% vs. 14.4% at 75 µM; 34.3% vs. 14.7% at 100 µM; 52.2% vs. 23.2% at 200 µM, respectively. * $p = 0.03$, ** $p = 0.02$, *** $p = 0.01$, respectively (Figure 2A).

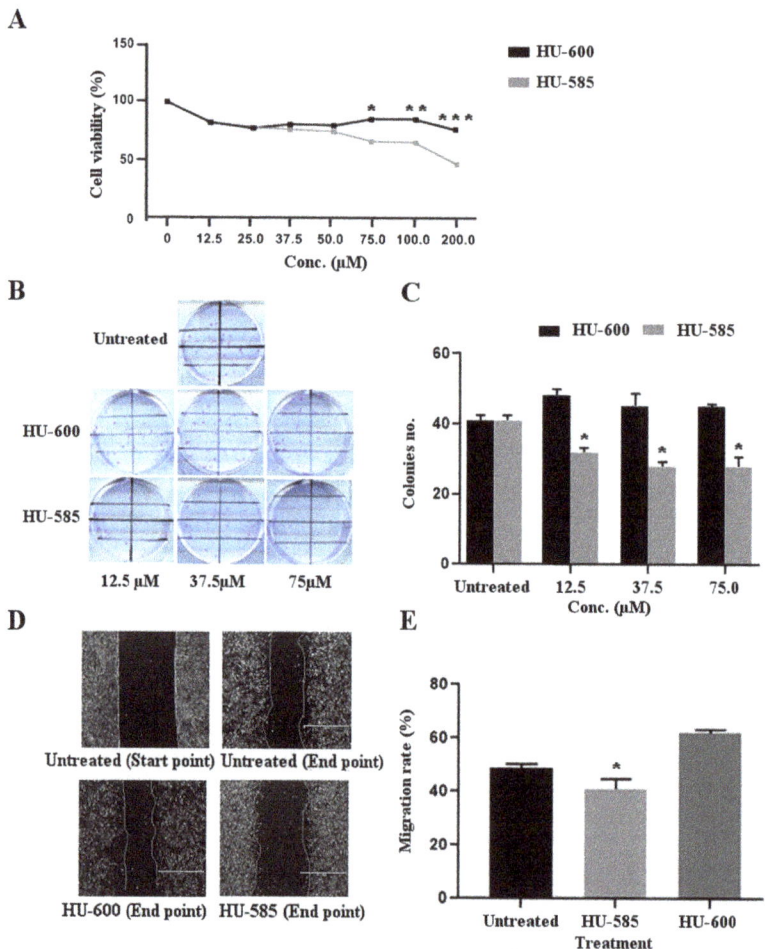

Figure 2. Anti-tumorigenic effects of HU-585 and HU-600. (A) Cell viability, measured with MTT assay in SK-N-SH cell line following treatment with HU-585 and HU-600. The cells were plated in 96-well plates and treated with increasing concentrations of HU-600 or HU-585 for 72 h. A significant decrease in cell viability was detected for both compounds at concentration of 12.5 μM (16.7%, $p < 0.05$). A better effect in cell viability reduction was obtained for HU-585 at concentration 75 μM and above. The cell viability reduction for HU-585 and HU-600 at 75 μM was 33.5% and 14.4%, respectively (* $p = 0.03$), at 100 μM, 34.3% and 14.7%, respectively (** $p = 0.02$), and at 200 μM, 52.2% and 23.2%, respectively (*** $p = 0.01$). Data are expressed as percentage of the vehicle control and are the mean of pooled results from several experiments ($n = 6$) performed in triplicate. Statistical significance was determined by GEE test. * $p < 0.05$ compared to HU-585 (1.15 < SE values < 1.99). (B,C) The effect of HU-585 and HU-600 on the colony formation ability of SK-N-SH cells showing a better effect of HU-585. The cells were plated in 6-well plates and treated with 12.5 μM, 37.5 μM and 75 μM of HU-585 or HU-600. Cells were fixed and stained with crystal violet 14 days later. Colonies were counted using ImageJ software. (B) Scanned image of representative wells showing different levels of colony formation in SK-N-SH treated cells. (C) Representation of the quantified number of colonies in increasing concentrations of the treatment used. Statistical significance was determined by GEE test, * $p < 0.05$ ($n = 3$, performed in duplicates). (D,E) Migration rate of SK-N-SH cells was

decreased following treatment with HU-585. Using ImageJ software, pre-migration (0 h) and post-migration (24 h) images of untreated and following treatment with 75 µM of HU-585 or 75 µM of HU-600 were taken (**D**). Treatment with HU-585 resulted in a better inhibitory effect of the migration rate in comparison to untreated and to HU-600 treated cells. Migration rate of the cells was quantified as the average percentage of gap closure following treatment (**E**). Data is reported as mean ± SE of triplicates. Statistical significance was determined by GEE test, * $p \leq 0.05$ compared to the two other group (n = 3, performed in duplicates).

Cologenic assay was used to determine the effect of HU-600 and HU-585 treatment on the cellular cologenic potential of SK-N-SH cells (Figure 2B,C). The results show a significant reduction in the number of colonies formed following HU-585 treatment in comparison to untreated cells (mean 29.2 colonies/field vs. 40.55 colonies/field respectively, $p < 0.001$). The significant difference between HU-585 treatment and untreated cells was observed in all concentrations used (12.5 µM, 37.5 µM & 75.5 µM, $p < 0.05$) (Figure 2C). A similar effect of reduction in colony formation was not obtained following treatment with HU-600.

Finally, to assess the effect of HU-600 and HU-585 treatment on SK-N-SH cell migration ability, a wound healing assay was performed. The results show a significant reduction in migration rate of cells treated with 75.5 µM of HU-585 in comparison to untreated cells. Decrease in migration rate following treatment with HU-600 was not observed (Figure 2D,E).

Taken together, these results provide evidence that both HU-585 and HU-600 have antitumorigenic effects as demonstrated by reduced cells viability following treatment. However, the new compound HU-585 obtained by structural modification of HU-600, has a better anti-tumorigenic effect in the MTT assay at concentration of 75 µM and above and in all the additional in vitro studies that were performed.

3.3. Apoptotic Cell Death and Senescence Following HU-585 Treatment in SK-N-SH Cells

To verify our hypothesis that HU-585 induced reduction in NB cell viability was indeed due to apoptotic cell death, we first examined the morphological changes following HU-585 treatment. Microscopic analysis showed that treatment with 75 µM and 100 µM of HU-585 affected cell morphology and increased the number of cells that had lost their normal shape and became rounded, swollen and floated in the medium (data not shown). These results confirmed that HU-585 treatment might induce the appearance of typical features of apoptosis. Next, we used caspase assay and Bcl-2 levels following treatment to better evaluate the apoptotic activity of HU-585. Staurosporine-treated cells were used as the positive control to apoptosis.

Treatment of SK-N-SH cells with 100 µM of HU-585 induced apoptosis as demonstrated by cleavage of caspase-3 represented by the appearance of activated 17 kDa and 19 kDa fragments on western blot (Figure 3A). The apoptotic effect was observed at 24 h and peaked at 48 h (Figure 3B). In order to evaluate Bcl-2 levels following treatment, we first determined its baseline levels in SK-N-SH cells in comparison to fibroblasts and human astrocyte cell line. Western blot revealed a high baseline level of Bcl-2 protein in the SK-N-SH cells in comparison to normal controls (Figure 3C). Treatment with 100 µM of HU-585 resulted in a decreased level of Bcl-2 with a better and significant effect at 48 h in comparison to 24 h (Figure 3D,E).

As senescence is generally regarded as a tumor suppressive process that evolves alongside apoptosis to suppress tumorigenesis, we next assessed the effect of treatment with HU-600 and HU-585 on cell senescence. β-Galactosidase activity was measured by blue-colored cell counting (Figure 3F). Results show that cellular senescence occurred at 48 h following treatment with HU-585, but not with HU-600 (Figure 3G).

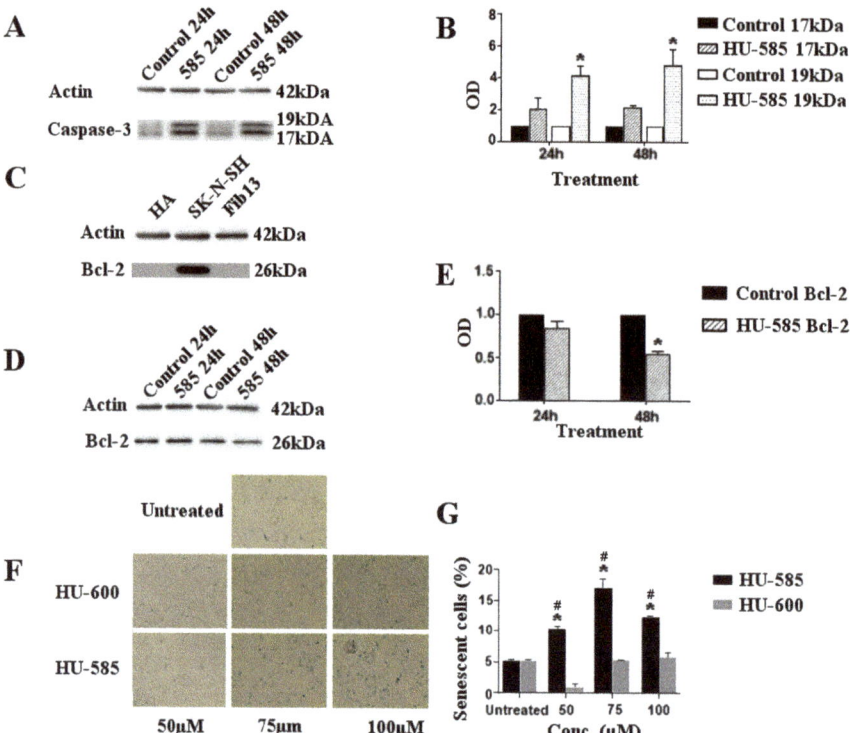

Figure 3. Growth suppression by HU-585 is mediated by apoptosis and senescence. (**A–E**) Apoptotic effects of HU-585. (**A**) Caspase-3 assay. Western blot of caspase-3 (35 kDa) cleavage to 19 kDa and 17 kDa represents the apoptotic effect of HU-585. SK-N-SH cells were treated with 100 µM of HU-585 for 24 h and 48 h. (**B**) Quantification of cleaved caspase-3. Quantification was done by Image Lab software and representation for 24 h and 48 h of incubation are shown. Cleaved 19 kDa level increased significantly in a time-dependent manner in comparison to its control following treatment with HU-585. Statistical differences at 24 h and 48 h were determined by two-way ANOVA (* $p < 0.01$). (**C**) Bcl-2 protein levels. Western blot of Bcl-2 protein levels determination for human astrocyte cell line (HA), SK-N-SH cells and fibroblast cell line (as a "normal control"). High levels of Bcl-2 protein were detected in SK-N-SH cells compared to the other cell lines. (**D,E**) Apoptotic effects of HU-585 analyzed by Bcl-2 levels following treatment. (**D**) Western blot of Bcl-2 protein levels in SK-N-SH cells following treatment with 100 µM HU-585 for 24 h and 48 h. (**E**) Quantification of Bcl-2 protein. Quantification was done by Image Lab software following treatment with 100 µM of HU-585 for 24 h and 48 h. Results revealed that the level of Bcl-2 protein decreased in a time-dependent manner, reaching maximal and significant effect at 48 h. Statistical significance was determined by Unpaired t-Test (* $p < 0.001$). (**F,G**) Senescence effect of HU-585 analyzed by β-galactosidase staining. (**F**) Activity of β-galactosidase in SK-N-SH cells following HU-600 and HU-585 treatment was measured by β-galactosidase staining. SK-N-SH cells were plated in 6-well plates and treated with 50 µM, 75 µM and 100 µM of HU-600, HU-585 or no treatment as control. Positivity for β-galactosidase following 48 h of treatment represents the cells that are in senescence. (**G**) Representation of the quantified percentages of senescent cells. Results show an increased number of senescent cells following HU-585 treatment compared to HU-600 treatment and untreated cells. Data is reported as mean ± SE of triplicates. Statistical significance was determined by GEE test. * $p < 0.05$ compared to HU-600 and # $p < 0.05$ compared to untreated cells.

Overall, these results provide evidence that treatment with HU-585 induces apoptosis and cellular senescence in SK-N-SH cells, while no such effect is demonstrated for HU-600 treatment.

3.4. Combined Treatment of HU-585 with Anti Bcl-2 Compounds ABT-263 or ABT-737 Results in Cell Growth Inhibition In Vitro and in Tumor Growth Delay In Vivo

As we have shown that SK-N-SH cells express high levels of Bcl-2 (Figure 3C), which have been shown to be important for neuroblastoma survival, we wished to study the effect of combined treatment of HU-585 with anti Bcl-2 compounds. First, MTT assay was performed to evaluate the in vitro effect of combined treatment of ABT-263 with HU-585 or HU-600. The reduction in SK-N-SH cell viability treated with the combination of HU-600 with 2.5 µM of ABT-263 was not significantly different in comparison to HU-600 alone (Figure 4A). In contrast, treatment of the cells with combination of HU-585 and 2.5 µM of ABT-263 resulted in a significantly reduced viability when compared to treatment with HU-585 alone. This effect was dose-dependent, with maximal effect observed in doses of 75 µM and 100 µM of HU-585 (Figure 4B).

Given the observed differential sensitivity of SK-N-SH cells to the various tested compounds, we further examined the in vivo antitumor effect using the nude mice Xn model. Nude immunodeficient mice bearing SK-N-SH Xns expressing mCherry were treated once daily for 21 days with HU-585, ABT-737, a combination of HU-585 and ABT-737 or with a vehicle control. For in vivo studies of senolytic compounds, ABT-737 (75 mg/kg) was used as previously described [23]. It was specifically chosen to be given IP in contrast to its closely related compound ABT-263 used in the in vitro tests that is an orally bioavailable agent. Based on the results of the in vitro studies that demonstrated a better efficacy of HU585 in comparison to its parent compound HU600 at lower doses, the doses selected for HU585 for the in vivo studies (120 mg/kg) were lower than the doses reported for HU600 treatment (200 mg/kg) in animal experiments [21]. Body weight change was assessed as an indicator of side effects and treatment toxicities. No significant weight loss was observed in any treatment group, indicating that this dosing strategy and the dosing intervals used were well tolerated and safe (Data not shown). The average total radiant efficiency signal as measured by IVIS was used to evaluate Xn response to treatment and tumor volume. At the end of treatment, the growth rate and volume of the Xns in the mice that were treated with the combination of HU-585 and ABT-737 were significantly lower in comparison to control or HU585 alone as shown in Figure 4C,D ($p < 0.05$). Moreover, the regression in tumor volume that was observed in the combined treatment group contrasted with the other groups in which progression was demonstrated. Together, the results suggest additive in vitro and in vivo anti-tumorigenic effect of combined treatment of HU-585 with the anti Bcl-2 compounds ABT-263 and ABT-737.

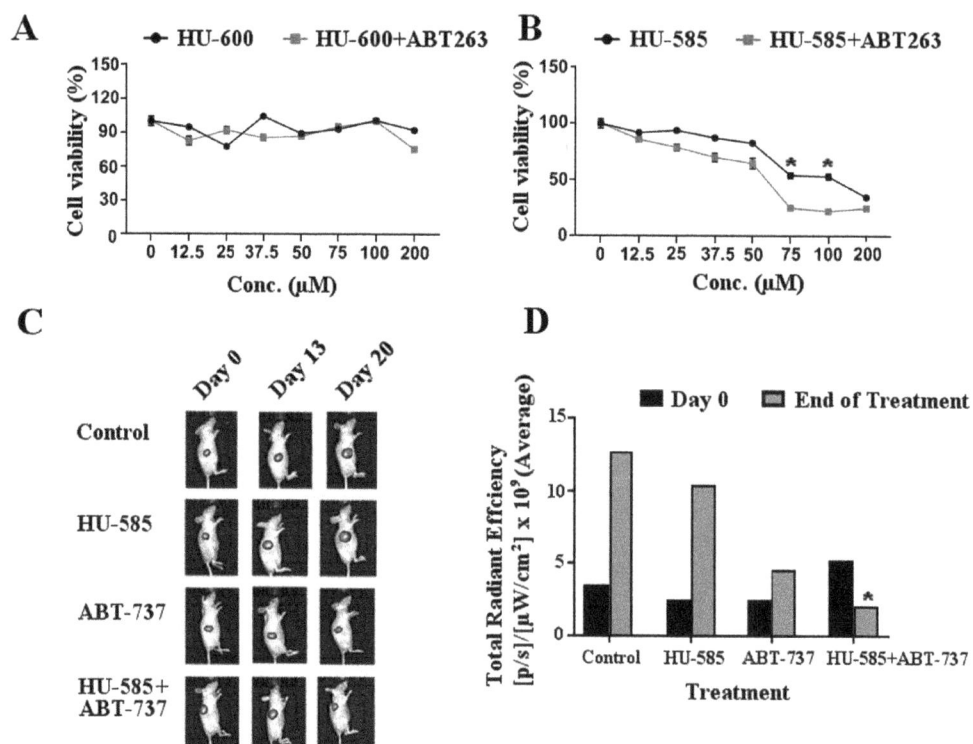

Figure 4. The combination of HU-585 with anti Bcl-2 compounds results in enhanced tumor growth delay in vitro and in vivo. (**A,B**) The effect of combination therapy of ABT-263 with HU-600 or HU-585 on SK-N-SH cells viability. The cells were plated in 96-well plate and treated with increasing concentrations of HU-600 (**A**) or HU-585 (**B**) for 72 h, with or without 2.5 μM of ABT-263. Viability measurements are shown by MTT assay and demonstrate a better effect of ABT-263 treatment combined with HU-585 in comparison to HU-585 alone. A similar effect was not obtained following combination of ABT-263 with HU-600. All values are normalized to control. Data are expressed as percentage of the vehicle control and are the mean of pooled results from several experiments performed in triplicate. Statistical significance was determined by GEE test, * $p < 0.05$ compared to HU-585 + ABT263 (0.86 < SE values < 4.22). (**C,D**) Combined treatment of ABT-737 with HU-585 inhibited tumor growth in mice model. A total of 5×10^6 SK-N-SH expressing mCherry cells were subcutaneously inoculated in the right flank of nude mice. The mice were divided into four groups and given vehicle, HU-585 (120 mg/kg), ABT-737 (75 mg/kg) or combination of HU-585 with ABT-737 (120 mg/kg, 75 mg/kg, respectively) once daily by IP injections for 21 days. (**C**) Tumor burden was followed by IVIS system once a week during treatment. (**D**) Average total radiant efficiency signal was significantly lower following combined treatment with HU-585 and ABT-737 compared to control or HU585 alone. The Kruskal-Wallis test and the post hoc Dunn's multiple comparisons test were used to evaluate significant differences in the growth rate of xenografts between treatment groups, * $p < 0.05$ compared to control and HU-585.

4. Discussions

The endocannabinoid system is currently under intense investigation due to the therapeutic potential of endocannabinoids as treatment options for cancer. Structural modifications of these substances are under investigation and synthesis of novel derivatives with better properties is being explored. Therefore, the aim of this study was to investigate the anti-tumorigenic effect of HU-585, a novel compound obtained by a combination of features of the endocannabinoid anandamide and the drug Minerval (HU-600), expecting to potentiate the antitumorigenic effects of HU-600 against neuroblastoma, an aggressive and resistant pediatric tumor in which identification of new therapeutic strategies are needed.

Minerval, a nontoxic synthetic analog of oleic acid (OA), represents a new class of orally bioavailable lipids used for membrane lipid therapy (MLT). MLT is a new rapidly evolving approach for treating cancer, in which the cellular membranes rather than specific proteins constitute the therapeutic target [22].

In the search for molecules capable of regulating membrane lipid structure, oleic acid was found to be the most active in many types of cancers [24]. However, the therapeutic effect of oleic acid is limited due to its rapid metabolism [25]. In contrast, its synthetic analog, Minerval, is believed to have a more long-lasting pharmacological effect, which favors its therapeutic effect [26]. Minerval has been shown to restore the normal membrane lipid structure and composition in certain tumor cells [27] and by this to inhibit membrane protein-associated aberrant signaling pathways, such as RAS/MAPK and PI3K/AKT pathways [28]. By contrast, Minerval does not significantly alter membrane lipid composition in non-tumor cells, which explains its specificity for cancer cells and the lack of undesired side effects [29]. Moreover, the difference in IC50 values between normal cells (>5000 µM) and cancer cells (30–200 µM) and minimum lethal dose >3000 mg/kg in rats indicate that the therapeutic window for this drug is far below the maximum tolerated dose (or minimum lethal dose), unlike most anticancer drugs currently used. These facts support the specificity of Minerval and its use as a therapy agent to treat cancer. This efficacy and lack of toxicity at therapeutic doses has been acknowledged by the European Medicines Agency (EMA) to designate 2OHOA orphan drug for the treatment of glioma [16].

In a similar way, endocannabinoids, such as AEA are lipid-based derivatives that demonstrate anti-tumorigenic effects mediated by modulation of the ERK and AKT signaling pathways [30,31]. We have previously shown that the ethanolamides of fatty acids have a better anticancer profile than the acids themselves [32]; hence, we synthesized and tested the ethanolamide derivative of Minerval. The novel compound, chemically closely related to Minerval, also resembles the endocannabinoid anandamide (AEA) found in the mammalian body [33]. As Minerval and AEA exert similar protective effects against cancer, we assumed that a molecule that is a derivative of both may have a better anticancer effect while maintaining the high safety profile typical of these two compounds.

To investigate the anti-tumorigenic effects and the mechanisms behind the effects of Minerval (HU-600) and the novel derivate HU-585 on SK-N-SH NBL cell line, cell viability, CFU, and migration in response to treatment were first analyzed followed by apoptosis and senescence studies.

We found that treatment with either HU-600 and HU-585 had an antiproliferative effect as demonstrated by MTT and by CFU assays. HU-600 had only a modest effect on the viability of these cells with a significantly better effect of the derivate HU-585. In addition, as membrane lipid composition has been shown to influence cancer cell migration abilities [34–36] we next explored whether HU-600 and its derivative HU-585 can disrupt the migratory ability of NBL cells, a crucial step in the metastatic process and in tumor dissemination. Using migration assay, we found that HU-585 had a better antimigratory effect on NBL cells in comparison to HU-600. Therefore, the conversion of HU-600 to its ethanolamide, leading to HU-585, increases the pharmacological potency of this drug, regarding viability and migration ability of NBL cells.

Impaired apoptosis plays an important role in tumorigenesis and tumor resistance to oncologic treatment [37]. The mechanism of apoptosis is evolutionarily conserved and is executed by a family of proteins called caspases, whose activation is mainly regulated by the anti- apoptotic Bcl-2 family proteins, including Bcl-2, Bcl-XL, Bcl-w, Mcl-,1 and Bfl-1/A1 [38]. HU-600 has been shown to induce apoptosis in several cancer cell lines [39], hence we sought to explore apoptosis as a possible anti-tumorigenic mechanism of its derivative

HU-585. We showed that HU-585 induces apoptosis as demonstrated by increased levels of active caspase-3 and a decreased expression of Bcl-2, both markers of apoptosis [40–42].

Bcl-2 expression was reported to be strongly increased in most NBL tumors, supporting that Bcl-2 antagonists may have clinical utility for a large subset of patients [43]. Indeed, preclinical studies using Bcl-2-specific inhibitors have demonstrated anti-tumor activity in neuroblastoma tumors with high Bcl-2 levels. Currently, Bcl-2 inhibitors in combination with classical cytostatic drugs are being investigated in clinical trials for the treatment of relapsed or refractory neuroblastoma [44].

Many oncogenic stimuli leading to apoptosis can also induce senescence, which is a special state of durable cell cycle arrest. Hence, further to our observation related to the proapoptotic properties of HU-585, we decided to explore whether HU-600 and HU-585 also induce senescence in SK-N-SH NBL cell line. Our results demonstrate that cells treated with HU-585 exhibited senescence in contrast to cells treated with HU-600. Senescence is generally regarded as a tumor suppressive process which evolved alongside apoptosis to suppress tumorigenesis and tumor progression and is considered as an important alternative cell fate to apoptosis [45,46]. Thus, one way to enhance anti-cancer treatment is to use compounds that induce senescence. To this end, senescence-inducing compounds have been developed, including CDK4/6 inhibitors, such as abemaciclib, palbociclib, and ribociclib [47,48]. With respect to neuroblastoma, LEE011, a highly specific CDK4/6 inhibitor caused cell-cycle arrest and cellular senescence in a large subset of neuroblastoma cell line and Xn models [49]. Because this class of drugs has shown promise in treating several cancers in pre-clinical and clinical studies [47–49], high-throughput screens have been employed to find additional drug targets that trigger senescence in cancer cells [50]. Based on our present findings, we think that HU-585 can also be considered as a senescence-inducing compound and is a promising candidate for further testing and implementation in current treatment protocols of neuroblastoma patients.

Paradoxically, senescence has also been proposed to have pro-tumorigenic effects. Accumulating evidence indicates that, following treatment, senescent tumor cells promote tumor relapse, aggressiveness, and metastases via upregulation of antiapoptotic mechanisms [51] and by secretion of cytokines and growth factors that may promote the proliferation of tumor cells [52]. In contrast to apoptosis, senescent cells are stably viable and have the potential to influence neighboring cells through secreted soluble factors, known as the senescence-associated secretory phenotype (SASP), which may have proneoplastic properties, including angiogenesis, epithelial—mesenchymal transitions, and differentiation within the local microenvironment [53–56].

Although senescence induction in cancer cells is a potential therapeutic option to reduce initial tumor growth, it seems to be an imperfect tumor-suppressive treatment. Hence, we assume that chronically persisting senescent cells should be removed by senolytic drugs, which selectively destroy such cells. These drugs can presumably be given in combination with other cancer therapies in order to minimize progression risk and avoid deleterious side effects [57].

It has been shown that overexpression of Bcl-2 counteracts the pro-apoptotic genes during senescence [58]. Senolytic drugs, which target the anti-apoptotic signaling through Bcl-2 family members, (Navitoclax/ABT-263 and ABT-737), were shown to be effective in inducing cell death in senescent cells [59]. As manipulation of the anti-apoptotic Bcl-2 family proteins can influence the choice between senescence and apoptosis, we decided to explore whether treatment with the combination of HU-585 with anti Bcl-2 compounds can have a better anti-tumorigenic effect compared with each drug alone in vitro and in vivo. We have shown that treatment of SK-N-SH NBL cells with a combination of anti Bcl-2 compounds and HU-585 resulted in enhanced anti-proliferative effect in vitro and reduced Xns growth in vivo in comparison to treatment with HU-585 alone.

5. Conclusions

In the search for novel therapeutic options in cancer treatment, it has become increasingly clear that in addition to targeting specific proteins, the cellular membrane constitutes an attractive target. In accordance with our findings, we conclude that the endocannabinoid-like substance HU-585, used for MLT, can halt the growth and dissemination of neuroblastoma cancer cells through apoptosis and senescence induction. Although senescence is beneficial for arresting apoptosis-resistant cancer cells, inducing senescence in other situations promotes cancer relapse and secondary tumors. Based on our present findings of enhanced anti-tumorigenic effects of combination therapy by HU-585 with senolytic drugs, we propose that this approach might provide a novel complementary and less toxic therapeutic strategy for the treatment of refractory neuroblastomas. Further studies are needed to validate the efficacy of this novel approach and to explore its advantage over current established treatments.

Author Contributions: Conceptualization, R.M., A.T., H.G. and T.F.; methodology, T.F. and H.G.; software, D.D.B.-L., T.F. and H.G.; validation, T.F. and H.G.; formal analysis, E.C.-Z., S.W., S.P.-C., T.F. and H.G.; investigation, E.C.-Z., S.W., S.P.-C., T.F. and H.G.; resources, R.M., R.S., C.G.H. and D.D.B.-L.; data curation, E.C.-Z., S.W., S.P.-C., T.F. and H.G.; writing—original draft preparation, T.F. and H.G.; writing review and editing, R.S.; A.T. and R.M.; visualization, I.G.; supervision, T.F. and H.G. All authors have read and agreed to the published version of the manuscript.

Funding: This research received no external funding.

Institutional Review Board Statement: The study was conducted according to the guidelines of the Declaration of Helsinki and approved by the Institutional Review Board of Sheba Medical Center (IRB No. ANIM/803/12, since 10 February 2012).

Informed Consent Statement: Informed consent was obtained from all subjects involved in the study.

Data Availability Statement: Data is contained within the article.

Conflicts of Interest: The authors declare no conflict of interest.

References

1. Matthay, K.K.; Maris, J.M.; Schleiermacher, G.; Nakagawara, A.; Mackall, C.L.; Diller, L.; Weiss, W.A. Neuroblastoma. *Nat. Rev. Dis. Primers* **2016**, *2*, 16078. [CrossRef] [PubMed]
2. Whittle, S.B.; Smith, V.; Doherty, E.; Zhao, S.; McCarty, S.; Zage, P.E. Overview and Recent Advances in the Treatment of Neuroblastoma. *Expert Rev. Anticancer Ther.* **2017**, *17*, 369–386. [CrossRef] [PubMed]
3. Speckhart, B.; Antony, R.; Fernandez, K.S. Long-Term Side Effects of High-Risk Neuroblastoma Survivors in a Referral Center in Central Illinois. *JCO* **2017**, *35*, 129. [CrossRef]
4. Hinz, B.; Ramer, R. Cannabinoids as Anticancer Drugs: Current Status of Preclinical Research. *Br. J. Cancer* **2022**, *126*, 1–13. [CrossRef]
5. Andre, C.M.; Hausman, J.-F.; Guerriero, G. *Cannabis sativa*: The Plant of the Thousand and One Molecules. *Front. Plant Sci.* **2016**, *7*, 19. [CrossRef]
6. Shahbazi, F.; Grandi, V.; Banerjee, A.; Trant, J.F. Cannabinoids and Cannabinoid Receptors: The Story so Far. *iScience* **2020**, *23*, 101301. [CrossRef] [PubMed]
7. Wu, J. Cannabis, Cannabinoid Receptors, and Endocannabinoid System: Yesterday, Today, and Tomorrow. *Acta Pharm. Sin.* **2019**, *40*, 297–299. [CrossRef] [PubMed]
8. Sainz-Cort, A.; Müller-Sánchez, C.; Espel, E. Anti-Proliferative and Cytotoxic Effect of Cannabidiol on Human Cancer Cell Lines in Presence of Serum. *BMC Res. Notes* **2020**, *13*, 389. [CrossRef]
9. Hosami, F.; Ghadimkhah, M.H.; Salimi, V.; Ghorbanhosseini, S.S.; Tavakoli-Yaraki, M. The Strengths and Limits of Cannabinoids and Their Receptors in Cancer: Insights into the Role of Tumorigenesis-Underlying Mechanisms and Therapeutic Aspects. *Biomed. Pharmacother.* **2021**, *144*, 112279. [CrossRef]
10. Ramer, R.; Schwarz, R.; Hinz, B. Modulation of the Endocannabinoid System as a Potential Anticancer Strategy. *Front. Pharmacol.* **2019**, *10*, 430. [CrossRef]
11. Huang, L.; Ramirez, J.C.; Frampton, G.A.; Golden, L.E.; Quinn, M.A.; Pae, H.Y.; Horvat, D.; Liang, L.; DeMorrow, S. Anandamide Exerts Its Antiproliferative Actions on Cholangiocarcinoma by Activation of the GPR55 Receptor. *Lab. Investig.* **2011**, *91*, 1007–1017. [CrossRef]
12. Pagano, E.; Borrelli, F. Targeting Cannabinoid Receptors in Gastrointestinal Cancers for Therapeutic Uses: Current Status and Future Perspectives. *Expert Rev. Gastroenterol. Hepatol.* **2017**, *11*, 871–873. [CrossRef] [PubMed]

13. Hsu, S.-S.; Huang, C.-J.; Cheng, H.-H.; Chou, C.-T.; Lee, H.-Y.; Wang, J.-L.; Chen, I.-S.; Liu, S.-I.; Lu, Y.-C.; Chang, H.-T.; et al. Anandamide-Induced Ca^{2+} Elevation Leading to P38 MAPK Phosphorylation and Subsequent Cell Death via Apoptosis in Human Osteosarcoma Cells. *Toxicology* 2007, *231*, 21–29. [CrossRef] [PubMed]
14. Ma, C.; Wu, T.-T.; Jiang, P.-C.; Li, Z.-Q.; Chen, X.-J.; Fu, K.; Wang, W.; Gong, R. Anti-carcinogenic Activity of Anandamide on Human Glioma In Vitro and In Vivo. *Mol. Med. Rep.* 2016, *13*, 1558–1562. [CrossRef] [PubMed]
15. Massalha, W.; Markovits, M.; Pichinuk, E.; Feinstein-Rotkopf, Y.; Tarshish, M.; Mishra, K.; Llado, V.; Weil, M.; Escriba, P.V.; Kakhlon, O. Minerval (2-Hydroxyoleic Acid) Causes Cancer Cell Selective Toxicity by Uncoupling Oxidative Phosphorylation and Compromising Bioenergetic Compensation Capacity. *Biosci. Rep.* 2019, *39*, BSR20181661. [CrossRef]
16. Terés, S.; Lladó, V.; Higuera, M.; Barceló-Coblijn, G.; Martin, M.L.; Noguera-Salvà, M.A.; Marcilla-Etxenike, A.; García-Verdugo, J.M.; Soriano-Navarro, M.; Saus, C.; et al. 2-Hydroxyoleate, a Nontoxic Membrane Binding Anticancer Drug, Induces Glioma Cell Differentiation and Autophagy. *Proc. Natl. Acad. Sci. USA* 2012, *109*, 8489. [CrossRef]
17. Torgersen, M.L.; Klokk, T.I.; Kavaliauskiene, S.; Klose, C.; Simons, K.; Skotland, T.; Sandvig, K. The Anti-Tumor Drug 2-Hydroxyoleic Acid (Minerval) Stimulates Signaling and Retrograde Transport. *Oncotarget* 2016, *7*, 86871–86888. [CrossRef]
18. Martin, M.L.; Barceló-Coblijn, G.; de Almeida, R.F.M.; Noguera-Salvà, M.A.; Terés, S.; Higuera, M.; Liebisch, G.; Schmitz, G.; Busquets, X.; Escribá, P.V. The Role of Membrane Fatty Acid Remodeling in the Antitumor Mechanism of Action of 2-Hydroxyoleic Acid. *Biochim. Biophys. Acta (BBA)-Biomembr.* 2013, *1828*, 1405–1413. [CrossRef]
19. Fisher, T.; Golan, H.; Schiby, G.; Prichen, S.; Smoum, R.; Moshe, I.; Peshes-Yaloz, N.; Castiel, A.; Waldman, D.; Gallily, R.; et al. In Vitro and in Vivo Efficacy of Non-Psychoactive Cannabidiol in Neuroblastoma. *Curr. Oncol.* 2016, *23*, 15–22. [CrossRef]
20. Adam, W.; Lazarus, M.; Schmerder, A.; Humpf, H.-U.; Saha-Möller, C.R.; Schreier, P. Synthesis of Optically Active α-Hydroxy Acids by Kinetic Resolution Through Lipase-Catalyzed Enantioselective Acetylation. *Eur. J. Org. Chem.* 1998, *1998*, 2013–2018. [CrossRef]
21. Jang, E.-J.; Choi, W.R.; Kim, S.-Y.; Hong, S.-S.; Rhee, I.; Lee, S.-J.; Choi, S.W.; Choi, H.-G.; Lim, S.-J. 2-Hydroxyoleic Acid-Inserted Liposomes as a Multifunctional Carrier of Anticancer Drugs. *Drug Deliv.* 2017, *24*, 1587–1597. [CrossRef] [PubMed]
22. Escribá, P.V. Membrane-Lipid Therapy: A Historical Perspective of Membrane-Targeted Therapies—From Lipid Bilayer Structure to the Pathophysiological Regulation of Cells. *Biochim. Biophys. Acta (BBA)-Biomembr.* 2017, *1859*, 1493–1506. [CrossRef] [PubMed]
23. Mason, K.D.; Vandenberg, C.J.; Scott, C.L.; Wei, A.H.; Cory, S.; Huang, D.C.S.; Roberts, A.W. In Vivo Efficacy of the Bcl-2 Antagonist ABT-737 against Aggressive Myc-Driven Lymphomas. *Proc. Natl. Acad. Sci. USA* 2008, *105*, 17961–17966. [CrossRef] [PubMed]
24. Jiang, L.; Wang, W.; He, Q.; Wu, Y.; Lu, Z.; Sun, J.; Liu, Z.; Shao, Y.; Wang, A. Oleic Acid Induces Apoptosis and Autophagy in the Treatment of Tongue Squamous Cell Carcinomas. *Sci. Rep.* 2017, *7*, 11277. [CrossRef] [PubMed]
25. Yang, Q.; Alemany, R.; Casas, J.; Kitajka, K.; Lanier, S.M.; Escriba, P.V. Influence of the Membrane Lipid Structure on Signal Processing via G Protein-Coupled Receptors. *Mol. Pharmacol.* 2005, *68*, 210–217. [CrossRef] [PubMed]
26. Wȩder, K.; Mach, M.; Hąc-Wydro, K.; Wydro, P. Studies on the Interactions of Anticancer Drug-Minerval—with Membrane Lipids in Binary and Ternary Langmuir Monolayers. *Biochim. Biophys. Acta (BBA)-Biomembr.* 2018, *1860*, 2329–2336. [CrossRef]
27. Piotto, S.; Concilio, S.; Bianchino, E.; Iannelli, P.; López, D.J.; Terés, S.; Ibarguren, M.; Barceló-Coblijn, G.; Martin, M.L.; Guardiola-Serrano, F.; et al. Differential Effect of 2-Hydroxyoleic Acid Enantiomers on Protein (Sphingomyelin Synthase) and Lipid (Membrane) Targets. *Biochim. Biophys. Acta* 2014, *1838*, 1628–1637. [CrossRef]
28. Ibarguren, M.; López, D.J.; Encinar, J.A.; González-Ros, J.M.; Busquets, X.; Escribá, P.V. Partitioning of Liquid-Ordered/Liquid-Disordered Membrane Microdomains Induced by the Fluidifying Effect of 2-Hydroxylated Fatty Acid Derivatives. *Biochim. Biophys. Acta (BBA)-Biomembr.* 2013, *1828*, 2553–2563. [CrossRef] [PubMed]
29. Barceló-Coblijn, G.; Martin, M.L.; de Almeida, R.F.; Noguera-Salvà, M.A.; Marcilla-Etxenike, A.; Guardiola-Serrano, F.; Lüth, A.; Kleuser, B.; Halver, J.E.; Escribá, P.V. Sphingomyelin and Sphingomyelin Synthase (SMS) in the Malignant Transformation of Glioma Cells and in 2-Hydroxyoleic Acid Therapy. *Proc. Natl. Acad. Sci. USA* 2011, *108*, 19569–19574. [CrossRef] [PubMed]
30. Patsos, H.A.; Greenhough, A.; Hicks, D.J.; Al Kharusi, M.; Collard, T.J.; Lane, J.D.; Paraskeva, C.; Williams, A.C. The Endogenous Cannabinoid, Anandamide, Induces COX-2-Dependent Cell Death in Apoptosis-Resistant Colon Cancer Cells. *Int. J. Oncol.* 2010, *37*, 187–193. [CrossRef]
31. Orellana-Serradell, O.; Poblete, C.E.; Sanchez, C.; Castellón, E.A.; Gallegos, I.; Huidobro, C.; Llanos, M.N.; Contreras, H.R. Proapoptotic Effect of Endocannabinoids in Prostate Cancer Cells. *Oncol. Rep.* 2015, *33*, 1599–1608. [CrossRef]
32. Brown, I.; Cascio, M.G.; Wahle, K.W.J.; Smoum, R.; Mechoulam, R.; Ross, R.A.; Pertwee, R.G.; Heys, S.D. Cannabinoid Receptor-Dependent and -Independent Anti-Proliferative Effects of Omega-3 Ethanolamides in Androgen Receptor-Positive and -Negative Prostate Cancer Cell Lines. *Carcinogenesis* 2010, *31*, 1584–1591. [CrossRef] [PubMed]
33. Devane, W.A.; Hanus, L.; Breuer, A.; Pertwee, R.G.; Stevenson, L.A.; Griffin, G.; Gibson, D.; Mandelbaum, A.; Etinger, A.; Mechoulam, R. Isolation and Structure of a Brain Constituent That Binds to the Cannabinoid Receptor. *Science* 1992, *258*, 1946–1949. [CrossRef] [PubMed]
34. Szlasa, W.; Zendran, I.; Zalesińska, A.; Tarek, M.; Kulbacka, J. Lipid Composition of the Cancer Cell Membrane. *J. Bioenerg. Biomembr.* 2020, *52*, 321–342. [CrossRef] [PubMed]
35. Li, Y.C.; Park, M.J.; Ye, S.-K.; Kim, C.-W.; Kim, Y.-N. Elevated Levels of Cholesterol-Rich Lipid Rafts in Cancer Cells Are Correlated with Apoptosis Sensitivity Induced by Cholesterol-Depleting Agents. *Am. J. Pathol.* 2006, *168*, 1107–1118. [CrossRef]

36. Guerra, F.S.; da Sampaio, L.; Konig, S.; Bonamino, M.; Rossi, M.I.D.; Costa, M.L.; Fernandes, P.; Mermelstein, C. Membrane Cholesterol Depletion Reduces Breast Tumor Cell Migration by a Mechanism That Involves Non-Canonical Wnt Signaling and IL-10 Secretion. *Transl. Med. Commun.* **2016**, *1*, 3. [CrossRef]
37. Zhang, X.; Liu, X.; Zhou, D.; Zheng, G. Targeting Anti-Apoptotic BCL-2 Family Proteins for Cancer Treatment. *Future Med. Chem.* **2020**, *12*, 563–565. [CrossRef]
38. Walensky, L.D. BCL-2 in the Crosshairs: Tipping the Balance of Life and Death. *Cell Death Differ.* **2006**, *13*, 1339–1350. [CrossRef]
39. Llado, V.; Gutierrez, A.; Martínez, J.; Casas, J.; Terés, S.; Higuera, M.; Galmés, A.; Saus, C.; Besalduch, J.; Busquets, X.; et al. Minerval Induces Apoptosis in Jurkat and Other Cancer Cells. *J. Cell. Mol. Med.* **2010**, *14*, 659–670. [CrossRef]
40. Ashkenazi, A.; Fairbrother, W.J.; Leverson, J.D.; Souers, A.J. From Basic Apoptosis Discoveries to Advanced Selective BCL-2 Family Inhibitors. *Nat. Rev. Drug Discov.* **2017**, *16*, 273–284. [CrossRef]
41. Edison, N.; Curtz, Y.; Paland, N.; Mamriev, D.; Chorubczyk, N.; Haviv-Reingewertz, T.; Kfir, N.; Morgenstern, D.; Kupervaser, M.; Kagan, J.; et al. Degradation of Bcl-2 by XIAP and ARTS Promotes Apoptosis. *Cell Rep.* **2017**, *21*, 442–454. [CrossRef]
42. Kirsch, D.G.; Doseff, A.; Chau, B.N.; Lim, D.-S.; de Souza-Pinto, N.C.; Hansford, R.; Kastan, M.B.; Lazebnik, Y.A.; Hardwick, J.M. Caspase-3-Dependent Cleavage of Bcl-2 Promotes Release of Cytochrome c. *J. Biol. Chem.* **1999**, *274*, 21155–21161. [CrossRef] [PubMed]
43. Lestini, B.J.; Goldsmith, K.C.; Fluchel, M.N.; Liu, X.; Chen, N.L.; Goyal, B.; Pawel, B.R.; Hogarty, M.D. Mcl1 Downregulation Sensitizes Neuroblastoma to Cytotoxic Chemotherapy and Small Molecule Bcl2-Family Antagonists. *Cancer Biol. Ther.* **2009**, *8*, 1587–1595. [CrossRef]
44. Place, A.E.; Goldsmith, K.; Bourquin, J.-P.; Loh, M.L.; Gore, L.; Morgenstern, D.A.; Sanzgiri, Y.; Hoffman, D.; Zhou, Y.; Ross, J.A.; et al. Accelerating Drug Development in Pediatric Cancer: A Novel Phase I Study Design of Venetoclax in Relapsed/Refractory Malignancies. *Future Oncol.* **2018**, *14*, 2115–2129. [CrossRef] [PubMed]
45. Childs, B.G.; Baker, D.J.; Kirkland, J.L.; Campisi, J.; van Deursen, J.M. Senescence and Apoptosis: Dueling or Complementary Cell Fates? *EMBO Rep.* **2014**, *15*, 1139–1153. [CrossRef]
46. Wyld, L.; Bellantuono, I.; Tchkonia, T.; Morgan, J.; Turner, O.; Foss, F.; George, J.; Danson, S.; Kirkland, J.L. Senescence and Cancer: A Review of Clinical Implications of Senescence and Senotherapies. *Cancers* **2020**, *12*, 2134. [CrossRef]
47. Turner, N.C.; Ro, J.; André, F.; Loi, S.; Verma, S.; Iwata, H.; Harbeck, N.; Loibl, S.; Huang Bartlett, C.; Zhang, K.; et al. Palbociclib in Hormone-Receptor-Positive Advanced Breast Cancer. *N. Engl. J. Med.* **2015**, *373*, 209–219. [CrossRef]
48. Goldman, J.W.; Shi, P.; Reck, M.; Paz-Ares, L.; Koustenis, A.; Hurt, K.C. Treatment Rationale and Study Design for the JUNIPER Study: A Randomized Phase III Study of Abemaciclib with Best Supportive Care Versus Erlotinib with Best Supportive Care in Patients with Stage IV Non-Small-Cell Lung Cancer with a Detectable KRAS Mutation Whose Disease Has Progressed After Platinum-Based Chemotherapy. *Clin. Lung Cancer* **2016**, *17*, 80–84. [CrossRef] [PubMed]
49. Rader, J.; Russell, M.R.; Hart, L.S.; Nakazawa, M.S.; Belcastro, L.T.; Martinez, D.; Li, Y.; Carpenter, E.L.; Attiyeh, E.F.; Diskin, S.J.; et al. Dual CDK4/CDK6 Inhibition Induces Cell-Cycle Arrest and Senescence in Neuroblastoma. *Clin. Cancer Res.* **2013**, *19*, 6173–6182. [CrossRef]
50. Wang, L.; Leite de Oliveira, R.; Wang, C.; Fernandes Neto, J.M.; Mainardi, S.; Evers, B.; Lieftink, C.; Morris, B.; Jochems, F.; Willemsen, L.; et al. High-Throughput Functional Genetic and Compound Screens Identify Targets for Senescence Induction in Cancer. *Cell Rep.* **2017**, *21*, 773–783. [CrossRef]
51. Milanovic, M.; Fan, D.N.Y.; Belenki, D.; Däbritz, J.H.M.; Zhao, Z.; Yu, Y.; Dörr, J.R.; Dimitrova, L.; Lenze, D.; Monteiro Barbosa, I.A.; et al. Senescence-Associated Reprogramming Promotes Cancer Stemness. *Nature* **2018**, *553*, 96–100. [CrossRef]
52. Llanos, S.; Serrano, M. Senescence and Cancer: In the Name of Immunosuppression. *Cancer Cell* **2016**, *30*, 507–508. [CrossRef] [PubMed]
53. Canino, C.; Mori, F.; Cambria, A.; Diamantini, A.; Germoni, S.; Alessandrini, G.; Borsellino, G.; Galati, R.; Battistini, L.; Blandino, R.; et al. SASP Mediates Chemoresistance and Tumor-Initiating-Activity of Mesothelioma Cells. *Oncogene* **2012**, *31*, 3148–3163. [CrossRef]
54. Coppé, J.-P.; Kauser, K.; Campisi, J.; Beauséjour, C.M. Secretion of Vascular Endothelial Growth Factor by Primary Human Fibroblasts at Senescence. *J. Biol. Chem.* **2006**, *281*, 29568–29574. [CrossRef]
55. Coppé, J.-P.; Patil, C.K.; Rodier, F.; Sun, Y.; Muñoz, D.P.; Goldstein, J.; Nelson, P.S.; Desprez, P.-Y.; Campisi, J. Senescence-Associated Secretory Phenotypes Reveal Cell-Nonautonomous Functions of Oncogenic RAS and the P53 Tumor Suppressor. *PLoS Biol.* **2008**, *6*, 2853–2868. [CrossRef] [PubMed]
56. Parrinello, S.; Coppe, J.-P.; Krtolica, A.; Campisi, J. Stromal-Epithelial Interactions in Aging and Cancer: Senescent Fibroblasts Alter Epithelial Cell Differentiation. *J. Cell Sci.* **2005**, *118*, 485–496. [CrossRef] [PubMed]
57. Demaria, M.; O'Leary, M.N.; Chang, J.; Shao, L.; Liu, S.; Alimirah, F.; Koenig, K.; Le, C.; Mitin, N.; Deal, A.M.; et al. Cellular Senescence Promotes Adverse Effects of Chemotherapy and Cancer Relapse. *Cancer Discov.* **2017**, *7*, 165–176. [CrossRef] [PubMed]
58. Czabotar, P.E.; Lessene, G.; Strasser, A.; Adams, J.M. Control of Apoptosis by the BCL-2 Protein Family: Implications for Physiology and Therapy. *Nat. Rev. Mol. Cell Biol.* **2014**, *15*, 49–63. [CrossRef]
59. Paez-Ribes, M.; González-Gualda, E.; Doherty, G.J.; Muñoz-Espín, D. Targeting Senescent Cells in Translational Medicine. *EMBO Mol. Med.* **2019**, *11*, e10234. [CrossRef]

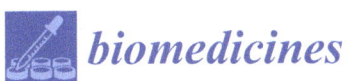

Article

Impact of Δ⁹-Tetrahydrocannabinol on Rheumatoid Arthritis Synovial Fibroblasts Alone and in Co-Culture with Peripheral Blood Mononuclear Cells

Torsten Lowin *, Christina Kok, Sophie Smutny and Georg Pongratz

Poliklinik, Funktionsbereich & Hiller Forschungszentrum für Rheumatologie, University Hospital Duesseldorf, 40225 Duesseldorf, Germany; christina.Kok@uni-duesseldorf.de (C.K.); sophie.Smutny@hhu.de (S.S.); georg.pongratz@hhu.de (G.P.)
* Correspondence: torsten.lowin@med.uni-duesseldorf.de; Tel.: +49-211-8106150

Abstract: δ9-Tetrahydrocannabinol (THC) has demonstrated anti-inflammatory effects in animal models of arthritis, but its mechanism of action and cellular targets are still unclear. The purpose of this study is to elucidate the effects of THC (0.1–25 µM) on synovial fibroblasts from patients with rheumatoid arthritis (RASF) and peripheral blood mononuclear cells (PBMC) from healthy donors in respect to proliferation, calcium mobilization, drug uptake, cytokine and immunoglobulin production. Intracellular calcium and drug uptake were determined by fluorescent dyes Cal-520 and PoPo3, respectively. Cytokine and immunoglobulin production were evaluated by ELISA. Cannabinoid receptors 1 and 2 (CB_1 and CB_2) were detected by flow cytometry. RASF express CB_1 and CB_2 and the latter was increased by tumor necrosis factor (TNF). In RASF, THC (≥5 µM) increased intracellular calcium levels/PoPo3 uptake in a TRPA1-dependent manner and reduced interleukin-8 (IL-8) and matrix metalloprotease 3 (MMP-3) production at high concentrations (25 µM). Proliferation was slightly enhanced at intermediate THC concentrations (1–10 µM) but was completely abrogated at 25 µM. In PBMC alone, THC decreased interleukin-10 (IL-10) production and increased immunoglobulin G (IgG). In PBMC/RASF co-culture, THC decreased TNF production when cells were stimulated with interferon-γ (IFN-γ) or CpG. THC provides pro- and anti-inflammatory effects in RASF and PBMC. This is dependent on the activating stimulus and concentration of THC. Therefore, THC might be used to treat inflammation in RA but it might need titrating to determine the effective concentration.

Keywords: synovial fibroblast; rheumatoid arthritis; cannabis; tetrahydrocannabinol; cytokines; calcium; PBMC; cannabinoid receptors; TRPA1

1. Introduction

Cannabis sativa contains over 400 compounds, with tetrahydrocannabinol (THC) and cannabidiol (CBD) being the most thoroughly investigated [1]. THC binds to classical cannabinoid receptors (CB_1 and CB_2) with high affinity but also targets other receptors, enzymes and transporters at higher concentrations [2–4]. While CB_1 is the most abundant G-protein-coupled receptor in the brain [5], CB_2 is mainly located peripherally [6,7]. Anti-inflammatory effects of cannabinoids occur directly via CB_2 activation [8], but also by modulation of sympathetic nervous system activity [9]. THC, an agonist at CB_1 and CB_2, resembles the effect of endogenous cannabinoids (endocannabinoids), which are produced by a wide variety of cells [10]. Of note, endocannabinoids control the tone of nervous system activity, including the sympathetic nervous system [11]. THC mediates its effects via several mechanisms: (1) directly on cells that carry target receptors for THC (e.g., CB_1 and CB_2) [12], (2) indirectly by modulation of neurotransmitter release via CB_1 on nerve terminals (e.g., acetylcholine and norepinephrine) in the periphery [13], and (3) indirectly by binding to fatty acid binding proteins, which releases endocannabinoids from these binding sites and increases their endogenous concentration [4]. THC has analgesic properties, but

also demonstrates antiedema and anti-inflammatory effects [14–18] in animal models of arthritis. However, it is still unclear what receptors and pathways are engaged by THC to elicit these effects.

Rheumatoid arthritis (RA) is an autoimmune inflammatory disorder that is characterized by joint destruction, elevated cytokine burden and several comorbidities such as depression, cachexia, insulin resistance and fatigue [19–22]. Cannabinoids might reduce pain and inflammation in RA [15,16] but they might also have beneficial effects on RA comorbidities, since these are often mediated by alterations in sympathetic nervous system activity [23–26]. One major mediator of joint pathology in RA is synovial fibroblasts (SF), which not only produce cytokines and matrix metalloproteinases, but also actively engage in cartilage invasion [27]. Rheumatoid arthritis synovial fibroblasts (RASF) express cannabinoid receptors, and activation of CB_1 or CB_2 initiates MAP kinase signaling [28]. While CB_1 mediates adhesion of RASF to extracellular matrix [29], CB_2 activation was described as anti-inflammatory in several studies [30,31] but, in contrast, it was also identified as proinflammatory by initiating transforming growth factor beta-activated kinase 1 kinase signaling [32]. In addition, inhibitory effects of synthetic cannabinoids on cytokine production were cannabinoid-receptor-independent [31,33]. In peripheral blood mononuclear cells (PBMC), similar results regarding the effects of cannabinoids have been documented. Springs et al. showed a reduction in splenocyte cytokine production by THC, which was independent of cannabinoid receptors [34]. CB_2, in general, affects many aspects of the immune response but, in most models of experimental arthritis in rodents, CB_2 reduces inflammation and arthritis severity by inhibiting immune cell migration to sites of inflammation [35–39].

In this study, we investigate the effects of THC (0.1–25 µM) on RASF in respect to intracellular calcium levels, drug uptake, proliferation and cytokine production. In addition, we perform RASF/PBMC co-cultures and PBMC monocultures under the influence of THC (1 and 10 µM) and determine cytokine and immunoglobulin production. This study might help to pinpoint the effects of cannabis and THC on arthritic disease and establish a rationale for why medical cannabis might be an appropriate adjunct therapy in RA.

2. Materials and Methods

2.1. Patients

A total of 14 patients with long-standing RA fulfilling the American College of Rheumatology revised criteria for RA [40] were included in this study. The RA group comprised of 14 females with a mean age of 68 years ± 10 years. C-reactive protein was 7.1 mg/dL ± 9.2 mg/dL 3 out of 14 glucocorticoids, 4 out of 14 methotrexate, 1 out of 14 sulfasalazine, 3 out of 14 biologicals and 1 out of 14 JAK inhibitor. All patients underwent elective knee joint replacement surgery, and they were informed about the purpose of the study and gave written consent. The study was approved by the Ethics Committees of the University of Düsseldorf (approval numbers 2018-87-KFogU and 2018-296-KFogU). We confirm that all experiments were performed in accordance with relevant guidelines and regulations.

2.2. Compounds

THC (Dronabinol) was obtained from THC Pharm, Frankfurt, Germany. A967079, COR170, HC030031, ruthenium red (RR) and rimonabant were obtained from Tocris/Biotechne, Wiesbaden, Germany. 1,1'-Diethyl-2,2'-cyanine iodide (Decynium-22; D22) was obtained from Sigma Aldrich, Taufkirchen, Germany. THC is a partial agonist at CB_1 and CB_2 receptors, but also at several TRP channels. It is the major psychoactive constituent of the plant *cannabis sativa*. A967079 and HC030031 are lipophilic antagonists at the TRPA1 ion channel, whereas RR unselectively blocks TRP channels at the plasma membrane. Rimonabant and COR170 are inverse agonists at CB_1 and CB_2, respectively. D22 is an inhibitor of organic cation transporters and monoamine transport.

2.3. Synovial Fibroblast and Tissue Preparation

Samples from RA synovial tissue were collected immediately after opening the knee joint capsule, and tissue was prepared for cell isolation thereafter [41]. Synovial tissue was cut into small fragments and treated with liberase (Roche Diagnostics, Mannheim, Germany) at 37 °C overnight. The cell suspension was filtered (70 µM) and centrifuged at 300 g for 10 min. After that, the pellet was treated with erythrocyte lysis buffer (20.7 g NH_4Cl, 1.97 g NH_4HCO_3, 0.09 g EDTA ad 1 L H_2O) for 5 min, recentrifuged for 10 min, and then resuspended in RPMI-1640 (Sigma Aldrich, Taufkirchen, Germany) with 10% FCS. After overnight incubation, RPMI medium was replaced with fresh medium to wash off dead cells and debris.

2.4. Intracellular Calcium and PoPo3 Uptake

In black 96-well plates, RASF were incubated with 4 µM of calcium dye Cal-520 (ab171868, Abcam, Cambridge, UK) in PBS with 0.02% Pluoronic F127 (Thermo Fisher scientific, Waltham, MA, USA, # P6866) for 60 min at 37 °C, followed by 30 min at room temperature. After washing, HBSS or PBS containing 1 µM PoPo3 iodide (Thermo Fisher scientific, # P3584) and respective antagonists/ligands/inhibitors were added for 30 min at room temperature. After that, THC was added and the intracellular Ca^{2+} concentration as well as PoPo3 uptake were evaluated with a TECAN multimode reader over 90 min.

2.5. Flow Cytometry

RASF were primed with TNF (10 ng/mL) (PeproTech, Hamburg, Germany) or left untreated for 72 h in RPMI medium with 2% FCS. Then, cells were analyzed for surface and intracellular expression of cannabinoid receptors. The following antibodies were used: CB_1 (FAB3834R, 0.2 mg/mL, 1:10, R&D Systems/Biotechne, Wiesbaden, Germany), CB_2 (FAB36551G, 0.2 mg/mL, 1:40, R&D Systems/Biotechne), Isotype MsIgG2a-Alexa 488 (IC003G, 5 µL/test, R&D Systems/Biotechne), and Isotype MsIgG2a-Alexa 647 (IC003R, 5 µL/test, R&D Systems/Biotechne5 µL/test); RASF were detached from culture dishes with citrate buffer (135 mM KCl, 15 mM $Na_3C_6H_5O_7$) and centrifuged at $300\times g$. Cells were resuspended in PBS with 10% FCS and incubated with antibodies for 30 min in the dark at room temperature. For intracellular staining, the inside stain kit was used (#130-090-477, Miltenyi biotec, Bergisch Gladbach, Germany) according to the manufacturer's instructions.

2.6. Isolation of PBMC from Peripheral Blood

PBMC were isolated using the Greiner LeucoSep Tubes (#227290, Greiner bio-one, Kremsmünster, Austria) according to manufacturer's instructions.

2.7. RASF Co-Culture with PBMC

Co-culture experiments were performed in 96-well plates (Cellstar, Greiner bio-one, Kremsmünster, Austria). In brief, 5.000 RASF were seeded in 200 µL RPMI-1640 with 10% FCS (Sigma-Aldrich) and grown for 72 h. Then, growth medium was replaced by fresh RPMI with 10% FCS, and 250.000 isolated human PBMCs were added. Cells were stimulated with cytokines/THC as indicated for 7d in RPMI medium with 10% FCS. After that, supernatants were collected and cytokine and immunoglobulin production were assessed by ELISA.

2.8. ELISA and Stimulation of SF

ELISAs for IL-6 (#555220), IL-10 (#555157) and TNF (#555212) were obtained from BD, Franklin Lakes, NJ, USA and were conducted according to the manufacturer's protocol. Immunoglobulin M (IgM) and G (IgG) were detected by an in-house ELISA. A total of 5.000 RASF were seeded in 200 µL RPMI-1640 with 10% FCS and grown for 72 h. Then, growth medium was replaced by fresh RPMI (2% FCS) and SF were primed with TNF (10 ng/mL) for 3 days to induce TRPA1 protein. After that, culture medium was replaced with RPMI (2% FCS) and THC was added for an additional 24 h. After that, supernatants were collected and analyzed.

2.9. RASF Cell Viability

Cell viability was assessed by the cell titer blue viability assay (Promega, Madison, WI, USA, # G8080) according to manufacturer's instructions.

2.10. Statistical Analysis

Statistical analysis was performed with SPSS 25 (IBM, Armonk, NY, USA). The statistic tests used were chosen according to previous reports and are given in the figure legends [42–44]. Normal distribution was determined using the Shapiro–Wilk test; equal variance was determined by Levene's test. In the case of equal variance, the Bonferroni post hoc test was used, otherwise the Dunnet's post hoc test was employed. When data are presented as box plots, the boxes represent the 25th to 75th percentiles, the lines within the boxes represent the median, and the lines outside the boxes represent the 10th and 90th percentiles. When data are presented as line plots, the line represents the mean. When data are presented as bar charts, the top of the bar represents the mean and error bars depict the standard error of the mean (sem). The level of significance was $p < 0.05$.

3. Results

3.1. RASF Express CB_1 and CB_2

In our experiments, RASF were treated with TNF (10 ng/mL) for 72 h before we conducted our experiments and, although the expression of CB_1 and CB_2 in SF was already documented [28], their regulation by TNF was only investigated by our group but under different experimental conditions [45]. We found little CB_1 expression at the cell surface but high intracellular levels that were not significantly regulated by TNF (Figure 1). CB_2 was exclusively found at the plasma membrane and it was upregulated by TNF ($p = 0.05$) (Figure 1).

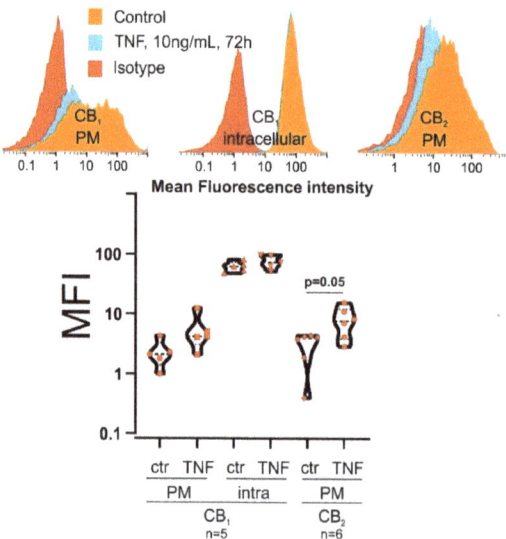

Figure 1. Flow cytometric detection of CB_1 and CB_2 in and on RASF. RASF were incubated with TNF (10 ng/mL) for 72 h, and CB_1 and CB_2 levels were determined thereafter. Upper panel: histogram; detection of CB_1 at the plasma membrane (PM) and intracellularly and CB_2 at the plasma membrane. Lower panel: violin plots; quantification of CB_1 and CB_2. *t*–test was used for comparisons. $p = 0.05$ was the level of significance.

3.2. THC Increases Intracellular Calcium in RASF Primed with TNF

Target receptors for THC include TRP ion channels [3] and CB_1 and activation [46] of either is coupled to elevations or reductions in intracellular calcium levels, respectively. Without TNF priming, THC (0.1–25 µM) did not modulate intracellular calcium levels (Figure 2A). However, when RASF were treated with TNF 72 h prior to THC addition, we detected a significant increase (up to ~200%) in intracellular calcium levels in response to THC ($p < 0.001$; 5–25 µM) (Figure 2B). This increase was not inhibited by the CB_1 antagonist/inverse agonist rimonabant (Figure 2C) and slightly modulated by the CB_2 antagonist COR170 (Figure 2D). TRPA1 is strongly upregulated by TNF [47] and, since it is also a receptor for THC, we inhibited this channel with ruthenium red (RR) (Figure 2E). RR not only increased basal intracellular calcium levels ($p < 0.001$), but also reduced THC-induced intracellular calcium levels (5 µM and 10 µM THC; $p = 0.032$ and $p < 0.001$, respectively). Previous results from our group suggest that TRPA1 is located intracellularly [45,47] and, since RR cannot actively cross the plasma membrane [48], we also employed specific lipophilic TRPA1 antagonists (Figure 2F,G). We found that both HC030031 (Figure 2F) and A967079 (Figure 2G) inhibited the stimulatory effects of THC ($p < 0.001$ for 5 µM and 10 µM THC (Figure 2F); $p < 0.001$ for 5 µM–25 µM THC (Figure 2G)) on intracellular calcium levels over a wide range of THC concentrations. The latter was more potent, since, in contrast to HC030031, it also reduced calcium elevations in response to the highest concentration of THC (25 µM, $p < 0.001$). We also conducted these experiments with PBS (Figure 2H–M) instead of HBSS, establishing a calcium-free extracellular environment. Under these conditions, alterations in intracellular calcium levels can only be elicited by emptying intracellular stores. Similar results compared to the HBSS groups were obtained but, under these conditions, the TRPA1 antagonist A967079 (Figure 2M) completely abrogated all effects of THC on intracellular calcium.

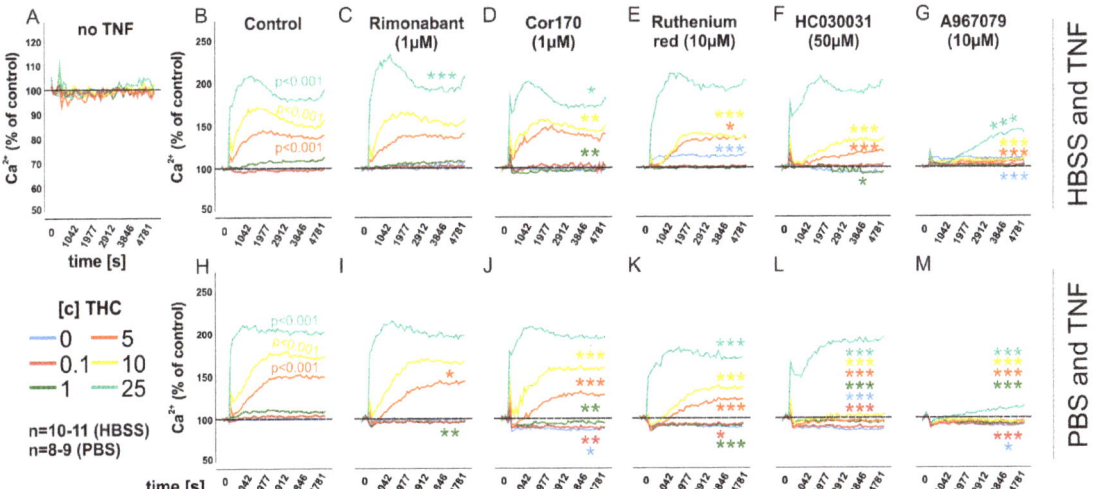

Figure 2. Mean intracellular calcium level changes in RASF in response to THC. (**A**) Intracellular calcium mobilization without TNF pre–stimulation. (**B,C**) Intracellular calcium level regulated by THC (0.1–25 µM) with TNF (10 ng/mL) pre–stimulation for 72 h and extracellular calcium (HBSS; (**B–G**)) or without calcium (PBS; (**H–M**)). *** $p < 0.001$, ** $p < 0.01$, * $p < 0.05$ for differences between antagonist treatment and control (THC only). (**B,H**) Comparisons of different THC concentrations versus control (no THC). Significant values are given in the graph. ANOVA with Bonferroni post hoc test was used for all comparisons. Rimonanbant, CB_1 inverse agonist; COR170, CB_2 inverse agonist; A967079, TRPA1 antagonist; HC-030031, TRPA1 antagonist; RR = Ruthenium Red, general TRP inhibitor.

3.3. THC Enhances PoPo3 Uptake in RASF Primed with TNF

In a previous study, we established PoPo3 as a surrogate marker for drug uptake [47], which was coupled to intracellular calcium levels and, therefore, we also assessed the ability of THC (0.1–25 µM) to modulate PoPo3 uptake. Without TNF priming, PoPo3 uptake was only slightly increased by THC (Figure 3A), whereas, after TNF stimulation, THC robustly increased PoPo3 uptake (Figure 3B; $p < 0.001$ for [c] 1 µM–25 µM of THC). Rimonabant modulated PoPo3 uptake only at low THC concentrations (0.1–1 µM), but the magnitude of uptake at these concentrations was rather small (Figure 3C). The CB_2 inverse agonist COR170 also reduced PoPo3 uptake by THC (Figure 3D; $p < 0.001$; 1 µM, 10 µM, 25 µM THC). RR modulated PoPo3 levels to all but the highest concentration of THC (Figure 3E), but increased rather than decreased its uptake. Like intracellular calcium, PoPo3 uptake was almost completely inhibited by the TRPA1 antagonists HC030031 (Figure 3F; $p < 0.001$ for all [c] of THC except 0.1 µM) and A967079 (Figure 3G, $p < 0.001$ for all [c] of THC except 0.1 µM). Decynium-22 (D22), an inhibitor of organic cation transporters [47], inhibited PoPo3 uptake alone (Figure 3H, blue line, $p = 0.018$) and together with THC (Figure 3H, $p < 0.001$ for all [c] of THC). Lastly, we investigated whether THC itself can block subsequent effects of added THC in higher concentrations and we found that it indeed inhibited further PoPo3 uptake by higher concentrations of THC (Figure 3I; $p < 0.001$, 10 µM and 25 µM). We also assessed the ability of THC to induce PoPo3 uptake without extracellular calcium in PBS (Figure 3J–Q). We confirmed our findings from the HBSS groups, but the CB_2 antagonist COR170 showed a higher efficacy in calcium-free conditions (Figure 3L; $p < 0.001$, for all [c] of THC). RR, HC030031, A967079 and D22 also inhibited Popo3 uptake almost completely (Figure 3M–O; $p < 0.001$ for all [c] of THC, except 0 µM and 0.1 µM in the A967079 and D22 group). THC itself also reduced PoPo3 uptake, but the effect was attenuated compared to the conditions with extracellular calcium (Figure 3Q).

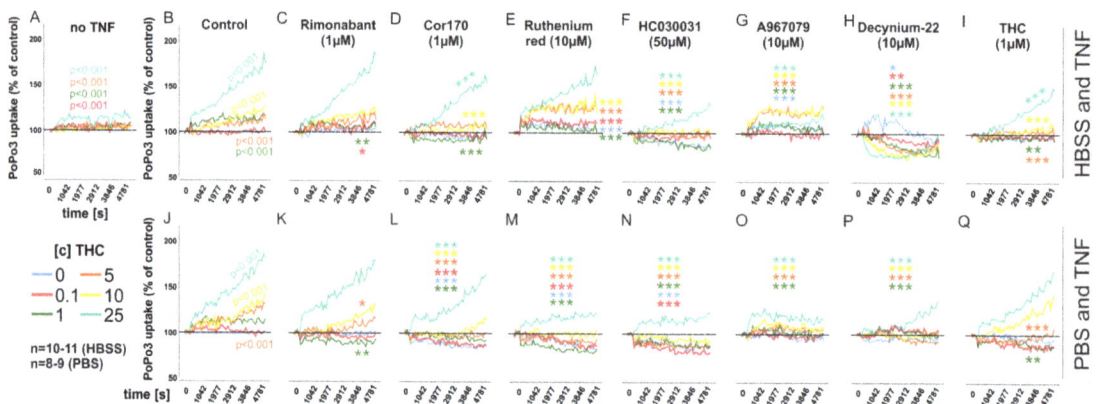

Figure 3. Mean PoPo3 uptake by RASF in response to THC. (A) PoPo3 uptake without TNF pre-stimulation, (B,C) by THC with TNF (10 ng/mL) pre-stimulation for 72 h and extracellular calcium (HBSS; (B–I)) or without calcium (PBS; (J–Q)). *** $p < 0.001$, ** $p < 0.01$, * $p < 0.05$ for differences between antagonist treatment and control (THC only, Figure 2B,J). (B,J) Comparisons of different THC concentrations versus control (no THC). Significant values are given in the graph. ANOVA with Bonferroni post hoc test was used for all comparisons. Rimonabant, CB_1 inverse agonist; COR170, CB_2 inverse agonist; A967079, TRPA1 antagonist; HC-030031, TRPA1 antagonist; RR = Ruthenium Red, general TRP inhibitor, Decynium-22, organic cation transport inhibitor.

3.4. THC Reduces Cytokine Production Only at High Concentrations

Besides intracellular calcium and PoPo3 uptake, we assessed whether THC (0.1–25 µM) also modulates cytokine production by RASF. We identified TRPA1 as an important target receptor for THC and, therefore, we induced its expression by stimulating RASF for 72 h with TNF before adding THC. THC did not modulate IL-6 or IL-8 production significantly but it blunted MMP-3 levels either alone or in combination with A967079 or rimonabant at 25 µM (Figure 4C, $p < 0.001$). IL-8 production was only reduced by THC (25 µM) when combined with A967079 ($p < 0.001$) or rimonabant ($p = 0.005$). Cell viability was slightly enhanced by THC at 5 µM ($p = 0.022$) but extensive cell death occurred at 25 µM ($p < 0.001$) (Figure 4D). In addition, cell viability was slightly increased when THC (1 µM, 5 µM and 10 µM) was combined with rimonabant or A967079, but the magnitude was small.

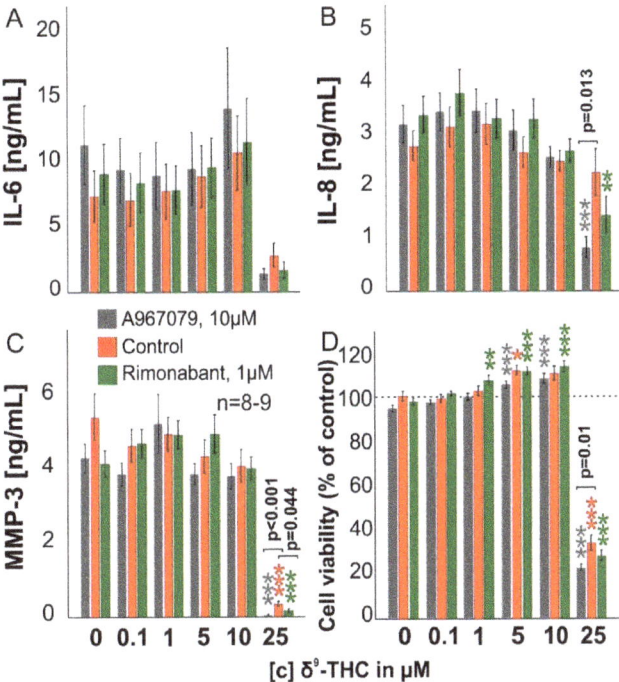

Figure 4. IL-6, IL-8, and MMP-3 production and live cell number after 72 h incubation with TNF and an additional 24 h of THC. RASF were incubated for 72 h with TNF (10 ng/mL). After wash-off, RASF were challenged with antagonists for 30 min, followed by THC (0.1–25 µM) addition for 24 h. ANOVA was used for all comparisons vs. control w/o THC. (**A**–**C**) IL-6, IL-8, and MMP-3 production after 24 h challenge with THC. (**D**) RASF cell number after 24 h challenge with THC. Significant differences between THC in different concentrations are depicted as * $p < 0.05$, ** $p < 0.01$, *** $p < 0.001$. ANOVA with Bonferroni post hoc test was used for all comparisons. Differences between THC with or without rimonabant or A9607079 are shown in the graph.

3.5. THC Has Negligible Effects on PBMC Cytokine, IgM and IgG Production

In synovial tissue, endocannabinoids are abundantly produced not only by RASF, but immune cells are also capable of producing anandamide and 2-AG [28,29,49]. Since lymphocytes and macrophages are also present in RA synovial tissue where these cells closely interact with RASF [27], we investigated the impact of THC (1 and 10 µM) on peripheral blood mononuclear cells (PBMC) alone or in co-culture with RASF (Figure 5). In co-culture with RASF, THC did not modulate IL-6 and IL-10 production but decreased TNF production when PBMC/RASF were stimulated with CpG or IFN-γ (1 µM THC, $p = 0.027$ and $p = 0.010$, respectively) (Figure 5C). Immunoglobulin G production induced by CpG was further enhanced by 1 µM and 10 µM THC, but it did not reach significance ($p = 0.077$ and $p = 0.085$, respectively) (Figure 5E). Without RASF, 10 µM THC reduced IL-10 levels in response to IFN-γ ($p = 0.011$) and CpG ($p = 0.03$) in PBMC (Figure 5G). Immunoglobulin

G production was fostered by 1 μM THC without any additional stimulus ($p = 0.026$) (Figure 5J).

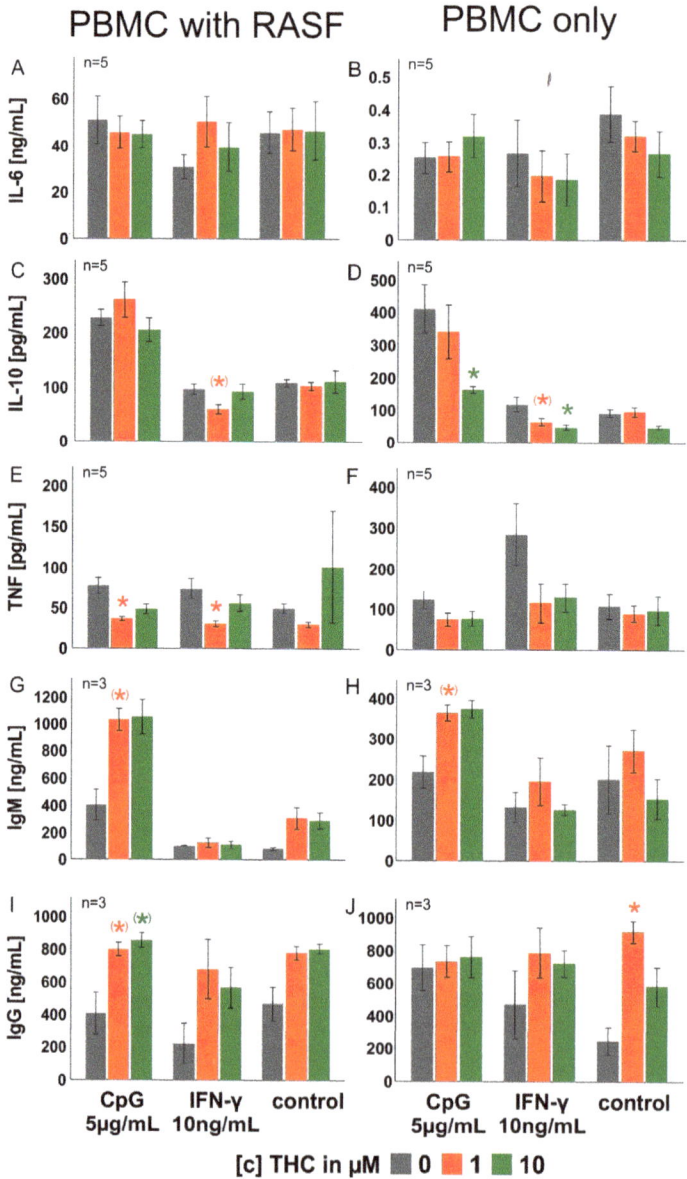

Figure 5. Cytokine production by human PBMC monoculture and co-culture with RASF in response to THC. (A,B) IL-6; (C,D) IL-10; (E,F) TNF; (G,H) immunoglobulin M (IgM) and (I,J) immunoglobulin G (IgG) production by PBMC and PBMC/RASF co-culture over 7 days. Cells were concomitantly stimulated with THC and the respective activation stimulus (IFN-γ or CpG). In co-culture experiments, RASF were stimulated with 10 ng/mL IFN-γ 72 h prior to PBMC addition to induce MHC II expression and induce an allogeneic T cell response. ANOVA with Bonferroni post hoc test was used for all comparisons. * $p < 0.05$.

4. Discussion

In this study, we show for the first time the effects of THC treatment on the function of RASF and PBMC. Firstly, we determined the expression of the main target receptors for THC, but also for endocannabinoids produced in the joint [28], CB_1 and CB_2, in and on RASF, and found CB_1 in intracellular compartments, whereas CB_2 was located at the plasma membrane. The latter was also upregulated by TNF. However, we demonstrated that THC elevates intracellular calcium and PoPo3 uptake by a TRPA1, rather than a CB receptor-dependent mechanism. RASF IL-6, IL-8 and MMP-3 production was reduced by THC only at the highest concentration investigated, and this effect was not antagonized by either TRPA1 or CB_1 antagonists, suggesting a receptor-independent effect. In addition, we showed that THC had only a minor influence on PBMC (alone or in co-culture with RASF) cytokine and immunoglobulin production.

We detected CB_1 protein intracellularly in RASF, which is line with our previous results [45]. In that study, we utilized a different antibody but it also detected CB_1 protein at the nuclear membrane, suggesting that signals initiated by this receptor are spatially confined, as already confirmed by other intracellular G-protein-coupled receptors (GPCRs) [50]. Another study showed that membrane GPCRs might "communicate" with its fraction of intracellular receptors by β-arrestin eliciting a combined response [51]. This might also be the case in RASF, since we found little but detectable cell surface expression of CB_1. CB_2 was exclusively located at the plasma membrane and its levels were regulated by TNF. In a previous study, we already demonstrated CB_2 upregulation in response to TNF, but these experiments were conducted under hypoxic conditions and CB_2 was detected by cell-based ELISA rather than flow cytometry [45].

In a next step, we investigated the effects of THC on intracellular calcium since it has been shown that CB_1, CB_2 and TRPA1 are able to modulate calcium levels [52–54]. We found that THC via TRPA1 activation elevates calcium levels and we already demonstrated that only TNF pre-stimulated RASF responded to TRPA1 agonism [54], which was confirmed in this study. In contrast to cannabidiol (CBD), THC is specific for TRPA1 and does not engage in significant off-target effects. Although both THC and CBD bind to TRPA1, CBD increased intracellular calcium levels mainly by disrupting mitochondrial calcium homeostasis with little TRPA1 contribution [47].

In previous studies, we revealed that elevations in intracellular calcium are coupled to the uptake of the cationic dye PoPo3 [47,54]. Therefore, we also investigated this uptake in response to THC and we found that intracellular PoPo3 levels increased. PoPo3 was identified as a surrogate marker for drug uptake [47], since its uptake is likely controlled by organic cation transporters that are also responsible for the uptake of several therapeutic compounds and drugs [47]. This finding might be relevant in RA therapy, since a combination of THC with an antiarthritic compound might have synergistic effects and, due to increased cellular uptake, lower drug concentrations might be necessary to elicit similar effects. In fact, this has already been demonstrated with CBD, and, in their study, the authors showed a higher efficacy of the chemotherapeutic drug doxorubicin when combined with CBD [55].

TRPA1 was identified as target receptor of THC and this channel is usually expressed at high levels in sensory nerve fibers where activation mediates the release of pain transmitters, calcitonin gene-related peptide and substance P [56]. While TRP channels are also ionotropic target receptors for endocannabinoids [57], they are also signaling partners with G-protein-coupled receptors [58]. After the identification of TRPA1 as a target receptor for THC, we investigated IL-6, IL-8, and MMP-3 production and proliferation of RASF in response to THC. We found that THC reduced cytokine levels only at the highest concentration and this effect was not antagonized by a TRPA1 inhibitor. This suggests an off-target effect, since the CB_1 antagonist rimonabant did not reverse the reduction induced by THC. CB_2 was also not involved, as we previously screened several CB_2 agonists and antagonists (data not shown) for their ability to modulate cytokine expression in SF and found no effect. This is in line with results from Fechtner et al., who showed that CB_2 ligands had negligible effects but deletion of the receptor had a proinflammatory impact on SF [32]. In addition, cell viability was impaired at high THC concentrations and we also observed extensive cell death, suggesting a cytotoxic effect by THC. Furthermore, given the affinity of THC at CB_1 and CB_2 [59], it is unlikely that only high micromolar concentrations of THC would affect cytokine production. Similar to THC, we already showed a reduction in cytokine production and cell viability by CBD [47]. At high CBD concentrations, this cannabinoid elicited the assembly of the mitochondrial permeability transition pore, which entailed cell death [47], and such a mechanism might also be employed by THC. Concomitantly with the reduction in cytokine levels, we also found reduced proliferation of RASF in response to THC, which demonstrates that cell death at least contributes to reduced cytokine levels.

In RA, lymphocytes and macrophages activate SF in synovial tissue, promoting them from a bystander to an active participant in the inflammatory process [60] and, therefore, we investigated the impact of THC on healthy PBMC alone or in co-culture with RASF. While IL-6 was increased in PBMC co-culture compared to monoculture, IL-10 and TNF levels were lower in co-culture. While IL-6 is mainly produced by RASF, IL-10 and TNF are exclusively produced by PBMC, and RASF have an inhibitory influence on production of these cytokines. A functional repression of B lymphocytes by RASF has also been confirmed in a study by Storch et al. [61]. We found that THC reduced TNF production by PBMC only in co-culture, suggesting a combined inhibitory influence of RASF and THC, while IL-10 was reduced in monoculture. Many studies showed an inhibitory effect of THC on lymphocyte function, but these studies did not investigate cytokine production [62–65]. In PBMC monoculture, THC had a significant effect on immunoglobulin G production without an activating stimulus (e.g., CpG). This suggests that THC in high concentrations is able to support T or B cell activation directly. In fact, it has been shown that T cells express TRPA1, and activation increased T cell activation and calcium influx [66]. This is in contrast to published findings that CB_2 mediates the immunosuppressive function of cannabinoids and THC via several different mechanisms [67–69], but necessary THC concentrations to activate CB_2 are much lower than those needed for TRPA1 activation. In line with this, THC in high concentrations has been found to modulate cytokine levels independent of cannabinoid receptors [34]. In general, it is yet unclear whether immunoglobulin production is enhanced or suppressed by cannabinoids. In mice, it has been shown that antigen-specific immunoglobulin M (IgM) and G (IgG) production are not affected by CB_1 and CB_2 deficiency [70]. Immunoglobulin E (IgE) production was enhanced by THC in a non-cannabinoid-receptor-dependent fashion [71], and class switching from IgM to IgE was supported by CB_2 activation in isolated murine B cells [72]. Due to these differential effects of cannabinoids on immune cells, it is difficult to predict whether THC has a stimulatory or inhibitory effect on the immune response in general. In fact, THC impairs the differentiation of monocyte-derived dendritic cells [65], regulates micro RNA relevant for T cell differentiation [73] or inhibits STAT3 phosphorylation [74], and none of these effects might regulate cytokine production in our experimental setting. In addition, THC has several cannabinoid-receptor-independent effects [34,64] and these might be different in every cell type. Single-cell transcriptomic analyses of PBMC revealed that THC does not suppress immune reactions in general but interferes with pro- and anti-inflammatory innate and adaptive pathways of the immune system [75], which might be counterbalanced in our setting.

5. Conclusions

Besides CB_1 and CB_2, we identified TRPA1 as a target receptor of THC that increases intracellular calcium levels and drug uptake in RASF. Although RASF cytokine production was not altered at relevant concentrations, THC might nevertheless be an important adjunct therapy option in RA, although endocannabinoid degradation inhibitors might be even more suitable, since endocannabinoids only elicit psychotropic effects at high concentrations [76], making the side effect profile more benign compared to THC. THC, on the one hand, might increase effective drug concentrations in target cells when administered with an antirheumatic drug (as demonstrated by PoPo3 uptake). On the other hand, THC might be used to treat comorbidities in RA and, in fact, it has been shown that THC ameliorates depression, sleep disturbances and pain [77,78]. The influence of THC on RA comorbidities might be mediated by the sympathetic nervous system, since CB_1 receptors control sympathetic outflow centrally and peripherally [9,79]. TRP channels in the nervous system increase excitability and neurotransmission [80], and, therefore, it might be possible that these channels also mediate the release of soluble mediators by peripheral cells, such as fibroblasts or tyrosine hydroxylase positive cells [81] that are increased in chronic inflammation. Although speculative, THC might trigger the release of catecholamines from tyrosine-hydroxylase-positive cells or RASF via TRPA1 activation, which would increase the sympathetic tone and provide anti-inflammatory effects via β adrenoceptor signaling [82,83]. While TRPA1 activation is the main mechanism by which RASF are modulated by THC, PBMC also respond to CB_1 or CB_2 stimulation [84]. Since THC reduced TNF at a physiological concentration of 1 μM [85], it might be a cannabinoid-receptor-driven effect. In addition, endocannabinoid levels might be increased by THC [86] in co-culture, since RASF and lymphocytes contribute to their production [29,49] and they might also be responsible for the observed inhibitory effects. In addition, THC's complex effects on the immune response (e.g., differentiation, intracellular signaling and activation of immune cells) might also support its use in chronic inflammatory conditions, such as RA.

Author Contributions: Conceptualization, T.L.; methodology, T.L., S.S. and C.K.; validation, T.L., S.S., C.K. and G.P.; formal analysis, T.L., S.S., C.K. and G.P.; investigation, T.L., C.K. and S.S.; resources, G.P.; data curation, T.L., S.S., C.K. and G.P.; writing—original draft preparation, T.L.; writing—review and editing, T.L. and G.P.; visualization, T.L.; supervision, T.L. and G.P.; project administration, T.L. All authors have read and agreed to the published version of the manuscript.

Funding: This research was funded by an unlimited grant by the HILLER foundation.

Institutional Review Board Statement: The study was conducted in accordance with the Declaration of Helsinki and approved by the local ethics committee of Düsseldorf (2018-87-KFogU and 2018-296-KFogU).

Informed Consent Statement: Informed consent was obtained from all subjects involved in the study.

Data Availability Statement: The datasets used and/or analyzed during the current study are available from the corresponding author on reasonable request.

Acknowledgments: We thank Birgit Opgenoorth for excellent technical assistance.

Conflicts of Interest: The authors declare no conflict of interest. The funders had no role in the design of the study; in the collection, analyses, or interpretation of data; in the writing of the manuscript, or in the decision to publish the results.

References

1. Atakan, Z. Cannabis, a complex plant: Different compounds and different effects on individuals. *Ther. Adv. Psychopharmacol.* **2012**, *2*, 241–254. [CrossRef] [PubMed]
2. Grotenhermen, F. Pharmacology of cannabinoids. *Neuro. Endocrinol. Lett.* **2004**, *25*, 14–23. [PubMed]
3. Muller, C.; Morales, P.; Reggio, P.H. Cannabinoid Ligands Targeting TRP Channels. *Front. Mol. Neurosci.* **2018**, *11*, 487. [CrossRef] [PubMed]
4. Deutsch, D.G. A Personal Retrospective: Elevating Anandamide (AEA) by Targeting Fatty Acid Amide Hydrolase (FAAH) and the Fatty Acid Binding Proteins (FABPs). *Front. Pharmacol.* **2016**, *7*, 370. [CrossRef] [PubMed]
5. Busquets-Garcia, A.; Bains, J.; Marsicano, G. CB1 Receptor Signaling in the Brain: Extracting Specificity from Ubiquity. *Neuropsychopharmacology* **2018**, *43*, 4–20. [CrossRef]
6. Munro, S.; Thomas, K.L.; Abu-Shaar, M. Molecular characterization of a peripheral receptor for cannabinoids. *Nature* **1993**, *365*, 61–65. [CrossRef]
7. Galiegue, S.; Mary, S.; Marchand, J.; Dussossoy, D.; Carriere, D.; Carayon, P.; Bouaboula, M.; Shire, D.; Le Fur, G.; Casellas, P. Expression of central and peripheral cannabinoid receptors in human immune tissues and leukocyte subpopulations. *Eur. J. Biochem.* **1995**, *232*, 54–61. [CrossRef]
8. Kinsey, S.G.; Naidu, P.S.; Cravatt, B.F.; Dudley, D.T.; Lichtman, A.H. Fatty acid amide hydrolase blockade attenuates the development of collagen-induced arthritis and related thermal hyperalgesia in mice. *Pharmacol. Biochem. Behav.* **2011**, *99*, 718–725. [CrossRef]

9. Mnich, S.J.; Hiebsch, R.R.; Huff, R.M.; Muthian, S. Anti-inflammatory properties of CB1-receptor antagonist involves beta2 adrenoceptors. *J. Pharmacol. Exp. Ther.* **2010**, *333*, 445–453. [CrossRef]
10. De Laurentiis, A.; Fernandez Solari, J.; Mohn, C.; Zorrilla Zubilete, M.; Rettori, V. Endocannabinoid system participates in neuroendocrine control of homeostasis. *Neuroimmunomodulation* **2010**, *17*, 153–156. [CrossRef]
11. Peters, K.Z.; Cheer, J.F.; Tonini, R. Modulating the Neuromodulators: Dopamine, Serotonin, and the Endocannabinoid System. *Trends Neurosci.* **2021**, *44*, 464–477. [CrossRef] [PubMed]
12. Watzl, B.; Scuderi, P.; Watson, R.R. Marijuana components stimulate human peripheral blood mononuclear cell secretion of interferon-gamma and suppress interleukin-1 alpha in vitro. *Int. J. Immunopharmacol.* **1991**, *13*, 1091–1097. [CrossRef]
13. Deis, S.; Srivastava, R.K.; Ruiz de Azua, I.; Bindila, L.; Baraghithy, S.; Lutz, B.; Bab, I.; Tam, J. Age-related regulation of bone formation by the sympathetic cannabinoid CB1 receptor. *Bone* **2018**, *108*, 34–42. [CrossRef] [PubMed]
14. Sofia, R.D.; Nalepa, S.D.; Harakal, J.J.; Vassar, H.B. Anti-edema and analgesic properties of delta9-tetrahydrocannabinol (THC). *J. Pharmacol. Exp. Ther.* **1973**, *186*, 646–655.
15. Ismail, M.; Hasan, H.; El-Orfali, Y.; Ismail, H.; Khawaja, G. Anti-Inflammatory, Antioxidative, and Hepatoprotective Effects of Trans Delta9-Tetrahydrocannabinol/Sesame Oil on Adjuvant-Induced Arthritis in Rats. *Evid. Based Complement. Alternat. Med* **2018**, *2018*, 9365464. [CrossRef]
16. Cox, M.L.; Welch, S.P. The antinociceptive effect of Delta9-tetrahydrocannabinol in the arthritic rat. *Eur. J. Pharmacol.* **2004**, *493*, 65–74. [CrossRef]
17. Cox, M.L.; Haller, V.L.; Welch, S.P. The antinociceptive effect of Delta9-tetrahydrocannabinol in the arthritic rat involves the CB(2) cannabinoid receptor. *Eur. J. Pharmacol.* **2007**, *570*, 50–56. [CrossRef]
18. Smith, F.L.; Fujimori, K.; Lowe, J.; Welch, S.P. Characterization of delta9-tetrahydrocannabinol and anandamide antinociception in nonarthritic and arthritic rats. *Pharmacol. Biochem. Behav.* **1998**, *60*, 183–191. [CrossRef]
19. Pezzato, S.; Bonetto, C.; Caimmi, C.; Tomassi, S.; Montanari, I.; Gnatta, M.G.; Fracassi, E.; Cristofalo, D.; Rossini, M.; Carletto, A.; et al. Depression is associated with increased disease activity and higher disability in a large Italian cohort of patients with rheumatoid arthritis. *Adv. Rheumatol.* **2021**, *61*, 57. [CrossRef]
20. Dey, M.; Parodis, I.; Nikiphorou, E. Fatigue in Systemic Lupus Erythematosus and Rheumatoid Arthritis: A Comparison of Mechanisms, Measures and Management. *J. Clin. Med.* **2021**, *10*, 3566. [CrossRef]
21. Ruscitti, P.; Cipriani, P.; Liakouli, V.; Iacono, D.; Pantano, I.; Margiotta, D.P.E.; Navarini, L.; Destro Castaniti, G.M.; Maruotti, N.; Di Scala, G.; et al. Occurrence and predictive factors of high blood pressure, type 2 diabetes, and metabolic syndrome in rheumatoid arthritis: Findings from a 3-year, multicentre, prospective, observational study. *Clin. Exp. Rheumatol.* **2021**, *39*, 995–1002. [PubMed]
22. Kemble, S.; Croft, A.P. Critical Role of Synovial Tissue-Resident Macrophage and Fibroblast Subsets in the Persistence of Joint Inflammation. *Front. Immunol.* **2021**, *12*, 715894. [CrossRef] [PubMed]
23. Lowin, T.; Straub, R.H. Cannabinoid-based drugs targeting CB1 and TRPV1, the sympathetic nervous system, and arthritis. *Arthritis Res. Ther.* **2015**, *17*, 226. [CrossRef] [PubMed]
24. Lowin, T.; Schneider, M.; Pongratz, G. Joints for joints: Cannabinoids in the treatment of rheumatoid arthritis. *Curr. Opin. Rheumatol.* **2019**, *31*, 271–278. [CrossRef]
25. Straub, R.H. Interaction of the endocrine system with inflammation: A function of energy and volume regulation. *Arthritis Res. Ther.* **2014**, *16*, 203. [CrossRef]
26. Pongratz, G.; Straub, R.H. The sympathetic nervous response in inflammation. *Arthritis Res. Ther.* **2014**, *16*, 504. [CrossRef]
27. Nygaard, G.; Firestein, G.S. Restoring synovial homeostasis in rheumatoid arthritis by targeting fibroblast-like synoviocytes. *Nat. Rev. Rheumatol.* **2020**, *16*, 316–333. [CrossRef]
28. Richardson, D.; Pearson, R.G.; Kurian, N.; Latif, M.L.; Garle, M.J.; Barrett, D.A.; Kendall, D.A.; Scammell, B.E.; Reeve, A.J.; Chapman, V. Characterisation of the cannabinoid receptor system in synovial tissue and fluid in patients with osteoarthritis and rheumatoid arthritis. *Arthritis Res. Ther.* **2008**, *10*, R43. [CrossRef]
29. Lowin, T.; Zhu, W.; Dettmer-Wilde, K.; Straub, R.H. Cortisol-mediated adhesion of synovial fibroblasts is dependent on the degradation of anandamide and activation of the endocannabinoid system. *Arthritis Rheum.* **2012**, *64*, 3867–3876. [CrossRef]
30. Gui, H.; Liu, X.; Wang, Z.W.; He, D.Y.; Su, D.F.; Dai, S.M. Expression of cannabinoid receptor 2 and its inhibitory effects on synovial fibroblasts in rheumatoid arthritis. *Rheumatology* **2014**, *53*, 802–809. [CrossRef]
31. Lowin, T.; Pongratz, G.; Straub, R.H. The synthetic cannabinoid WIN55,212-2 mesylate decreases the production of inflammatory mediators in rheumatoid arthritis synovial fibroblasts by activating CB2, TRPV1, TRPA1 and yet unidentified receptor targets. *J. Inflamm.* **2016**, *13*, 15. [CrossRef] [PubMed]
32. Fechtner, S.; Singh, A.K.; Ahmed, S. Role of cannabinoid receptor 2 in mediating interleukin-1beta-induced inflammation in rheumatoid arthritis synovial fibroblasts. *Clin. Exp. Rheumatol.* **2019**, *37*, 1026–1035. [PubMed]
33. Selvi, E.; Lorenzini, S.; Garcia-Gonzalez, E.; Maggio, R.; Lazzerini, P.E.; Capecchi, P.L.; Balistreri, E.; Spreafico, A.; Niccolini, S.; Pompella, G.; et al. Inhibitory effect of synthetic cannabinoids on cytokine production in rheumatoid fibroblast-like synoviocytes. *Clin. Exp. Rheumatol.* **2008**, *26*, 574–581. [PubMed]
34. Springs, A.E.; Karmaus, P.W.; Crawford, R.B.; Kaplan, B.L.; Kaminski, N.E. Effects of targeted deletion of cannabinoid receptors CB1 and CB2 on immune competence and sensitivity to immune modulation by Delta9-tetrahydrocannabinol. *J. Leukoc. Biol.* **2008**, *84*, 1574–1584. [CrossRef] [PubMed]

35. Montecucco, F.; Burger, F.; Mach, F.; Steffens, S. CB2 cannabinoid receptor agonist JWH-015 modulates human monocyte migration through defined intracellular signaling pathways. *Am. J. Physiol. Heart Circ. Physiol.* **2008**, *294*, H1145–H1155. [CrossRef]
36. Lunn, C.A.; Fine, J.; Rojas-Triana, A.; Jackson, J.V.; Lavey, B.; Kozlowski, J.A.; Hipkin, R.W.; Lundell, D.J.; Bober, L. Cannabinoid CB(2)-selective inverse agonist protects against antigen-induced bone loss. *Immunopharmacol. Immunotoxicol.* **2007**, *29*, 387–401. [CrossRef]
37. McDougall, J.J.; Yu, V.; Thomson, J. In vivo effects of CB2 receptor-selective cannabinoids on the vasculature of normal and arthritic rat knee joints. *Br. J. Pharmacol.* **2008**, *153*, 358–366. [CrossRef]
38. Zhu, M.; Yu, B.; Bai, J.; Wang, X.; Guo, X.; Liu, Y.; Lin, J.; Hu, S.; Zhang, W.; Tao, Y.; et al. Cannabinoid Receptor 2 Agonist Prevents Local and Systemic Inflammatory Bone Destruction in Rheumatoid Arthritis. *J. Bone Miner. Res.* **2019**, *34*, 739–751. [CrossRef]
39. Bai, J.; Ge, G.; Wang, Y.; Zhang, W.; Wang, Q.; Wang, W.; Guo, X.; Yu, B.; Xu, Y.; Yang, H.; et al. A selective CB2 agonist protects against the inflammatory response and joint destruction in collagen-induced arthritis mice. *Biomed. Pharmacother.* **2019**, *116*, 109025. [CrossRef]
40. Arnett, F.C.; Edworthy, S.M.; Bloch, D.A.; McShane, D.J.; Fries, J.F.; Cooper, N.S.; Healey, L.A.; Kaplan, S.R.; Liang, M.H.; Luthra, H.S.; et al. The American Rheumatism Association 1987 revised criteria for the classification of rheumatoid arthritis. *Arthritis Rheum.* **1988**, *31*, 315–324. [CrossRef]
41. Miller, L.E.; Justen, H.P.; Scholmerich, J.; Straub, R.H. The loss of sympathetic nerve fibers in the synovial tissue of patients with rheumatoid arthritis is accompanied by increased norepinephrine release from synovial macrophages. *FASEB J.* **2000**, *14*, 2097–2107. [CrossRef] [PubMed]
42. Panda, A.; Chen, S.; Shaw, A.C.; Allore, H.G. Statistical approaches for analyzing immunologic data of repeated observations: A practical guide. *J. Immunol. Methods* **2013**, *398–399*, 19–26. [CrossRef] [PubMed]
43. Skinner, J. Statistics for Immunologists. *Curr. Protoc. Immunol.* **2018**, *122*, 54. [CrossRef] [PubMed]
44. Lew, M. Good statistical practice in pharmacology. Problem 2. *Br. J. Pharmacol.* **2007**, *152*, 299–303. [CrossRef] [PubMed]
45. Lowin, T.; Apitz, M.; Anders, S.; Straub, R.H. Anti-inflammatory effects of N-acylethanolamines in rheumatoid arthritis synovial cells are mediated by TRPV1 and TRPA1 in a COX-2 dependent manner. *Arthritis Res. Ther.* **2015**, *17*, 321. [CrossRef]
46. Kim, D.J.; Thayer, S.A. Activation of CB1 cannabinoid receptors inhibits neurotransmitter release from identified synaptic sites in rat hippocampal cultures. *Brain Res.* **2000**, *852*, 398–405. [CrossRef]
47. Lowin, T.; Tingting, R.; Zurmahr, J.; Classen, T.; Schneider, M.; Pongratz, G. Cannabidiol (CBD): A killer for inflammatory rheumatoid arthritis synovial fibroblasts. *Cell Death Dis.* **2020**, *11*, 714. [CrossRef]
48. Viele, D.; Betz, E. Effect of the calcium entry blocker, flunarizine, on ruthenium red uptake by endothelial cells following acute electrical stimulation of rabbit carotid arteries. *Basic Res. Cardiol.* **1985**, *80*, 59–65. [CrossRef]
49. Sido, J.M.; Nagarkatti, P.S.; Nagarkatti, M. Production of endocannabinoids by activated T cells and B cells modulates inflammation associated with delayed-type hypersensitivity. *Eur. J. Immunol.* **2016**, *46*, 1472–1479. [CrossRef]
50. Goncalves-Monteiro, S.; Ribeiro-Oliveira, R.; Vieira-Rocha, M.S.; Vojtek, M.; Sousa, J.B.; Diniz, C. Insights into Nuclear G-Protein-Coupled Receptors as Therapeutic Targets in Non-Communicable Diseases. *Pharmaceuticals* **2021**, *14*, 429. [CrossRef]
51. DeNies, M.S.; Smrcka, A.V.; Schnell, S.; Liu, A.P. beta-arrestin mediates communication between plasma membrane and intracellular GPCRs to regulate signaling. *Commun. Biol.* **2020**, *3*, 789. [CrossRef] [PubMed]
52. Qian, W.J.; Yin, N.; Gao, F.; Miao, Y.; Li, Q.; Li, F.; Sun, X.H.; Yang, X.L.; Wang, Z. Cannabinoid CB1 and CB2 receptors differentially modulate L- and T-type Ca^{2+} channels in rat retinal ganglion cells. *Neuropharmacology* **2017**, *124*, 143–156. [CrossRef] [PubMed]
53. Laguerre, A.; Keutler, K.; Hauke, S.; Schultz, C. Regulation of Calcium Oscillations in beta-Cells by Co-activated Cannabinoid Receptors. *Cell Chem. Biol.* **2021**, *28*, 88–96.e3. [CrossRef] [PubMed]
54. Lowin, T.; Bleck, J.; Schneider, M.; Pongratz, G. Selective killing of proinflammatory synovial fibroblasts via activation of transient receptor potential ankyrin (TRPA1). *Biochem. Pharmacol.* **2018**, *154*, 293–302. [CrossRef]
55. Neumann-Raizel, H.; Shilo, A.; Lev, S.; Mogilevsky, M.; Katz, B.; Shneor, D.; Shaul, Y.D.; Leffler, A.; Gabizon, A.; Karni, R.; et al. 2-APB and CBD-Mediated Targeting of Charged Cytotoxic Compounds Into Tumor Cells Suggests the Involvement of TRPV2 Channels. *Front. Pharmacol.* **2019**, *10*, 1198. [CrossRef]
56. Silverman, H.A.; Chen, A.; Kravatz, N.L.; Chavan, S.S.; Chang, E.H. Involvement of Neural Transient Receptor Potential Channels in Peripheral Inflammation. *Front. Immunol.* **2020**, *11*, 590261. [CrossRef]
57. Storozhuk, M.V.; Zholos, A.V. TRP Channels as Novel Targets for Endogenous Ligands: Focus on Endocannabinoids and Nociceptive Signalling. *Curr. Neuropharmacol.* **2018**, *16*, 137–150. [CrossRef]
58. Dall'Acqua, M.C.; Bonet, I.J.; Zampronio, A.R.; Tambeli, C.H.; Parada, C.A.; Fischer, L. The contribution of transient receptor potential ankyrin 1 (TRPA1) to the in vivo nociceptive effects of prostaglandin E(2). *Life Sci.* **2014**, *105*, 7–13. [CrossRef]
59. Gamage, T.F.; Farquhar, C.E.; Lefever, T.W.; Marusich, J.A.; Kevin, R.C.; McGregor, I.S.; Wiley, J.L.; Thomas, B.F. Molecular and Behavioral Pharmacological Characterization of Abused Synthetic Cannabinoids MMB- and MDMB-FUBINACA, MN-18, NNEI, CUMYL-PICA, and 5-Fluoro-CUMYL-PICA. *J. Pharmacol. Exp. Ther.* **2018**, *365*, 437–446. [CrossRef]
60. Bottini, N.; Firestein, G.S. Duality of fibroblast-like synoviocytes in RA: Passive responders and imprinted aggressors. *Nat. Rev. Rheumatol.* **2013**, *9*, 24–33. [CrossRef]
61. Storch, H.; Zimmermann, B.; Resch, B.; Tykocinski, L.O.; Moradi, B.; Horn, P.; Kaya, Z.; Blank, N.; Rehart, S.; Thomsen, M.; et al. Activated human B cells induce inflammatory fibroblasts with cartilage-destructive properties and become functionally suppressed in return. *Ann. Rheum. Dis.* **2016**, *75*, 924–932. [CrossRef] [PubMed]

62. Petersen, B.H.; Graham, J.; Lemberger, L. Marihuana, tetrahydrocannabinol and T-cell function. *Life Sci.* **1976**, *19*, 395–400. [CrossRef]
63. Rachelefsky, G.S.; Opelz, G. Normal lymphocyte function in the presence of delta-9-tetrahydrocannabinol. *Clin. Pharmacol. Ther.* **1977**, *21*, 44–46. [CrossRef] [PubMed]
64. Karmaus, P.W.; Chen, W.; Kaplan, B.L.; Kaminski, N.E. Delta9-tetrahydrocannabinol suppresses cytotoxic T lymphocyte function independent of CB1 and CB 2, disrupting early activation events. *J. Neuroimmune Pharmacol.* **2012**, *7*, 843–855. [CrossRef] [PubMed]
65. Roth, M.D.; Castaneda, J.T.; Kiertscher, S.M. Exposure to Delta9-Tetrahydrocannabinol Impairs the Differentiation of Human Monocyte-derived Dendritic Cells and their Capacity for T cell Activation. *J. Neuroimmune Pharmacol.* **2015**, *10*, 333–343. [CrossRef] [PubMed]
66. Sahoo, S.S.; Majhi, R.K.; Tiwari, A.; Acharya, T.; Kumar, P.S.; Saha, S.; Kumar, A.; Goswami, C.; Chattopadhyay, S. Transient receptor potential ankyrin1 channel is endogenously expressed in T cells and is involved in immune functions. *Biosci. Rep.* **2019**, *39*, BSR20191437. [CrossRef]
67. Gardner, B.; Zu, L.X.; Sharma, S.; Liu, Q.; Makriyannis, A.; Tashkin, D.P.; Dubinett, S.M. Autocrine and paracrine regulation of lymphocyte CB2 receptor expression by TGF-beta. *Biochem. Biophys. Res. Commun.* **2002**, *290*, 91–96. [CrossRef]
68. Eisenstein, T.K.; Meissler, J.J.; Wilson, Q.; Gaughan, J.P.; Adler, M.W. Anandamide and Delta9-tetrahydrocannabinol directly inhibit cells of the immune system via CB2 receptors. *J. Neuroimmunol.* **2007**, *189*, 17–22. [CrossRef]
69. Buckley, N.E.; McCoy, K.L.; Mezey, E.; Bonner, T.; Zimmer, A.; Felder, C.C.; Glass, M.; Zimmer, A. Immunomodulation by cannabinoids is absent in mice deficient for the cannabinoid CB(2) receptor. *Eur. J. Pharmacol.* **2000**, *396*, 141–149. [CrossRef]
70. Basu, S.; Ray, A.; Dittel, B.N. Cannabinoid Receptor 2 (CB2) Plays a Role in the Generation of Germinal Center and Memory B Cells, but Not in the Production of Antigen-Specific IgG and IgM, in Response to T-dependent Antigens. *PLoS ONE* **2013**, *8*, e67587. [CrossRef]
71. Newton, C.A.; Klein, T.W. Cannabinoid 2 (CB2) receptor involvement in the down-regulation but not up-regulation of serum IgE levels in immunized mice. *J. Neuroimmune Pharmacol.* **2012**, *7*, 591–598. [CrossRef] [PubMed]
72. Agudelo, M.; Newton, C.; Widen, R.; Sherwood, T.; Nong, L.; Friedman, H.; Klein, T.W. Cannabinoid receptor 2 (CB2) mediates immunoglobulin class switching from IgM to IgE in cultures of murine-purified B lymphocytes. *J. Neuroimmune Pharmacol.* **2008**, *3*, 35–42. [CrossRef] [PubMed]
73. Sido, J.M.; Jackson, A.R.; Nagarkatti, P.S.; Nagarkatti, M. Marijuana-derived Delta-9-tetrahydrocannabinol suppresses Th1/Th17 cell-mediated delayed-type hypersensitivity through microRNA regulation. *J. Mol. Med.* **2016**, *94*, 1039–1051. [CrossRef] [PubMed]
74. Ngaotepprutaram, T.; Kaplan, B.L.; Carney, S.; Crawford, R.; Kaminski, N.E. Suppression by Delta(9)-tetrahydrocannabinol of the primary immunoglobulin M response by human peripheral blood B cells is associated with impaired STAT3 activation. *Toxicology* **2013**, *310*, 84–91. [CrossRef] [PubMed]
75. Hu, Y.; Ranganathan, M.; Shu, C.; Liang, X.; Ganesh, S.; Osafo-Addo, A.; Yan, C.; Zhang, X.; Aouizerat, B.E.; Krystal, J.H.; et al. Single-cell Transcriptome Mapping Identifies Common and Cell-type Specific Genes Affected by Acute Delta9-tetrahydrocannabinol in Humans. *Sci. Rep.* **2020**, *10*, 3450. [CrossRef]
76. Ghosh, S.; Kinsey, S.G.; Liu, Q.S.; Hruba, L.; McMahon, L.R.; Grim, T.W.; Merritt, C.R.; Wise, L.E.; Abdullah, R.A.; Selley, D.E.; et al. Full Fatty Acid Amide Hydrolase Inhibition Combined with Partial Monoacylglycerol Lipase Inhibition: Augmented and Sustained Antinociceptive Effects with Reduced Cannabimimetic Side Effects in Mice. *J. Pharmacol. Exp. Ther.* **2015**, *354*, 111–120. [CrossRef]
77. Habib, G.; Khazin, F.; Artul, S. The Effect of Medical Cannabis on Pain Level and Quality of Sleep among Rheumatology Clinic Outpatients. *Pain. Res. Manag.* **2021**, *2021*, 1756588. [CrossRef]
78. Graczyk, M.; Lukowicz, M.; Dzierzanowski, T. Prospects for the Use of Cannabinoids in Psychiatric Disorders. *Front. Psychiatry* **2021**, *12*, 620073. [CrossRef]
79. Mendiguren, A.; Aostri, E.; Pineda, J. Regulation of noradrenergic and serotonergic systems by cannabinoids: Relevance to cannabinoid-induced effects. *Life Sci.* **2018**, *192*, 115–127. [CrossRef]
80. Luo, Y.; Sun, W.; Feng, X.; Ba, X.; Liu, T.; Guo, J.; Xiao, L.; Jiang, J.; Hao, Y.; Xiong, D.; et al. (-)-menthol increases excitatory transmission by activating both TRPM8 and TRPA1 channels in mouse spinal lamina II layer. *Biochem. Biophys. Res. Commun.* **2019**, *516*, 825–830. [CrossRef]
81. Capellino, S.; Weber, K.; Gelder, M.; Harle, P.; Straub, R.H. First appearance and location of catecholaminergic cells during experimental arthritis and elimination by chemical sympathectomy. *Arthritis Rheum.* **2012**, *64*, 1110–1118. [CrossRef] [PubMed]
82. Jenei-Lanzl, Z.; Capellino, S.; Kees, F.; Fleck, M.; Lowin, T.; Straub, R.H. Anti-inflammatory effects of cell-based therapy with tyrosine hydroxylase-positive catecholaminergic cells in experimental arthritis. *Ann Rheum. Dis.* **2015**, *74*, 444–451. [CrossRef] [PubMed]
83. Wu, H.; Chen, J.; Wang, C.; Liu, L.; Wu, Y.; Zhang, Y.; Zhou, A.; Zhang, L.; Wei, W. beta2-adrenoceptor signaling reduction is involved in the inflammatory response of fibroblast-like synoviocytes from adjuvant-induced arthritic rats. *Inflammopharmacology* **2019**, *27*, 271–279. [CrossRef] [PubMed]
84. Makda, A.A.; Elmore, M.A.; Hill, M.E.; Stamps, A.; Tejura, S.; Finnen, M.J. Differential effects of CB1 and CB2 agonists on cAMP levels and MAP kinase activation in human peripheral blood mononuclear cells. *Biochem. Soc. Trans.* **1997**, *25*, 217S. [CrossRef]
85. Kraemer, M.; Madea, B.; Hess, C. Detectability of various cannabinoids in plasma samples of cannabis users: Indicators of recent cannabis use? *Drug Test. Anal.* **2019**, *11*, 1498–1506. [CrossRef]
86. Maia, J.; Midao, L.; Cunha, S.C.; Almada, M.; Fonseca, B.M.; Braga, J.; Goncalves, D.; Teixeira, N.; Correia-da-Silva, G. Effects of cannabis tetrahydrocannabinol on endocannabinoid homeostasis in human placenta. *Arch. Toxicol.* **2019**, *93*, 649–658. [CrossRef]

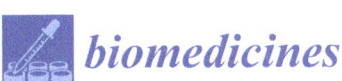

Review

The Endocannabinoid System as a Target for Neuroprotection/Neuroregeneration in Perinatal Hypoxic–Ischemic Brain Injury

Andrea Duranti [1,*], Gorane Beldarrain [2], Antonia Álvarez [2], Matilde Sbriscia [1], Silvia Carloni [1], Walter Balduini [1] and Daniel Alonso-Alconada [2,*]

[1] Department of Biomolecular Sciences, University of Urbino Carlo Bo, 61029 Urbino, Italy
[2] Department of Cell Biology and Histology, School of Medicine and Nursing, University of the Basque Country (UPV/EHU), 48940 Leioa, Spain
* Correspondence: andrea.duranti@uniurb.it (A.D.); daniel.alonsoa@ehu.eus (D.A.-A.); Tel.: +39-0722-303501 (A.D.); +34-946-013294 (D.A.-A.)

Abstract: The endocannabinoid (EC) system is a complex cell-signaling system that participates in a vast number of biological processes since the prenatal period, including the development of the nervous system, brain plasticity, and circuit repair. This neuromodulatory system is also involved in the response to endogenous and environmental insults, being of special relevance in the prevention and/or treatment of vascular disorders, such as stroke and neuroprotection after neonatal brain injury. Perinatal hypoxia–ischemia leading to neonatal encephalopathy is a devastating condition with no therapeutic approach apart from moderate hypothermia, which is effective only in some cases. This overview, therefore, gives a current description of the main components of the EC system (including cannabinoid receptors, ligands, and related enzymes), to later analyze the EC system as a target for neonatal neuroprotection with a special focus on its neurogenic potential after hypoxic–ischemic brain injury.

Keywords: endocannabinoid system; cannabinoid receptors; FAAH inhibitors; MGL inhibitors; neonatal brain injury; hypoxia–ischemia; neuroprotection; neurogenesis

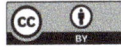

1. The Endocannabinoid System

The endocannabinoid (EC) system is a cell-signaling system consisting mainly of at least two cannabinoid (CB) receptors, namely CB_1 and CB_2, their endogenous ligands, and the enzymes responsible for the synthesis, transport, and degradation of endocannabinoids (ECs) [1]. Changes in the expression or activity of CB receptors, ligands, or enzymes are implicated in many pathological conditions [2]. Neurological disorders such as anxiety, depression, schizophrenia, neurodegenerative (e.g., Parkinson's and Huntington's disease), and stroke-related disorders, together with osteoporosis, multiple sclerosis, neuropathic pain, cancer, glaucoma, hypertension, and obesity/metabolic syndrome are just the major diseases associated with perturbations of the EC system [3]. Recently, it has been hypothesized that CB_2 receptor activation may be also useful to reduce the inflammatory response induced by SARS-CoV-2 infection, due to its capacity to ameliorate the production of cytokines responsible for the pathological phenomenon [4].

However, changes in EC tone are sometimes transient and likely part of the organism's compensatory response mainly aimed at reducing symptoms or slowing the progression of pathological conditions. In the nervous system, the activity of the EC system also appears related to neuroprotection, because of its ability to modulate the intensity and extent of a series of dangerous biological events involved in the neurodegenerative process. These include modulation of glutamate excitotoxicity [5] and oxidative stress [6], and a reduction in the inflammatory response [7]. This scenario led to considering the EC system as a potential target for developing new neuroprotective therapies [3]. However, it is not always clear whether an increased activity of the EC system can be consequent to a higher biosynthetic activity or a reduction in the metabolic degradation of the endogenous ligands. Therefore, a better understanding of the role and mechanisms underlying EC tone alterations during the neurodegenerative process represents key factors for developing new therapeutic agents acting through this important modulatory system.

Overall, despite the vast amount of knowledge acquired over time, the exploration of the EC system still represents a stimulating goal. Indeed, the complexity of its structures, the species variability of its characteristics, and the overlapping of pharmacological targets, still leave open many questions and scientific opportunities. This review aims to highlight the potential role of the EC system in the neurodegenerative and neuro-reparative processes resulting from hypoxic–ischemic insults occurring during brain development. A summary of CB receptors, ligands, and related enzymes is also reported.

1.1. Cannabinoid Receptors

The effects associated with the endo and exocannabinoid compounds are primarily related to their interaction with the CB_1 and CB_2 receptors, discovered some decades ago [8–10] and characterized based on their neurobiology signaling [11]. Their involvement in many physiological and pathological events justifies the central role that they play as a possible therapeutic key for many diseases. CB receptors can be stimulated or antagonized by different ligands and can also be modulated through the inhibition of the enzymes responsible for the degradation of their endogenous ligands [12]. Unfortunately, the interaction of exocannabinoids with these receptors, especially with the CB_1 subtype, is also associated with the psychotropic effects of many recreational drugs, including *Cannabis*, the so-called new psychoactive substances [13], and smart drugs (SPICE and K2 ...) [14], or to other undesirable serious effects of synthetic agonist or antagonist drugs [15–17].

CB_1 receptors are abundantly expressed in the central nervous system (CNS), particularly in the cerebral cortex, hippocampus, basal ganglia, and cerebellum. CB_2 receptors, instead, are mostly expressed in the immune system, particularly in B and natural killer cells. However, CB_2 receptors have been also found in some districts of the CNS [18] and the CB_1 also peripherally, albeit at low levels [11]. More detailed information on the origin, structural aspects, and signaling processes mediated by CB_1 and CB_2 receptors are reported in [19,20].

Generally, the activation of CB receptors determines the inhibition of adenylate cyclase, with a consequent decrease in the levels of cyclic adenosine monophosphate (cAMP), a second messenger involved in numerous intracellular signaling and essential for the regulation of many cell functions. There is also evidence that the CB_1 receptor, in addition to acting on adenylate cyclase, can be coupled to ion channels [21], confirming the key role of CBs in inducing activation or depression of neurotransmission [11].

Recent studies have also revealed the existence of "atypical" EC receptors, i.e., the transient receptor potential vanilloid (TRPV) channels, involved in the nociceptive signaling; the GRP55, G-protein coupled receptors responsible for some independent CB_1 and CB_2 responses; the peroxisome proliferator-activated receptor gamma (PPAR-γ) receptors, which are physiologically involved in glucose metabolism and insulin signaling, and also in inflammation and pain; and the dopamine, adenosine, opioid, and 5-HT_{1A} receptors [22].

1.2. Endocannabinoids

Endocannabinoids (ECs) are endogenous lipidic compounds formed by a long-chain polyunsaturated fatty acid tail and a polar head containing functional groups such as amide, ester, ether, or hydroxy one. They bind to CB receptors but, unlike most neurotransmitters that are synthesized and stored in vesicles; their synthesis from membrane phospholipids is on-demand and use-dependent [23,24].

ECs are released from postsynaptic terminals in a Ca^{2+}-dependent manner. After their release, they activate presynaptic CB receptors usually through retrograde signaling, although non-retrograde signaling may occur [24]. The retrograde signaling mechanism is responsible for modulating both short-term and long-term neuroplasticity [25]. The short-term type of modulation (seconds) participates in processes, such as depolarization-induced suppression of inhibition and depolarization-induced suppression of excitation. This may occur through the inhibition of Ca^{2+} voltage-gated channels and the modulation of the synaptic release of various neurotransmitters, including glutamate and γ-aminobutyric acid (GABA) [26,27]. In addition, ECs are also involved in long-term synaptic plasticity (in the order of minutes) through a CB_1 repeated stimulation of these brain circuits [24]. This process leads to the long-term depression phenomenon, with the final decrease in the glutamatergic and GABAergic synaptic activity [28]. Thus, ECs may function as a polymodal signal integrator to allow the diversification of synaptic plasticity in a single neuron [29]. EC receptors, in particular those in the CNS, can, therefore, be potential drug targets for the prevention and treatment of neurologic disorders, such as brain ischemia [30].

The best-studied ECs are N-arachidonoylethanolamine (anandamide and AEA, as seen in Figure 1) [31] and 2-arachidonoyl-sn-glycerol (2-AG, as seen in Figure 1) [32,33], but other arachidonic acid derivatives (e.g., noladin ether, virodhamine, and N-arachidonoyldopamine) can bind CB_1 and/or CB_2 receptors, although their physiological role is not yet clear.

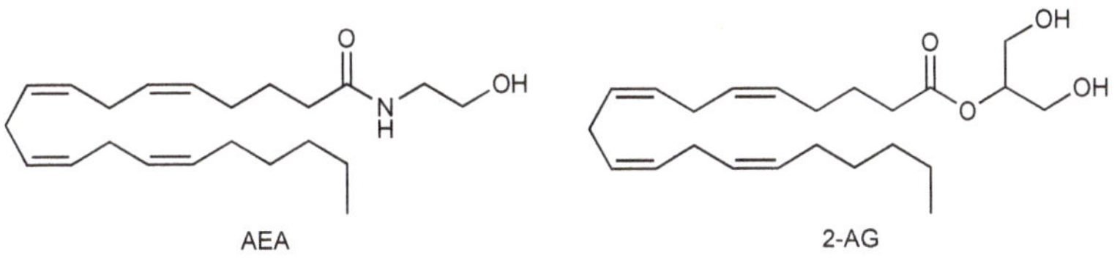

Figure 1. Chemical structures of AEA and 2-AG.

AEA is a full or partial agonist of the CB_1 receptor but also shows low activity towards the CB_2 receptor [34–38], whereas 2-AG is a full agonist of both CB_1 and CB_2 receptors [39].

Differences between AEA and 2-AG occur also in the biosynthetic pathways responsible for their formation and degradation. With reference to the synthetic step, N-acyl phosphatidylethanolamine phospholipase D (NAPE-PLD) [40,41] or diacylglycerol lipase (DGL) [42,43] are the enzymes directly involved, whereas fatty acid amide hydrolase (FAAH) [44–47] or monoglyceride lipase (MGL) [48–50] are the main enzymes responsible for their metabolism, leading to the formation of arachidonic acid and ethanolamine [51] or glycerol [52] following a cellular internalization process carried out by specific transporters [53–55].

1.3. Cannabis, Phytocannabinoids, and Synthetic Cannabinoids

Cannabis contains more than 500 compounds, of which at least 100 are known to be phytocannabinoids [56] owing to pharmacological properties [57]; they are described in detail in [58]. Paleobotanical studies attest that *Cannabis* was already present during the Holocene epoch about 11,700 years ago, more likely in the territories of Central Asia near the Altai Mountains [59]. The first written testimony on the use of *Cannabis* for therapeutic purposes dates back to 2700 BC, when the Chinese emperor Shen-Nung reported a detailed description of it in a book that later became the Chinese compendium of drugs [60]. Chinese people used this plant for diseases such as rheumatic pain, malaria, constipation, etc. [61]. Despite their long history, the phytocannabinoids contained in *Cannabis* were identified only a few decades ago and progressively studied both as single molecules and as their derivatives, and also based on structure–activity relationship studies [62].

The most studied and characterized phytocannabinoids have been Δ^9-tetrahydrocannabinol (Δ^9-THC, Figure 2) [63], which constitutes the main psychoactive compound of *Cannabis*, and the non-psychotropic cannabidiol (CBD, Figure 2) [64]. Despite similar structures, their pharmacodynamic properties deeply differ.

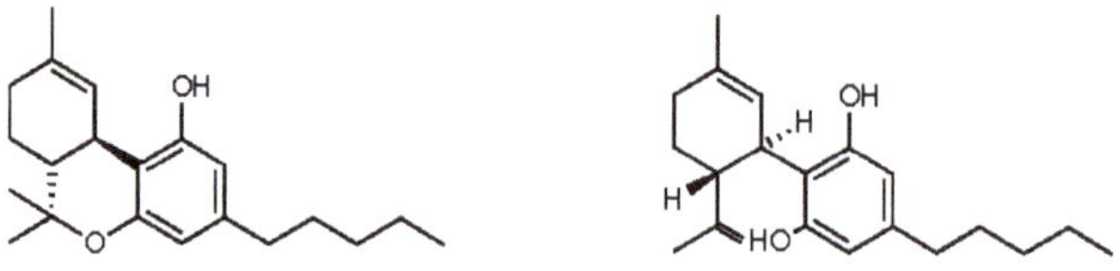

Figure 2. Chemical structures of Δ^9-THC and CBD.

Δ^9-THC acts as a partial agonist of the CB_1 receptor, which explains its strong psychoactive outcomes inducing the tetrad effects (hypothermia, catalepsy, hypolocomotion, and analgesia). These unwanted effects make the medical use of the Δ^9-THC strongly restricted despite its beneficial action (neuroprotective, anti-inflammatory, and antispasmodic), which depends on the activation of CB_2 and PPAR-γ receptors [56]. In addition, the activity of the molecule is dependent on cell type, receptor expression, and the presence of ECs or other agonists [56,65].

For its part, CBD has a high affinity on a series of targets, including CB_1 and CB_2, GPR55, TRPV, PPAR-γ, 5-HT$_{1A}$, dopamine, and opioid receptors, and also on ion channels, which contributes to the beneficial effects of *Cannabis* in diseases related to a wide range of pathologies (neurological, ischemic stroke, inflammatory, pain, etc.) [22,66,67].

Although Δ^9-THC and CBD are the best-known and studied phytocannabinoids, other compounds have been relieved in *Cannabis* owing to their therapeutic potential. Among these, the main ones are reported below. (1) Cannabigerol (CBG), which is a non-psychotropic derivative with a low affinity for the CB_1 and CB_2, but it is able to interact with other receptors, such as α_2-adrenergic, TRPs superfamily, and 5-HT$_{1A}$, and to possess various properties (antiproliferative, antibacterial, antioxidant, etc.) [56]. (2) Cannabichromene (CBC), which acts weakly with CB_1 and CB_2 receptors and is able to inhibit AEA uptake, is the most potent agonist of TRPA1 channels and possesses antinociceptive and anti-inflammatory properties in vitro and in vivo [56]. (3) Δ^9-Tetrahydrocannabivarine (Δ^9-THCV), which is the *n*-propyl analogue of Δ^9-THC and acts weakly with CB_1 receptors and more potently with the CB_2 ones. However, it is also able to act with other targets such as TRP, GPR6, GPR55, and D_2 receptors and to exert related pharmacological actions [56]. (4) Cannabinol (CBN), which is the first phytocannabinoid structurally characterized; its derivatives are considered as the oxidative by-product of the degradation process of Δ^9-THC and CBD [62,68]. It acts as a partial agonist of CB_1 and CB_2 and exerts neuroprotective, antiepileptic, and analgesic properties [68,69].

Synthetic cannabinoids are ligands that bind to CB receptors and modulate their activity. Their design and the studies aimed to acquire information on the structural requirements to establish interactions with CB receptors. Moreover, the goal was also related to the understanding of the role played by molecules that bind with these targets, the role of the targets themselves, and, more generally, the role of the EC system, since synthetic cannabinoids can be considered tools to increase knowledge in the field. As for natural ligands, the role of synthetic cannabinoids must always be contextualized within the situation of a risk/benefit ratio that would derive from their use. In spite of the large effort in synthesizing and characterizing the pharmacological profile of these molecules, apart from nabilone, there are currently no drugs on the market containing a synthetic cannabinoid, but many of them are used for recreational purposes and are included in the list of substances of abuse [15,70–73].

The structural requirements that allow synthetic cannabinoids to interact with CB receptors are highly variable, a situation that strongly influences their pharmacological activity, in particular for what concern agonism, antagonism, and, more rarely, inverse agonism. It is interesting to consider, however, that their activity sometimes depends on the experimental model used for their characterization (e.g., antagonism vs. inverse agonism). An overview of these features and the therapeutic potential of CB ligands are presented in Refs. [74–79].

The therapeutic interest of the drugs that bind to CB receptors is also proved by the marketed drugs mentioned above. Cesamet® (nabilone—the synthetic dibenzopyran-9-one analog of Δ^9-THC), administered for the improvement of chemotherapy-induced nausea and vomiting (CINV) states in patients not responding to conventional antiemetic therapies. Marinol® (dronabinol—the synthetic pure isomer (−)-*trans*-Δ^9-THC) is prescribed for the same purposes as the former and also for appetite stimulation in patients with AIDS (acquired immune deficiency syndrome). Sativex® (Δ^9-THC and cannabidiol in an approximate 1:1 fixed ratio) is used for the symptomatic relief of the pain and/or the management of neuropathic pain and spasticity in adults with multiple sclerosis and is not responsive to other antispasticity therapies. More recently, a new drug containing > 98% CBD and less than 0.15% Δ^9-THC (Epidiolex®) has been approved for the treatment of seizures associated with two rare and severe forms of epilepsy (Lennox–Gastaut and Dravet syndromes) in patients two years of age and older [56,66,80,81].

An intriguing and interesting feature of CB receptor ligands is that they are able to exert a neuroprotective role after ischemic injuries [82–85]. The CB_1 and CB_2 agonists (−)-CP-55,940 [86] and (R)-(+)-WIN-55212-2 [87], the CB_1 inverse agonists SR141716A [88] and AM 251 [89], the CB_1 antagonists LY320135 [90], and the CB_2 agonist/CB_1 antagonist URB447 [91] (Figure 3) are the related tools studied.

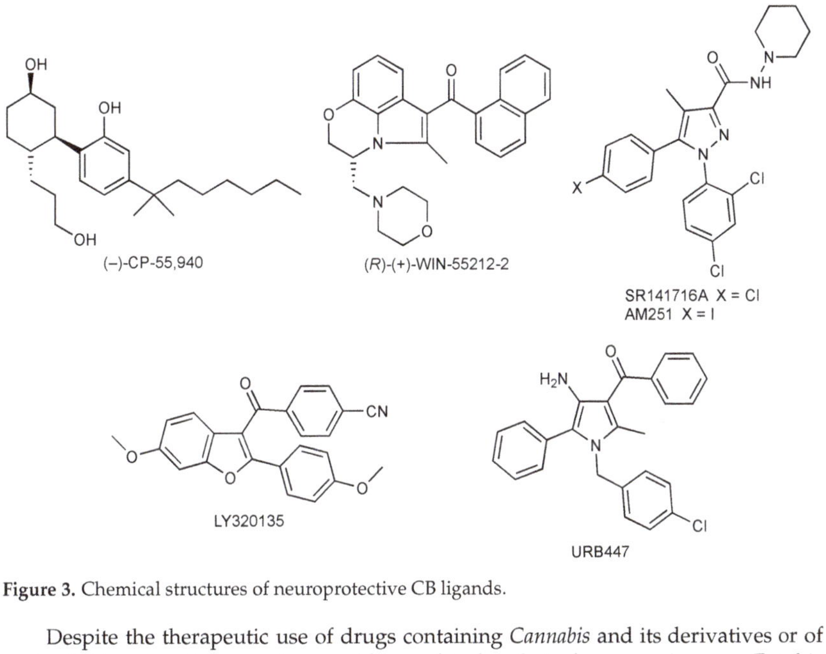

Figure 3. Chemical structures of neuroprotective CB ligands.

Despite the therapeutic use of drugs containing *Cannabis* and its derivatives or of synthetic ligands of CB receptors, problems related to their abuse remain open. For this reason, molecules inhibiting the degradation of endogenous ligands may represent an interesting alternative for modulating the EC system [92].

1.4. FAAH and MGL Inhibitors

These compounds increase AEA and 2-AG levels by inhibiting their intracellular degradation. The hypothesis leading to the design and development of EC metabolism inhibitors is based on the fact that, by blocking the degradation of these endogenous mediators, we can increase their concentrations in the physiological districts where they are formed. By using this approach, it may be possible to obtain pharmacological agents characterized by the absence of the psychotropic side effects typical of CB_1 exogenous ligands. Indeed, ECs are synthesized and released *on-demand* in a tissue-specific and time-dependent manner and inhibitors of their metabolic enzymes will cause an increase in EC levels only where and when it is physiologically required. In this way, the activation of CB receptors is obtained through endogenous ligands, but it is prolonged over time. Several pieces of evidence support this approach. For example, it has been reported that FAAH knockdown mice show increased levels of AEA in the brain and other tissues leading to CB_1 receptor-mediated analgesia [93,94], or a reduction in anxiety symptoms without the appearance of catalepsy [95].

The possibility of targeting the FAAH and MGL enzymes, therefore, may represent an important therapeutic approach for different pathologies [2,96–99] and, even if there are no drugs on the market yet, studies carried out in this regard are promising. Disorders related to anxiety, pain, and cigarette and cannabis smoking are the main pathological states in which EC metabolism inhibitors have been studied [2], and clinical studies are in progress. FAAH and MGL inhibitors have also been considered pharmacological tools to increase information on the role of the EC system in neurodegeneration/neuroprotection after ischemic injuries [100–105]. The FAAH inhibitor URB597 [95,106–113] and MGL inhibitors URB602 [101,114–116], JZL184 [117], KML29 [118], and MJN110 [119] (Figure 4) are the main experimental molecules assessed in these studies.

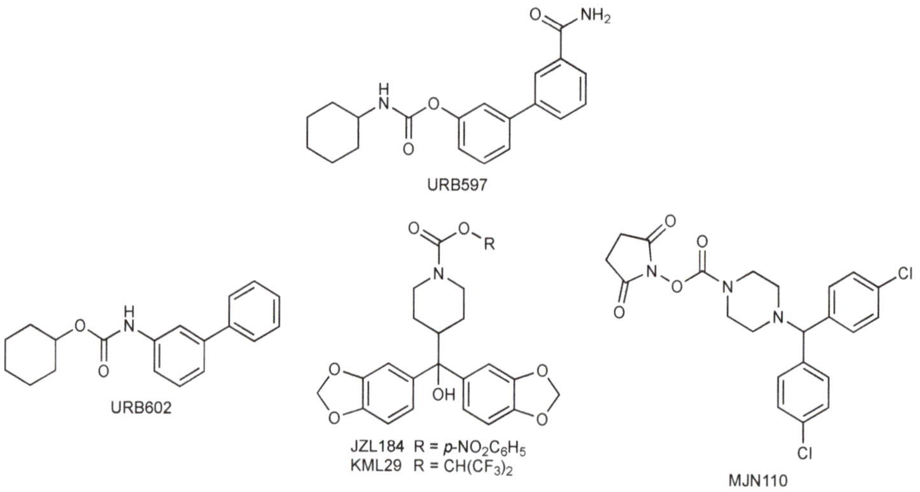

Figure 4. Chemical structures of neuroprotective FAAH and MGL inhibitors.

2. The Endocannabinoid System in Prenatal and Postnatal Development

During prenatal and postnatal brain development, the EC system may play an active role in the control of the cell cycle, proliferation, survival, and differentiation of neural stem cells [120], as well as in the maturation of the nervous system and its functions. The modulation of some of these processes appears regulated by the CB_1 receptor, which is expressed in the very early stages of neural development. Indeed, the expression of members of the EC system has been described during early developmental and postnatal stages [121–123], and in the embryonic rat brain, its presence was found around day 11 of gestation [124]. In 1998, Berrendero et al. [121] not only demonstrated the existence of CB_1 receptors, but they also showed that these receptors were already functional in embryonic stages. In humans, the presence of CB_1 receptors has been documented as soon as at week 14 of gestation in the embryo [125].

The regions in which CB_1 receptors are expressed in these early stages, i.e., the corpus callosum, stria terminalis, stria medullaris, fasciculus retroflexum, or anterior commissure, are related to processes such as cell proliferation, migration, axonal elongation and synaptogenesis [121–123,126]. The later modifications in CB_1 receptors' location during neural development (becoming different in the adult brain), suggest that their expression in the brain changes once their contribution to neural development finishes [121,123].

In murine cell cultures, CB_1 receptors appear in several cell types, including stem-like cells, astrocytes, and immature neurons [127]. It has also been observed that the agonist (R)-(+)-methanandamide promoted self-renewal, multipotency, and neuronal differentiation via CB_1 activation. When ECs are produced or exogenously administered with bind CB_1 receptors, the α_i subunit linked to the protein inhibits the activity of adenylyl cyclase and the synthesis of cAMP. Low levels of cAMP reduce the activity of the protein kinase-A and, consequently, the type-A potassium channels are activated and lead to membrane hyperpolarization. The α_o subunit of the G protein associated with the CB_1 receptor, instead, inhibits voltage-dependent Ca^{2+} channels causing cell depolarization. The β and γ subunits, moreover, interact with pathways, such as PI3K or PKB/Akt, that have been shown to induce the expression of transcription factors associated with cell proliferation (CREB, STAT-3, PAX-6, and β-catenin). CB receptors are also closely related to neutral sphingomyelinase, which generates ceramide from sphingomyelin located in the plasma membrane, thus activating the synthesis of transcription factors, such as ERK or p38, that control cell fate and survival [128,129]. The involvement of factors, such as ERK or PI3K, in neurogenesis associated with CB_1 activation was also observed by Xapelli et al. [127].

The processes of migration and path-finding during neurogenesis appear also partially regulated by the CB_1 receptor. Their blockage with a selective antagonist caused a decrease of 50% in migration in a scratch wound assay in mouse fetal cortex-derived cells [130]. The same authors also labeled the rostral migratory stream explants embedded in Matrigel using the migrating neuroblast markers PSA-NCAM and DCX, and observed a significant reduction (30%) in the migratory distance after the treatment with a CB_1 receptor antagonist. The role of the EC system in the path-finding function also became evident when EC signals were proven to be behind axon direction cues, helping neurons find their path [131].

Together with CB receptors, the ECs AEA and 2-AG also make their appearance in the prenatal period. Despite the presence of AEA levels having been detected from the early stages of the embryo [132], 2-AG seems to be predominant in the fetal period, as this molecule has been found in higher concentrations than AEA [133]. Conversely, AEA levels increase gradually during brain development until an adult level is reached, while the concentration of 2-AG remains more or less stable than in the fetal, young, and adult brains [122].

3. The Endocannabinoid System as a Target for Neuroprotection in Hypoxic–Ischemic Encephalopathy

Perinatal HI leading to neonatal encephalopathy (NE) represents a major cause of death and long-term disability in neonates [134]. Each year, up to 20,000 infants are affected by NE in Europe and even more in regions with a lower level of perinatal care [135]. Whereas the incidence of NE in Western Europe and North America is around 1.6/1000 term births [136], neonatal mortality is 6 times higher in developing or low-resourced countries compared with developed or middle-to-high-resourced countries.

Current treatment options for HI are extremely limited, making the management of long-term outcomes or its prevention difficult. Actually, the only approved therapy is therapeutic hypothermia, consisting in lowering the body temperature of patients to 33.5 °C for 72 h through cooling of either the whole body or just the head [137]. Therapeutic hypothermia is routinely implemented in the majority of first-world hospitals to treat term infants with moderate to severe NE; however, cooling is only partially effective as a neuroprotective therapy (>45% of infants have adverse neurodevelopmental outcomes despite treatment) [138]. At the same time, hypothermia can develop some potential side effects due to the slowing of the mechanisms of clearance and metabolism, the induced immunosuppressive activity, and the increase in energy expenditure resulting from the thermoregulatory response [139]. As the current cooling therapy protocols appear to be optimal [140], there is an urgent need to improve neonatal neuroprotection by developing additional safe and effective neuroprotective treatments [141,142].

The EC system is able to limit the deleterious effects caused by multiple toxic stimuli such as glutamate excitotoxicity, oxidative stress, and inflammation, thus providing neuroprotection in different paradigms of brain injury [84,143]. Therefore, compounds that modulate the EC system could be promising neuroprotective and/or neurogenic agents for the treatment of CNS pathologies, including NE.

The first cannabinoid tested in cerebral ischemic models was the synthetic CB_1/CB_2 agonist (R)-(+)-WIN-55,212-2 [144]. The authors showed that the exogenous administration of this CB agonist significantly reduced the infarct volume and the loss of hippocampal neurons. They also studied the neuroprotective effect of cannabinoids during brain development and showed that exogenous administration of the ECs AEA and 2-AG reduced brain infarction in newborn rats subjected to HI [145]. Later, some of the co-authors described the neuroprotective and long-lasting beneficial effect of URB602, an inhibitor of the degradation of 2-AG [101] in the same murine model. The neuroprotective effect of cannabinoids was also confirmed in an experimental model closer to the human condition, i.e., in the fetal lamb. In this model, the synthetic cannabinoid agonist (R)-(+)-WIN-55,212-2 protected the neonatal brain at very low doses to maintain mitochondrial integrity and functionality [146], to reduce apoptotic cell death [147], and to ameliorate the inflammatory response [148].

The classical way to modulate the EC system is through the activation or blockade of CB_1 and CB_2 receptors, as described in the first part of this review. However, CB_1 receptors seem to play a dual role in post-ischemic neuronal damage, as the decrease in glutamate release due to CB_1 activation is accompanied by a parallel decrease in GABA release, resulting in neurotoxicity instead of neuroprotection [149]. Moreover, CB_1 overactivation in the perinatal period could be harmful [150] and this can limit the translational interest of CB_1 agonists. In addition, CB_1-mediated psychoactive effects [151], which are unwanted in clinical treatments, should also be considered.

Activation of the other CB receptor, the CB_2, results in potent anti-inflammatory effects [143], and the CB_2 antagonism has no described beneficial effect. A therapeutic approach with drugs interacting with CB_2 receptors can be developed using either indirect (e.g., cannabidiol) or selective (e.g., GW405833) CB_2 agonists. Nevertheless, cannabidiol can induce severe hypotension [152] despite being neuroprotective in different experimental paradigms [153], whereas GW405833 showed no protection after HI [154]. This evidence together with the finding that the CB_1 antagonist/inverse agonist rimonabant also exerts a neuroprotective effect, which adds further complexity to the effect of cannabinoid-interacting compounds in neurodegeneration.

Recently, some of the co-authors evaluated the neuroprotective potential of the synthetic cannabinoid URB447 [85]. URB447 is the first mixed CB_1 antagonist and CB_2 agonist that binds to both CB_1 and CB_2 receptors with submicromolar affinity and good stereoselectivity [91]. URB447 strongly reduced brain injury when administered before HI in neonatal rats, but more interestingly, the compound was effective also when administered 30 min or 3 h after the initial insult. URB447 reduced cerebral infarction by 95.7% (30 min) and 88% (at 3 h) in the whole ipsilateral (damaged) hemisphere.

Since a pharmacological intervention within 3 h after the injury is considered a clinically feasible therapeutic window to treat perinatal brain injury in humans [155], we characterized the effect of URB447 administered at this time point, focusing on the consequences of HI and URB447 administration on the activation of glial cells and white matter injury. Together with a reduction in astrogliosis and microglial activation, URB447 decreased white matter damage restoring myelin basic protein levels 7 days after HI, confirming the important role played by the EC system in the neurodegenerative and neuroreparative processes after HI.

As commented above, nowadays, the only clinical therapy against HI-induced NE is moderate hypothermia, which exerts a number of neuroprotective responses through the reduction in excitotoxicity, free radical exposure, blood–brain barrier dysfunction, and delayed cell death [156]. Leker et al. [157] observed that a single injection of the CB_1 synthetic agonist HU-210 significantly reduced body temperature, conferring a strong neuroprotective effect to the hypoxic–ischemic rats, a beneficial effect that was lost when animals were treated with the selective CB_1 antagonist SR141716. The enhancement of hypothermia by stimulating the EC system or by the combined therapy EC system plus hypothermia may have beneficial outcomes in neonates, so these responses are currently under investigation in preclinical models [158,159].

4. Can Endocannabinoid System Interacting Drugs Modulate Neurogenesis after HI?

The discovery of stem cells in the postnatal and adult mammalian brain changed the previously believed assertion that the adult brain is unable to replace lost neurons [160,161]. Although still unknown with certainty in other regions of the CNS, two neurogenic areas persist after birth: the subventricular zone (SVZ) of the lateral ventricles and the subgranular zone (SGZ) of the dentate gyrus of the hippocampus [162–164].

The ability to generate new neurons and glial cells from these niches may contribute to the plasticity of the newborn brain and tissue remodeling after damage [165–169]. Based on their regenerative potential, cells from the SVZ of the ventricles can be molecularly manipulated in situ to induce their proliferation and migration to damaged sites or stimulated in vitro for later transplantation [162,170–173]. However, the processes of proliferation, migration, differentiation, and survival will depend on a wide range of factors, including the type, intensity, duration, and/or location of the damage [174]. Thus, it is not yet known whether these newly formed neurons are properly integrated into the existing neural network and if they can represent a fully functional microenvironment after a brain injury [175]. It has been estimated that 85% of the new neurons generated in response to the insult do not survive after reaching maturation [176].

The global damage induced by perinatal HI may also affect the neurogenic niches and their neuro-proliferative capacity. After 24–48 h from moderate/severe hypoxic–ischemic damage, the SVZ may show extensive cell death, primarily affecting neuronal stem cells and also oligodendrocyte progenitors [177,178]. Interestingly, the neurogenic potential of this area can be affected independently from cell death [179]. Indeed, in a preclinical model close to the human condition, i.e., newborn piglets, it has been shown that a decreased cellularity is associated with a reduction in cell proliferation and neurogenesis in the SVZ [179]. These effects occurred without necrotic or apoptotic cell death 48 h after hypoxic–ischemic damage. Whether this discrepancy could be related to differences in the severity/duration of the insult or the experimental model employed (rodent vs. piglet) remains the subject of investigation. It should also be considered that the SVZ can present sub-regional sensitivity, with areas and cell types showing selective vulnerability to the insult. Higher rates of survival were observed in its medial zone [180] and in different responses of pre-oligodendrocytes and neuroblasts to hypoxic–ischemic damage [181].

Whereas several works pointed toward HI leading to decreased cell proliferation in the SVZ (for a review, see [182]), other authors have described that the injured ipsilateral SVZ has the ability to increase its size after a longer recovery interval [176,178,183,184], a phenomenon attributed to increased cell proliferation [176,185]. For its part, the undamaged contralateral SVZ can also suffer an expansion after HI [176], with the most undifferentiated precursors being responsible for this increase in its size [185].

The other neurogenic niche, the SGZ of the dentate gyrus of the hippocampus, also revealed conflicting results. Bartley et al. [186] showed that neuronal (together with microglial and endothelial) cell proliferation was significantly increased in the injured ipsilateral hippocampus. The authors used a postnatal day 7 (P7) neonatal mice model subjected to permanent unilateral carotid ligation plus 8% hypoxia for 75 min. Conversely, early after the publication of that work, Kadam et al. [187] described that total counts of new cells were significantly lower in both ipsilateral and contralateral hippocampi, which in turn correlated with lesion-induced atrophy. They used, however, a neonatal stroke model of unilateral carotid ligation alone to produce infarcts in P12 CD1 mice. In a more recent work by Ziemka-Nalecz et al. [188] using the HI permanent unilateral carotid ligation plus hypoxia (7.6% O_2 for 60 min) model of brain injury, the authors showed no signs of increased or decreased cell proliferation in the dentate gyrus of the hippocampi, with no differences between sham (non-operated), ipsilateral, or contralateral hippocampi, in none of the five timepoints evaluated (3, 6, 9, 11, or 14 days after HI). This usage of different experimental models of brain injury may add complexity to unraveling the neurogenic response of the neonatal hippocampal SGZ.

To better understand the modulation in cellular populations after HI, experiments have been carried out using flow cytometry with multi-markers in order to quantify the proportion of each cell type. It seems that neuronal stem cells decrease while multipotential, as well as the glial cell progenitors, increase [189]. The increase in the number of reactive astrocytes can be translated into greater production of components of the extracellular matrix, such as hyaluronic acid and chondroitin sulfate, which can, in turn, inhibit the differentiation of oligodendrocytes and limit myelin synthesis [190,191]. This suggests that hypoxia–ischemia may alter the cellular composition of the neurogenic niches [189].

As described, the effect of neonatal HI on the neurogenic response after brain injury remains far from clear [179]. The modulation of the proliferative capacity of the neurogenic niches might be enhanced by using CBs, as the EC system seems to play an important role in processes, such as cell proliferation and differentiation of neural stem cells, during normal brain development.

Aguado et al. [192] observed that stimulation of the EC system enhanced neurogenesis after kainic acid-induced excitotoxicity in neural progenitor cell cultures. The effect was revealed as increased expression of the progenitor markers nestin, Sox-2, and musashi-1, and also as a higher proliferation rate. They also examined whether neural progenitor cell division may result in effective neurogenesis. By immunostaining dividing cells with the mature neuron marker NeuN, the authors described the presence of newly generated neurons one month after injury, suggesting that long-term neurogenesis can be enhanced by EC system modulation [192].

In a model of HI in rodents, Fernández-López et al. [193] stimulated the CB_1 receptor by exogenous administration of the synthetic cannabinoid (R)-(+)-WIN-55,212-2, showing increased cell proliferation and doublecortin expression (a marker of neuroblasts) after HI and cannabinoid administration. However, the long-lasting effect described by Aguado et al. [192] here was lost. (R)-(+)-WIN-55,212-2 was able to promote neurogenesis up to 7 days after HI (P14), but the survival of the new neurons decreased shortly after the withdrawal of the treatment. It remains unclear whether prolonging the administration of cannabinoids could be beneficial regarding neurogenesis [193].

Therapeutic hypothermia (the only clinical therapy against HI-induced neonatal encephalopathy) is also able to modulate and enhance endogenous reparative processes. Bregy et al. [194] showed an increase in doublecortin-positive cells in the hippocampal dentate gyrus of cooled animals treated with therapeutic hypothermia after experimental traumatic brain injury. Works using models of ischemic and hypoxic–ischemic brain injury described similar results [195,196]. Rats treated with hypothermia increased their counts of neurogenesis markers compared to normothermic animals. As the activation of the EC system may decrease body temperature, it seems feasible that exogenous administration of CBs may indirectly modulate the neurogenic response after neonatal brain damage.

In addition to neurogenesis, cannabinoids may be of great benefit in white matter recovery after brain damage. The administration of the CB_1 agonist ACEA resulted in increased Olig2 (an oligodendrocyte progenitor marker) expressing cells in the SVZ and-myelination in the subcortical white matter [197]. (R)-(+)-WIN-55,212-2 administration after HI also promoted remyelination of the injured external capsule by increasing the number of early oligodendrocyte progenitors and mature oligodendrocytes [193]. The enhancement of oligodendrogenesis is of great interest when treating the developing brain, as increased remyelination is linked with the improvement of sensorimotor functions after hypoxic–ischemic injury [198].

5. Concluding Remarks and Perspectives

The ubiquitous lipid signaling-based EC system is involved in outstanding regulatory functions throughout the human body, including neural development under physiological conditions and neuroprotection, and repair after pathophysiological processes.

In the context of neonatal brain injury, the administration of endogenous or exogenous CBs, or the blockage of EC degradation, has revealed a strong neuroprotective response in different preclinical models after HI. Similarly, the possibility of tissue repair in the developing brain by enhancing the proliferative potential of the SVZ and SGZ neurogenic niches is currently under active investigation. Selective modulation of the EC system in the sites of damage by targeting the enzymes responsible for EC degradation may represent an important therapeutic approach in order to avoid non-desired widespread effects.

Despite the clinical use of CB-related drugs that must be taken with caution, the modulation of the EC system to ameliorate the neurological consequences after neonatal HI is currently an exciting field of research with enormous possibilities for clinical translation.

Author Contributions: Conceptualization A.D. and D.A.-A.; writing—original draft preparation A.D., G.B., A.Á., M.S., S.C., W.B. and D.A.-A.; writing—review and editing, A.D., W.B. and D.A.-A.; supervision A.D. and D.A.-A. All authors have read and agreed to the published version of the manuscript.

Funding: EITB Maratoia-BIOEF (BIO18/IC/003), the Spanish Ministry of Science and Innovation: (MINECOR20/P66/AEI/10.13039/501100011033).

Institutional Review Board Statement: Not applicable.

Informed Consent Statement: Not applicable.

Data Availability Statement: Data sharing not applicable.

Conflicts of Interest: The authors declare no conflict of interest.

References

1. Lu, H.-C.; Mackie, K. An introduction to the endogenous cannabinoid system. *Biol. Psychiatry* **2016**, *79*, 516–525. [CrossRef] [PubMed]
2. Piomelli, D.; Mabou Tagne, A. Endocannabinoid-based therapies. *Annu. Rev. Pharmacol. Toxicol.* **2022**, *62*, 483–507. [CrossRef] [PubMed]
3. Lowe, H.; Toyang, N.; Steele, B.; Bryant, J.; Ngwa, W. The endocannabinoid system: A potential target for the treatment of various diseases. *Int. J. Mol. Sci.* **2021**, *22*, 9472. [CrossRef]
4. Rossi, F.; Tortora, C.; Argenziano, M.; Di Paola, A.; Punzo, F. Cannabinoid receptor type 2: A possible target in SARS-CoV-2 (CoV-19) infection? *Int. J. Mol. Sci.* **2020**, *21*, 3809. [CrossRef] [PubMed]
5. Kim, S.H.; Won, S.J.; Mao, X.O.; Jin, K.; Greenberg, D.A. Molecular mechanisms of cannabinoid protection from neuronal excitotoxicity. *Mol. Pharmacol.* **2006**, *69*, 691–696. [CrossRef] [PubMed]
6. Waksman, Y.; Olson, J.M.; Carlisle, S.J.; Cabral, G.A. The central cannabinoid receptor (CB_1) mediates inhibition of nitric oxide production by rat microglial cells. *J. Pharmacol. Exp. Ther.* **1999**, *288*, 1357–1366.
7. Walter, L.; Stella, N. Cannabinoids and neuroinflammation. *Br. J. Pharmacol.* **2004**, *141*, 775–785. [CrossRef]
8. Devane, W.A.; Dysarz, F.A.; Johnson, M.R.; Melvin, L.S.; Howlett, A.C. Determination and characterization of a cannabinoid receptor in rat brain. *Mol. Pharmacol.* **1988**, *34*, 605–613.
9. Matsuda, L.A.; Lolait, S.J.; Brownstein, M.J.; Young, A.C.; Bonner, T.I. Structure of a cannabinoid receptor and functional expression of the cloned cDNA. *Nature* **1990**, *346*, 561–564. [CrossRef]
10. Munro, S.; Thomas, K.L.; Abu-Shaar, M. Molecular characterization of a peripheral receptor for cannabinoids. *Nature* **1993**, *365*, 61–65. [CrossRef]
11. Lutz, B. Neurobiology of cannabinoid receptor signaling. *Dialogues Clin. Neurosci.* **2020**, *22*, 207–222. [CrossRef] [PubMed]
12. Ren, S.; Wang, Z.; Zhang, Y.; Chen, N. Potential application of endocannabinoid system agents in neuropsychiatric and neurodegenerative diseases—Focusing on FAAH/MAGL inhibitors. *Acta Pharmacol. Sin.* **2020**, *41*, 1263–1271. [CrossRef] [PubMed]
13. UNODC. Early Warning Advisory on New Psychoactive Substances. What are NPS? December 2021. Available online: https://www.unodc.org/LSS/Page/NPS (accessed on 16 November 2022).
14. Auwärter, V.; Dresen, S.; Weinmann, W.; Müller, M.; Pütz, M.; Ferreirós, N. 'Spice' and other herbal blends: Harmless incense or cannabinoid designer drugs? *J. Mass Spectrom.* **2009**, *44*, 832–837. [CrossRef] [PubMed]

15. An, D.; Peigneur, S.; Hendrickx, L.A.; Tytgat, J. Targeting cannabinoid receptors: Current status and prospects of natural products. *Int. J. Mol. Sci.* **2020**, *21*, 5064. [CrossRef] [PubMed]
16. Deventer, M.H.; Van Uytfanghe, K.; Vinckier, I.M.J.; Reniero, F.; Guillou, C.; Stove, C.P. Cannabinoid receptor activation potential of the next generation, generic ban evading OXIZID synthetic cannabinoid receptor agonists. *Drug Test. Anal.* **2022**, *14*, 1565–1575. [CrossRef]
17. Markham, J.; Sparkes, E.; Boyd, R.; Chen, S.; Manning, J.J.; Finlay, D.; Lai, F.; McGregor, E.; Maloney, C.J.; Gerona, R.R.; et al. Defining steric requirements at CB_1 and CB_2 cannabinoid receptors using synthetic cannabinoid receptor agonists 5F-AB-PINACA, 5F-ADB-PINACA, PX-1, PX-2, NNL-1, and their analogues. *ACS Chem. Neurosci.* **2022**, *13*, 1281–1295. [CrossRef]
18. Van Sickle, M.D.; Duncan, M.; Kingsley, P.J.; Mouihate, A.; Urbani, P.; Mackie, K.; Stella, N.; Makriyannis, A.; Piomelli, D.; Davison, J.S.; et al. Identification and functional characterization of brainstem cannabinoid CB_2 receptors. *Science* **2005**, *310*, 329–332. [CrossRef]
19. Shahbazi, F.; Grandi, V.; Banerjee, A.; Trant, J.F. Cannabinoids and cannabinoid receptors: The story so far. *iScience* **2020**, *23*, 101301. [CrossRef]
20. Tang, X.; Liu, Z.; Li, X.; Wang, J.; Li, L. Cannabinoid receptors in myocardial injury: A brother born to rival. *Int. J. Mol. Sci.* **2021**, *22*, 6886. [CrossRef]
21. Felder, C.C.; Joyce, K.E.; Briley, E.M.; Mansouri, J.; Mackie, K.; Blond, O.; Lai, Y.; Ma, A.L.; Mitchell, R.L. Comparison of the pharmacology and signal transduction of the human cannabinoid CB_1 and CB_2 receptors. *Mol. Pharmacol.* **1995**, *48*, 443–450.
22. de Almeida, D.L.; Devi, L.A. Diversity of molecular targets and signaling pathways for CBD. *Pharmacol. Res. Perspect.* **2020**, *8*, e00682. [CrossRef]
23. Piomelli, D. The molecular logic of endocannabinoid signalling. *Nat. Rev. Neurosci.* **2003**, *4*, 873–884. [CrossRef] [PubMed]
24. Augustin, S.M.; Lovinger, D.M. Functional relevance of endocannabinoid-dependent synaptic plasticity in the central nervous system. *ACS Chem. Neurosci.* **2018**, *9*, 2146–2161. [CrossRef]
25. Alger, B.E. Retrograde signaling in the regulation of synaptic transmission: Focus on endocannabinoids. *Prog. Neurobiol.* **2002**, *68*, 247–286. [CrossRef] [PubMed]
26. Diana, M.A.; Marty, A. Endocannabinoid-mediated short-term synaptic plasticity: Depolarization-induced suppression of inhibition (DSI) and depolarization-induced suppression of excitation (DSE). *Br. J. Pharmacol.* **2004**, *142*, 9–19. [CrossRef] [PubMed]
27. Hohmann, A.G.; Suplita, R.L.; Bolton, N.M.; Neely, M.H.; Fegley, D.; Mangieri, R.; Krey, J.F.; Walker, J.M.; Holmes, P.V.; Crystal, J.D.; et al. An endocannabinoid mechanism for stress-induced analgesia. *Nature* **2005**, *435*, 1108–1112. [CrossRef]
28. Castillo, P.E.; Younts, T.J.; Chávez, A.E.; Hashimotodani, Y. Endocannabinoid signaling and synaptic function. *Neuron* **2012**, *76*, 70–81. [CrossRef]
29. Puente, N.; Cui, Y.; Lassalle, O.; Lafourcade, M.; Georges, F.; Venance, L.; Grandes, P.; Manzoni, O.J. Polymodal activation of the endocannabinoid system in the extended amygdala. *Nat. Neurosci.* **2011**, *14*, 1542–1547. [CrossRef]
30. Estrada, J.A.; Contreras, I. Endocannabinoid receptors in the CNS: Potential drug targets for the prevention and treatment of neurologic and psychiatric disorders. *Curr. Neuropharmacol.* **2020**, *18*, 769–787. [CrossRef]
31. Devane, W.A.; Hanus, L.; Breuer, A.; Pertwee, R.G.; Stevenson, L.A.; Griffin, G.; Gibson, D.; Mandelbaum, A.; Etinger, A.; Mechoulam, R. Isolation and structure of a brain constituent that binds to the cannabinoid receptor. *Science* **1992**, *258*, 1946–1949. [CrossRef]
32. Mechoulam, R.; Ben-Shabat, S.; Hanus, L.; Ligumsky, M.; Kaminski, N.E.; Schatz, A.R.; Gopher, A.; Almog, S.; Martin, B.R.; Compton, D.R. Identification of an endogenous 2-monoglyceride, present in canine gut, that binds to cannabinoid receptors. *Biochem. Pharmacol.* **1995**, *50*, 83–90. [CrossRef] [PubMed]
33. Sugiura, T.; Kondo, S.; Sukagawa, A.; Nakane, S.; Shinoda, A.; Itoh, K.; Yamashita, A.; Waku, K. 2-Arachidonoylglycerol: A possible endogenous cannabinoid receptor ligand in brain. *Biochem. Biophys. Res. Commun.* **1995**, *215*, 89–97. [CrossRef]
34. Hillard, C.J.; Campbell, W.B. Biochemistry and pharmacology of arachidonylethanolamide, a putative endogenous cannabinoid. *J. Lipid Res.* **1997**, *38*, 2383–2398. [CrossRef] [PubMed]
35. Vogel, Z.; Barg, J.; Levy, R.; Saya, D.; Heldman, E.; Mechoulam, R. Anandamide, a brain endogenous compound, interacts specifically with cannabinoid receptors and inhibits adenylate cyclase. *J. Neurochem.* **1993**, *61*, 352–355. [CrossRef]
36. Mackie, K.; Devane, W.A.; Hille, B. Anandamide, an endogenous cannabinoid, inhibits calcium currents as a partial agonist in N18 neuroblastoma cells. *Mol. Pharmacol.* **1993**, *44*, 498–503.
37. Facci, L.; Dal Toso, R.; Romanello, S.; Buriani, A.; Skaper, S.D.; Leon, A. Mast cells express a peripheral cannabinoid receptor with differential sensitivity to anandamide and palmitoylethanolamide. *Proc. Natl. Acad. Sci. USA* **1995**, *92*, 3376–3380. [CrossRef] [PubMed]
38. Bayewitch, M.; Avidor-Reiss, T.; Levy, R.; Barg, J.; Mechoulam, R.; Vogel, Z. The peripheral cannabinoid receptor: Adenylate cyclase inhibition and G protein coupling. *FEBS Lett.* **1995**, *375*, 143–147. [CrossRef]
39. Sugiura, T.; Waku, K. 2-Arachidonoylglycerol and the cannabinoid receptors. *Chem. Phys. Lipids* **2000**, *108*, 89–106. [CrossRef]
40. Di Marzo, V.; Fontana, A.; Cadas, H.; Schinelli, S.; Cimino, G.; Schwartz, J.C.; Piomelli, D. Formation and inactivation of endogenous cannabinoid anandamide in central neurons. *Nature* **1994**, *372*, 686–691. [CrossRef]
41. Cadas, H.; di Tomaso, E.; Piomelli, D. Occurrence and biosynthesis of endogenous cannabinoid precursor, N-arachidonoyl phosphatidylethanolamine, in rat brain. *J. Neurosci.* **1997**, *17*, 1226–1242. [CrossRef]

42. Farooqui, A.A.; Rammohan, K.W.; Horrocks, L.A. Isolation, characterization, and regulation of diacylglycerol lipases from the bovine brain. *Ann. N. Y. Acad. Sci.* **1989**, *559*, 25–36. [CrossRef] [PubMed]
43. Bisogno, T.; Howell, F.; Williams, G.; Minassi, A.; Cascio, M.G.; Ligresti, A.; Matias, I.; Schiano-Moriello, A.; Paul, P.; Williams, E.-J.; et al. Cloning of the first Sn1-DAG lipases points to the spatial and temporal regulation of endocannabinoid signaling in the brain. *J. Cell Biol.* **2003**, *163*, 463–468. [CrossRef] [PubMed]
44. Desarnaud, F.; Cadas, H.; Piomelli, D. Anandamide amidohydrolase activity in rat brain microsomes: Identification and partial characterization. *J. Biol. Chem.* **1995**, *270*, 6030–6035. [CrossRef] [PubMed]
45. Hillard, C.J.; Wilkison, D.M.; Edgemond, W.S.; Campbell, W.B. Characterization of the kinetics and distribution of N-Arachidonylethanolamine (Anandamide) hydrolysis by rat brain. *Biochim. Biophys. Acta Lipids Lipid Metab.* **1995**, *1257*, 249–256. [CrossRef] [PubMed]
46. Ueda, N.; Kurahashi, Y.; Yamamoto, S.; Tokunaga, T. Partial purification and characterization of the porcin brain enzyme hydrolyzing and synthesizing anandamide. *J. Biol. Chem.* **1995**, *270*, 23823–23827. [CrossRef]
47. Cravatt, B.F.; Giang, D.K.; Mayfield, S.P.; Boger, D.L.; Lerner, R.A.; Gilula, N.B. Molecular characterization of an enzyme that degrades neuromodulatory fatty-acid amides. *Nature* **1996**, *384*, 83–87. [CrossRef] [PubMed]
48. Tornqvist, H.; Belfrage, P. Purification and some properties of a monoacylglycerol hydrolyzing enzyme of rat adipose tissue. *J. Biol. Chem.* **1976**, *251*, 813–819. [CrossRef]
49. Prescott, S.M.; Majerus, P.W. Characterization of 1,2-diacylglycerol hydrolysis in human platelets. Demonstration of an arachidonoyl-monoacylglycerol intermediate. *J. Biol. Chem.* **1983**, *258*, 764–769. [CrossRef]
50. Farooqui, A.A.; Taylor, W.A.; Horrocks, L.A. Separation of bovine brain mono- and diacylglycerol lipases by heparin sepharose affinity chromatography. *Biochem. Biophys. Res. Commun.* **1984**, *122*, 1241–1246. [CrossRef]
51. Deutsch, D.G.; Chin, S.A. Enzymatic synthesis and degradation of anandamide, a cannabinoid receptor agonist. *Biochem. Pharmacol.* **1993**, *46*, 791–796. [CrossRef]
52. Dinh, T.P.; Carpenter, D.; Leslie, F.M.; Freund, T.F.; Katona, I.; Sensi, S.L.; Kathuria, S.; Piomelli, D. Brain monoglyceride lipase participating in endocannabinoid inactivation. *Proc. Natl. Acad. Sci. USA* **2002**, *99*, 10819–10824. [CrossRef] [PubMed]
53. Beltramo, M.; Stella, N.; Calignano, A.; Lin, S.Y.; Makriyannis, A.; Piomelli, D. Functional role of high affinity anandamide transport, as revelead by selective inhibition. *Science* **1997**, *277*, 1094–1097. [CrossRef] [PubMed]
54. Hillard, C.J.; Edgemond, W.S.; Jarrahian, A.; Campbell, W.B. Accumulation of N-arachidonylethanolamine (anandamide) into cerebellar granule cells occurs via facilitated diffusion. *J. Neurochem.* **1997**, *69*, 631–638. [CrossRef] [PubMed]
55. Beltramo, M.; Piomelli, D. Carrier-mediated Transport and enzymatic hydrolysis of the endogenous cannabinoid 2-arachidonoylglycerol. *Neuroreport* **2000**, *11*, 1231–1235. [CrossRef]
56. Pagano, C.; Navarra, G.; Coppola, L.; Avilia, G.; Bifulco, M.; Laezza, C. Cannabinoids: Therapeutic use in clinical practice. *Int. J. Mol. Sci.* **2022**, *23*, 3344. [CrossRef]
57. Kumar, P.; Mahato, D.K.; Kamle, M.; Borah, R.; Sharma, B.; Pandhi, S.; Tripathi, V.; Yadav, H.S.; Devi, S.; Patil, U.; et al. Pharmacological properties, therapeutic potential, and legal status of *Cannabis sativa* L.: An overview. *Phytother. Res.* **2021**, *35*, 6010–6029. [CrossRef]
58. Gülck, T.; Møller, B.L. Phytocannabinoids: Origins and biosynthesis. *Trends Plant Sci.* **2020**, *25*, 985–1004. [CrossRef]
59. Tarasov, P.; Bezrukova, E.; Karabanov, E.; Nakagawa, T.; Wagner, M.; Kulagina, N.; Letunova, P.; Abzaeva, A.; Granoszewski, W.; Riedel, F. Vegetation and climate dynamics during the holocene and eemian interglacials derived from lake baikal pollen records. *Palaeogeogr. Palaeoclimatol. Palaeoecol.* **2007**, *252*, 440–457. [CrossRef]
60. Pisanti, S.; Bifulco, M. Medical cannabis: A plurimillennial history of an evergreen. *J. Cell. Physiol.* **2019**, *234*, 8342–8351. [CrossRef]
61. Li, H.-L. The origin and use of cannabis in Eastern Asia linguistic-cultural implications. *Econ. Bot.* **1974**, *28*, 293–301. [CrossRef]
62. Prandi, C.; Blangetti, M.; Namdar, D.; Koltai, H. Structure-activity relationship of cannabis derived compounds for the treatment of neuronal activity-related diseases. *Molecules* **2018**, *23*, 1526. [CrossRef] [PubMed]
63. Gaoni, Y.; Mechoulam, R. Isolation, structure, and partial synthesis of an active constituent of hashish. *J. Am. Chem. Soc.* **1964**, *86*, 1646–1647. [CrossRef]
64. Adams, R.; Hunt, M.; Clark, J.H. Structure of cannabidiol, a product isolated from the marihuana extract of Minnesota wild hemp. I. *J. Am. Chem. Soc.* **1940**, *62*, 196–200. [CrossRef]
65. Morales, P.; Hurst, D.P.; Reggio, P.H. Molecular targets of the phytocannabinoids: A complex picture. *Prog. Chem. Org. Nat. Prod.* **2017**, *103*, 103–131. [CrossRef]
66. Peng, J.; Fan, M.; An, C.; Ni, F.; Huang, W.; Luo, J. A narrative review of molecular mechanism and therapeutic effect of cannabidiol (CBD). *Basic Clin. Pharmacol. Toxicol.* **2022**, *130*, 439–456. [CrossRef]
67. Hayakawa, K.; Mishima, K.; Fujiwara, M. Therapeutic potential of non-psychotropic cannabidiol in ischemic stroke. *Pharmaceuticals* **2010**, *3*, 2197–2212. [CrossRef]
68. Dos Santos, R.G.; Hallak, J.E.C.; Crippa, J.A.S. Neuropharmacological effects of the main phytocannabinoids: A narrative review. *Adv. Exp. Med. Biol.* **2021**, *1264*, 29–45. [CrossRef]
69. Stone, N.L.; Murphy, A.J.; England, T.J.; O'Sullivan, S.E. A systematic review of minor phytocannabinoids with promising neuroprotective potential. *Br. J. Pharmacol.* **2020**, *177*, 4330–4352. [CrossRef]
70. Alves, V.L.; Gonçalves, J.L.; Aguiar, J.; Teixeira, H.M.; Câmara, J.S. The synthetic cannabinoids phenomenon: From structure to toxicological properties. a review. *Crit. Rev. Toxicol.* **2020**, *50*, 359–382. [CrossRef]

71. Shafi, A.; Berry, A.J.; Sumnall, H.; Wood, D.M.; Tracy, D.K. New psychoactive substances: A review and updates. *Ther. Adv. Psychopharmacol.* **2020**, *10*, 2045125320967197. [CrossRef]
72. Brown, J.D.; Rivera Rivera, K.J.; Hernandez, L.Y.C.; Doenges, M.R.; Auchey, I.; Pham, T.; Goodin, A.J. Natural and synthetic cannabinoids: Pharmacology, uses, adverse drug events, and drug interactions. *J. Clin. Pharmacol.* **2021**, *61* (Suppl. 2), S37–S52. [CrossRef] [PubMed]
73. Chung, E.Y.; Cha, H.J.; Min, H.K.; Yun, J. Pharmacology and adverse effects of new psychoactive substances: Synthetic cannabinoid receptor agonists. *Arch. Pharm. Res.* **2021**, *44*, 402–413. [CrossRef] [PubMed]
74. Cinar, R.; Iyer, M.R.; Kunos, G. The therapeutic potential of second and third generation CB_1R antagonists. *Pharmacol. Ther.* **2020**, *208*, 107477. [CrossRef] [PubMed]
75. Sholler, D.J.; Huestis, M.A.; Amendolara, B.; Vandrey, R.; Cooper, Z.D. Therapeutic potential and safety considerations for the clinical use of synthetic cannabinoids. *Pharmacol. Biochem. Behav.* **2020**, *199*, 173059. [CrossRef] [PubMed]
76. Coronado-Álvarez, A.; Romero-Cordero, K.; Macías-Triana, L.; Tatum-Kuri, A.; Vera-Barrón, A.; Budde, H.; Machado, S.; Yamamoto, T.; Imperatori, C.; Murillo-Rodríguez, E. The synthetic CB_1 cannabinoid receptor selective agonists: Putative medical uses and their legalization. *Prog. Neuropsychopharmacol. Biol. Psychiatry* **2021**, *110*, 110301. [CrossRef]
77. Saldaña-Shumaker, S.L.; Grenning, A.J.; Cunningham, C.W. Modern approaches to the development of synthetic cannabinoid receptor probes. *Pharmacol. Biochem. Behav.* **2021**, *203*, 173119. [CrossRef]
78. Manning, J.J.; Green, H.M.; Glass, M.; Finlay, D.B. Pharmacological selection of cannabinoid receptor effectors: Signalling, allosteric modulation and bias. *Neuropharmacology* **2021**, *193*, 108611. [CrossRef]
79. Leo, L.M.; Abood, M.E. CB_1 Cannabinoid receptor signaling and biased signaling. *Molecules* **2021**, *26*, 5413. [CrossRef]
80. Manera, C.; Bertini, S. Cannabinoid-based medicines and Multiple Sclerosis. *Adv. Exp. Med. Biol.* **2021**, *1264*, 111–129. [CrossRef]
81. Products (Outside US). Jazz Pharmaceuticals. Available online: https://www.jazzpharma.com/medicines/our-medicines/ (accessed on 29 July 2022).
82. Landucci, E.; Scartabelli, T.; Gerace, E.; Moroni, F.; Pellegrini-Giampietro, D.E. CB_1 receptors and post-ischemic brain damage: Studies on the toxic and neuroprotective effects of cannabinoids in rat organotypic hippocampal slices. *Neuropharmacology* **2011**, *60*, 674–682. [CrossRef]
83. Benyó, Z.; Ruisanchez, É.; Leszl-Ishiguro, M.; Sándor, P.; Pacher, P. Endocannabinoids in cerebrovascular regulation. *Am. J. Physiol. Heart Circ. Physiol.* **2016**, *310*, H785–H801. [CrossRef] [PubMed]
84. Sagredo, O.; Palazuelos, J.; Gutierrez-Rodriguez, A.; Satta, V.; Galve-Roperh, I.; Martínez-Orgado, J. Cannabinoid signalling in the immature brain: Encephalopathies and neurodevelopmental disorders. *Biochem. Pharmacol.* **2018**, *157*, 85–96. [CrossRef] [PubMed]
85. Carloni, S.; Crinelli, R.; Palma, L.; Álvarez, F.J.; Piomelli, D.; Duranti, A.; Balduini, W.; Alonso-Alconada, D. The synthetic cannabinoid URB447 reduces brain injury and the associated white matter demyelination after hypoxia-ischemia in neonatal rats. *ACS Chem. Neurosci.* **2020**, *11*, 1291–1299. [CrossRef] [PubMed]
86. Melvin, L.S.; Johnson, M.R. Structure-activity relationships of tricyclic and nonclassical bicyclic cannabinoids. *NIDA Res. Monogr.* **1987**, *79*, 31–34.
87. Pacheco, M.; Childers, S.R.; Arnold, R.; Casiano, F.; Ward, S.J. Aminoalkylindoles: Actions on specific g-protein-linked receptors. *J. Pharmacol. Exp. Ther.* **1991**, *257*, 170–183. [PubMed]
88. Rinaldi-Carmona, M.; Barth, F.; Héaulme, M.; Shire, D.; Calandra, B.; Congy, C.; Martinez, S.; Maruani, J.; Néliat, G.; Caput, D. SR141716A, a potent and selective antagonist of the brain cannabinoid receptor. *FEBS Lett.* **1994**, *350*, 240–244. [CrossRef]
89. Lan, R.; Makriyannis, A.; Gatley, S.J. Preparation of iodine-123 labeled AM251: A potential SPECT radioligand for the brain cannabinoid CB_1 receptor. *J. Label. Compd. Radiopharm.* **1996**, *38*, 875–882. [CrossRef]
90. Felder, C.C.; Joyce, K.E.; Briley, E.M.; Glass, M.; Mackie, K.P.; Fahey, K.J.; Cullinan, G.J.; Hunden, D.C.; Johnson, D.W.; Chaney, M.O.; et al. LY320135, a novel cannabinoid CB_1 receptor antagonist, unmasks coupling of the CB_1 receptor to stimulation of cAMP accumulation. *J. Pharmacol. Exp. Ther.* **1998**, *284*, 291–297.
91. LoVerme, J.; Duranti, A.; Tontini, A.; Spadoni, G.; Mor, M.; Rivara, S.; Stella, N.; Xu, C.; Tarzia, G.; Piomelli, D. Synthesis and characterization of a peripherally restricted CB_1 cannabinoid antagonist, URB447, that reduces feeding and body-weight gain in mice. *Bioorg. Med. Chem. Lett.* **2009**, *19*, 639–643. [CrossRef]
92. De Luca, M.A.; Fattore, L. Therapeutic use of synthetic cannabinoids: Still an open issue? *Clin. Ther.* **2018**, *40*, 1457–1466. [CrossRef]
93. Cravatt, B.F.; Demarest, K.; Patricelli, M.P.; Bracey, M.H.; Giang, D.K.; Martin, B.R.; Lichtman, A.H. Supersensitivity to anandamide and enhanced endogenous cannabinoid signaling in mice lacking fatty acid amide hydrolase. *Proc. Natl. Acad. Sci. USA* **2001**, *98*, 9371–9376. [CrossRef] [PubMed]
94. Lichtman, A.H.; Shelton, C.C.; Advani, T.; Cravatt, B.F. Mice lacking fatty acid amide hydrolase exhibit a cannabinoid receptor-mediated phenotypic hypoalgesia. *Pain* **2004**, *109*, 319–327. [CrossRef] [PubMed]
95. Kathuria, S.; Gaetani, S.; Fegley, D.; Valiño, F.; Duranti, A.; Tontini, A.; Mor, M.; Tarzia, G.; La Rana, G.; Calignano, A.; et al. Modulation of anxiety through blockade of anandamide hydrolysis. *Nat. Med.* **2003**, *9*, 76–81. [CrossRef]
96. Tuo, W.; Leleu-Chavain, N.; Spencer, J.; Sansook, S.; Millet, R.; Chavatte, P. Therapeutic potential of fatty acid amide hydrolase, monoacylglycerol lipase, and *N*-acylethanolamine acid amidase inhibitors. *J. Med. Chem.* **2017**, *60*, 4–46. [CrossRef] [PubMed]

97. Tripathi, R.K.P. A perspective review on fatty acid amide hydrolase (FAAH) inhibitors as potential therapeutic agents. *Eur. J. Med. Chem.* **2020**, *188*, 111953. [CrossRef] [PubMed]
98. Van Egmond, N.; Straub, V.M.; van der Stelt, M. Targeting endocannabinoid signaling: FAAH and MAG lipase inhibitors. *Annu. Rev. Pharmacol. Toxicol.* **2021**, *61*, 441–463. [CrossRef]
99. Abhishek, K.; Suresh, K.; Rohit, D. A review on structurally diversified synthesized molecules as monoacyl-glycerol lipase inhibitors and their therapeutic uses. *Curr. Drug Res. Rev.* **2022**, *14*, 96–115. [CrossRef]
100. Wang, D.-P.; Jin, K.-Y.; Zhao, P.; Lin, Q.; Kang, K.; Hai, J. Neuroprotective effects of VEGF-A nanofiber membrane and FAAH inhibitor URB597 against oxygen-glucose deprivation-induced ischemic neuronal injury. *Int. J. Nanomedicine* **2021**, *16*, 3661–3678. [CrossRef]
101. Carloni, S.; Alonso-Alconada, D.; Girelli, S.; Duranti, A.; Tontini, A.; Piomelli, D.; Hilario, E.; Alvarez, A.; Balduini, W. Pretreatment with the monoacylglycerol lipase inhibitor URB602 protects from the long-term consequences of neonatal hypoxic–ischemic brain injury in rats. *Pediatr. Res.* **2012**, *72*, 400–406. [CrossRef]
102. Choi, S.-H.; Arai, A.L.; Mou, Y.; Kang, B.; Yen, C.C.-C.; Hallenbeck, J.; Silva, A.C. Neuroprotective effects of MAGL (Monoacylglycerol Lipase) inhibitors in experimental ischemic stroke. *Stroke* **2018**, *49*, 718–726. [CrossRef]
103. Piro, J.R.; Suidan, G.L.; Quan, J.; Pi, Y.; O'Neill, S.M.; Ilardi, M.; Pozdnyakov, N.; Lanz, T.A.; Xi, H.; Bell, R.D.; et al. Inhibition of 2-AG hydrolysis differentially regulates blood brain barrier permeability after injury. *J. Neuroinflammation* **2018**, *15*, 142. [CrossRef] [PubMed]
104. Xiong, Y.; Yao, H.; Cheng, Y.; Gong, D.; Liao, X.; Wang, R. Effects of monoacylglycerol lipase inhibitor URB602 on lung ischemia-reperfusion injury in mice. *Biochem. Biophys. Res. Commun.* **2018**, *506*, 578–584. [CrossRef] [PubMed]
105. Yamasaki, T.; Hatori, A.; Zhang, Y.; Mori, W.; Kurihara, Y.; Ogawa, M.; Wakizaka, H.; Rong, J.; Wang, L.; Liang, S.; et al. Neuroprotective effects of minocycline and KML29, a potent inhibitor of monoacylglycerol lipase, in an experimental stroke model: A small-animal positron emission tomography study. *Theranostics* **2021**, *11*, 9492–9502. [CrossRef] [PubMed]
106. Mor, M.; Rivara, S.; Lodola, A.; Plazzi, P.V.; Tarzia, G.; Duranti, A.; Tontini, A.; Piersanti, G.; Kathuria, S.; Piomelli, D. Cyclohexylcarbamic acid 3'- or 4'-Substituted Biphenyl-3-yl esters as fatty acid amide hydrolase inhibitors: Synthesis, quantitative structure-activity relationships, and molecular modeling studies. *J. Med. Chem.* **2004**, *47*, 4998–5008. [CrossRef]
107. Fegley, D.; Gaetani, S.; Duranti, A.; Tontini, A.; Mor, M.; Tarzia, G.; Piomelli, D. Characterization of the fatty acid amide hydrolase inhibitor cyclohexyl carbamic acid 3'-carbamoyl-biphenyl-3-yl ester (URB597): Effects on anandamide and oleoylethanolamide deactivation. *J. Pharmacol. Exp. Ther.* **2005**, *313*, 352–358. [CrossRef]
108. Gobbi, G.; Bambico, F.R.; Mangieri, R.; Bortolato, M.; Campolongo, P.; Solinas, M.; Cassano, T.; Morgese, M.G.; Debonnel, G.; Duranti, A.; et al. Antidepressant-like activity and modulation of brain monoaminergic transmission by blockade of anandamide hydrolysis. *Proc. Natl. Acad. Sci. USA* **2005**, *102*, 18620–18625. [CrossRef]
109. Piomelli, D.; Tarzia, G.; Duranti, A.; Tontini, A.; Mor, M.; Compton, T.R.; Dasse, O.; Monaghan, E.P.; Parrott, J.A.; Putman, D. Pharmacological profile of the selective FAAH inhibitor KDS-4103 (URB597). *CNS Drug Rev.* **2006**, *12*, 21–38. [CrossRef]
110. Russo, R.; Loverme, J.; La Rana, G.; Compton, T.R.; Parrott, J.; Duranti, A.; Tontini, A.; Mor, M.; Tarzia, G.; Calignano, A.; et al. The fatty acid amide hydrolase inhibitor URB597 (cyclohexylcarbamic acid 3'-carbamoylbiphenyl-3-yl ester) reduces neuropathic pain after oral administration in mice. *J. Pharmacol. Exp. Ther.* **2007**, *322*, 236–242. [CrossRef]
111. Bortolato, M.; Mangieri, R.A.; Fu, J.; Kim, J.H.; Arguello, O.; Duranti, A.; Tontini, A.; Mor, M.; Tarzia, G.; Piomelli, D. Antidepressant-like activity of the fatty acid amide hydrolase inhibitor URB597 in a rat model of chronic mild stress. *Biol. Psychiatry* **2007**, *62*, 1103–1110. [CrossRef]
112. Vacondio, F.; Silva, C.; Lodola, A.; Fioni, A.; Rivara, S.; Duranti, A.; Tontini, A.; Sanchini, S.; Clapper, J.R.; Piomelli, D.; et al. Structure-property relationships of a class of carbamate-based fatty acid amide hydrolase (FAAH) inhibitors: Chemical and biological stability. *ChemMedChem* **2009**, *4*, 1495–1504. [CrossRef]
113. Bambico, F.R.; Duranti, A.; Nobrega, J.N.; Gobbi, G. The fatty acid amide hydrolase inhibitor URB597 modulates serotonin-dependent emotional behaviour, and serotonin1A and serotonin2A/C activity in the hippocampus. *Eur. Neuropsychopharmacol.* **2016**, *26*, 578–590. [CrossRef] [PubMed]
114. Tarzia, G.; Duranti, A.; Tontini, A.; Piersanti, G.; Mor, M.; Rivara, S.; Plazzi, P.V.; Park, C.; Kathuria, S.; Piomelli, D. Design, synthesis, and structure-activity relationships of alkylcarbamic acid aryl esters, a new class of fatty acid amide hydrolase inhibitors. *J. Med. Chem.* **2003**, *46*, 2352–2360. [CrossRef] [PubMed]
115. Makara, J.K.; Mor, M.; Fegley, D.; Szabó, S.I.; Kathuria, S.; Astarita, G.; Duranti, A.; Tontini, A.; Tarzia, G.; Rivara, S.; et al. Selective inhibition of 2-AG hydrolysis enhances endocannabinoid signaling in hippocampus. *Nat. Neurosci.* **2005**, *8*, 1139–1141. [CrossRef] [PubMed]
116. King, A.R.; Duranti, A.; Tontini, A.; Rivara, S.; Rosengarth, A.; Clapper, J.R.; Astarita, G.; Geaga, J.A.; Luecke, H.; Mor, M.; et al. URB602 inhibits monoacylglycerol lipase and selectively blocks 2-arachidonoylglycerol degradation in intact brain slices. *Chem. Biol.* **2007**, *14*, 1357–1365. [CrossRef] [PubMed]
117. Long, J.Z.; Li, W.; Booker, L.; Burston, J.J.; Kinsey, S.G.; Schlosburg, J.E.; Pavón, F.J.; Serrano, A.M.; Selley, D.E.; Parsons, L.H.; et al. Selective blockade of 2-arachidonoylglycerol hydrolysis produces cannabinoid behavioral effects. *Nat. Chem. Biol.* **2009**, *5*, 37–44. [CrossRef] [PubMed]

118. Chang, J.W.; Niphakis, M.J.; Lum, K.M.; Cognetta, A.B., III; Wang, C.; Matthews, M.L.; Niessen, S.; Buczynski, M.W.; Parsons, L.H.; Cravatt, B.F. Highly selective inhibitors of monoacylglycerol lipase bearing a reactive group that is bioisosteric with endocannabinoid substrates. *Chem. Biol.* **2012**, *19*, 579–588. [CrossRef]
119. Niphakis, M.J.; Cognetta, A.B.; Chang, J.W.; Buczynski, M.W.; Parsons, L.H.; Byrne, F.; Burston, J.J.; Chapman, V.; Cravatt, B.F. Evaluation of NHS carbamates as a potent and selective class of endocannabinoid hydrolase inhibitors. *ACS Chem. Neurosci.* **2013**, *4*, 1322–1332. [CrossRef]
120. Gaffuri, A.-L.; Ladarre, D.; Lenkei, Z. Type-1 cannabinoid receptor signaling in neuronal development. *Pharmacology* **2012**, *90*, 19–39. [CrossRef]
121. Berrendero, F.; Garcia-Gil, L.; Hernandez, M.L.; Romero, J.; Cebeira, M.; de Miguel, R.; Ramos, J.A.; Fernández-Ruiz, J.J. Localization of MRNA expression and activation of signal transduction mechanisms for cannabinoid receptor in rat brain during fetal development. *Development* **1998**, *125*, 3179–3188. [CrossRef]
122. Berrendero, F.; Sepe, N.; Ramos, J.A.; Di Marzo, V.; Fernández-Ruiz, J.J. Analysis of cannabinoid receptor binding and mRNA expression and endogenous cannabinoid contents in the developing rat brain during late gestation and early postnatal period. *Synapse* **1999**, *33*, 181–191. [CrossRef]
123. Romero, J.; Garcia-Palomero, E.; Berrendero, F.; Garcia-Gil, L.; Hernandez, M.L.; Ramos, J.A.; Fernández-Ruiz, J.J. Atypical location of cannabinoid receptors in white matter areas during rat brain development. *Synapse* **1997**, *26*, 317–323. [CrossRef]
124. Buckley, N.E.; Hansson, S.; Harta, G.; Mezey, É. Expression of the CB_1 and CB_2 receptor messenger rnas during embryonic development in the rat. *Neuroscience* **1997**, *82*, 1131–1149. [CrossRef] [PubMed]
125. Biegon, A.; Kerman, I.A. Autoradiographic study of pre- and postnatal distribution of cannabinoid receptors in human brain. *NeuroImage* **2001**, *14*, 1463–1468. [CrossRef] [PubMed]
126. Mato, S.; Del Olmo, E.; Pazos, A. Ontogenetic development of cannabinoid receptor expression and signal transduction functionality in the human brain: Ontogeny of CB_1 receptors in human brain. *Eur. J. Neurosci.* **2003**, *17*, 1747–1754. [CrossRef]
127. Xapelli, S.; Agasse, F.; Sardà-Arroyo, L.; Bernardino, L.; Santos, T.; Ribeiro, F.F.; Valero, J.; Bragança, J.; Schitine, C.; de Melo Reis, R.A.; et al. Activation of type 1 cannabinoid receptor (CB_1R) promotes neurogenesis in murine subventricular zone cell cultures. *PLoS ONE* **2013**, *8*, e63529. [CrossRef]
128. Díaz-Alonso, J.; Guzmán, M.; Galve-Roperh, I. Endocannabinoids via CB_1 receptors act as neurogenic niche cues during cortical development. *Philos. Trans. R. Soc. B Biol. Sci.* **2012**, *367*, 3229–3241. [CrossRef]
129. Fernández-López, D.; Lizasoain, I.; Moro, M.; Martínez-Orgado, J. Cannabinoids: Well-suited candidates for the treatment of perinatal brain injury. *Brain Sci.* **2013**, *3*, 1043–1059. [CrossRef]
130. Oudin, M.J.; Gajendra, S.; Williams, G.; Hobbs, C.; Lalli, G.; Doherty, P. Endocannabinoids regulate the migration of subventricular zone-derived neuroblasts in the postnatal brain. *J. Neurosci.* **2011**, *31*, 4000–4011. [CrossRef]
131. Berghuis, P.; Rajnicek, A.M.; Morozov, Y.M.; Ross, R.A.; Mulder, J.; Urbán, G.M.; Monory, K.; Marsicano, G.; Matteoli, M.; Canty, A.; et al. Hardwiring the brain: Endocannabinoids shape neuronal connectivity. *Science* **2007**, *316*, 1212–1216. [CrossRef]
132. Paria, B.C.; Dey, S.K. Ligand-receptor signaling with endocannabinoids in preimplantation embryo development and implantation. *Chem. Phys. Lipids* **2000**, *108*, 211–220. [CrossRef]
133. Fernández-Ruiz, J.; Berrendero, F.; Hernández, M.L.; Ramos, J.A. The endogenous cannabinoid system and brain development. *Trends Neurosci.* **2000**, *23*, 14–20. [CrossRef] [PubMed]
134. Douglas-Escobar, M.; Weiss, M.D. Hypoxic-ischemic encephalopathy: A review for the clinician. *JAMA Pediatr.* **2015**, *169*, 397–403. [CrossRef]
135. Maiwald, C.A.; Annink, K.V.; Rüdiger, M.; Benders, M.J.N.L.; van Bel, F.; Allegaert, K.; Naulaers, G.; Bassler, D.; Klebermaß-Schrehof, K.; Vento, M.; et al. Effect of allopurinol in addition to hypothermia treatment in neonates for hypoxic-ischemic brain injury on neurocognitive outcome (ALBINO): Study protocol of a blinded randomized placebo-controlled parallel group multicenter trial for superiority (Phase III). *BMC Pediatr.* **2019**, *19*, 210. [CrossRef]
136. Lee, A.C.; Kozuki, N.; Blencowe, H.; Vos, T.; Bahalim, A.; Darmstadt, G.L.; Niermeyer, S.; Ellis, M.; Robertson, N.J.; Cousens, S.; et al. Intrapartum-related neonatal encephalopathy incidence and impairment at regional and global levels for 2010 with trends from 1990. *Pediatr. Res.* **2013**, *74*, 50–72. [CrossRef] [PubMed]
137. Davidson, J.O.; Wassink, G.; van den Heuij, L.G.; Bennet, L.; Gunn, A.J. Therapeutic hypothermia for neonatal hypoxic–ischemic encephalopathy—Where to from here? *Front. Neurol.* **2015**, *6*, 198. [CrossRef] [PubMed]
138. Edwards, A.D.; Brocklehurst, P.; Gunn, A.J.; Halliday, H.; Juszczak, E.; Levene, M.; Strohm, B.; Thoresen, M.; Whitelaw, A.; Azzopardi, D. Neurological outcomes at 18 months of age after moderate hypothermia for perinatal hypoxic ischaemic encephalopathy: Synthesis and meta-analysis of trial data. *BMJ* **2010**, *340*, c363. [CrossRef]
139. Tetorou, K.; Sisa, C.; Iqbal, A.; Dhillon, K.; Hristova, M. Current therapies for neonatal hypoxic–ischaemic and infection-sensitised hypoxic–ischaemic brain damage. *Front. Synaptic Neurosci.* **2021**, *13*, 709301. [CrossRef]
140. Alonso-Alconada, D.; Broad, K.D.; Bainbridge, A.; Chandrasekaran, M.; Faulkner, S.D.; Kerenyi, Á.; Hassell, J.; Rocha-Ferreira, E.; Hristova, M.; Fleiss, B.; et al. Brain cell death is reduced with cooling by 3.5 °C to 5 °C but increased with cooling by 8.5 °C in a piglet asphyxia model. *Stroke* **2015**, *46*, 275–278. [CrossRef]
141. Gonzalez, F.F. Neuroprotection strategies for term encephalopathy. *Semin. Pediatr. Neurol.* **2019**, *32*, 100773. [CrossRef]
142. Victor, S.; Rocha-Ferreira, E.; Rahim, A.; Hagberg, H.; Edwards, D. New possibilities for neuroprotection in neonatal hypoxic-ischemic encephalopathy. *Eur. J. Pediatr.* **2022**, *181*, 875–887. [CrossRef]

143. Fernández-Ruiz, J.; Moro, M.A.; Martínez-Orgado, J. Cannabinoids in neurodegenerative disorders and stroke/brain trauma: From preclinical models to clinical applications. *Neurotherapeutics* **2015**, *12*, 793–806. [CrossRef] [PubMed]
144. Nagayama, T.; Sinor, A.D.; Simon, R.P.; Chen, J.; Graham, S.H.; Jin, K.; Greenberg, D.A. Cannabinoids and neuroprotection in global and focal cerebral ischemia and in neuronal cultures. *J. Neurosci.* **1999**, *19*, 2987–2995. [CrossRef] [PubMed]
145. Lara-Celador, I.; Castro-Ortega, L.; Álvarez, A.; Goñi-de-Cerio, F.; Lacalle, J.; Hilario, E. Endocannabinoids reduce cerebral damage after hypoxic–ischemic injury in perinatal rats. *Brain Res.* **2012**, *1474*, 91–99. [CrossRef] [PubMed]
146. Alonso-Alconada, D.; Alvarez, F.J.; Alvarez, A.; Mielgo, V.E.; Goñi-de-Cerio, F.; Rey-Santano, M.C.; Caballero, A.; Martinez-Orgado, J.; Hilario, E. The cannabinoid receptor agonist WIN 55,212-2 reduces the initial cerebral damage after hypoxic–ischemic injury in fetal lambs. *Brain Res.* **2010**, *1362*, 150–159. [CrossRef] [PubMed]
147. Alonso-Alconada, D.; Álvarez, A.; Álvarez, F.J.; Martínez-Orgado, J.A.; Hilario, E. The cannabinoid WIN 55212-2 mitigates apoptosis and mitochondrial dysfunction after hypoxia ischemia. *Neurochem. Res.* **2012**, *37*, 161–170. [CrossRef]
148. Alonso-Alconada, D.; Álvarez, A.; Arteaga, O.; Martínez-Ibargüen, A.; Hilario, E. Neuroprotective effect of melatonin: A novel therapy against perinatal hypoxia-ischemia. *Int. J. Mol. Sci.* **2013**, *14*, 9379–9395. [CrossRef]
149. Pellegrini-Giampietro, D.E.; Mannaioni, G.; Bagetta, G. Post-ischemic brain damage: The endocannabinoid system in the mechanisms of neuronal death: The endocannabinoid system in cerebral ischemia. *FEBS J.* **2009**, *276*, 2–12. [CrossRef]
150. Lombard, C.; Hegde, V.L.; Nagarkatti, M.; Nagarkatti, P.S. Perinatal exposure to Δ^9-tetrahydrocannabinol triggers profound defects in T cell differentiation and function in fetal and postnatal stages of life, including decreased responsiveness to HIV antigens. *J. Pharmacol. Exp. Ther.* **2011**, *339*, 607–617. [CrossRef]
151. Turcotte, C.; Blanchet, M.-R.; Laviolette, M.; Flamand, N. The CB_2 receptor and its role as a regulator of inflammation. *Cell. Mol. Life Sci.* **2016**, *73*, 4449–4470. [CrossRef]
152. Garberg, H.T.; Solberg, R.; Barlinn, J.; Martinez-Orgado, J.; Løberg, E.-M.; Saugstad, O.D. High-dose cannabidiol induced hypotension after global hypoxia-ischemia in piglets. *Neonatology* **2017**, *112*, 143–149. [CrossRef]
153. Martínez-Orgado, J.; Villa, M.; del Pozo, A. Cannabidiol for the treatment of neonatal hypoxic-ischemic brain injury. *Front. Pharmacol.* **2021**, *11*, 584533. [CrossRef] [PubMed]
154. Rivers-Auty, J.R.; Smith, P.F.; Ashton, J.C. The cannabinoid CB_2 receptor agonist GW405833 does not ameliorate brain damage induced by hypoxia-ischemia in rats. *Neurosci. Lett.* **2014**, *569*, 104–109. [CrossRef] [PubMed]
155. Azzopardi, D.; Strohm, B.; Linsell, L.; Hobson, A.; Juszczak, E.; Kurinczuk, J.J.; Brocklehurst, P.; Edwards, A.D.; UK TOBY Cooling Register. Implementation and conduct of therapeutic hypothermia for perinatal asphyxial encephalopathy in the UK—Analysis of national data. *PLoS ONE* **2012**, *7*, e38504. [CrossRef] [PubMed]
156. Drury, P.P.; Gunn, E.R.; Bennet, L.; Gunn, A.J. Mechanisms of hypothermic neuroprotection. *Clin. Perinatol.* **2014**, *41*, 161–175. [CrossRef]
157. Leker, R.R.; Gai, N.; Mechoulam, R.; Ovadia, H. Drug-induced hypothermia reduces ischemic damage: Effects of the cannabinoid HU-210. *Stroke* **2003**, *34*, 2000–2006. [CrossRef]
158. Barata, L.; Arruza, L.; Rodríguez, M.-J.; Aleo, E.; Vierge, E.; Criado, E.; Sobrino, E.; Vargas, C.; Ceprián, M.; Gutiérrez-Rodríguez, A.; et al. Neuroprotection by cannabidiol and hypothermia in a piglet model of newborn hypoxic-ischemic brain damage. *Neuropharmacology* **2019**, *146*, 1–11. [CrossRef]
159. Lafuente, H.; Pazos, M.R.; Alvarez, A.; Mohammed, N.; Santos, M.; Arizti, M.; Alvarez, F.J.; Martinez-Orgado, J.A. Effects of cannabidiol and hypothermia on short-term brain damage in new-born piglets after acute hypoxia-ischemia. *Front. Neurosci.* **2016**, *10*, 323. [CrossRef]
160. Ihrie, R.A.; Álvarez-Buylla, A. Lake-front property: A unique germinal niche by the lateral ventricles of the adult brain. *Neuron* **2011**, *70*, 674–686. [CrossRef]
161. Spalding, K.L.; Bergmann, O.; Alkass, K.; Bernard, S.; Salehpour, M.; Huttner, H.B.; Boström, E.; Westerlund, I.; Vial, C.; Buchholz, B.A.; et al. Dynamics of hippocampal neurogenesis in adult humans. *Cell* **2013**, *153*, 1219–1227. [CrossRef]
162. Lois, C.; Alvarez-Buylla, A. Proliferating subventricular zone cells in the adult mammalian forebrain can differentiate into neurons and glia. *Proc. Natl. Acad. Sci. USA* **1993**, *90*, 2074–2077. [CrossRef]
163. Eriksson, P.S.; Perfilieva, E.; Björk-Eriksson, T.; Alborn, A.-M.; Nordborg, C.; Peterson, D.A.; Gage, F.H. Neurogenesis in the adult human hippocampus. *Nat. Med.* **1998**, *4*, 1313–1317. [CrossRef] [PubMed]
164. Kornack, D.R.; Rakic, P. Cell proliferation without neurogenesis in adult primate neocortex. *Science* **2001**, *294*, 2127–2130. [CrossRef] [PubMed]
165. Asrican, B.; Paez-Gonzalez, P.; Erb, J.; Kuo, C.T. Cholinergic circuit control of postnatal neurogenesis. *Neurogenesis* **2016**, *3*, e1127310. [CrossRef] [PubMed]
166. Benner, E.J.; Luciano, D.; Jo, R.; Abdi, K.; Paez-Gonzalez, P.; Sheng, H.; Warner, D.S.; Liu, C.; Eroglu, C.; Kuo, C.T. Protective astrogenesis from the SVZ niche after injury is controlled by notch modulator Thbs4. *Nature* **2013**, *497*, 369–373. [CrossRef]
167. Faiz, M.; Sachewsky, N.; Gascón, S.; Bang, K.W.A.; Morshead, C.M.; Nagy, A. Adult neural stem cells from the subventricular zone give rise to reactive astrocytes in the cortex after stroke. *Cell Stem Cell* **2015**, *17*, 624–634. [CrossRef]
168. Livneh, Y.; Adam, Y.; Mizrahi, A. Odor processing by adult-born neurons. *Neuron* **2014**, *81*, 1097–1110. [CrossRef]
169. Sakamoto, M.; Ieki, N.; Miyoshi, G.; Mochimaru, D.; Miyachi, H.; Imura, T.; Yamaguchi, M.; Fishell, G.; Mori, K.; Kageyama, R.; et al. Continuous postnatal neurogenesis contributes to formation of the olfactory bulb neural circuits and flexible olfactory associative learning. *J. Neurosci.* **2014**, *34*, 5788–5799. [CrossRef]

170. Gil-Perotín, S.; Duran-Moreno, M.; Cebrián-Silla, A.; Ramírez, M.; García-Belda, P.; García-Verdugo, J.M. Adult neural stem cells from the subventricular zone: A review of the neurosphere assay: A review of the neurosphere assay. *Anat. Rec.* **2013**, *296*, 1435–1452. [CrossRef]
171. Kukekov, V.G.; Laywell, E.D.; Suslov, O.; Davies, K.; Scheffler, B.; Thomas, L.B.; O'Brien, T.F.; Kusakabe, M.; Steindler, D.A. Multipotent stem/progenitor cells with similar properties arise from two neurogenic regions of adult human brain. *Exp. Neurol.* **1999**, *156*, 333–344. [CrossRef]
172. Ostenfeld, T.; Tai, Y.-T.; Martin, P.; Déglon, N.; Aebischer, P.; Svendsen, C.N. Neurospheres modified to produce glial cell line-derived neurotrophic factor increase the survival of transplanted dopamine neurons: GDNF-modified ns improve neuron survival. *J. Neurosci. Res.* **2002**, *69*, 955–965. [CrossRef]
173. Yu, S.-J.; Tseng, K.-Y.; Shen, H.; Harvey, B.K.; Airavaara, M.; Wang, Y. Local Administration of AAV-BDNF to subventricular zone induces functional recovery in stroke rats. *PLoS ONE* **2013**, *8*, e81750. [CrossRef] [PubMed]
174. Chang, E.H.; Adorjan, I.; Mundim, M.V.; Sun, B.; Dizon, M.L.V.; Szele, F.G. Traumatic brain injury activation of the adult subventricular zone neurogenic niche. *Front. Neurosci.* **2016**, *10*, 332. [CrossRef] [PubMed]
175. Yu, T.-S.; Washington, P.M.; Kernie, S.G. Injury-induced neurogenesis: Mechanisms and relevance. *Neuroscientist* **2016**, *22*, 61–71. [CrossRef] [PubMed]
176. Plane, J.M.; Liu, R.; Wang, T.-W.; Silverstein, F.S.; Parent, J.M. Neonatal hypoxic–ischemic injury increases forebrain subventricular zone neurogenesis in the mouse. *Neurobiol. Dis.* **2004**, *16*, 585–595. [CrossRef]
177. Levison, S.W.; Rothstein, R.P.; Romanko, M.J.; Snyder, M.J.; Meyers, R.L.; Vannucci, S.J. Hypoxia/ischemia depletes the rat perinatal subventricular zone of oligodendrocyte progenitors and neural stem cells. *Dev. Neurosci.* **2001**, *23*, 234–247. [CrossRef]
178. Niimi, Y.; Levison, S.W. Pediatric brain repair from endogenous neural stem cells of the subventricular zone. *Pediatr. Res.* **2018**, *83*, 385–396. [CrossRef]
179. Alonso-Alconada, D.; Gressens, P.; Golay, X.; Robertson, N.J. Neurogenesis is reduced at 48 h in the subventricular zone independent of cell death in a piglet model of perinatal hypoxia-ischemia. *Front. Pediatr.* **2022**, *10*, 793189. [CrossRef]
180. Brazel, C.Y.; Rosti III, R.T.; Boyce, S.; Rothstein, R.P.; Levison, S.W. Perinatal hypoxia/ischemia damages and depletes progenitors from the mouse subventricular zone. *Dev. Neurosci.* **2004**, *26*, 266–274. [CrossRef]
181. Romanko, M.J.; Rothstein, R.P.; Levison, S.W. Neural stem cells in the subventricular zone are resilient to hypoxia/ischemia whereas progenitors are vulnerable. *J. Cereb. Blood Flow Metab.* **2004**, *24*, 814–825. [CrossRef]
182. Visco, D.B.; Toscano, A.E.; Juárez, P.A.R.; Gouveia, H.J.C.B.; Guzman-Quevedo, O.; Torner, L.; Manhães-de-Castro, R. A systematic review of neurogenesis in animal models of early brain damage: Implications for cerebral palsy. *Exp. Neurol.* **2021**, *340*, 113643. [CrossRef]
183. Ong, J.; Plane, J.M.; Parent, J.M.; Silverstein, F.S. Hypoxic-ischemic injury stimulates subventricular zone proliferation and neurogenesis in the neonatal rat. *Pediatr. Res.* **2005**, *58*, 600–606. [CrossRef] [PubMed]
184. Yang, Z.; Levison, S.W. Hypoxia/ischemia expands the regenerative capacity of progenitors in the perinatal subventricular zone. *Neuroscience* **2006**, *139*, 555–564. [CrossRef] [PubMed]
185. Felling, R.J. Neural stem/progenitor cells participate in the regenerative response to perinatal hypoxia/ischemia. *J. Neurosci.* **2006**, *26*, 4359–4369. [CrossRef] [PubMed]
186. Bartley, J.; Soltau, T.; Wimborne, H.; Kim, S.; Martin-Studdard, A.; Hess, D.; Hill, W.; Waller, J.; Carroll, J. BrdU-positive cells in the neonatal mouse hippocampus following hypoxic-ischemic brain injury. *BMC Neurosci.* **2005**, *6*, 15. [CrossRef] [PubMed]
187. Kadam, S.D.; Mulholland, J.D.; McDonald, J.W.; Comi, A.M. Neurogenesis and neuronal commitment following ischemia in a new mouse model for neonatal stroke. *Brain Res.* **2008**, *1208*, 35–45. [CrossRef] [PubMed]
188. Ziemka-Nalecz, M.; Jaworska, J.; Sypecka, J.; Polowy, R.; Filipkowski, R.K.; Zalewska, T. Sodium butyrate, a histone deacetylase inhibitor, exhibits neuroprotective/neurogenic effects in a rat model of neonatal hypoxia-ischemia. *Mol. Neurobiol.* **2017**, *54*, 5300–5318. [CrossRef] [PubMed]
189. Buono, K.D.; Goodus, M.T.; Guardia Clausi, M.; Jiang, Y.; Loporchio, D.; Levison, S.W. Mechanisms of mouse neural precursor expansion after neonatal hypoxia-ischemia. *J. Neurosci.* **2015**, *35*, 8855–8865. [CrossRef]
190. Back, S.A.; Tuohy, T.M.F.; Chen, H.; Wallingford, N.; Craig, A.; Struve, J.; Luo, N.L.; Banine, F.; Liu, Y.; Chang, A.; et al. Hyaluronan accumulates in demyelinated lesions and inhibits oligodendrocyte progenitor maturation. *Nat. Med.* **2005**, *11*, 966–972. [CrossRef]
191. Pendleton, J.C.; Shamblott, M.J.; Gary, D.S.; Belegu, V.; Hurtado, A.; Malone, M.L.; McDonald, J.W. Chondroitin sulfate proteoglycans inhibit oligodendrocyte myelination through PTPσ. *Exp. Neurol.* **2013**, *247*, 113–121. [CrossRef]
192. Aguado, T.; Romero, E.; Monory, K.; Palazuelos, J.; Sendtner, M.; Marsicano, G.; Lutz, B.; Guzmán, M.; Galve-Roperh, I. The CB$_1$ cannabinoid receptor mediates excitotoxicity-induced neural progenitor proliferation and neurogenesis. *J. Biol. Chem.* **2007**, *282*, 23892–23898. [CrossRef]
193. Fernández-López, D.; Pradillo, J.M.; García-Yébenes, I.; Martínez-Orgado, J.A.; Moro, M.A.; Lizasoain, I. The cannabinoid WIN55212-2 promotes neural repair after neonatal hypoxia–ischemia. *Stroke* **2010**, *41*, 2956–2964. [CrossRef] [PubMed]
194. Bregy, A.; Nixon, R.; Lotocki, G.; Alonso, O.F.; Atkins, C.M.; Tsoulfas, P.; Bramlett, H.M.; Dietrich, W.D. Posttraumatic hypothermia increases doublecortin expressing neurons in the dentate gyrus after traumatic brain injury in the rat. *Exp. Neurol.* **2012**, *233*, 821–828. [CrossRef] [PubMed]
195. Silasi, G.; Colbourne, F. Therapeutic hypothermia influences cell genesis and survival in the rat hippocampus following global ischemia. *J. Cereb. Blood Flow Metab.* **2011**, *31*, 1725–1735. [CrossRef] [PubMed]

196. Xiong, M.; Cheng, G.-Q.; Ma, S.-M.; Yang, Y.; Shao, X.-M.; Zhou, W.-H. Post-ischemic hypothermia promotes generation of neural cells and reduces apoptosis by Bcl-2 in the striatum of neonatal rat brain. *Neurochem. Int.* **2011**, *58*, 625–633. [CrossRef] [PubMed]
197. Arévalo-Martín, Á.; García-Ovejero, D.; Rubio-Araiz, A.; Gómez, O.; Molina-Holgado, F.; Molina-Holgado, E. Cannabinoids modulate olig2 and polysialylated neural cell adhesion molecule expression in the subventricular zone of post-natal rats through cannabinoid receptor 1 and cannabinoid receptor 2: Cannabinoid receptors in post-natal SVZ. *Eur. J. Neurosci.* **2007**, *26*, 1548–1559. [CrossRef] [PubMed]
198. Iwai, M.; Stetler, R.A.; Xing, J.; Hu, X.; Gao, Y.; Zhang, W.; Chen, J.; Cao, G. Enhanced oligodendrogenesis and recovery of neurological function by erythropoietin after neonatal hypoxic/ischemic brain injury. *Stroke* **2010**, *41*, 1032–1037. [CrossRef] [PubMed]

Disclaimer/Publisher's Note: The statements, opinions and data contained in all publications are solely those of the individual author(s) and contributor(s) and not of MDPI and/or the editor(s). MDPI and/or the editor(s) disclaim responsibility for any injury to people or property resulting from any ideas, methods, instructions or products referred to in the content.

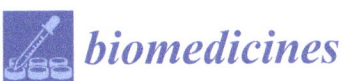

Review

Secondary Terpenes in *Cannabis sativa* L.: Synthesis and Synergy

Francisco T. Chacon [1], Wesley M. Raup-Konsavage [2], Kent E. Vrana [2] and Joshua J. Kellogg [1,3,*]

[1] Intercollege Graduate Degree Program in Plant Biology, Pennsylvania State University, University Park, State College, PA 16802, USA
[2] Department of Pharmacology, Penn State College of Medicine, Hershey, PA 17033, USA
[3] Department of Veterinary and Biomedical Sciences, Pennsylvania State University, University Park, State College, PA 16802, USA
* Correspondence: jjk6146@psu.edu; Tel.: +1-814-865-2887

Abstract: Cannabis is a complex biosynthetic plant, with a long history of medicinal use. While cannabinoids have received the majority of the attention for their psychoactive and pharmacological activities, cannabis produces a diverse array of phytochemicals, such as terpenes. These compounds are known to play a role in the aroma and flavor of cannabis but are potent biologically active molecules that exert effects on infectious as well as chronic diseases. Furthermore, terpenes have the potential to play important roles, such as synergistic and/or entourage compounds that modulate the activity of the cannabinoids. This review highlights the diversity and bioactivities of terpenes in cannabis, especially minor or secondary terpenes that are less concentrated in cannabis on a by-mass basis. We also explore the question of the entourage effect in cannabis, which studies to date have supported or refuted the concept of synergy in cannabis, and where synergy experimentation is headed, to better understand the interplay between phytochemicals within *Cannabis sativa* L.

Keywords: cannabis; phytochemistry; cannabinoids; terpenes; synergy; entourage effect; biosynthesis

1. Introduction

Cannabis sativa L. is a dioecious plant of the Cannabaceae family and is perhaps most famous for its production of the psychedelic metabolite delta-9 tetrahydrocannabinol (D9-THC). Cannabis has been used in traditional medicine for millennia across several continents; cannabis has been used in traditional Chinese medicine therapies for the treatment of gout, pain, convulsions, insomnia, cough, headache, itching, and anemia [1], while in traditional Aryuvedic practices, cannabis has been reported to stimulate digestion, function as an analgesic and sedative, and have aphrodisiac, anti-parasitic, and anti-viral properties [2]. Review articles covering the chemistry, pharmacology, botany, genomics, and ethnology of cannabis are regularly published as the plant's usage grows in prevalence [3–7]. In addition to THC, cannabis produces a number of other cannabinoid compounds with potent activities. Cannabidiol (CBD) is one non-psychedelic cannabinoid that has emerged as a popular botanical supplement ingredient [8]. A majority of Americans are aware of CBD, and ca. 18% have tried or are regular users of CBD products [9]. The US hemp-derived market in cannabidiol (CBD) topped $4.7 billion in 2021 and is expected to reach $12.0 billion by 2026 [10]. However, while many bioactivities can be ascribed to the presence of cannabinoids, cannabis is a prolific biosynthetic organism, producing over 750 known phytochemicals, including flavonoids and terpenoids, many of which possess putative medicinal properties [11], yet the majority of these phytochemical constituents and their mechanisms of action have not been fully explored.

Terpenes (also termed isoprenoids) are the most diverse class of natural products and are the most abundant by mass [12]; in cannabis, terpenes account for 3–5% of the dry mass of the inflorescence [13]. Terpenes have incredible potential for bioactivity against both

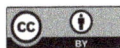

infectious and chronic health conditions [14–16] and have been employed for thousands of years for therapeutic purposes, including in anti-inflammatory, anti-microbial, antioxidant, antitumor, and antidiabetic capacities [17]. In addition, terpenes often provide the foundation for the flavor and aroma of numerous plants and food products [18–20], including cannabis [21], granting the plant earthy or herbal aromas that combine with hints of sweet, citrusy, or piney scents. The terpene profile and content of cannabis has been reviewed previously [13,22,23]; however, analytical profiling studies, as well as cannabis phytochemistry reviews, traditionally focus on the more prevalent, terpenes such as myrcene, α-pinene, limonene, β-caryophyllene, linalool, humulene, ocimene, bisabolol, and terpinolene. The presence of a vast array of terpenes highlights the additional complexity of cannabis, as well as the further potential for bioactivity within this complex plant.

In botanical samples, mixtures of phytochemicals are often more effective than their individual constituents in isolation due to additive or synergistic interactions among compounds. Indeed, many chronic and infectious diseases are not regulated by a single cellular target, but often have multiple regulating pathways [24,25]. As organisms in a complex and dynamic ecological environment, plants have evolved to address this multifactorial disease etiology through the synthesis of structurally and functionally diverse phytochemicals. Thus, cannabis may also exert its bioactive effects via a combination of multiple constituents. Originally hypothesized in the late 20th century and termed the "entourage effect" [26], synergy between different cannabinoids has been documented in several studies. However, the potential for synergy between cannabinoids and other chemical classes, especially terpenes, has remained underreported.

This review aims to synthesize recent studies and information regarding the compositional diversity of terpenes, especially 'minor' terpenoid structures (compounds that are less prevalent in the plant on a by-mass basis) that have not been the focus of other reviews, yet are found in diverse cultivars of cannabis and have unique and varied bioactivities as well. This is a unique feature of this review. In addition, we will build on the body of knowledge regarding how terpenes can potentially work in concert with cannabinoids to enhance bioactivity, as this is a timely topic given the upswing in interest in cannabis and potential synergy/entourage effects.

2. Terpene Biosynthesis

Terpenes originate from the 5-carbon precursor isopentenyl diphosphate (IPP), which is biosynthesized from either pyruvate and glyceraldehyde (via the methylerythritol phosphate (MEP) pathway in plastids) [27] or from acetyl-coA (via the mevalonic acid (MEV) pathway in the cytoplasm) [28] (Figure 1). One or more IPPs condense with dimethylallyl diphosphate (DMAPP) in a 1'–4 fashion to form geranyl diphosphate (GPP, C10), farnesyl diphosphate (FPP, C15), or geranylgeranyl diphosphate (GGPP, C20). GPP and FPP serve as substrates for a multitude of synthetic reactions, condensing together to form the precursors of carotenoids and steroids, or cyclizing to form a myriad of terpene natural products (e.g., monoterpenes (C10), sesquiterpenes (C15), and diterpenes (C20)) [12,29]. GPP also condenses with a diphenol with an alkyl chain (e.g., olivetolic acid) to form the cannabinoids [30]. In cannabis, over 200 terpenes have been published to date [31].

Terpenoid biosynthesis is governed by a family of homologous enzymes, the terpene synthases (TPS) [29,32], which catalyze the formation of different types of terpenes, including monoterpenes, diterpenes, hemiterpenes, and sesquiterpenes. These essential enzymes are encoded in large gene families that have been broken down into seven subfamilies based on phylogenetic analyses rendering, TPS-a, -b, -c, -d, -e/-f, -g, and -h, each based on amino acid length and location of emergence, such as angiosperms or gymnosperms [29,33]. In angiosperms, the TPS-a subfamily contains sesquiterpene synthases (sesqui-TPSs); the TPS-b subfamily contains monoterpenes synthases (mono-TPSs) and hemiterpene synthases [34].

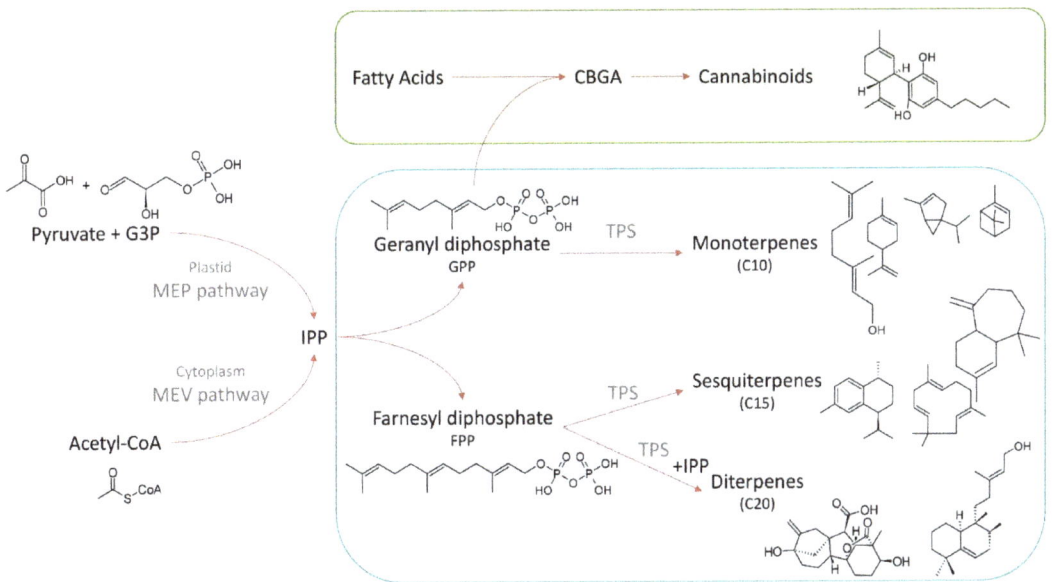

Figure 1. General scheme of terpene synthesis pathway in *Cannabis sativa* L.

Booth et al. analyzed the genome and transciptome of Purple Kush cannabis to identify more than 30 cannabis terpene synthases (CsTPS genes) [35], which has been expanded to over 14 cultivars, representing chemotypes I, II, and III [34,36,37]. The characterized TPS genes of cannabis are documented as being a part of the TPS-a and TPS-b subfamilies [29]. Only nine of the 30 CsTPS genes have been fully characterized with respect to their catalytic functions, eight of which are multi-product enzymes that can generate different terpene structures from either GPP or FPP substrates [35,38]. Interestingly, genetic variation in these CsTPS has been associated with differences in the Sativa-Indica scale of cannabis labeling. Genotyping 100 cannabis samples for >100,000 single nucleotide polymorphisms revealed that Sativa- and Indica-labelled samples were indistinguishable from a genome perspective; however, variation in CsTPS genes translated to shifts in the terpene profile and was correlated with the current dichotomous label system, suggesting terpenes (and genetic markers associated with terpene biosynthesis) could have a large role in governing the strain classification [39]. This biosynthetic plasticity could be one explanation for the diversity of terpenes found in cannabis; however, it is important to keep in mind that the CsTPS responsible for many cannabis terpenes remain unexplored. When considering the incredible diversity of cannabis terpenes, it is unknown how the expression levels of different CsTPS could vary with plant development stage, plant organ and cell-type, and environmental factors. In addition, non-enzymatic modifications of terpenes, such as cyclization and oxidation, can increase structural diversity independent of enzymatic biochemical reactions. Even post-harvest considerations can change the terpene profile, especially the smaller, more volatile hemiterpenes and monoterpenes [40]. More qualitative and quantitative studies are needed to comprehensively profile the terpenes found in cannabis and how those concentrations relate to expression levels and functionality of the CsTPS.

3. Terpene Diversity in Cannabis

Over 20,000 terpenes have been identified in the Plantae kingdom, making these highly volatile compounds one of the most structurally and functionally diverse groups of natural products [41]. Cannabis is widely known for its assorted terpene profiles.

To date, 200 terpenes/terpenoids have been detected in cannabis [42]. However, the complete identification and quantification of the vast majority of terpenes/terpenoids remains undetermined, blunting our knowledge of the impact of cannabis terpenes on plant and human health [43]. Thus, the complete identification of terpenes in cannabis may suggest a substantial assortment of cannabis terpenes unknown to current breeders and researchers.

With the tremendous diversity of compounds in cannabis, researchers seek to categorize the main chemical constituents of cannabis cultivars or 'strains' by establishing five classes of chemotypes based on cannabinoid ratios. These are classified as Chemotypes (I): high THCA:CBDA ratio; (II) intermediate ratios of THCA:CBDA; (III) low THCA:CBDA ratio; (IV) high CBGA content/low ratio of THCA:CBDA; and (V) containing almost no cannabinoids [44]. This classification has drawn researchers to further categorize cannabis chemical profiles by associating cannabinoid content with bioactive metabolites such as terpenes. Table 1 illustrates the concentration range (mg/g) of terpenes and terpene derivatives reported in published research articles investigating the terpene content of specific cannabis chemotypes. Chemical profiles of common cannabis cultivars continue to show that myrcene, β-caryophyllene, limonene, α-terpinene, and α-pinene are the most prominent terpenes that can be found in the first three chemotype varieties [34,45–48]. Terpene profiles of the remaining chemotypes are limited or have yet to be investigated. Conversely, the classification of secondary terpenes (terpenes found in lower concentrations) in cannabis chemotypes is limited, as they are often disregarded or unreported due to a lack of reference material. More studies on cannabis terpene chemotypes are required to identify the relationships between specific terpenes and cannabinoid content.

Birenboim et al., 2022, were the first to demonstrate a highly accurate classification of medicinal cannabis chemovars based on their cannabinoid and terpene profiles. Using a partial least-square discriminant analysis multivariate (PLS-DA) technique, Birenboim et al. were able to differentiate terpene content between the inflorescences of three major chemovars (high-THCA, high-CBGA, and a hybrid). They concluded that the terpenes of the three major classes were significantly different in their concentrations of different terpenes [49], providing evidence of the high-THCA class having a higher abundance of limonene, β-caryophyllene, β-pinene, α-humulene, γ-elemene, and seychellene. Within the hybrid class, α-pinene and β-myrcene are more pronounced, followed by a high abundance of γ-eudesmol, α-bisabolol, and guaiol in the high-CBGA class. However, these results represent 14 different cannabis chemovars, including seven high THC chemovars, five hybrid chemovars, and only two high-CBG chemovars. The plant material used was from commercial breeding lines that could not be affiliated to a specific subspecies because of crossings between different cultivars over many generations. Moreover, several factors have been shown to influence terpene diversity, such as plant genetics, pest presence, overall plant health, soil composition, proper drying, curing, and microbiology [34,50–55].

Variations in terpene expression can also be dependent upon the stage of growth. In 2016, Aizpurua-Olaizola et al. analyzed the terpene and cannabinoid content of the leaves and flowers of cannabis chemotypes I, II, and III. For 23 weeks, a chemical profile was generated on a weekly basis, providing the researchers with a total content of cannabinoids and terpenes at different stages of growth. Researchers found that chemotypes II and III required more time to reach their peak production of monoterpenes compared to chemotype I. Major terpene differences were also observed between chemotypes I and III. The distinct terpenes of chemotype I included γ-selinene, β-selinene, α-gurjunene, γ-elemene, Selina-3.7 (11) diene, and β-curcumene, while chemotype III displayed β-eudesmol, γ-eudesmol, guaiol, α-bisabolol, or eucalyptol. This suggests a chemotype-dependent terpene distribution, as the investigators describe the more prominent terpenes in chemotype III as having a higher correlation coefficient with CBDA and chemotype I terpenes having a higher correlation coefficient with THCA [53]. Despite the differences in terpene content at different stages of growth, limitations of terpenes and cannabinoid expression may be observed based on light exposure and select spectra.

A high abundance of terpenes and cannabinoids can be found on the surface of cannabis inflorescence and leaves in the glandular appendages known as trichomes [56,57]. Trichomes are believed to be a defense mechanism against several different stresses, including light stress [58,59]. This has led to the proposed ecological function of cannabinoids and terpenes aiding in protection against high light exposure [58]. Additionally, research has shown the altering effects LED light can have on THC and terpene concentrations, but not CBD [57,58]. One study provided evidence of supplemental green light increasing THC and terpene content in comparison to controls. However, quantification of IPP and DMAPP were not conducted, leaving the mechanistic implications undetermined [52]. With the increasing application of LED lighting for indoor cultivation, the chemical profiles of the desired chemotype may be susceptible based on light application. Nonetheless, with the information surrounding the factors that influence terpene concentrations, terpene biosynthesis, and genetic expression, new cultivars with desired cannabinoid and terpene profiles may become attainable as the research surrounding terpenes in cannabis continues.

Table 1. Concentrations of terpenes found in cannabis. Concentration range is given by chemotype where available; Tr—trace (<level of quantitation).

Compound	Chemotypes		Rage of Average Concentrations Reported per Chemotype (mg/g Dry Weight)	Reference
Agrospirol	I	I:	Tr–0.50	[45]
Alloaromandrene	I, II, III	I:	0.004–0.08	[53,60]
		II:	0.08–0.10	
		III:	0.05–0.10	
Aromadendrene	I	I:	0.02–0.13	[61]
α-Bisabolol	I, II, III	I:	Tr–1.10	[34,45,46,53,60,62–64]
		II:	0.57–1.22	
		III:	0.07–2.31	
α-Bisabolene	I, II, III	I:	0.13–0.50	[53,61]
		II:	0.11–0.29	
		III:	0.03–0.50	
β-Bisabolene	I, II, III	I:	0.05–0.17	[53]
		II:	0.18–0.51	
		III:	0.12–0.71	
Borneol	I, II, III	I:	0.01–0.03	[34,61,63,64]
		II:	0.05	
		III:	0.009–0.02	
α-bergamotene	I, II, III	I:	0.024–1.18	[34,53]
		II:	0.45–0.81	
		III:	0.018–0.68	
Cis-bergamotene	I, III	I:	0.07–0.11	[61]
		III:	0.21	
Trans-bergamotene	I, III	I:	0.12–0.28	[61]
		III:	0.04	
Bulnesol	I, II, III	I:	0.10–0.50	[34,45,53]
		II:	0.090–0.19	
		III:	0.070–0.49	
γ-cadinene	I, III	I:	0.41–0.60	[61]
		III:	0.02	
Camphene	I, III	I:	0.002–0.09	[34,60,63,64]
		III:	0.001–0.48	
Camphor	I	I:	0.001–0.01	[61,64]
P-Cimene	I, III	I:	0.016	[64]
		III:	0.01	
β-Caryophyllene	I, II, III	I:	0.24–8.20	[34,45,46,60–65]
		II:	0.86–3.90	
		III:	0.16–3.17	

Table 1. Cont.

Compound	Chemotypes	Rage of Average Concentrations Reported per Chemotype (mg/g Dry Weight)		Reference
β-Caryophyllene oxide	I, II, III	I: II: III:	0.005–0.06 0.02 0.09	[60,61,63]
Trans-β-caryophyllene	I, III	I: III:	0.02–0.06 0.06	[53,61]
δ-3-carene	I, II, III	I: II: III:	Tr–0.60 Tr 0.065–0.070	[45,46,61,64,65]
α-Cedrene	I, III	I: III:	0.038 0.023	[64]
β-Citronellol	I, III	I: III:	0.002 0.001–0.003	[60,64]
α-curcumene	I, III	I: III:	0.008 0.017	[60]
β-Curcumene	I, II, III	I: II: III:	0.014–0.61 0.061–0.16 0.016–0.09	[53,60]
Cyclounatriene	I, III	I: III:	0.02–0.13 0.086	[34]
Elemene	I, II	I: II:	Tr–2.70 Tr	[45,65]
γ-elemene	I, III	I: III:	0.104–1.89 0.04–0.068	[34,53,61]
δ-elemene	I, III	I: III:	Tr–0.392 0.005	[34]
Eucalyptol	II, III	II: III:	0.010–0.07 0.052–0.14	[53,60,63]
Eudesma-3,7(11)-diene	I, III	I: III:	Tr–0.80 0.05	[34,61,65]
Eudesmane	I, III	I: III:	0.33–0.55 0.04	[34]
A-eudesmol	I, II	I: II:	0.02 0.26	[63]
β-Eudesmol	I, II, III	I: II: III:	Tr–0.92 0.23–0.65 0.085–1.01	[45,53,61,63,64]
γ-Eudesmol	I, III	I: II: III:	Tr–0.80 0.30–0.78 0.010–1.03	[34,45,53,61]
α-farnesene	I, II, III	I: II: III:	0.02–0.06 0.24 0.002	[34,63]
β-farnesene	I, II, III	I: II: III:	0.019–1.96 0.73–1.6 0.008–1.4	[34,53,65]
Trans-β-farnesene	I, III	I: II: III:	0.31–1.06 0.35 0.05	[61,63]
Fenchone	I, II, III	I: II: III:	0.005–0.03 0.02 0.007–0.008	[60,63,64]
Fenchol	I, II, III	I: II: III:	0.047–1.09 0.09–0.31 0.028–0.138	[34,46,60–64]
Germacrene B	I, III	I: III:	0.25–1.27 0.34	[34]

Table 1. Cont.

Compound	Chemotypes	Rage of Average Concentrations Reported per Chemotype (mg/g Dry Weight)		Reference
Geraniol	I, III	I: III:	0.01 0.004	[63,64]
Geranyl Acetate	I	I:	Tr–0.70	[46]
Guaiol	I, II, III	I: II: III:	Tr–1.09 0.27–0.87 0.010–1.21	[34,45,53,61,63,65]
α-guaiene	I, III	I: II: III:	Tr–0.50 Tr Tr	[45,65]
δ-guaiene	I, II	I: II:	Tr–0.80 0.8	[45,61,65]
α-gurjunene	I	I:	0.1–0.46	[53]
Humulene	I, II, III	I: II: III:	Tr–4.00 0.64–1.11 0.26–0.93	[45,46,53,64]
α-Humulene	I, II, III	I: II: III:	0.09–1.93 0.32–0.36 0.14–0.27	[34,60,62,63,65]
Isopulegol	I, II	I: II:	0.02–0.04 0.02	[63]
Ledene	I, II	I: II:	0.11–0.13 0.05	[63]
Limonene	I, II, III	I: II: III:	Tr–9.1 0.079–1.14 0.022–1.44	[34,45,46,53,60–64]
Linalool	I, II, III	I: II: III:	Tr–3.10 0.27–0.35 Tr–0.36	[34,45,46,53,60–64]
Cis-linalool oxide	I, III	I: III:	0.002 0.005	[60]
Trans-linalool oxide	I, III	I: III:	0.002 0.002	[60]
Menthol	I, III	I: III:	0.001 0.001	[60]
β-Myrcene	I, II, III	I: II: III:	0.12–14.8 0.20–3.02 0.18–7.60	[34,45,46,53,60–65]
Nerolidol	I, II, III	I: III:	0.02 0.01	[61]
Trans-nerolidol	I, III	I: II: III:	0.019–1.66 0.09 0.005–0.07	[60,63,64]
β-Ocimene	I, III	I: II: III:	0.21–1.38 0.02 0.19	[34,53,63]
Cis-Ocimene	I, II, III	I: II: III:	0.006–3.9 1 1	[45,60,61,64,65]
Trans-Ocimene	I, III	I: III:	Tr–3.8 0.007–0.01	[46,60,64]
α-phellandrene	I, II, III	I: II: III:	Tr–0.60 Tr Tr	[65]
β-phellandrene	I, III	I: II: III:	Tr–2.1 0.7 0.097–0.50	[34,65]

Table 1. Cont.

Compound	Chemotypes	Rage of Average Concentrations Reported per Chemotype (mg/g Dry Weight)		Reference
α-pinene	I, II, III	I:	Tr–6.70	[34,45,46,53,60–65]
		II:	0.068–4.63	
		III:	0.004–1.40	
β-pinene	I, II, III	I:	Tr–2.00	[34,45,46,53,60–65]
		II:	0.054–0.80	
		III:	0.001–0.50	
α-phellandrene	I, II, III	I:	0.003–0.7	[46,60,61]
		II:	Tr	
		III:	0.001	
2-pinanol	I, III	I:	0.036–0.16	[34]
		III:	0.047	
Sabinene	I, III	I:	0.005	[60]
		III:	0.001	
Cis-sabinene hydrate	I, II	I:	0.015–0.08	[60,61,63]
		II:	0.003–0.03	
α-selinene	I, II, III	I:	0.04–1.36	[34,53,63]
		II:	0.26–0.65	
		III:	0.094–0.79	
β-selinene	I, II, III	I:	0.093–0.61	[53,63]
		II:	0.09–0.34	
		III:	0.10–0.22	
γ-selinene	I, II, III	I:	0.09–0.63	[53,61,65]
		II:	0.06–0.09	
		III:	0.03–0.14	
δ-selinene	I, III	I:	0.10–0.36	[34]
		III:	0.09	
Selina-3.7 (11) diene	I, II, III	I:	0.03–1.89	[53]
		II:	0.05–0.07	
		III:	0.06–0.092	
β-Sesquiphellanderene	I, II, III	I:	0.09–0.48	[53]
		II:	0.14–0.23	
		III:	0.074–0.19	
α-Terpinene	I, II, III	I:	Tr–0.10	[45,60,64]
		II:	Tr	
		III:	Tr–0.068	
γ-Terpinene	I, III	I:	0.02–0.06	[46,60,61,64]
		III:	0.01–0.06	
Terpineol	I, II, III	I:	Tr–0.70	[45]
		II:	0.6	
		III:	Tr	
Terpinen-4-ol	I, III	I:	0.02	[60]
		III:	0.01	
α-Terpineol	I, III	I:	0.04–0.9	[34,46,60,62,64,65]
		II:	0.29	
		III:	0.11–0.22	
Terpinolene	I, II, III	I:	Tr–13.9	[34,45,46,53,60,63–65]
		II:	0.010–3.70	
		III:	0.019–2.90	
Valencene	I, II	I:	0.001–0.06	[34,60,63]
		II:	0.01	
		III:	0.16	

4. Potential Roles of Secondary Terpenes

The biological activity of cannabis terpenes is a growing topic that been extensively covered in multiple reviews [13,23,66–71]. These reviews on the therapeutic properties of cannabis terpenes primarily cover the commonly encountered mono- and sesquiterpenes (e.g., β-caryophyllene, β-myrcene, α- and β-pinene, α-humulene, limonene, terpenoline, and linalool). For this reason, this review aims to further investigate nine secondary terpenes of cannabis, based on their abundance in the plant and their therapeutic potential (Figure 2). Regardless of their minor presence, the significant therapeutic value could point towards stronger or novel synergistic effects. The following is a summary of the more uncommon but notable secondary terpenes/terpenoids in cannabis and their potential therapeutic value; it is impossible to describe all the pharmacological effects of terpenes/terpenoids in this paper, but we shall give some examples of how these compounds possess multi-functional bioactivity. It is worth noting that the compounds often have multiple potential activities, and there is overlap of activities between terpene compounds.

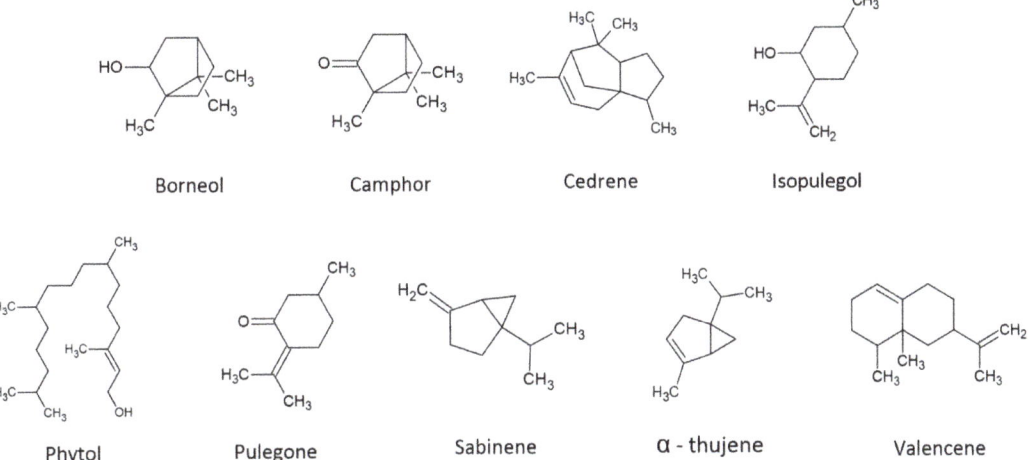

Figure 2. Structures of secondary terpenes present in *Cannabis sativa* L.

4.1. Borneol

Identified as a monoterpene, borneol is a terpene derivative that can be found in several plant species, including *Cannabis sativa* L. [34,61,64]. The scent of this aromatic compound has been equated to a woody balsam aroma. Traditional Chinese medicine has employed the therapeutic properties of borneol for thousands of years as a resuscitation drug due to its active orifice-opening effects [72,73]. These effects are hypothesized to enhance blood–brain barrier (BBB) permeability [72–74], allowing for improved drug delivery to the central nervous system [73]. On top of its enhancement of BBB permeability, borneol also possesses anti-microbial, anti-inflammatory, anti-nociceptive, antithrombotic, neuroprotective, and genoprotective effects [75–81].

4.2. Camphor

This cyclic monoterpene ketone has been described as producing a strong mothball-like scent [82]. Like borneol, camphor has a long history of being used for its repellent and biological effects [83,84]. The medicinal properties of camphor oil include antibacterial, antiviral, antitussive, antimutagenic, anti-cancer, anti-inflammatory, antioxidant, and antidiabetic activity [85–91]. Studies evaluating camphor's biological effects typically involve wood extracts of *Cinnamomum camphora*, the camphor laurel tree that primarily consists of high levels of camphor and its derivatives [92].

4.3. Cedrene

Cedrene is a sesquiterpenoid that is classified as a secondary terpene of cannabis as only small amounts of the terpenoid have been identified in select cultivars. This sesquiterpenoid is commonly found in cedar and juniper trees [93,94]. The aroma produced by cedrene has been described as a woody, crisp scent. Like many aromatic compounds, the biological activities of cedrene have been explored primarily through extracts of cedarwood oil, which has been characterized as having copious amounts of the sesquiterpenoid [95]. Although many of the studies report the effects of full cedarwood oil, cedrene is a primary constituent of this oil and thus leads to speculation that the biological activity of cedarwood oil is due to cedrene, with activities including antifungal, anti-microbial, and anti-cancer [96–98]. A few studies have been performed on isolated α-cedrene, suggesting potential anti-obesity properties [99,100].

4.4. Isopulegol

Identified as a monoterpene alcohol, isopulegol can be found at different concentrations in a variety of plants, including lemongrass, mint, eucalyptus, and several others [101–103]. The scent of isopulegol has been described as a minty fragrance [104]. Because of its presence in a diversity of plants, researchers have described its potential bioactivity, including antidepressant [105], antianxiety [105], anticonvulsant [106], gastroprotective [107], and anti-inflammatory activity [108]. Though isopulegol is said to contain several diverse bioactive properties, more research is required to characterize the mechanism in play.

4.5. Phytol

Phytol is a diterpenoid that has been described as having a grassy-fresh aroma [104]. Phytol is a common terpenoid of highly aromatic plants such as green tea, mint, tarragon, basil, and cannabis cultivars [109,110]. This terpenoid has been speculated to hold antioxidant [111,112], anti-inflammatory [113], analgesic [112], anti-cancer [111,114], anti-anxiety [115], anti-convulsant [116], and sedative [117] properties. Phytol and its derivatives have also been explored for toxicity in immune-compromised mice, suggesting non-toxic effects [118–120].

4.6. Pulegone

As a monoterpene, pulegone can be found in various aromatic herbs, but is commonly associated with the mint family, such as catnip and peppermint [121,122]. Known for its minty fragrance, pulegone has been identified at low concentrations in cannabis [22,123]. Researchers have suggested that pulegone contains anti-microbial [124], anti-anxiety [125], antipyretic [126], sedative [126,127], and anti-inflammatory [128] properties.

4.7. Sabinene

This bicyclic monoterpene can be found in a variety of different plant species and is often associated with a spicy flavor and aroma. Cannabis cultivars typically contain small concentrations of sabinene; however, some cultivars have been characterized as having more sabinene than others, such as Super Silver Haze and Arjan's Ultra Haze [104]. The medical benefits of this monoterpene suggest anti-inflammatory [129], antioxidant [130], and anti-microbial [131] properties. The known benefits of this terpene are limited, requiring more research and exploration of the effects of sabinene in cannabis.

4.8. Thujene

Like many monoterpenes, thujene can be found in a variety of plant-derived essential oils such as eucalyptus [132], frankincense [133], and dill [134]. Similar to humulene, α-thujene produces a woody, spicy aroma [135]. Researchers have tested the bioactivity of essential oils that consist of high levels of thujene, such as the essential oil of *Boswellia serrata*, which has been reported to consist of 61.36% α-thujene [136]. Investigations exploring the bioactivity of essential oils containing α-thujene suggest antioxidant [137], anti-inflammatory [138], anti-microbial [139], and analgesic [140] properties. Although these studies provide insight into the bioactivity of essential oils containing this compound, more research is required to delineate the therapeutic properties of isolated α-thujene.

4.9. Valencene

The sesquiterpene valencene produces an aroma that is often associated with citrus fruits such as Valencia oranges [141]. In cannabis, valencene has been reported in several different cultivars, but only at low concentrations [70]. Aside from its appealing scent, valencene's bioactivity has been explored through various essential oil profiles, speculating anti-inflammatory [142], neuroprotective [143], anti-allergic [144], and anti-microbial [145] properties.

While minor terpenes may not be the most abundant in cannabis, they have the potential to aid in the biological activities of cannabis. These terpenes demonstrate overlapping activity with each other, often targeting the same biological function (even if mechanism of action remains unknown) (Figure 3). Likewise, an overlap of therapeutic benefit between cannabinoids and these secondary terpenes may be inferred based on current cannabinoid research [60], suggesting a potential to increase the efficacy of these cannabinoids in an additive or synergistic manner.

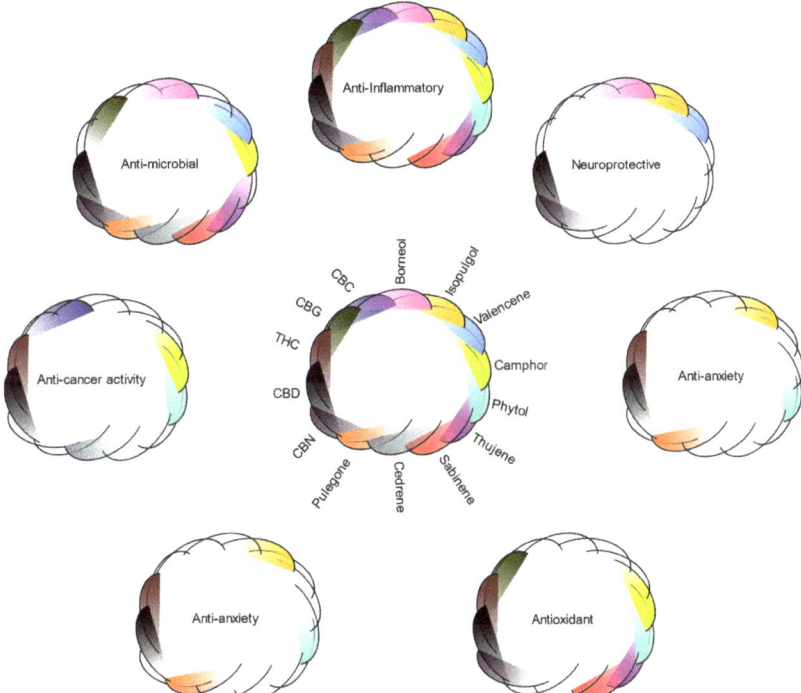

Figure 3. Bioactivities of the nine secondary terpenes covered in this review, along with cannabis's principal cannabinoids (CBD, cannabidiol; THC, tetrahydrocannabinol; CBG, cannabigerol; CBN, cannabinol; CBC, cannabichromene). Bioactivity circles are color-coded to match the legend in the middle; the presence of a particular shading in the circle is indicative that the terpene or cannabinoid has been reported to possess that bioactivity. The figure demonstrates that not only do terpenes have multiple potential bioactivities, but different compounds possess overlapping activities, suggesting their potential to exert combination effects.

5. Mechanism of Action for Terpenes—Pharmacologic Receptor Targets (TRPs)

Several studies have investigated the pharmacodynamics of the receptors for the major terpenoids found in cannabis (e.g., β-caryophyllene, β-myrcene, β-pinene, α-humulene, linalool). For instance, β-caryophyllene has been found to be an agonist at the cannabinoid receptor 2 (CB2), peroxisome proliferator-activated receptor gamma (PPARγ), and the toll-like receptor 4 (TLR4)/CD14/MD2 complex, while β-myrcene is an agonist at α2-adrenergic receptors and transient receptor potential cation channel subfamily V member 1 (TRPV1) [13,146–149]. The information on the receptors modulated by the minor terpenes found in cannabis is much more variable and will be the focus of the discussion below.

Borneol is an agonist of TRPM8. This activation of TRPM8 by borneol has been found to be temperature sensitive and dose-dependent across a range of concentrations, from 10 μM to 2 mM; however, no EC_{50} was reported because the study failed to reach a maximal response [150,151]. The activation of TRPM8 receptors by borneol has been found to activate glutamatergic and GABAergic transmission in the spinal cord, leading to anti-nociceptive activity [152,153]. The activation of TRPM8 by borneol has also been shown to enhance the chemosensitivity of lung cancer cell lines to doxycycline [151]. Borneol is also an agonist of TRPV3 (EC_{50} = 3.45 mM) channels [154]. Furthermore, borneol is an antagonist of the TRPA1 channel, with an IC_{50} of 0.2–0.3 mM in cell-based assays [155,156]. The activation of TRPV3 and inhibition of TRPA1 also likely contribute to the antinociceptive properties of borneol. Of note, the antagonist/agonist profile of borneol at these receptors matches that of several cannabinoids, including CBD, CBG, and THC; however, these effects occur at relatively high levels.

Camphor is a major terpenoid constituent of cannabis but is best known as an isolate from the camphor laurel (*Cinnamomum camphora*). This compound is FDA-approved as an additive to soothing creams and ointments and as a component of over-the-counter respiratory treatments. Camphor has been found to act as an agonist at TRPM8 and TRPV3 and an antagonist at TRPA1, which is perhaps not surprising considering the structural similarity of camphor to borneol. Despite this structural similarity, camphor is less potent at both TRPV3 (EC_{50} = 6.03 mM) and TRPA1 (IC_{50} = 1.26 mM) compared to borneol [154,156]. At TRPM8, camphor has an EC_{50} of approximately 4.5 mM [157]. Additionally, camphor has been shown to be a partial agonist at TRPV1, with similar potency as at TRPV3 and TRPA1 (EC_{50} > 3 mM) [158,159]. The action of camphor at these receptors likely accounts for its analgesic activities. In addition, activation of the TRPV family of receptors has been linked to the ability of camphor to relax the trachea in rats, which may help explain its anti-congestive activities [160].

Cedrene has been identified as a potent agonist of the olfactory receptor 10J5 (OR10J5), a GPCR that is also found in liver and muscle tissue [161]. In human hepatocytes, cedrane has been shown to lower lipid levels through OR10J5. Furthermore, cedrane has been shown to reduce muscle atrophy induced by a high fat diet in mice, this action is mediated through the mouse ortholog of OR10J5, MOR23 [162]. This study also found that cedrane increased muscle mass and strength, possibly through increasing expression of IGF1.

Isopulegol has been identified as an agonist of the most abundant $GABA_AR$ in the brain, α1β2γ2, with an EC_{50} of approximately 3.25 μM. Activation of the GABAR produces sedative effects, and these receptors are targets for both analgesics and anticonvulsant medications [163]. Isopulegol is also an agonist at TRPM8 and may also antagonize the TRPV1 receptor [164,165]. Either of these actions may account for the anti-nociceptive properties of isopulegol that have been described in mice [165].

Phytol and its metabolites can act as natural ligands for a variety of transcription factor receptors. This list includes the peroxisome proliferator-activated receptor (PPAR) α and γ; however, an EC_{50} was not reported because the assay did not reach a plateau at 100 μM, the highest concentration tested [166,167]. Additionally, phytol has been shown to be an agonist of retinoid X receptors (RXR), with EC_{50} estimates ranging from 41.9 to 67.2 μM, depending upon the isotype [168]. Through activation of these receptors, phytol has been shown to reduce cancer cell viability in a number of cancer cell lines. Indeed, it has been found to have a lower IC_{50} in the lung adenocarcinoma cell line, A549, than the chemotherapeutic agent methotrexate [169]. Phytol induced apoptosis in this system through the activation of the TNF receptor, TRAIL, and FAS. Additionally, the authors used molecular docking to suggest that phytol may bind to glucose-6-phosphate dehydrogenase to inhibit tumor progression. In vitro, phytol has also been shown to increase the release of CA^{2+} reserves via activation of GPR40, a G-protein-coupled receptor that normally binds to free fatty acids, with an EC_{50} of 34.5 µM [170]. The activation of PPARs, RXRs, and GPR40 by phytol may also be of potential therapeutic benefit for the treatment of diabetes, and because of the ability to activate RXR receptors, phytol is also being pursued by the cosmeceutical industry as an anti-aging treatment in lieu of retinol (which is not well tolerated by all individuals due to its activation of TRPV1) [171,172].

Using a recently developed in vitro receptor binding assay, pulegone was shown to be the component in *Ziziphora clinopodioides* that binds and potentially activates β_1-adrenoceptors [173]. Pulegone has been found to be an agonist of avian TRPM8 at low concentrations; however, it antagonizes this receptor at higher concentrations [174]. This study also found that pulegone is an antagonist of TRPA1 at both low and high concentrations. Taken together, these data suggest that pulegone may have anti-nociceptive and analgesic utility.

Computer-based molecular docking research predicted that sabinene may be a potent interactor with L-asparginase from the bacterial pathogen, *Salmonella typhimurium* [175]. This study found that sabinene had a higher docking score than the antibiotic ciprofloxacin, suggesting that sabinene may have antibacterial properties and may be a good candidate for antibiotic development. Additionally, sabinene has been found to reduce levels of the inflammatory marker nitric oxide in cells exposed to lipopolysaccharide [129]. Another molecular docking study suggested that sabinene may interact with the spike protein on the SARS-CoV2 (COVID-19) virus along with three cell membrane proteins (transmembrane serine protease 2, cathepsin B, and cathepsin L) that play a role in mediating viral entry into cells [176]. Additional studies will be needed to determine if any of these interactions occur in vivo, as well as which receptors might mediate the decrease in nitric oxide production caused by sabinene. An in silico study suggested that thujene may have a modest binding affinity for the SARS-CoV2 main protease and papain-like protease, but further work will be needed to confirm these findings [177]. Additionally, no studies could be located that identified potential human receptors for this terpene.

Valencene has been reported to be cardioprotective following myocardial infarction in rats, and this protection is mediated through the inhibition of the NF-κB pathway, oxidative stress, and cardiac hypertrophy; however, the receptors that mediate this inhibition were not examined [178]. Valencene has been found to be an antagonist of the calcium ion channel TRPV1 and the slow release calcium release-activated calcium channel protein 1 (ORAI1), which inhibited the melanin content in UVB exposed melanoma cells, and may therefore be useful for treating photo-aging of the skin [179]. This inhibition, may also mediate the ability of valencene to potentially treat atopic dermatitis [180].

6. Synergy and the Entourage Effect: Beyond Cannabinoids

Natural product discovery efforts are traditionally reductionist in nature, devoted to condensing a complex botanical extract down to a single bioactive agent for drug development purposes. This is true for cannabis research and development, where the single molecule approach remains the dominant approach [181]. However, botanical medicines, including cannabis, are in fact complex diverse concoctions of phytochemicals that have the potential of exerting differing and potentially complementary biological effects. Indeed, it is often observed that these mixtures work in concert to achieve a specific physiological effect [182]. Compounds can work in a synergistic manner, in which each active compound potentiates the other to achieve a greater than expected benefit when combined (i.e., 1 + 1 > 2). If one compound, having no activity of its own, impacts the efficacy of an active molecule to increase activity (i.e., 1 + 0 > 1), this is known as an entourage effect [26]. As cannabis research has evolved, there has been a growing body of evidence that cannabinoids beyond THC demonstrate efficacy in humans [183,184] and that synergy/entourage could potentially play a large role in the bioactivity of cannabis extracts and products [22,185].

Botanical synergy and entourage have been demonstrated in cannabis, first in the combination of THC with other, "minor", cannabinoids. Johnson et al. (2010) tested a cannabis-based extract for patients with intractable pain and found that, while the THC dominant extract did not improve patient outcome versus the placebo (the mean pain Numerical Rating Scale (NRS) was a nonsignificant change of -1.01 vs. -0.69), a whole plant extract (the only difference being the presence of CBD) demonstrated a significant improvement in pain outcome (mean NRS of -1.37 vs. -0.69) compared to the placebo [186]. Animal studies focusing on analgesia also evidenced greater response from a full-spectrum cannabis extract as compared to pure CBD dosing [187]. Recently, experiments with a seizure mouse model looked at the effects of different strains of cannabis that all contained an equivalent CBD concentration. While all were effective, there were noticeable differences between the strains, and profiling 94 phytocannabinoids across 36 of the most commonly used *Cannabis* plants prescribed to patients in Israel led to the conclusion that these other cannabinoids have an impact on the overall efficacy of cannabis plant extracts [188]. In one in vitro study, one study of breast cancer cell lines revealed that the extract of the whole cannabis was more effective than a preparation featuring THC by itself; the boost in activity was attributed to the presence of "minor" cannabinoids cannabigerol (CBG) and tetrahydrocannabinolic acid (THCA) [189]. Complex fractions from cannabis extracts demonstrated synergistic interactions on colorectal cancer cell lines [190].

Cannabinoids have been widely studied for the treatment of epilepsy [191,192]; complex extracts containing multiple cannabinoids were found to treat severe epilepsy, such as Dravet and Lennox-Gastaut syndromes, at lower doses than trials using purer preparations (e.g., Epidiolex, which contains 97% CBD) [66,193]. A 2018 meta-analysis by Pamplona et al. of 11 studies demonstrated that the response rate at 50% improvement of seizure frequency was similar between the two groups, but the average daily doses were significantly different: 27.1 mg/kg/d for purified CBD as opposed to 6.1 mg/kg/d. for cannabis extracts [194]. Moreover, the incidence of adverse events was discernably higher in the CBD versus complex extract treatments ($p < 0.0001$), a result that the authors attributed to the lower dose utilized, which was achieved in their opinion by the synergistic contributions of other entourage compounds.

Most synergy studies have focused primarily on the interactions between cannabinoid structures, despite the fact that the original definition of the entourage effect arose from the interaction of 2-acyl-glycerol esters with cannabinoids [26]. As terpenes are a large and diverse family of phytochemicals found in cannabis, they have the potential to serve as potentiating agents working in concert with cannabinoids. Terpenes, broadly speaking, have been found to be broadly synergistic, helping modulate the activity of a number of other botanicals, pharmaceuticals, and compounds. The terpenes highlighted in this review also have a strong history of synergistic activity with other compounds. Borneol was shown to synergize with curcumin to induce apoptosis in human melanoma cells [195], potentiate the activity of berberine and baicalein in inhibiting in vitro and in vivo fungal growth [196], and function as a potentiating agent to sensitize cancer cells to doxorubicin treatment [151]. Sabinene [197] and pulegone [198] each indicated the potential for synergistic interactions with prescription antibiotics in treating bacterial infections, and β-caryophyllene and phytol demonstrated combination effects inducing apoptosis in skin epidermoid cancer cells [199]. Terpenes have also demonstrated efficacy in the treatment of mood and anxiety disorders, suggesting the possibility of combination effects with cannabinoids for more effective treatments [200]. Thus, while the potential of cannabis terpenes to possess additive or synergistic properties was originally posited as hypothetical based upon similar bioactivities [23], more recent studies have explored this possibility in earnest.

A 2021 study by LaVigne et al. found that α-humulene, geraniol, linalool, and β-pinene were cannabimimetic at the CB_1 receptor and produced cannabinoid-like behaviors in a mouse model. Furthermore, the terpenes potentiated the effects of a cannabinoid agonist, suggesting synergistic activity [201]. Di Giacomo et al. treated triple negative breast cancer cells (MDA-MB-468) with hemp inflorescences and pure compounds of CBD, caryophyllene and cannabichromene. The presence of these other compounds induced the potentiating effects of CBD, likely mediated through CB2 activation [202]. However, separate studies observed that none of the terpenes α-pinene, β-pinene, β-caryophyllene, linalool, limonene, and β-myrcene were found to alter potassium channel signaling in AtT20 cells expressing CB_1 and CB_2 receptors, and did not interact with THC at the receptor [203], nor did they affect changes in intracellular calcium at the human transient receptor potential ankyrin 1 (hTRPA1) or human transient receptor potential vanilloid 1 (hTRPV1) channels [204]. Using a radioligand ([^{3}H]-CP55,940) to measure binding at the CB1 and CB2 receptors, none of the tested terpenes (myrcene, α-pinene, β-pinene, β-caryophyllene, and limonene) had interactions with receptors, nor did they modulate the binding of THC or CBD [205]. Similarly, no synergy was detected between myrcene and CBD in modulating inflammation and analgesic properties in a rat adjuvant monoarthritis model [206]. Research on colorectal cancer cells did not detect any enhancement of activity when terpenes were included as part of a complex CBD oil compared to the effect of CBD alone [207].

The divergence of results involving potential synergy or entourage effects has led to doubt surrounding the entourage effect in cannabis and whether it really holds pharmaceutical potential. Cogan (2020) references several studies where individual cannabinoids did not improve the clinical performance of THC or CBD [208]. However, the intellectual leap to label cannabis potential synergistic interactions as "questionable" is perhaps premature. Botanicals or combinations exhibiting synergy or entourage does not necessitate that the effects take place at the same target to elicit a heightened response; compounds can exhibit "pharmacodynamic synergism" by acting at multiple cellular targets (seen in both antibiotic and cancer synergistic therapies) [209,210] and "pharmacokinetic synergism" by increasing the solubility or disposition (absorption, distribution, metabolism) of active constituents [211,212], and can limit side effects of the active constituent [213,214] or disrupt resistance mechanisms [215,216]. Indeed, the study Santiago et al. that purported the "absence of entourage" nevertheless suggested that synergy could still be taking place at a different molecular target than the CB receptors [203]. Therefore, as further studies are developed, it would be prudent to also employ phenotypic assays that encompass more than a single receptor/enzyme/target and can better deduce the combination effects at complementary sites and pathways to deliver heightened results. Thus, the heightened skepticism or dismissal of synergism in cannabis is perhaps unwarranted at this time, as there exists a growing body of evidence suggestive that not only do multiple cannabinoids work in concert to produce heightened effects (or potentially lower deleterious side effects), as seen in the prescription drugs that utilize multi-component cannabis extracts (Sativex® and Epidolex®) [186], but that terpenes/terpenoids can also potentially function as synergists with cannabinoids to deliver amplified results. Furthermore, studies from our own group, using an animal model of chemotherapeutic induced peripheral neuropathy, demonstrated an enhanced effect at reducing mechanical hypersensitivity by an extract containing equal parts CBG and CBD, in addition to other cannabinoids and terpenes, compared to pure CBG [217]. Additionally, in the same animal model we found that pure CBD was without an effect; however, when animals were treated with a complex hemp extract at the same CBD concentration, a reduction in mechanical sensitivity was observed [218]. These studies suggest that there is a potential interaction between cannabinoids and terpenes that can enhance the effect of pure cannabinoids alone. Moreover, the lack of synergy in vitro may not hold true for results in intact organisms, and the entourage effect does not have to be present or absent in all systems or biomedical indications. The search for synergy and entourage effects within the diverse phytochemical landscape of cannabis remains in its infancy; to better understand these combination effects, further research on the potential combination effects of cannabis's polypharmacy is essential to establish mechanisms of interaction, cellular targets of interest, and adverse events.

7. Conclusions and Future Directions

While commonly thought of as a psychoactive plant producing one of the most famous mind-altering chemicals discovered by humans, cannabis is a biosynthetic engine, producing hundreds of diverse phytochemicals that have the potential to impact a wide variety of human health conditions. In particular, cannabis produces 200 terpene structures that are of interest, both as independently bioactive molecules as well as by modulating or potentiating the effects of cannabinoids or other phytochemicals from cannabis. Terpenes are already widely implemented in traditional medicines and pharmaceuticals, as well as in industrial processes, perfumery, cosmetics, and food additives. They demonstrate generally low toxic profiles and high bioavailability and are highly selective to TRP channels, among other targets. There are known cannabimimetic activities of some terpenes, and they already have shown synergy amongst each other in other in vitro and in vivo studies. Thus, there is a firm foundation for cannabis synergy and the involvement of terpenes in the flavor, aroma, and bioactivity of cannabis. Investigations into potential combination effects in cannabis is a growing field, one which requires rigorous experimental design and execution but has the possibility to evolve our understanding of cannabis's diverse pharmaceutical effects.

Author Contributions: Conceptualization, F.T.C., W.M.R.-K., K.E.V. and J.J.K.; writing—original draft preparation, F.T.C., K.E.V. and J.J.K.; writing—review and editing, F.T.C., W.M.R.-K., K.E.V. and J.J.K.; visualization, F.T.C.; supervision, J.J.K. All authors have read and agreed to the published version of the manuscript.

Funding: J.J.K. is supported in part by the USDA National Institute of Food and Agriculture's Hatch Appropriations (PEN04772). K.E.V. (and the Penn State College of Medicine) is the recipient of research support from PA Options for Wellness (a state-approved medical marijuana clinical registrant). The funding sources were not involved in: study design; providing any experimental materials; data collection, analysis and interpretation; writing of the report; or the decision to submit the article for publication.

Conflicts of Interest: The authors declare no conflict of interest.

References

1. Brand, E.J.; Zhao, Z. Cannabis in Chinese Medicine: Are Some Traditional Indications Referenced in Ancient Literature Related to Cannabinoids? *Front. Pharmacol.* **2017**, *8*, 108. [CrossRef]
2. Ranade, A.; Tavhare, S.D.; Acharya, R.; Pawar, S.D. Cannabis (Bhanga) in Classical Text of Ayurveda: An Evidence-Based Rationale. In *Cannabis/Marijuana for Healthcare*; Agrawal, D.C., Kumar, R., Dhanasekaran, M., Eds.; Springer Nature: Singapore, 2022; pp. 235–251. ISBN 9789811688225.
3. Bonini, S.A.; Premoli, M.; Tambaro, S.; Kumar, A.; Maccarinelli, G.; Memo, M.; Mastinu, A. Cannabis Sativa: A Comprehensive Ethnopharmacological Review of a Medicinal Plant with a Long History. *J. Ethnopharmacol.* **2018**, *227*, 300–315. [CrossRef]
4. Kumar, P.; Mahato, D.K.; Kamle, M.; Borah, R.; Sharma, B.; Pandhi, S.; Tripathi, V.; Yadav, H.S.; Devi, S.; Patil, U.; et al. Pharmacological Properties, Therapeutic Potential, and Legal Status of *Cannabis sativa* L.: An Overview. *Phytother. Res.* **2021**, *35*, 6010–6029. [CrossRef]
5. Hurgobin, B.; Tamiru-Oli, M.; Welling, M.T.; Doblin, M.S.; Bacic, A.; Whelan, J.; Lewsey, M.G. Recent Advances in *Cannabis Sativa* Genomics Research. *New Phytol.* **2021**, *230*, 73–89. [CrossRef]
6. Monthony, A.S.; Page, S.R.; Hesami, M.; Jones, A.M.P. The Past, Present and Future of Cannabis Sativa Tissue Culture. *Plants* **2021**, *10*, 185. [CrossRef]
7. Radwan, M.M.; Chandra, S.; Gul, S.; ElSohly, M.A. Cannabinoids, Phenolics, Terpenes and Alkaloids of Cannabis. *Molecules* **2021**, *26*, 2774. [CrossRef]
8. Smith, T.; May, G.; Eckl, V.; Reynolds, C.M. US Sales of Herbal Supplements Increase by 8.6% in 2019. *HerbalGram* **2020**, 54–69.
9. Avins, D.; Kopf, J. New Data Show Americans Are Turning to CBD as a Cure-All for the Modern Condition. Available online: https://qz.com/1590765/survey-shows-americans-use-cbd-to-treat-anxiety-and-stress/ (accessed on 2 February 2022).
10. The Brightfield Group. *US CBD Market Industry Update*; The Brightfield Group: Chicago, IL, USA, 2022.
11. Hartsel, J.A.; Eades, J.; Hickory, B.; Makriyannis, A. Cannabis Sativa and Hemp. In *Nutraceuticals*; Elsevier: Amsterdam, The Netherlands, 2016; pp. 735–754. ISBN 978-0-12-802147-7.

12. Oldfield, E.; Lin, F.-Y. Terpene Biosynthesis: Modularity Rules. *Angew. Chem. Int. Ed.* **2012**, *51*, 1124–1137. [CrossRef]
13. Nuutinen, T. Medicinal Properties of Terpenes Found in Cannabis Sativa and Humulus Lupulus. *Eur. J. Med. Chem.* **2018**, *157*, 198–228. [CrossRef]
14. Cox-Georgian, D.; Ramadoss, N.; Dona, C.; Basu, C. Therapeutic and Medicinal Uses of Terpenes. In *Medicinal Plants: From Farm to Pharmacy*; Joshee, N., Dhekney, S.A., Parajuli, P., Eds.; Springer International Publishing: Cham, Switzerland, 2019; pp. 333–359. ISBN 978-3-030-31269-5.
15. Greay, S.J.; Hammer, K.A. Recent Developments in the Bioactivity of Mono- and Diterpenes: Anticancer and Antimicrobial Activity. *Phytochem. Rev.* **2015**, *14*, 1–6. [CrossRef]
16. Masyita, A.; Mustika Sari, R.; Dwi Astuti, A.; Yasir, B.; Rahma Rumata, N.; Emran, T.B.; Nainu, F.; Simal-Gandara, J. Terpenes and Terpenoids as Main Bioactive Compounds of Essential Oils, Their Roles in Human Health and Potential Application as Natural Food Preservatives. *Food Chem. X* **2022**, *13*, 100217. [CrossRef]
17. Koziol, A.; Stryjewska, A.; Librowski, T.; Salat, K.; Gawel, M.; Moniczewski, A.; Lochynski, S. An Overview of the Pharmacological Properties and Potential Applications of Natural Monoterpenes. *Mini Rev. Med. Chem.* **2014**, *14*, 1156–1168. [CrossRef]
18. Lasekan, O.; Abbas, K.A. Distinctive Exotic Flavor and Aroma Compounds of Some Exotic Tropical Fruits and Berries: A Review. *Crit. Rev. Food Sci. Nutr.* **2012**, *52*, 726–735. [CrossRef]
19. Marais, J. Terpenes in the Aroma of Grapes and Wines: A Review. *SAJEV* **2017**, *4*, 49–58. [CrossRef]
20. Mele, M.A.; Kang, H.-M.; Lee, Y.-T.; Islam, M.Z. Grape Terpenoids: Flavor Importance, Genetic Regulation, and Future Potential. *Crit. Rev. Food Sci. Nutr.* **2021**, *61*, 1429–1447. [CrossRef]
21. Roell, M.-S. Terpenes in Cannabis: Solving the Puzzle of How to Predict Taste and Smell. *Plant Physiol.* **2020**, *184*, 8–9. [CrossRef]
22. McPartland, J.M.; Russo, E.B. Cannabis and Cannabis Extracts. *J. Cannabis Ther.* **2001**, *1*, 103–132. [CrossRef]
23. Russo, E.B. Taming THC: Potential Cannabis Synergy and Phytocannabinoid-Terpenoid Entourage Effects. *Br. J. Pharmacol.* **2011**, *163*, 1344–1364. [CrossRef]
24. Efferth, T.; Koch, E. Complex Interactions between Phytochemicals. The Multi-Target Therapeutic Concept of Phytotherapy. *Curr. Drug Targets* **2011**, *12*, 122–132. [CrossRef]
25. Wagner, H.; Ulrich-Merzenich, G. Synergy Research: Approaching a New Generation of Phytopharmaceuticals. *Phytomedicine* **2009**, *16*, 97–110. [CrossRef]
26. Ben-Shabat, S.; Fride, E.; Sheskin, T.; Tamiri, T.; Rhee, M.-H.; Vogel, Z.; Bisogno, T.; De Petrocellis, L.; Di Marzo, V.; Mechoulam, R. An Entourage Effect: Inactive Endogenous Fatty Acid Glycerol Esters Enhance 2-Arachidonoyl-Glycerol Cannabinoid Activity. *Eur. J. Pharmacol.* **1998**, *353*, 23–31. [CrossRef]
27. Rohmer, M. From Molecular Fossils of Bacterial Hopanoids to the Formation of Isoprene Units: Discovery and Elucidation of the Methylerythritol Phosphate Pathway. *Lipids* **2008**, *43*, 1095–1107. [CrossRef]
28. Miziorko, H.M. Enzymes of the Mevalonate Pathway of Isoprenoid Biosynthesis. *Arch. Biochem. Biophys.* **2011**, *505*, 131–143. [CrossRef]
29. Jiang, S.-Y.; Jin, J.; Sarojam, R.; Ramachandran, S. A Comprehensive Survey on the Terpene Synthase Gene Family Provides New Insight into Its Evolutionary Patterns. *Genome Biol. Evol.* **2019**, *11*, 2078–2098. [CrossRef]
30. Degenhardt, F.; Stehle, F.; Kayser, O. Chapter 2—The Biosynthesis of Cannabinoids. In *Handbook of Cannabis and Related Pathologies*; Preedy, V.R., Ed.; Academic Press: San Diego, CA, USA, 2017; pp. 13–23. ISBN 978-0-12-800756-3.
31. Hanuš, L.O.; Hod, Y. Terpenes/Terpenoids in Cannabis: Are They Important? *MCA* **2020**, *3*, 25–60. [CrossRef]
32. McGarvey, D.J.; Croteau, R. Terpenoid Metabolism. *Plant Cell* **1995**, *7*, 1015–1026. [CrossRef]
33. Chen, F.; Tholl, D.; Bohlmann, J.; Pichersky, E. The Family of Terpene Synthases in Plants: A Mid-Size Family of Genes for Specialized Metabolism That Is Highly Diversified throughout the Kingdom. *Plant J.* **2011**, *66*, 212–229. [CrossRef]
34. Booth, J.K.; Yuen, M.M.S.; Jancsik, S.; Madilao, L.L.; Page, J.E.; Bohlmann, J. Terpene Synthases and Terpene Variation in Cannabis Sativa. *Plant Physiol.* **2020**, *184*, 130–147. [CrossRef]
35. Booth, J.K.; Page, J.E.; Bohlmann, J. Terpene Synthases from Cannabis Sativa. *PLoS ONE* **2017**, *12*, e0173911. [CrossRef]
36. Livingston, S.J.; Quilichini, T.D.; Booth, J.K.; Wong, D.C.J.; Rensing, K.H.; Laflamme-Yonkman, J.; Castellarin, S.D.; Bohlmann, J.; Page, J.E.; Samuels, A.L. Cannabis Glandular Trichomes Alter Morphology and Metabolite Content during Flower Maturation. *Plant J.* **2020**, *101*, 37–56. [CrossRef]
37. Zager, J.J.; Lange, I.; Srividya, N.; Smith, A.; Lange, B.M. Gene Networks Underlying Cannabinoid and Terpenoid Accumulation in Cannabis. *Plant Physiol.* **2019**, *180*, 1877–1897. [CrossRef]
38. Günnewich, N.; Page, J.E.; Köllner, T.G.; Degenhardt, J.; Kutchan, T.M. Functional Expression and Characterization of Trichome-Specific (-)-Limonene Synthase and (+)-α-Pinene Synthase from Cannabis Sativa. *Nat. Prod. Commun.* **2007**, *2*, 223–232. [CrossRef]
39. Watts, S.; McElroy, M.; Migicovsky, Z.; Maassen, H.; van Velzen, R.; Myles, S. Cannabis Labelling Is Associated with Genetic Variation in Terpene Synthase Genes. *Nat. Plants* **2021**, *7*, 1330–1334. [CrossRef]
40. Ross, S.A.; ElSohly, M.A. The Volatile Oil Composition of Fresh and Air-Dried Buds of Cannabis Sativa. *J. Nat. Prod.* **1996**, *59*, 49–51. [CrossRef]
41. Tholl, D. Terpene Synthases and the Regulation, Diversity and Biological Roles of Terpene Metabolism. *Curr. Opin. Plant Biol.* **2006**, *9*, 297–304. [CrossRef]
42. Lewis, M.A.; Russo, E.B.; Smith, K.M. Pharmacological Foundations of Cannabis Chemovars. *Planta Med.* **2018**, *84*, 225–233. [CrossRef]

43. Brown, A.K.; Xia, Z.; Bulloch, P.; Idowu, I.; Francisco, O.; Stetefeld, J.; Stout, J.; Zimmer, J.; Marvin, C.; Letcher, R.J.; et al. Validated Quantitative Cannabis Profiling for Canadian Regulatory Compliance—Cannabinoids, Aflatoxins, and Terpenes. *Anal. Chim. Acta* **2019**, *1088*, 79–88. [CrossRef]
44. Pacifico, D.; Miselli, F.; Carboni, A.; Moschella, A.; Mandolino, G. Time Course of Cannabinoid Accumulation and Chemotype Development during the Growth of *Cannabis sativa* L. *Euphytica* **2008**, *160*, 231–240. [CrossRef]
45. Fischedick, J.T.; Hazekamp, A.; Erkelens, T.; Choi, Y.H.; Verpoorte, R. Metabolic Fingerprinting of Cannabis Sativa L., Cannabinoids and Terpenoids for Chemotaxonomic and Drug Standardization Purposes. *Phytochemistry* **2010**, *71*, 2058–2073. [CrossRef]
46. Fischedick, J.T. Identification of Terpenoid Chemotypes Among High (−)-Trans-Δ9- Tetrahydrocannabinol-Producing *Cannabis sativa* L. Cultivars. *Cannabis Cannabinoid Res.* **2017**, *2*, 34–47. [CrossRef]
47. Richins, R.D.; Rodriguez-Uribe, L.; Lowe, K.; Ferral, R.; O'Connell, M.A. Accumulation of Bioactive Metabolites in Cultivated Medical Cannabis. *PLoS ONE* **2018**, *13*, e0201119. [CrossRef]
48. Reimann-Philipp, U.; Speck, M.; Orser, C.; Johnson, S.; Hilyard, A.; Turner, H.; Stokes, A.J.; Small-Howard, A.L. Cannabis Chemovar Nomenclature Misrepresents Chemical and Genetic Diversity; Survey of Variations in Chemical Profiles and Genetic Markers in Nevada Medical Cannabis Samples. *Cannabis Cannabinoid Res.* **2020**, *5*, 215–230. [CrossRef]
49. Birenboim, M.; Chalupowicz, D.; Maurer, D.; Barel, S.; Chen, Y.; Fallik, E.; Paz-Kagan, T.; Rapaport, T.; Sadeh, A.; Kengisbuch, D.; et al. Multivariate Classification of Cannabis Chemovars Based on Their Terpene and Cannabinoid Profiles. *Phytochemistry* **2022**, *200*, 113215. [CrossRef]
50. Lemay, J.; Zheng, Y.; Scott-Dupree, C. Factors Influencing the Efficacy of Biological Control Agents Used to Manage Insect Pests in Indoor Cannabis (*Cannabis sativa*) Cultivation. *Front. Agron.* **2022**, *4*, 795989. [CrossRef]
51. Whipker, B.E. Put Your Fertilizer Program to the Test. Available online: https://www.cannabisbusinesstimes.com/article/cultivation-matters-ncsu-north-carolina-cannabis-fertilization-program-management-npk-nitrogen-phosphorus-potassium/ (accessed on 28 September 2022).
52. Hawley, D.; Graham, T.; Stasiak, M.; Dixon, M. Improving Cannabis Bud Quality and Yield with Subcanopy Lighting. *HortScience* **2018**, *53*, 1593–1599. [CrossRef]
53. Aizpurua-Olaizola, O.; Soydaner, U.; Öztürk, E.; Schibano, D.; Simsir, Y.; Navarro, P.; Etxebarria, N.; Usobiaga, A. Evolution of the Cannabinoid and Terpene Content during the Growth of Cannabis Sativa Plants from Different Chemotypes. *J. Nat. Prod.* **2016**, *79*, 324–331. [CrossRef]
54. AL Ubeed, H.M.S.; Wills, R.B.H.; Chandrapala, J. Post-Harvest Operations to Generate High-Quality Medicinal Cannabis Products: A Systemic Review. *Molecules* **2022**, *27*, 1719. [CrossRef]
55. Pagnani, G.; Pellegrini, M.; Galieni, A.; D'Egidio, S.; Matteucci, F.; Ricci, A.; Stagnari, F.; Sergi, M.; Lo Sterzo, C.; Pisante, M.; et al. Plant Growth-Promoting Rhizobacteria (PGPR) in Cannabis Sativa 'Finola' Cultivation: An Alternative Fertilization Strategy to Improve Plant Growth and Quality Characteristics. *Ind. Crops Prod.* **2018**, *123*, 75–83. [CrossRef]
56. Hudson, J.R. Humulones, Lupulones and Other Constituents of Hops. In *Modern Methods of Plant Analysis/Moderne Methoden der Pflanzenanalyse*; Linskens, H.F., Tracey, M.V., Beiss, U., Bendall, F., Björk, W., Bohlmann, F., Boman, H.G., Braun, R., Heinen, W., Hesse, M., et al., Eds.; Springer: Berlin/Heidelberg, Germany, 1963; pp. 135–154. ISBN 978-3-642-94878-7.
57. Desaulniers Brousseau, V.; Wu, B.-S.; MacPherson, S.; Morello, V.; Lefsrud, M. Cannabinoids and Terpenes: How Production of Photo-Protectants Can Be Manipulated to Enhance *Cannabis sativa* L. Phytochemistry. *Front. Plant Sci.* **2021**, *12*, 620021. [CrossRef]
58. Lydon, J.; Teramura, A.H.; Coffman, C.B. UV-B RADIATION EFFECTS ON PHOTOSYNTHESIS, GROWTH and CANNABINOID PRODUCTION OF TWO *Cannabis sativa* CHEMOTYPES. *Photochem. Photobiol.* **1987**, *46*, 201–206. [CrossRef] [PubMed]
59. Eichhorn Bilodeau, S.; Wu, B.-S.; Rufyikiri, A.-S.; MacPherson, S.; Lefsrud, M. An Update on Plant Photobiology and Implications for Cannabis Production. *Front. Plant Sci.* **2019**, *10*, 296. [CrossRef] [PubMed]
60. Milay, L.; Berman, P.; Shapira, A.; Guberman, O.; Meiri, D. Metabolic Profiling of Cannabis Secondary Metabolites for Evaluation of Optimal Postharvest Storage Conditions. *Front. Plant Sci.* **2020**, *11*, 583605. [CrossRef] [PubMed]
61. Hazekamp, A.; Tejkalová, K.; Papadimitriou, S. Cannabis: From Cultivar to Chemovar II—A Metabolomics Approach to Cannabis Classification. *Cannabis Cannabinoid Res.* **2016**, *1*, 202–215. [CrossRef]
62. Sexton, M.; Shelton, K.; Haley, P.; West, M. Evaluation of Cannabinoid and Terpenoid Content: Cannabis Flower Compared to Supercritical CO_2 Concentrate. *Planta Med.* **2018**, *84*, 234–241. [CrossRef] [PubMed]
63. Jin, D.; Dai, K.; Xie, Z.; Chen, J. Secondary Metabolites Profiled in Cannabis Inflorescences, Leaves, Stem Barks, and Roots for Medicinal Purposes. *Sci. Rep.* **2020**, *10*, 3309. [CrossRef] [PubMed]
64. Dei Cas, M.; Arnoldi, S.; Monguzzi, L.; Casagni, E.; Morano, C.; Vieira de Manincor, E.; Bolchi, C.; Pallavicini, M.; Gambaro, V.; Roda, G. Characterization of Chemotype-Dependent Terpenoids Profile in Cannabis by Headspace Gas-Chromatography Coupled to Time-of-Flight Mass Spectrometry. *J. Pharm. Biomed. Anal.* **2021**, *203*, 114180. [CrossRef]
65. Hazekamp, A.; Fischedick, J.T. Cannabis—From Cultivar to Chemovar. *Drug Test. Anal.* **2012**, *4*, 660–667. [CrossRef]
66. Russo, E.B.; Marcu, J. Cannabis Pharmacology: The Usual Suspects and a Few Promising Leads. In *Advances in Pharmacology*; Elsevier: Amsterdam, The Netherlands, 2017; Volume 80, pp. 67–134. ISBN 978-0-12-811232-8.
67. Baron, E.P. Medicinal Properties of Cannabinoids, Terpenes, and Flavonoids in Cannabis, and Benefits in Migraine, Headache, and Pain: An Update on Current Evidence and Cannabis Science. *Headache J. Head Face Pain* **2018**, *58*, 1139–1186. [CrossRef]
68. Sommano, S.R.; Chittasupho, C.; Ruksiriwanich, W.; Jantrawut, P. The Cannabis Terpenes. *Molecules* **2020**, *25*, 5792. [CrossRef]

69. Weston-Green, K.; Clunas, H.; Jimenez Naranjo, C. A Review of the Potential Use of Pinene and Linalool as Terpene-Based Medicines for Brain Health: Discovering Novel Therapeutics in the Flavours and Fragrances of Cannabis. *Front. Psychiatry* **2021**, *12*, 583211. [CrossRef]
70. Lowe, H.; Steele, B.; Bryant, J.; Toyang, N.; Ngwa, W. Non-Cannabinoid Metabolites of *Cannabis sativa* L. with Therapeutic Potential. *Plants* **2021**, *10*, 400. [CrossRef]
71. Pattnaik, F.; Nanda, S.; Mohanty, S.; Dalai, A.K.; Kumar, V.; Ponnusamy, S.K.; Naik, S. Cannabis: Chemistry, Extraction and Therapeutic Applications. *Chemosphere* **2022**, *289*, 133012. [CrossRef] [PubMed]
72. Wang, L.-P.; Feng, J.-F.; Hu, K.-L. Progress in regulation effect of aromatic refreshing traditional Chinese medicine on BBB permeability and its mechanism. *Zhongguo Zhong Yao Za Zhi* **2014**, *39*, 949–954.
73. Zhang, Q.-L.; Fu, B.M.; Zhang, Z.-J. Borneol, a Novel Agent That Improves Central Nervous System Drug Delivery by Enhancing Blood–Brain Barrier Permeability. *Drug Deliv.* **2017**, *24*, 1037–1044. [CrossRef] [PubMed]
74. Xiong, Z.-Y.; Xiao, F.-M.; Xu, X.; Wu, Y.-F.; Jiang, X.-M. Studies on pharmacological activity of borneol. *Zhongguo Zhong Yao Za Zhi* **2013**, *38*, 786–790. [PubMed]
75. da Silva Almeida, J.R.G.; Souza, G.R.; Silva, J.C.; de Lima Saraiva, S.R.G.; de Oliveira Júnior, R.G.; de Souza Siqueira Quintans, J.; de Souza Siqueira Barreto, R.; Bonjardim, L.R.; de Holanda Cavalcanti, S.C.; Junior, L.J.Q. Borneol, a Bicyclic Monoterpene Alcohol, Reduces Nociceptive Behavior and Inflammatory Response in Mice. *Sci. World J.* **2013**, *2013*, e808460. [CrossRef]
76. Li, Y.-H.; Sun, X.-P.; Zhang, Y.-Q.; Wang, N.-S. The Antithrombotic Effect of Borneol Related to Its Anticoagulant Property. *Am. J. Chin. Med.* **2008**, *36*, 719–727. [CrossRef]
77. Liu, R.; Zhang, L.; Lan, X.; Li, L.; Zhang, T.-T.; Sun, J.-H.; Du, G.-H. Protection by Borneol on Cortical Neurons against Oxygen-Glucose Deprivation/Reperfusion: Involvement of Anti-Oxidation and Anti-Inflammation through Nuclear Transcription Factor KappaB Signaling Pathway. *Neuroscience* **2011**, *176*, 408–419. [CrossRef]
78. Chen, X.; Lin, Z.; Liu, A.; Ye, J.; Luo, Y.; Luo, Y.; Mao, X.; Liu, P.; Pi, R. The Orally Combined Neuroprotective Effects of Sodium Ferulate and Borneol against Transient Global Ischaemia in C57 BL/6J Mice. *J. Pharm. Pharmacol.* **2010**, *62*, 915–923. [CrossRef]
79. Horvathova, E.; Mastihubova, M.; Karnisova Potocka, E.; Kis, P.; Galova, E.; Sevcovicova, A.; Klapakova, M.; Hunakova, L.; Mastihuba, V. Comparative Study of Relationship between Structure of Phenylethanoid Glycopyranosides and Their Activities Using Cell-Free Assays and Human Cells Cultured in Vitro. *Toxicol. Vitr.* **2019**, *61*, 104646. [CrossRef]
80. Corrêa, P.R.C.; Miranda, R.R.S.; Duarte, L.P.; Silva, G.D.F.; Filho, S.A.V.; Okuma, A.A.; Carazza, F.; Morgado-Díaz, J.A.; Pinge-Filho, P.; Yamauchi, L.M.; et al. Antimicrobial Activity of Synthetic Bornyl Benzoates against Trypanosoma Cruzi. *Pathog. Glob. Health* **2012**, *106*, 107–112. [CrossRef]
81. Vasconcelos, R.M.C.; Leite, F.C.; Leite, J.A.; Rodrigues Mascarenhas, S.; Rodrigues, L.C.; Piuvezam, M.R. Synthesis, Acute Toxicity and Anti-Inflammatory Effect of Bornyl Salicylate, a Salicylic Acid Derivative. *Immunopharmacol. Immunotoxicol.* **2012**, *34*, 1028–1038. [CrossRef]
82. PubChem Camphor. Available online: https://pubchem.ncbi.nlm.nih.gov/compound/2537 (accessed on 4 October 2022).
83. Chen, W.; Vermaak, I.; Viljoen, A. Camphor—A Fumigant during the Black Death and a Coveted Fragrant Wood in Ancient Egypt and Babylon—A Review. *Molecules* **2013**, *18*, 5434–5454. [CrossRef]
84. Hamidpour, R.; Hamidpour, S.; Hamidpour, M.; Shahlari, M. Camphor (*Cinnamomum Camphora*), a Traditional Remedy with the History of Treating Several Diseases. *Int. J. Case Rep. Images (IJCRI)* **2013**, *4*, 86–89. [CrossRef]
85. Wang, L.; Zhang, K.; Zhang, K.; Zhang, J.; Fu, J.; Li, J.; Wang, G.; Qiu, Z.; Wang, X.; Li, J. Antibacterial Activity of Cinnamomum Camphora Essential Oil on Escherichia Coli During Planktonic Growth and Biofilm Formation. *Front. Microbiol.* **2020**, *11*, 561002. [CrossRef]
86. Zarubaev, V.V.; Garshinina, A.V.; Tretiak, T.S.; Fedorova, V.A.; Shtro, A.A.; Sokolova, A.S.; Yarovaya, O.I.; Salakhutdinov, N.F. Broad Range of Inhibiting Action of Novel Camphor-Based Compound with Anti-Hemagglutinin Activity against Influenza Viruses in Vitro and in Vivo. *Antivir. Res.* **2015**, *120*, 126–133. [CrossRef]
87. Kumar, N.; Nepali, K.; Sapra, S.; Bijjem, K.R.V.; Kumar, R.; Suri, O.P.; Dhar, K.L. Effect of Nitrogen Insertion on the Antitussive Properties of Menthol and Camphor. *Med. Chem. Res.* **2012**, *21*, 531–537. [CrossRef]
88. Nikolić, B.; Vasilijević, B.; Mitić-Ćulafić, D.; Vuković-Gačić, B.; Knežević-Vukćević, J. Comparative Study of Genotoxic, Antigenotoxic and Cytotoxic Activities of Monoterpenes Camphor, Eucalyptol and Thujone in Bacteria and Mammalian Cells. *Chem.-Biol. Interact.* **2015**, *242*, 263–271. [CrossRef]
89. Moayedi, Y.; Greenberg, S.A.; Jenkins, B.A.; Marshall, K.L.; Dimitrov, L.V.; Nelson, A.M.; Owens, D.M.; Lumpkin, E.A. Camphor White Oil Induces Tumor Regression through Cytotoxic T Cell-Dependent Mechanisms. *Mol. Carcinog.* **2019**, *58*, 722–734. [CrossRef]
90. Shata, F.Y.H.; Eldebaky, H.A.A. Effects of Camphor on Hepatic Enzymes, Steroids and Antioxidant Capacity of Male Rats Intoxicated with Atrazine. *Middle-East J. of Sci. Res.* **2014**, *22*, 553–560.
91. Drikvandi, P.; Bahramikia, S.; Alirezaei, M. Modulation of the Antioxidant Defense System in Liver, Kidney, and Pancreas Tissues of Alloxan-Induced Diabetic Rats by Camphor. *J. Food Biochem.* **2020**, *44*, e13527. [CrossRef]
92. Poudel, D.K.; Rokaya, A.; Ojha, P.K.; Timsina, S.; Satyal, R.; Dosoky, N.S.; Satyal, P.; Setzer, W.N. The Chemical Profiling of Essential Oils from Different Tissues of Cinnamomum Camphora L. and Their Antimicrobial Activities. *Molecules* **2021**, *26*, 5132. [CrossRef]

93. Baker, B.P.; Grant, J.A.; Malakar-Kuenen, R. *Cedarwood Oil Profile. Cornell Cooperative Extension Integrated Pest Management Program*; Cornell University: Ithaca, NY, USA, 2018; pp. 1–8. Available online: https://ecommons.cornell.edu/handle/1813/56116 (accessed on 15 September 2022).
94. Johnston, W.H.; Karchesy, J.J.; Constantine, G.H.; Craig, A.M. Antimicrobial Activity of Some Pacific Northwest Woods against Anaerobic Bacteria and Yeast. *Phytother. Res.* **2001**, *15*, 586–588. [CrossRef] [PubMed]
95. National Toxicology Program (NTP). *NTP Technical Report on the Toxicity Studies of Cedarwood Oil (Virginia) (CASRN 8000-27-9) Administered Dermally to F344/N Rats and B6C3F1/N Mice*; National Toxicology Program: Research Triangle Park, NC, USA, 2019; p. 86.
96. Al-Daghri, N.M.; Alokail, M.S.; Alkharfy, K.M.; Mohammed, A.K.; Abd-Alrahman, S.H.; Yakout, S.M.; Amer, O.E.; Krishnaswamy, S. Fenugreek Extract as an Inducer of Cellular Death via Autophagy in Human T Lymphoma Jurkat Cells. *BMC Complement. Altern. Med.* **2012**, *12*, 202. [CrossRef] [PubMed]
97. Al-Rahmah, A.N.; Mostafa, A.A.; Abdel-Megeed, A.; Yakout, S.M.; Hussein, S.A. Fungicidal Activities of Certain Methanolic Plant Extracts against Tomato Phytopathogenic Fungi. *Afr. J. Microbiol. Res.* **2013**, *7*, 517–524.
98. Su, Y.-C.; Hsu, K.-P.; Wang, E.I.-C.; Ho, C.-L. Composition, Anticancer, and Antimicrobial Activities in Vitro of the Heartwood Essential Oil of Cunninghamia Lanceolata Var. Konishii from Taiwan. *Nat. Prod. Commun.* **2012**, *7*, 1245–1247. [CrossRef]
99. Kim, T.H.; Yoo, S.D.; Lee, H.S.; Lee, K.M.; Seok, S.H.; Kim, M.G.; Jung, B.H.; Kim, M.G.; Shin, B.S. In Vivo Absorption and Disposition of α-Cedrene, a Sesquiterpene Constituent of Cedarwood Oil, in Female and Male Rats. *Drug Metab. Pharmacokinet.* **2015**, *30*, 168–173. [CrossRef]
100. Tong, T.; Yu, R.; Park, T. α-Cedrene Protects Rodents from High-Fat Diet-Induced Adiposity via Adenylyl Cyclase 3. *Int. J. Obes.* **2019**, *43*, 202–216. [CrossRef]
101. Haque, A.N.M.A.; Remadevi, R.; Naebe, M. Lemongrass (Cymbopogon): A Review on Its Structure, Properties, Applications and Recent Developments. *Cellulose* **2018**, *25*, 5455–5477. [CrossRef]
102. Spencer, J.S.; Dowd, E.; Faas, W.; Company, A.T. The Genuineness of Two Mint Essential Oils. *Perfum. Flavorist* **1997**, *22*, 37–45.
103. Rajeswara Rao, B.R.; Kaul, P.N.; Syamasundar, K.V.; Ramesh, S. Comparative Composition of Decanted and Recovered Essential Oils of Eucalyptus Citriodora Hook. *Flavour Fragr. J.* **2003**, *18*, 133–135. [CrossRef]
104. Leafly Cannabis Glossary. Available online: https://www.leafly.com/learn/cannabis-glossary (accessed on 15 September 2022).
105. Silva, M.I.G.; de Aquino Neto, M.R.; Teixeira Neto, P.F.; Moura, B.A.; do Amaral, J.F.; de Sousa, D.P.; Vasconcelos, S.M.M.; de Sousa, F.C.F. Central Nervous System Activity of Acute Administration of Isopulegol in Mice. *Pharmacol. Biochem. Behav.* **2007**, *88*, 141–147. [CrossRef]
106. Silva, M.I.G.; Silva, M.A.G.; de Aquino Neto, M.R.; Moura, B.A.; de Sousa, H.L.; de Lavor, E.P.H.; de Vasconcelos, P.F.; Macêdo, D.S.; de Sousa, D.P.; Vasconcelos, S.M.M.; et al. Effects of Isopulegol on Pentylenetetrazol-Induced Convulsions in Mice: Possible Involvement of GABAergic System and Antioxidant Activity. *Fitoterapia* **2009**, *80*, 506–513. [CrossRef] [PubMed]
107. Silva, M.I.G.; Moura, B.A.; de Aquino Neto, M.R.; da Rocha Tomé, A.; Rocha, N.F.M.; de Carvalho, A.M.R.; Macêdo, D.S.; Vasconcelos, S.M.M.; de Sousa, D.P.; de Barros Viana, G.S.; et al. Gastroprotective Activity of Isopulegol on Experimentally Induced Gastric Lesions in Mice: Investigation of Possible Mechanisms of Action. *Naunyn-Schmied Arch Pharm.* **2009**, *380*, 233–245. [CrossRef] [PubMed]
108. Bounihi, A.; Hajjaj, G.; Alnamer, R.; Cherrah, Y.; Zellou, A. In Vivo Potential Anti-Inflammatory Activity of *Melissa Officinalis* L. Essential Oil. *Adv. Pharmacol. Pharm. Sci.* **2013**, *2013*, e101759. [CrossRef]
109. Guo, X.; Ho, C.-T.; Schwab, W.; Wan, X. Aroma Profiles of Green Tea Made with Fresh Tea Leaves Plucked in Summer. *Food Chem.* **2021**, *363*, 130328. [CrossRef]
110. Hossain, M.A.; Al-Hdhrami, S.S.; Weli, A.M.; Al-Riyami, Q.; Al-Sabahi, J.N. Isolation, Fractionation and Identification of Chemical Constituents from the Leaves Crude Extracts of Mentha Piperita L Grown in Sultanate of Oman. *Asian Pac. J. Trop. Biomed.* **2014**, *4*, S368–S372. [CrossRef]
111. Kim, C.-W.; Lee, H.J.; Jung, J.H.; Kim, Y.H.; Jung, D.-B.; Sohn, E.J.; Lee, J.H.; Woo, H.J.; Baek, N.-I.; Kim, Y.C.; et al. Activation of Caspase-9/3 and Inhibition of Epithelial Mesenchymal Transition Are Critically Involved in Antitumor Effect of Phytol in Hepatocellular Carcinoma Cells. *Phytother. Res.* **2015**, *29*, 1026–1031. [CrossRef]
112. Santos, C.C.d.M.P.; Salvadori, M.S.; Mota, V.G.; Costa, L.M.; de Almeida, A.A.C.; de Oliveira, G.A.L.; Costa, J.P.; de Sousa, D.P.; Freitas, R.M.; de Almeida, R.N. Antinociceptive and Antioxidant Activities of Phytol In Vivo and In Vitro Models. *Neurosci. J.* **2013**, *2013*, 949452. [CrossRef]
113. Silva, R.O.; Sousa, F.B.M.; Damasceno, S.R.B.; Carvalho, N.S.; Silva, V.G.; Oliveira, F.R.M.A.; Sousa, D.P.; Aragão, K.S.; Barbosa, A.L.R.; Freitas, R.M.; et al. Phytol, a Diterpene Alcohol, Inhibits the Inflammatory Response by Reducing Cytokine Production and Oxidative Stress. *Fundam. Clin. Pharmacol.* **2014**, *28*, 455–464. [CrossRef]
114. Pejin, B.; Kojic, V.; Bogdanovic, G. An Insight into the Cytotoxic Activity of Phytol at in Vitro Conditions. *Nat. Prod. Res.* **2014**, *28*, 2053–2056. [CrossRef] [PubMed]
115. Costa, J.P.; de Oliveira, G.A.L.; de Almeida, A.A.C.; Islam, M.T.; de Sousa, D.P.; de Freitas, R.M. Anxiolytic-like Effects of Phytol: Possible Involvement of GABAergic Transmission. *Brain Res.* **2014**, *1547*, 34–42. [CrossRef] [PubMed]
116. Costa, J.P.; Ferreira, P.B.; De Sousa, D.P.; Jordan, J.; Freitas, R.M. Anticonvulsant Effect of Phytol in a Pilocarpine Model in Mice. *Neurosci. Lett.* **2012**, *523*, 115–118. [CrossRef] [PubMed]

117. Moniruzzaman, M.; Mannan, M.A.; Hossen Khan, M.F.; Abir, A.B.; Afroze, M. The Leaves of Crataeva Nurvala Buch-Ham. Modulate Locomotor and Anxiety Behaviors Possibly through GABAergic System. *BMC Complement. Altern. Med.* **2018**, *18*, 283. [CrossRef] [PubMed]
118. de Moraes, J.; de Oliveira, R.N.; Costa, J.P.; Junior, A.L.G.; de Sousa, D.P.; Freitas, R.M.; Allegretti, S.M.; Pinto, P.L.S. Phytol, a Diterpene Alcohol from Chlorophyll, as a Drug against Neglected Tropical Disease Schistosomiasis Mansoni. *PLOS Negl. Trop. Dis.* **2014**, *8*, e2617. [CrossRef]
119. Chowdhury, R.; Ghosh, S. Phytol-Derived Novel Isoprenoid Immunostimulants. *Front. Immunol.* **2012**, *3*, 49. [CrossRef]
120. Aachoui, Y.; Chowdhury, R.R.; Fitch, R.W.; Ghosh, S.K. Molecular Signatures of Phytol-Derived Immunostimulants in the Context of Chemokine–Cytokine Microenvironment and Enhanced Immune Response. *Cell. Immunol.* **2011**, *271*, 227–238. [CrossRef]
121. Liu, C.; Srividya, N.; Parrish, A.N.; Yue, W.; Shan, M.; Wu, Q.; Lange, B.M. Morphology of Glandular Trichomes of Japanese Catnip (Schizonepeta Tenuifolia Briquet) and Developmental Dynamics of Their Secretory Activity. *Phytochemistry* **2018**, *150*, 23–30. [CrossRef]
122. Farley, D.R.; Howland, V. The Natural Variation of the Pulegone Content in Various Oils of Peppermint. *J. Sci. Food Agric.* **1980**, *31*, 1143–1151. [CrossRef]
123. Turner, C.E.; Elsohly, M.A.; Boeren, E.G. Constituents of Cannabis Sativa L. XVII. A Review of the Natural Constituents. *J. Nat. Prod.* **1980**, *43*, 169–234. [CrossRef]
124. Formisano, C.; Rigano, D.; Napolitano, F.; Senatore, F.; Arnold, N.A.; Piozzi, F.; Rosselli, S. Volatile Constituents of Calamintha Origanifolia Boiss. Growing Wild in Lebanon. *Nat. Prod. Commun.* **2007**, *2*, 1253–1256. [CrossRef]
125. da Silveira, N.S.; de Oliveira-Silva, G.L.; de Freitas Lamanes, B.; da Silva Prado, L.C.; Bispo-da-Silva, L.B. The Aversive, Anxiolytic-Like, and Verapamil-Sensitive Psychostimulant Effects of Pulegone. *Biol. Pharm. Bull.* **2014**, *37*, 771–778. [CrossRef] [PubMed]
126. Ortiz de Urbina, A.V.; Martín, M.L.; Montero, M.J.; Morán, A.; San Román, L. Sedating and Antipyretic Activity of the Essential Oil of Calamintha Sylvatica Subsp. Ascendens. *J. Ethnopharmacol.* **1989**, *25*, 165–171. [CrossRef]
127. Božović, M.; Ragno, R. *Calamintha nepeta* (L.) Savi and Its Main Essential Oil Constituent Pulegone: Biological Activities and Chemistry. *Molecules* **2017**, *22*, 290. [CrossRef]
128. Hilfiger, L.; Triaux, Z.; Marcic, C.; Héberlé, E.; Emhemmed, F.; Darbon, P.; Marchioni, E.; Petitjean, H.; Charlet, A. Anti-Hyperalgesic Properties of Menthol and Pulegone. *Front. Pharmacol.* **2021**, *12*, 753873. [CrossRef]
129. Valente, J.; Zuzarte, M.; Gonçalves, M.J.; Lopes, M.C.; Cavaleiro, C.; Salgueiro, L.; Cruz, M.T. Antifungal, Antioxidant and Anti-Inflammatory Activities of Oenanthe Crocata L. Essential Oil. *Food Chem. Toxicol.* **2013**, *62*, 349–354. [CrossRef]
130. Quiroga, P.R.; Asensio, C.M.; Nepote, V. Antioxidant Effects of the Monoterpenes Carvacrol, Thymol and Sabinene Hydrate on Chemical and Sensory Stability of Roasted Sunflower Seeds. *J. Sci. Food Agric.* **2015**, *95*, 471–479. [CrossRef]
131. Sela, F.; Karapandzova, M.; Stefkov, G.; Cvetkovikj, I.; Kulevanova, S. Chemical Composition and Antimicrobial Activity of Essential Oils of Juniperus Excelsa Bieb. (Cupressaceae) Grown in R. Macedonia. *Pharmacogn. Res.* **2015**, *7*, 74–80. [CrossRef]
132. Maghsoodlou, M.T.; Kazemipoor, N.; Valizadeh, J.; Falak Nezhad Seifi, M.; Rahneshan, N. Essential Oil Composition of Eucalyptus Microtheca and Eucalyptus Viminalis. *Avicenna J. Phytomed.* **2015**, *5*, 540–552.
133. Johnson, S.; DeCarlo, A.; Satyal, P.; Dosoky, N.S.; Sorensen, A.; Setzer, W.N. The Chemical Composition of Single-Tree Boswellia Frereana Resin Samples. *Nat. Prod. Commun.* **2021**, *16*, 1934578X211043727. [CrossRef]
134. Hao, Y.; Kang, J.; Guo, X.; Yang, R.; Chen, Y.; Li, J.; Shi, L. Comparison of Nutritional Compositions and Essential Oil Profiles of Different Parts of a Dill and Two Fennel Cultivars. *Foods* **2021**, *10*, 1784. [CrossRef]
135. Aros, D.; Garrido, N.; Rivas, C.; Medel, M.; Müller, C.; Rogers, H.; Úbeda, C. Floral Scent Evaluation of Three Cut Flowers Through Sensorial and Gas Chromatography Analysis. *Agronomy* **2020**, *10*, 131. [CrossRef]
136. Verghese, J.; Joy, M.T.; Retamar, J.A.; Malinskas, G.G.; Catalán, C.A.N.; Gros, E.G. A Fresh Look at the Constituents of Indian Olibanum Oil. *Flavour Fragr. J.* **1987**, *2*, 99–102. [CrossRef]
137. Ali, N.A.A.; Wurster, M.; Arnold, N.; Teichert, A.; Schmidt, J.; Lindequist, U.; Wessjohann, L. Chemical Composition and Biological Activities of Essential Oils from the Oleogum Resins of Three Endemic Soqotraen Boswellia Species. *Rec. Nat. Prod.* **2008**, *8*, 6–12.
138. Siddiqui, M.Z. Boswellia Serrata, a Potential Antiinflammatory Agent: An Overview. *Indian J. Pharm. Sci.* **2011**, *73*, 255–261. [CrossRef]
139. Sadhasivam, S.; Palanivel, S.; Ghosh, S. Synergistic Antimicrobial Activity of Boswellia Serrata Roxb. Ex Colebr. (Burseraceae) Essential Oil with Various Azoles against Pathogens Associated with Skin, Scalp and Nail Infections. *Lett. Appl. Microbiol.* **2016**, *63*, 495–501. [CrossRef]
140. Prabhavathi, K.; Chandra, U.S.J.; Soanker, R.; Rani, P.U. A Randomized, Double Blind, Placebo Controlled, Cross over Study to Evaluate the Analgesic Activity of Boswellia Serrata in Healthy Volunteers Using Mechanical Pain Model. *Indian J. Pharmacol.* **2014**, *46*, 475. [CrossRef]
141. Elston, A.; Lin, J.; Rouseff, R. Determination of the Role of Valencene in Orange Oil as a Direct Contributor to Aroma Quality. *Flavour Fragr. J.* **2005**, *20*, 381–386. [CrossRef]
142. Marques, F.M.; Figueira, M.M.; Schmitt, E.F.P.; Kondratyuk, T.P.; Endringer, D.C.; Scherer, R.; Fronza, M. In Vitro Anti-Inflammatory Activity of Terpenes via Suppression of Superoxide and Nitric Oxide Generation and the NF-KB Signalling Pathway. *Inflammopharmacology* **2019**, *27*, 281–289. [CrossRef]

143. Sánchez-Martínez, J.D.; Alvarez-Rivera, G.; Gallego, R.; Fagundes, M.B.; Valdés, A.; Mendiola, J.A.; Ibañez, E.; Cifuentes, A. Neuroprotective Potential of Terpenoid-Rich Extracts from Orange Juice by-Products Obtained by Pressurized Liquid Extraction. *Food Chem. X* **2022**, *13*, 100242. [CrossRef]
144. Jin, J.H.; Lee, D.-U.; Kim, Y.S.; Kim, H.P. Anti-Allergic Activity of Sesquiterpenes from the Rhizomes of Cyperus Rotundus. *Arch. Pharm. Res.* **2011**, *34*, 223–228. [CrossRef]
145. Muthaiyan, A.; Biswas, D.; Crandall, P.G.; Wilkinson, B.J.; Ricke, S.C. Application of Orange Essential Oil as an Antistaphylococcal Agent in a Dressing Model. *BMC Complement. Altern. Med.* **2012**, *12*, 125. [CrossRef]
146. Rao, V.S.N.; Menezes, A.M.S.; Viana, G.S.B. Effect of Myrcene on Nociception in Mice. *J. Pharm. Pharmacol.* **1990**, *42*, 877–878. [CrossRef] [PubMed]
147. Gertsch, J.; Leonti, M.; Raduner, S.; Racz, I.; Chen, J.-Z.; Xie, X.-Q.; Altmann, K.-H.; Karsak, M.; Zimmer, A. Beta-Caryophyllene Is a Dietary Cannabinoid. *Proc. Natl. Acad. Sci. USA* **2008**, *105*, 9099–9104. [CrossRef] [PubMed]
148. Bento, A.F.; Marcon, R.; Dutra, R.C.; Claudino, R.F.; Cola, M.; Pereira Leite, D.F.; Calixto, J.B. β-Caryophyllene Inhibits Dextran Sulfate Sodium-Induced Colitis in Mice through CB2 Receptor Activation and PPARγ Pathway. *Am. J. Pathol.* **2011**, *178*, 1153–1166. [CrossRef]
149. Jansen, C.; Shimoda, L.M.N.; Kawakami, J.K.; Ang, L.; Bacani, A.J.; Baker, J.D.; Badowski, C.; Speck, M.; Stokes, A.J.; Small-Howard, A.L.; et al. Myrcene and Terpene Regulation of TRPV1. *Channels* **2019**, *13*, 344–366. [CrossRef]
150. Chen, G.-L.; Lei, M.; Zhou, L.-P.; Zeng, B.; Zou, F. Borneol Is a TRPM8 Agonist That Increases Ocular Surface Wetness. *PLoS ONE* **2016**, *11*, e0158868. [CrossRef]
151. Lai, H.; Liu, C.; Hou, L.; Lin, W.; Chen, T.; Hong, A. TRPM8-Regulated Calcium Mobilization Plays a Critical Role in Synergistic Chemosensitization of Borneol on Doxorubicin. *Theranostics* **2020**, *10*, 10154–10170. [CrossRef]
152. Granger, R.E.; Campbell, E.L.; Johnston, G.A.R. (+)- And (−)-Borneol: Efficacious Positive Modulators of GABA Action at Human Recombinant Alpha1beta2gamma2L GABA(A) Receptors. *Biochem. Pharmacol.* **2005**, *69*, 1101–1111. [CrossRef]
153. Jiang, J.; Shen, Y.Y.; Li, J.; Lin, Y.H.; Luo, C.X.; Zhu, D.Y. (+)-Borneol Alleviates Mechanical Hyperalgesia in Models of Chronic Inflammatory and Neuropathic Pain in Mice. *Eur. J. Pharmacol.* **2015**, *757*, 53–58. [CrossRef]
154. Vogt-Eisele, A.K.; Weber, K.; Sherkheli, M.A.; Vielhaber, G.; Panten, J.; Gisselmann, G.; Hatt, H. Monoterpenoid Agonists of TRPV3. *Br. J. Pharmacol.* **2007**, *151*, 530–540. [CrossRef]
155. Takaishi, M.; Uchida, K.; Fujita, F.; Tominaga, M. Inhibitory Effects of Monoterpenes on Human TRPA1 and the Structural Basis of Their Activity. *J. Physiol. Sci.* **2014**, *64*, 47–57. [CrossRef]
156. Sherkheli, M.A.; Schreiner, B.; Haq, R.; Werner, M.; Hatt, H. Borneol Inhibits TRPA1, a Proinflammatory and Noxious Pain-Sensing Cation Channel. *Pak. J. Pharm. Sci.* **2015**, *28*, 1357–1363.
157. Selescu, T.; Ciobanu, A.C.; Dobre, C.; Reid, G.; Babes, A. Camphor Activates and Sensitizes Transient Receptor Potential Melastatin 8 (TRPM8) to Cooling and Icilin. *Chem. Senses* **2013**, *38*, 563–575. [CrossRef]
158. Marsakova, L.; Touska, F.; Krusek, J.; Vlachova, V. Pore Helix Domain Is Critical to Camphor Sensitivity of Transient Receptor Potential Vanilloid 1 Channel. *Anesthesiology* **2012**, *116*, 903–917. [CrossRef]
159. Nguyen, T.H.D.; Itoh, S.G.; Okumura, H.; Tominaga, M. Structural Basis for Promiscuous Action of Monoterpenes on TRP Channels. *Commun. Biol.* **2021**, *4*, 293. [CrossRef]
160. Freitas, M.M.; Cavalcante, P.M.; Duarte-Filho, L.A.M.S.; Macedo, C.A.F.; Brito, M.C.; Menezes, P.M.N.; Ribeiro, T.F.; Costa, S.M.; Carvalho, B.A.G.; Ribeiro, F.P.R.A.; et al. Investigation of the Relaxing Effect of a Camphor Nanoemulsion on Rat Isolated Trachea. *Chem. Biol. Interact.* **2021**, *348*, 109656. [CrossRef]
161. Tong, T.; Ryu, S.E.; Min, Y.; de March, C.A.; Bushdid, C.; Golebiowski, J.; Moon, C.; Park, T. Olfactory Receptor 10J5 Responding to α-Cedrene Regulates Hepatic Steatosis via the CAMP–PKA Pathway. *Sci. Rep.* **2017**, *7*, 9471. [CrossRef] [PubMed]
162. Tong, T.; Kim, M.; Park, T. α-Cedrene, a Newly Identified Ligand of MOR23, Increases Skeletal Muscle Mass and Strength. *Mol. Nutr. Food Res.* **2018**, *62*, e1800173. [CrossRef] [PubMed]
163. Kessler, A.; Sahin-Nadeem, H.; Lummis, S.C.R.; Weigel, I.; Pischetsrieder, M.; Buettner, A.; Villmann, C. GABAA Receptor Modulation by Terpenoids from Sideritis Extracts. *Mol. Nutr. Food Res.* **2014**, *58*, 851–862. [CrossRef]
164. Chuang, H.; Neuhausser, W.M.; Julius, D. The Super-Cooling Agent Icilin Reveals a Mechanism of Coincidence Detection by a Temperature-Sensitive TRP Channel. *Neuron* **2004**, *43*, 859–869. [CrossRef] [PubMed]
165. Andrade Próspero, D.F.; Reis Filho, A.C.; Piauilino, C.A.; Lopes, E.M.; de Sousa, D.P.; de Castro Almeida, F.R. Effects of Isopulegol in Acute Nociception in Mice: Possible Involvement of Muscarinic Receptors, Opioid System and l-Arginine/NO/CGMP Pathway. *Chem. Biol. Interact.* **2018**, *293*, 55–60. [CrossRef] [PubMed]
166. Ellinghaus, P.; Wolfrum, C.; Assmann, G.; Spener, F.; Seedorf, U. Phytanic Acid Activates the Peroxisome Proliferator-Activated Receptor Alpha (PPARalpha) in Sterol Carrier Protein 2-/ Sterol Carrier Protein x-Deficient Mice. *J. Biol. Chem.* **1999**, *274*, 2766–2772. [CrossRef]
167. Zomer, A.W.; van Der Burg, B.; Jansen, G.A.; Wanders, R.J.; Poll-The, B.T.; van Der Saag, P.T. Pristanic Acid and Phytanic Acid: Naturally Occurring Ligands for the Nuclear Receptor Peroxisome Proliferator-Activated Receptor Alpha. *J. Lipid Res.* **2000**, *41*, 1801–1807. [CrossRef]
168. Kitareewan, S.; Burka, L.T.; Tomer, K.B.; Parker, C.E.; Deterding, L.J.; Stevens, R.D.; Forman, B.M.; Mais, D.E.; Heyman, R.A.; McMorris, T.; et al. Phytol Metabolites Are Circulating Dietary Factors That Activate the Nuclear Receptor RXR. *Mol. Biol. Cell* **1996**, *7*, 1153–1166. [CrossRef]

169. Thakor, P.; Subramanian, R.B.; Thakkar, S.S.; Ray, A.; Thakkar, V.R. Phytol Induces ROS Mediated Apoptosis by Induction of Caspase 9 and 3 through Activation of TRAIL, FAS and TNF Receptors and Inhibits Tumor Progression Factor Glucose 6 Phosphate Dehydrogenase in Lung Carcinoma Cell Line (A549). *Biomed. Pharmacother.* **2017**, *92*, 491–500. [CrossRef]
170. Kruska, N.; Reiser, G. Phytanic Acid and Pristanic Acid, Branched-Chain Fatty Acids Associated with Refsum Disease and Other Inherited Peroxisomal Disorders, Mediate Intracellular Ca2+ Signaling through Activation of Free Fatty Acid Receptor GPR40. *Neurobiol. Dis.* **2011**, *43*, 465–472. [CrossRef]
171. Elmazar, M.M.; El-Abhar, H.S.; Schaalan, M.F.; Farag, N.A. Phytol/Phytanic Acid and Insulin Resistance: Potential Role of Phytanic Acid Proven by Docking Simulation and Modulation of Biochemical Alterations. *PLoS ONE* **2013**, *8*, e45638. [CrossRef]
172. Sadgrove, N.J.; Oblong, J.E.; Simmonds, M.S.J. Inspired by Vitamin A for Anti-ageing: Searching for Plant-derived Functional Retinoid Analogues. *Skin Health Dis.* **2021**, *1*, e36. [CrossRef]
173. Shayiranbieke, A.; Liang, Q.; Wang, T.; Ma, J.; Li, G.; Du, X.; Zhang, G.; Wang, C.; Zhao, X. Development of Immobilized Beta1-Adrenoceptor Chromatography for Rapid Discovery of Ligands Specifically Binding to the Receptor from Herbal Extract. *J. Chromatogr. A* **2022**, *1677*, 463298. [CrossRef]
174. Majikina, A.; Takahashi, K.; Saito, S.; Tominaga, M.; Ohta, T. Involvement of Nociceptive Transient Receptor Potential Channels in Repellent Action of Pulegone. *Biochem. Pharmacol.* **2018**, *151*, 89–95. [CrossRef]
175. Vimal, A.; Pal, D.; Tripathi, T.; Kumar, A. Eucalyptol, Sabinene and Cinnamaldehyde: Potent Inhibitors of Salmonella Target Protein l-Asparaginase. *3 Biotech* **2017**, *7*, 258. [CrossRef]
176. İstİflİ, E.S.; ŞihoĞlu Tepe, A.; SarikÜrkcÜ, C.; Tepe, B. Interaction of Certain Monoterpenoid Hydrocarbons with the Receptor Binding Domain of 2019 Novel Coronavirus (2019-NCoV), Transmembrane Serine Protease 2 (TMPRSS2), Cathepsin B, and Cathepsin L (CatB/L) and Their Pharmacokinetic Properties. *Turk. J. Biol.* **2020**, *44*, 242–264. [CrossRef]
177. Lakhera, S.; Devlal, K.; Ghosh, A.; Chowdhury, P.; Rana, M. Modelling the DFT Structural and Reactivity Study of Feverfew and Evaluation of Its Potential Antiviral Activity against COVID-19 Using Molecular Docking and MD Simulations. *Chem. Zvesti* **2022**, *76*, 2759–2776. [CrossRef]
178. Shervin Prince, S.; Stanely Mainzen Prince, P.; Berlin Grace, V.M. Valencene Post-Treatment Exhibits Cardioprotection via Inhibiting Cardiac Hypertrophy, Oxidative Stress, Nuclear Factor- KB Inflammatory Pathway, and Myocardial Infarct Size in Isoproterenol-Induced Myocardial Infarcted Rats; A Molecular Study. *Eur. J. Pharmacol.* **2022**, *927*, 174975. [CrossRef]
179. Nam, J.H.; Nam, D.-Y.; Lee, D.-U. Valencene from the Rhizomes of Cyperus Rotundus Inhibits Skin Photoaging-Related Ion Channels and UV-Induced Melanogenesis in B16F10 Melanoma Cells. *J. Nat. Prod.* **2016**, *79*, 1091–1096. [CrossRef]
180. Yang, I.J.; Lee, D.-U.; Shin, H.M. Inhibitory Effect of Valencene on the Development of Atopic Dermatitis-Like Skin Lesions in NC/Nga Mice. *Evid. -Based Complement. Altern. Med.* **2016**, *2016*, 1–11. [CrossRef]
181. Bonn-Miller, M.O.; ElSohly, M.A.; Loflin, M.J.E.; Chandra, S.; Vandrey, R. Cannabis and Cannabinoid Drug Development: Evaluating Botanical versus Single Molecule Approaches. *Int. Rev. Psychiatry* **2018**, *30*, 277–284. [CrossRef]
182. Caesar, L.K.; Cech, N.B. Synergy and Antagonism in Natural Product Extracts: When 1 + 1 Does Not Equal 2. *Nat. Prod. Rep.* **2019**, *36*, 869–888. [CrossRef]
183. Russo, E.B.; McPartland, J.M. Cannabis Is More than Simply Δ9-Tetrahydrocannabinol. *Psychopharmacology* **2003**, *165*, 431–432. [CrossRef]
184. Wilkinson, J.D.; Whalley, B.J.; Baker, D.; Pryce, G.; Constanti, A.; Gibbons, S.; Williamson, E.M. Medicinal Cannabis: Is Δ9–Tetrahydrocannabinol Necessary for All Its Effects? *J. Pharm. Pharmacol.* **2003**, *55*, 1687–1694. [CrossRef] [PubMed]
185. McPartland, J.M.; Pruitt, P.L. Side Effects of Pharmaceuticals Not Elicited By Comparable Herbal Medicines: The Case of Tetrahydrocannabinol and Marijuana. *Altern. Ther. Health Med.* **1999**, *5*, 57–62. [PubMed]
186. Johnson, J.R.; Burnell-Nugent, M.; Lossignol, D.; Ganae-Motan, E.D.; Potts, R.; Fallon, M.T. Multicenter, Double-Blind, Randomized, Placebo-Controlled, Parallel-Group Study of the Efficacy, Safety, and Tolerability of THC:CBD Extract and THC Extract in Patients with Intractable Cancer-Related Pain. *J. Pain Symptom Manag.* **2010**, *39*, 167–179. [CrossRef]
187. Gallily, R.; Yekhtin, Z.; Hanuš, L.O. Overcoming the Bell-Shaped Dose-Response of Cannabidiol by Using *Cannabis* Extract Enriched in Cannabidiol. *Pharmacol. Pharm.* **2015**, *6*, 75. [CrossRef]
188. Berman, P.; Futoran, K.; Lewitus, G.M.; Mukha, D.; Benami, M.; Shlomi, T.; Meiri, D. A New ESI-LC/MS Approach for Comprehensive Metabolic Profiling of Phytocannabinoids in Cannabis. *Sci. Rep.* **2018**, *8*, 14280. [CrossRef]
189. Blasco-Benito, S.; Seijo-Vila, M.; Caro-Villalobos, M.; Tundidor, I.; Andradas, C.; García-Taboada, E.; Wade, J.; Smith, S.; Guzmán, M.; Pérez-Gómez, E.; et al. Appraising the "Entourage Effect": Antitumor Action of a Pure Cannabinoid versus a Botanical Drug Preparation in Preclinical Models of Breast Cancer. *Biochem. Pharmacol.* **2018**, *157*, 285–293. [CrossRef]
190. Nallathambi, R.; Mazuz, M.; Namdar, D.; Shik, M.; Namintzer, D.; Vinayaka, A.C.; Ion, A.; Faigenboim, A.; Nasser, A.; Laish, I.; et al. Identification of Synergistic Interaction Between Cannabis-Derived Compounds for Cytotoxic Activity in Colorectal Cancer Cell Lines and Colon Polyps That Induces Apoptosis-Related Cell Death and Distinct Gene Expression. *Cannabis Cannabinoid Res.* **2018**, *3*, 120–135. [CrossRef]
191. Reddy, D.S.; Golub, V.M. The Pharmacological Basis of Cannabis Therapy for Epilepsy. *J. Pharmacol. Exp. Ther.* **2016**, *357*, 45–55. [CrossRef]
192. Russo, E.B. Cannabis and Epilepsy: An Ancient Treatment Returns to the Fore. *Epilepsy Behav.* **2017**, *70*, 292–297. [CrossRef]
193. Sulak, D.; Saneto, R.; Goldstein, B. The Current Status of Artisanal Cannabis for the Treatment of Epilepsy in the United States. *Epilepsy Behav.* **2017**, *70*, 328–333. [CrossRef]

194. Pamplona, F.A.; da Silva, L.R.; Coan, A.C. Potential Clinical Benefits of CBD-Rich Cannabis Extracts Over Purified CBD in Treatment-Resistant Epilepsy: Observational Data Meta-Analysis. *Front. Neurol.* **2018**, *9*, 759. [CrossRef] [PubMed]
195. Chen, J.; Li, L.; Su, J.; Li, B.; Chen, T.; Wong, Y.-S. Synergistic Apoptosis-Inducing Effects on A375 Human Melanoma Cells of Natural Borneol and Curcumin. *PLoS ONE* **2014**, *9*, e101277. [CrossRef] [PubMed]
196. Liu, Y.; Zhao, Y.; Guo, D.; Liu, W.; Liu, Y. Synergistic Antimicrobial Activity of Berberine Hydrochloride, Baicalein and Borneol against Candida Albicans. *Chin. Herb. Med.* **2017**, *9*, 353–357. [CrossRef]
197. Rocha, P.M.d.M.; Rodilla, J.M.; Díez, D.; Elder, H.; Guala, M.S.; Silva, L.A.; Pombo, E.B. Synergistic Antibacterial Activity of the Essential Oil of Aguaribay (*Schinus molle* L.). *Molecules* **2012**, *17*, 12023–12036. [CrossRef]
198. Farhanghi, A.; Aliakbarlu, J.; Tajik, H.; Mortazavi, N.; Manafi, L.; Jalilzadeh-Amin, G. Antibacterial Interactions of Pulegone and 1,8-Cineole with Monolaurin Ornisin against Staphylococcus Aureus. *Food Sci. Nutr.* **2022**, *10*, 2659–2666. [CrossRef]
199. Pavithra, P.S.; Mehta, A.; Verma, R.S. Synergistic Interaction of β-Caryophyllene with Aromadendrene Oxide 2 and Phytol Induces Apoptosis on Skin Epidermoid Cancer Cells. *Phytomedicine* **2018**, *47*, 121–134. [CrossRef]
200. Ferber, S.G.; Namdar, D.; Hen-Shoval, D.; Eger, G.; Koltai, H.; Shoval, G.; Shbiro, L.; Weller, A. The "Entourage Effect": Terpenes Coupled with Cannabinoids for the Treatment of Mood Disorders and Anxiety Disorders. *Curr. Neuropharmacol.* **2020**, *18*, 87–96. [CrossRef]
201. LaVigne, J.E.; Hecksel, R.; Keresztes, A.; Streicher, J.M. Cannabis Sativa Terpenes Are Cannabimimetic and Selectively Enhance Cannabinoid Activity. *Sci. Rep.* **2021**, *11*, 8232. [CrossRef]
202. Di Giacomo, S.; Mariano, A.; Gullì, M.; Fraschetti, C.; Vitalone, A.; Filippi, A.; Mannina, L.; Scotto d'Abusco, A.; Di Sotto, A. Role of Caryophyllane Sesquiterpenes in the Entourage Effect of Felina 32 Hemp Inflorescence Phytocomplex in Triple Negative MDA-MB-468 Breast Cancer Cells. *Molecules* **2021**, *26*, 6688. [CrossRef]
203. Santiago, M.; Sachdev, S.; Arnold, J.C.; McGregor, I.S.; Connor, M. Absence of Entourage: Terpenoids Commonly Found in *Cannabis Sativa* Do Not Modulate the Functional Activity of Δ^9-THC at Human CB$_1$ and CB$_2$ Receptors. *Cannabis Cannabinoid Res.* **2019**, *4*, 165–176. [CrossRef]
204. Heblinski, M.; Santiago, M.; Fletcher, C.; Stuart, J.; Connor, M.; McGregor, I.S.; Arnold, J.C. Terpenoids Commonly Found in Cannabis Sativa Do Not Modulate the Actions of Phytocannabinoids or Endocannabinoids on TRPA1 and TRPV1 Channels. *Cannabis Cannabinoid Res.* **2020**, *5*, 305–317. [CrossRef] [PubMed]
205. Finlay, D.B.; Sircombe, K.J.; Nimick, M.; Jones, C.; Glass, M. Terpenoids From Cannabis Do Not Mediate an Entourage Effect by Acting at Cannabinoid Receptors. *Front. Pharmacol.* **2020**, *11*, 359. [CrossRef] [PubMed]
206. McDougall, J.J.; McKenna, M.K. Anti-Inflammatory and Analgesic Properties of the Cannabis Terpene Myrcene in Rat Adjuvant Monoarthritis. *Int. J. Mol. Sci.* **2022**, *23*, 7891. [CrossRef]
207. Raup-Konsavage, W.M.; Carkaci-Salli, N.; Greenland, K.; Gearhart, R.; Vrana, K.E. Cannabidiol (CBD) Oil Does Not Display an Entourage Effect in Reducing Cancer Cell Viability in Vitro. *Med. Cannabis Cannabinoids* **2020**, *3*, 95–102. [CrossRef] [PubMed]
208. Cogan, P.S. The 'Entourage Effect' or 'Hodge-Podge Hashish': The Questionable Rebranding, Marketing, and Expectations of Cannabis Polypharmacy. *Expert Rev. Clin. Pharmacol.* **2020**, *13*, 835–845. [CrossRef] [PubMed]
209. Brooks, B.D.; Brooks, A.E. Therapeutic Strategies to Combat Antibiotic Resistance. *Adv. Drug Deliv. Rev.* **2014**, *78*, 14–27. [CrossRef] [PubMed]
210. Hu, C.-M.J.; Zhang, L. Nanoparticle-Based Combination Therapy toward Overcoming Drug Resistance in Cancer. *Biochem. Pharmacol.* **2012**, *83*, 1104–1111. [CrossRef]
211. Ma, X.H.; Zheng, C.J.; Han, L.Y.; Xie, B.; Jia, J.; Cao, Z.W.; Li, Y.X.; Chen, Y.Z. Synergistic Therapeutic Actions of Herbal Ingredients and Their Mechanisms from Molecular Interaction and Network Perspectives. *Drug Discov. Today* **2009**, *14*, 579–588. [CrossRef]
212. Spinella, M. The Importance of Pharmacological Synergy in Psychoactive Herbal Medicines. *Altern. Med. Rev. J. Clin. Ther.* **2002**, *7*, 9.
213. Wang, S.; Zhu, F.; Marcone, M.F. Staghorn Sumac Reduces 5-Fluorouracil-Induced Toxicity in Normal Cells. *J. Med. Food* **2015**, *18*, 938–940. [CrossRef]
214. McCune, L.M.; Johns, T. Antioxidant Activity in Medicinal Plants Associated with the Symptoms of Diabetes Mellitus Used by the Indigenous Peoples of the North American Boreal Forest. *J. Ethnopharmacol.* **2002**, *82*, 197–205. [CrossRef] [PubMed]
215. Leyte-Lugo, M.; Britton, E.R.; Foil, D.H.; Brown, A.R.; Todd, D.A.; Rivera-Chávez, J.; Oberlies, N.H.; Cech, N.B. Secondary Metabolites from the Leaves of the Medicinal Plant Goldenseal (Hydrastis Canadensis). *Phytochem. Lett.* **2017**, *20*, 54–60. [CrossRef] [PubMed]
216. Britton, E.R.; Kellogg, J.J.; Kvalheim, O.M.; Cech, N.B. Biochemometrics to Identify Synergists and Additives from Botanical Medicines: A Case Study with Hydrastis Canadensis (Goldenseal). *J. Nat. Prod.* **2018**, *81*, 484–493. [CrossRef]
217. Sepulveda, D.E.; Morris, D.P.; Raup-Konsavage, W.M.; Sun, D.; Vrana, K.E.; Graziane, N.M. Cannabigerol (CBG) Attenuates Mechanical Hypersensitivity Elicited by Chemotherapy-Induced Peripheral Neuropathy. *Eur. J. Pain* **2022**, *26*, 1950–1966. [CrossRef]
218. Sepulveda, D.E.; Vrana, K.E.; Graziane, N.M.; Raup-Konsavage, W.M. Combinations of Cannabidiol and Δ9-Tetrahydrocannabinol in Reducing Chemotherapeutic Induced Neuropathic Pain. *Biomedicines* **2022**, *10*, 2548. [CrossRef]

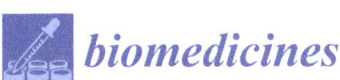

Review

The Therapeutic Potential of the Endocannabinoid System in Age-Related Diseases

Ivona Maria Tudorancea [1], Mitică Ciorpac [1], Gabriela Dumitrița Stanciu [1], Cătălin Caratașu [1], Alina Săcărescu [2,3], Bogdan Ignat [4], Alexandra Burlui [5,6], Elena Rezuș [5,6], Ioana Creangă [1,7], Teodora Alexa-Stratulat [7,8], Ionuț Tudorancea [9,10,*] and Bogdan Ionel Tamba [1,11]

- [1] Advanced Research and Development Center for Experimental Medicine (CEMEX), "Grigore T. Popa" University of Medicine and Pharmacy, 16 Universității Street, 700115 Iași, Romania
- [2] Department of Medical Specialties II, "Grigore T. Popa" University of Medicine and Pharmacy, 16 Universității, 700115 Iași, Romania
- [3] Department of Neurology, Clinical Rehabilitation Hospital, 14 Pantelimon Halipa, 700661 Iași, Romania
- [4] Department of Neurology, "Grigore T. Popa" University of Medicine and Pharmacy, 700115 Iași, Romania
- [5] Department of Rheumatology and Rehabilitation, "Grigore T. Popa" University of Medicine and Pharmacy, 700115 Iași, Romania
- [6] Clinical Rehabilitation Hospital, 700661 Iași, Romania
- [7] Oncology Department, "Grigore T. Popa" University of Medicine and Pharmacy, 700115 Iași, Romania
- [8] Oncology Department, Regional Institute of Oncology, 700483 Iași, Romania
- [9] Department of Morpho-Functional Sciences II, Discipline of Physiology, "Grigore T. Popa" University of Medicine and Pharmacy, 700115 Iași, Romania
- [10] Cardiology Clinic "St. Spiridon" County Clinical Emergency Hospital, 700111 Iași, Romania
- [11] Department of Pharmacology, Clinical Pharmacology and Algesiology, "Grigore T. Popa" University of Medicine and Pharmacy, 16 Universității Street, 700115 Iași, Romania
- * Correspondence: ionut.tudorancea@umfiasi.ro

Citation: Tudorancea, I.M.; Ciorpac, M.; Stanciu, G.D.; Caratașu, C.; Săcărescu, A.; Ignat, B.; Burlui, A.; Rezuș, E.; Creangă, I.; Alexa-Stratulat, T.; et al. The Therapeutic Potential of the Endocannabinoid System in Age-Related Diseases. *Biomedicines* **2022**, *10*, 2492. https://doi.org/10.3390/biomedicines10102492

Academic Editor: Wesley M. Raup-Konsavage

Received: 21 August 2022
Accepted: 3 October 2022
Published: 6 October 2022

Publisher's Note: MDPI stays neutral with regard to jurisdictional claims in published maps and institutional affiliations.

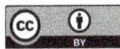

Copyright: © 2022 by the authors. Licensee MDPI, Basel, Switzerland. This article is an open access article distributed under the terms and conditions of the Creative Commons Attribution (CC BY) license (https://creativecommons.org/licenses/by/4.0/).

Abstract: The endocannabinoid system (ECS) dynamically regulates many aspects of mammalian physiology. ECS has gained substantial interest since growing evidence suggests that it also plays a major role in several pathophysiological conditions due to its ability to modulate various underlying mechanisms. Furthermore, cannabinoids, as components of the cannabinoid system (CS), have proven beneficial effects such as anti-inflammatory, immunomodulatory, neuromodulatory, antioxidative, and cardioprotective effects. In this comprehensive review, we aimed to describe the complex interaction between CS and most common age-related diseases such as neuro-degenerative, oncological, skeletal, and cardiovascular disorders, together with the potential of various cannabinoids to ameliorate the progression of these disorders. Since chronic inflammation is postulated as the pillar of all the above-mentioned medical conditions, we also discuss in this paper the potential of CS to ameliorate aging-associated immune system dysregulation.

Keywords: cannabinoids; aging; endocannabinoid system; cannabinoid receptors; age-related diseases

1. Introduction

It is well established that the endocannabinoid system (ECS) is involved in the modulation of various physiological processes such as memory, pain, cognition, temperature, mood, feeding, and pregnancy [1,2]. In the past decades, ECS has gained substantial interest since growing evidence suggests that ECS also plays a major role in several physiopathological conditions due to its ability to modulate various underlying mechanisms [3]. For example, a neuromodulatory effect induced by ECS was recently described in neurodegenerative disorders such as Alzheimer's and Parkinson's disease. Additionally, ECS has been shown to play a significant role in inflammation associated with these medical conditions [4–6].

The ECS is comprised of endocannabinoids, cannabinoid receptors, and the proteins that are involved in the transport, degradation, and synthesis of cannabinoids, such as diacylglycerol (DAG) lipase isozymes α and β, fatty acid amide hydrolase (FAAH), monoacylglycerol lipase (MAGL), and N-acylphosphatidylethanolamine-selective phospholipase D (NAPE-PLD) [3,7]. Recent studies focusing on the modulation of the ECS have demonstrated that multiple signaling pathways are involved in its modulation. This particular feature is proven by the multifunctionality of its components [7]. It is well known that cannabinoids interact mainly, but without excluding other classes, with three classes of receptors: (1) G-Coupled Protein Receptors (GPCRs)—Cannabinoid receptors 1 and 2 (rCB1 and rCB2), (2) Ligand-sensitive ion channels (e.g., Transient Receptor Potential Vanilloid 1—TRPV1), and (3) nuclear receptors (e.g., nuclear receptor peroxisome proliferator-activated receptor gamma (PPAR-γ)) [3]. CB1 receptor was initially discovered and characterized in rat brain and thereafter in the human central nervous system [8,9]. Unlike rCB1, the second cannabinoid receptor (CB2) was initially cloned and characterized in two type of cells: in a human promyelocytic leukemic cell line and in rodent spleen cells [10]. In the past years, the main structural features of cannabinoid receptors CB1 and CB2 were clarified by using X-ray crystallography [11,12]. These modern methods paved the way for the synthetization of agonists and/or antagonists with a high selectivity for cannabinoid receptors leading thus to a complete description of various underlying rCB-related pathways [13]. The most important modulators of cannabinoid receptors, their mechanism of action, and the main findings in various experimental models are summarized in Table 1.

Table 1. The most important modulators of cannabinoid receptors, their mechanism of action, and the main findings in various experimental models.

Cannabinoids	Cannabinoid Origin	Mechanism of Action on Cannabinoids Receptors	Experimental Model	Main Findings	Ref.
CP 55.940	→ synthetic	→ rCB1 and CB2 agonist	→ acute pain models in mice; → neuropathic pain models induced by paclitaxel in CB1, CB2 knockout and wild-type mice.	→ CP 55.940 combined with a μ opioid agonist displayed synergism in two experimental pain test; → antiallodynic dose-dependent effects.	[14,15]
Rimonabant (SR-141716A)	→ synthetic	→ rCB1 selective → antagonist	→ obese Zucker (fa/fa) rats model; → non-obese Wistar rats.	→ reduction of hyperinsulinemia; → dose-dependent reduction of both food intake and body weight.	[16,17]
AM251	→ synthetic	→ neutral antagonist	→ acute foot-shock stress in mice; → neurodevelopmental animal model based on a social isolation procedure; → 129/SVE and C57BL/6 male mice.	→ antidepressant-like effect through interaction of opioid and cannabinoid pathways; → long-lasting effect on psychotic-like symptoms; reduction in neuronal activity induced by isolation; → antidepressant-like and anorectic effect.	[18–20]
WIN 55212-2	→ synthetic	→ rCB1/CB2 → agonist with a slightly higher CB2R selectivity	→ neuropathic pain models; → autoimmune encephalomyelitis model; → behavioral changes induced by trauma exposure; → post-traumatic stress disorder models; → animal model of hypoxia-ischemia in fetal lambs.	→ analgesic effect; → reduction of the increased leukocyte rolling and firm adhesion in the brain; → restoring normal social behavior by modulating the stress response; → reduction of anxiety-like behavior; → reduction of the pro-inflammatory cytokines tumor necrosis factor (TNF)-α and interleukin (IL)-1β and IL-6 (interleukin 6).	[21–25]

Table 1. Cont.

Cannabinoids	Cannabinoid Origin	Mechanism of Action on Cannabinoids Receptors	Experimental Model	Main Findings	Ref.
Δ9-THC (Δ9-tetrahydrocannabinol)	→ natural	→ rCB1/ CB2 → partial agonist	→ male Sprague–Dawley rats exposed to chronic treatment with Δ9-THC.	→ neuroadaptive responses to cannabinoids via the increased expression of brain-derived neurotrophic factor.	[26,27]
CBD (cannabidiol)	→ natural	→ rCB1 antagonist/ inverse agonist; CB2 partial agonist	→ Alzheimer's disease mouse model; → rat model of neuropathic pain; → epilepsy mice model; → Parkinson's disease rat model.	→ reversed cognitive deficits in object recognition memory and social recognition memory; → modulates chronic neuropathic pain and depression-specific behavior; → reduces seizures and associated behavioral comorbidities; → neuroprotective and symptomatic effects.	[28–31]
JWH-015	→ synthetic	→ rCB2 selective → agonist	→ mice model of induced neuropathic pain; → rat model of induced arthritis; → acute and persistent inflammatory pain model.	→ antiallodynic effect; → anti-inflammatory effect; → antinociceptive effects.	[32–34]
JWH-133	→ synthetic	→ rCB2 selective → agonist	→ rat model of spinal cord ischemia reperfusion injury; → wild-type and knockout mice lacking CB2 in neurons, monocytes or constitutively, exploring spontaneous neuropathic pain.	→ attenuated neurological deficit and blood-spinal cord barrier disruption via toll-like receptors 4 (TLR4)/matrix metalloproteinase 9 (MMP9) signal pathway; → alleviates spontaneous pain and anxiety-associated behavior.	[35,36]

The cannabinoid receptors 1 and 2 are found in a variety of tissues and organs and are the pillar of the ECS signaling complexity. Both rCB1 and rCB2 are G protein coupled receptors but they are characterized by structural differences and thus, the affinity for various endogenous or exogenous ligands vary accordingly. rCB1 is mainly found in the central nervous system into axons and presynaptic terminals in the amygdala and cortex, in GABAergic interneurons in the hippocampus, glial cells (astrocytes, oligodendrocytes), and microglia [37–39]. Interestingly, rCB1 are also involved in neurotransmission since they were found in glutamatergic, cholinergic, dopaminergic, and serotonergic systems. Remarkably, significant differences in receptor density were reported in these regions depending on physiological or pathological conditions [40]. rCB2 are found in different populations of circulating immune cells and cellular elements in the spleen and thymus and are mainly involved in the immune reactions [41,42]. Moreover, recent evidence advocates that rCB2 play a pivotal role in the reduction of progression of neurodegenerative disorders such as multiple sclerosis, Alzheimer's, and Parkinson's disease [43–45].

All the compounds which have either a natural or synthetic source, as well as an endogenous origin and are able to interact with abovementioned cannabinoid receptors are generally known as cannabinoids. The recent advances in the field of spectrometric methods made possible the isolation and extraction of Δ9-tetrahydrocannabinol (Δ9-THC) and cannabidiol (CBD)—the 2 main phytocannabinoids found in highest concentration in the *Cannabis sativa* [40,46]. Given the vast history of empirical use of *Cannabis* sp. due to its analgesic, anti-inflammatory, and anxiolytic properties, experimental studies have focused on identifying new potential therapeutic effects of Δ9-THC and CBD. For example, in animal models of multiple sclerosis, CBD has been shown to have a significant anti-inflammatory effect since it was able to decrease the concentration of proinflammatory cytokines interleukin 6 (IL-6), interleukin 12 (IL-12), tumor necrosis factor α (TNF-α), and interleukin 1 (IL-1) [47]. Moreover, recent evidence has shown additional benefits such as analgesic effects in rheumatoid arthritis, fibromyalgia, and oncological conditions [40].

The extensive research on phytocannabinoids have led to the discovery of two endocannabinoids: anandamide or N-arachidonoyl ethanolamine (AEA) and 2-arachidonoylglycerol (2-AG) [48]. Together with the enzymes involved in their metabolism such as FAAH, monoacylglycerol lipase, and NAPE-PLD, they represent the basis of the well-known ECS [49]. AEA and 2-AG represent the main signaling lipids for cannabinoid receptors and share many features such as structural similarity and synthesis mechanism. Interestingly, both of them are synthesized "on demand" as a result of increased intracellular Ca^{2+} concentration. The enzymes involved in the synthesis and degradation of AEA and 2-AG are sensitive to both intra- and extracellular calcium ions [50]. The biosynthesis of AEA is carried out under the action of NAPE-PLD, from the precursor N-arachidonoylphosphatidylethanolamine (NAPE) [51]. The enzyme involved in AEA degradation is FAAH which transforms AEA into arachidonic acid and ethanolamine. Some authors suggest the possibility that FAAH also metabolize 2-AG [52,53]. 2-Arachidonoylglycerol is generated into a two-step synthesis pathway by removal of inositol triphosphate (IP3) from arachidonoyl-containing phosphatidyl inositol biphosphate (PIP2), followed by removal of the acyl group at position 1 by a diacylglycerol (DAG) lipase [54]. 2-AG degradation is primarily carried out by MAGL and secondary by serine hydrolase α-β-hydrolase domain 6 (ABHD6) [7,55].

Endocannabinoids are implicated in various physiological and pathological processes. Changes in endocannabinoids concentration, as well as dysregulation of the ECS have been associated with pathological conditions, including, but not limited to: cancer, osteoporosis, neuromotor, neuropsychological, and neurodegenerative diseases, respiratory diseases such as asthma, cardiovascular diseases such as stroke, atherosclerosis, myocardial infarction, metabolic disorders, arrhythmias, and hypertension [3,56].

Synthetic cannabinoids (SC) were synthetized to overcome the undesirable effects of phytocannabinoids by optimizing and/or improving the pharmacological profile. For example, current research is focusing on obtaining new classes of analgesics based on SC. As we have previously concluded, replacing opioids with SC for pain management will present not only mechanistic benefits, but it will also reduce health costs and deaths associated with excessive opioid use [57].

Aging is a complex physiological process which is under the influence of different genetic and biological factors and is generally characterized by a progressive loss of functional integrity. Epidemiological studies predict that 1 out of 6 individuals will be over the age of 65 in 2050 and the number of the elderlies is likely to double in the next 3 decades with the biggest increase among the population of east and southeast Asia. In these regions, the number of people is expected to increase from 261 million to >570 million in 2050. Furthermore, the least developed countries will host an average of about 2/3 of the world's population [58]. It is well known that population aging will significantly increase the incidence and prevalence of the disorders that associate an increased mortality and morbidity. Neurodegenerative and cardiovascular diseases, cancer, and diabetes are the most common aging-associated disorders which significantly increase the risk of death [59,60]. At the same time, aging is one of the most significant risk factors for the aforementioned pathologies.

Growing evidence suggests that CS may represent a promising therapeutic approach for these disorders. Moreover, all the encouraging results from experimental studies focusing on the role of both classical and newly described cannabinoid receptors pave the way for the use of cannabinoids in a variety of medical conditions. The most representative clinical studies focusing on cannabinoids effect in various age related-diseases are summarized in Table 2.

Table 2. The most representative clinical studies focusing on cannabinoids effect in various age related-diseases.

Cannabinoid	Specific Cannabinoid Studied	Disease	Number of Patients Enrolled	Inclusion Criteria	Main Findings	Ref.
Synthetic Δ9-tetrahy-drocanna-binol	Dronabinol	Multiple Sclerosis	240	→ McDonald criteria [61]; → age: 18–70 years old; → stable multiple sclerosis (MS) symptoms; → moderate to severe central neuropathic pain (CNP).	→ clinically significant reduction of mean pain intensities but without reaching a statistical significant difference between treatment and placebo groups; → dronabinol is safe over the long term; → positive influence on patients' overall Quality of Life (QoF).	[62]
Synthetic Δ9-tetrahy-drocanna-binol	ECP002A (oral formulation of Δ9-tetrahydro-cannabinol)	Multiple Sclerosis	24	→ age: ≥18 years old → progressive MS according to the revised McDonald criteria; → disease >1 year → clinically stable for at least 30 days before the inclusion; → moderate spasticity as defined by an Ashworth score of ≥2 (range, 0–4) and a Kurtzke Expanded Disability Status Scale score between 4.5 and 7.5 at baseline (range, 0–10).	→ ECP002A is well tolerated with a stable pharmacokinetic profile; → significant reduction of pain after ECP002A administration; → subjective MS related spasticity improved after 2 and 4 weeks of treatment.	[63]
Synthetic Tetrahydro-canna-binol:Canna-bidiol spray	Nabiximols	Multiple Sclerosis	106	→ age: ≥18 years old; → moderate to severe MS spasticity defined as a score of ≥4 on the MS spasticity 0–10 numerical rating scale; → spasticity symptoms for at least 12 months; → resistant MS spasticity.	→ THC:CBD spray significantly improved resistant MS spasticity when compared with first-line medication alone; → THC:CBD spray was significantly superior to placebo for spasms severity, sleep disruption and modified Ashworth scale (MAS) score.	[64]
Synthetic Cannabidiol	ZYN002 (transdermal synthetic cannabidiol gel)	Osteoarthritis	320	→ fulfil of American College of Rheumatology criteria for knee osteoarthritis; → 7 days wash-out of current anti-inflammatory and analgesic drugs, except paracetamol.	→ although ZYN002 was not statistically different from placebo, post-hoc analyses showed that men treated with ZYN002 had statistically significant reductions from baseline in average worst knee pain scores when compared with placebo group.	[65]
Synthetic Δ9-tetrahy-drocanna-binol	Nabilone	Alzheimer disease	38	→ patients with moderate to severe Alzheimer disease (AD); → age ≥55 years old; → fulfil of Diagnostic and Statistical Manual of Mental Disorders (DSM)-5 criteria for Major Neurocognitive Disorder due to AD, or met both Major Neurocognitive Disorder due to AD and Major Vascular Neurocognitive Disorder; → patients with a score of ≤24 on the standardized Mini-Mental Status Examination (sMMSE) and clinically significant agitation/aggression (Neuropsychiatric Inventory (NPI)-agitation/aggression subscore ≥3).	→ nabilone administration significantly reduced agitation over 6 weeks; → nabilone as associated with improvements on overall neuropsychiatric symptom; → nabilone showed greater improvements in agitation when compared to other cannabinoids; → nabilone was associated with significant improvements on the short-form mini-nutritional assessment (MNA-SF), suggesting potential benefits on nutritional status.	[66]

Table 2. Cont.

Cannabinoid	Specific Cannabinoid Studied	Disease	Number of Patients Enrolled	Inclusion Criteria	Main Findings	Ref.
Synthetic Δ9-tetrahydrocannabinol	Donabinol	Pancreatic cancer	104 estimated	→ patients ≥55 years od → locally advanced, inoperable or metastatic pancreatic cancer, eligible for first-line chemotherapy; → life expectancy of >4 months at screening; → female patients must either be post-menopausal or surgically sterilized or use a highly effective method of birth control (hormonal contraceptives, intra-uterine devices, or diaphragms with spermicide).	→ ongoing phase III clinical trial assessing the efficacy and safety of dronabinol in the improvement of chemotherapy-induced and tumor-related symptoms in advanced pancreatic cancer; → estimated completion date later in 2023 (NCT03984214).	

However, to narrow the scope of the present paper we aimed to describe only the interaction between CS and most common age-related diseases such as neurodegenerative, oncological, skeletal, and cardiovascular disorders, together with the potential of various cannabinoids to ameliorate the progression of these disorders, as summarized in Figure 1. Since chronic inflammation is postulated as the pillar of all the above-mentioned conditions, we will also discuss in this paper the potential of CS to ameliorate aging-associated immune system dysregulation.

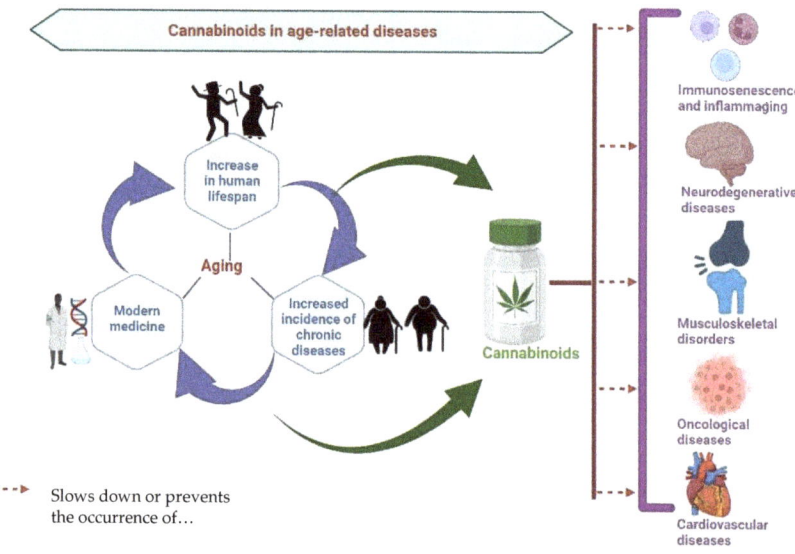

Figure 1. Schematic representation of the potential positive influence of cannabinoids use in various aging-related diseases.

The Physiology of Aging

The remarkable achievements of modern civilization in terms of living conditions together with the development of modern medicine have generated a considerable increase in humans' lifespan. It is predicted that the abolition of pathological factors that are responsible for the main causes of death will increase the life expectancy from 50 to about 95 years [67]. It is clear now that the population aging will lead to a significant increase of the incidence and prevalence of chronic diseases that associate the highest mortality and morbidity rates. Among them, ischemic cerebro-cardiovascular diseases, neurodegenerative, oncological, and respiratory pathologies associate a continuously rising mortality rate and also have the biggest impact on overall prognosis and survival rate [68]. Thus, the abovementioned diseases clearly represent a challenge for the research community to improve the interrelation between chronic diseases and the increase in lifespan and aging.

Aging involves degenerative processes and functional changes at molecular, cellular, tissue, and whole body levels [69,70]. Understanding both the physiological and pathophysiological alterations that contribute to aging will provide a solid basis not only for the treatment, but also for the development of novel biomarkers which may reflect the risk of developing these age-related diseases.

The etiology of aging is complex and multifactorial. Experimental and clinical studies have failed to reveal until now the main mechanisms of aging and a plethora of theories have emerged in the past years [71]. We will discuss the most postulated theories of aging together with the potential of the CS to ameliorate various underlying mechanisms of the progression of aging-related diseases. One of the hypotheses proposed as the basic mechanism of aging is known as the telomeres theory of aging [72]. Telomeres have specialized deoxyribonucleic acid (DNA) protein structures that are found at the ends of all mammalian chromosomes and play a major role in covering the ends of the chromosomes to reduce DNA loss during cell replication. Telomere shortening may cause end-to-end fusion and chromosomal instability. The shortening phenomenon of telomeres to a critically short length during cell division has been associated with the finite replication capacity of somatic cells up to a certain critical point named the Hayflick limit, which precedes cellular senescence and apoptosis. Interestingly, telomere length decreases with age in somatic cells leading thus to the loss of the cell ability to divide [73]. On the other hand, this mechanism represents also a physiological response of the organism that prevents genomic instability due to the accumulation of damaged DNA [73–77]. Taken together, the length of the telomers may be considered as a key biomarker of the onset of senescence in human cell [78]. However, the telomere-dependent replicative senescence mechanism may differ between species and cell types leading to multiple limitations in translating the results from animals to humans [79,80]. Among the phenomenon of progressive shortening of telomers, other factors such as telomere dysfunction, genetic mutations, radiation and the presence of alkylating agents lead to the development and accumulation of senescent cells at different organism's levels [81].

Emerging evidence indicates that senescent cells are characterized by a state of irreversible cell-cycle arrest together with a series of progressive and phenotypically diverse cellular states acquired after the initial growth arrest [82]. In addition, senescent cells release proinflammatory cytokines, chemokines, growth factors and proteases. This phenotype is known as the senescence-associated secretory phenotype (SASP) which generates both positive and negative effects [69]. For example, SASP may be effective in liver fibrosis and wound healing by interfering with remodeling processes of fibrous tissue. On the other hand, SASP may stimulate tumorigenesis by promoting angiogenesis or tumor growth [70,77,82]. Additionally, due to its paracrine mechanism of action, SASP may negatively impact adjacent cells by locally promoting a chronic state of inflammation, i.e., inflammaging, which is closely linked to several aging associated diseases such as rheumatoid arthritis, cancer, atherosclerosis, and neurodegenerative diseases [83,84]. Recent studies have shown that senescent cells may also induce a progressive functional deterioration in the tissues in which they accumulate contributing thus to the development of several age-related pathologies such as osteoarthritis, fibrosis, Alzheimer's disease, pancreatitis, metabolic disorders, and atherosclerosis [70,71,77,83].

Additionally, cellular senescence is induced by high levels of reactive oxygen and nitrogen species (RONS) that further influence various components of SASP. The accumulation of altered macromolecules induced by RONS during oxidative processes that trigger the initiation of cellular senescence led to the elaboration of another theory of aging called the oxidative stress theory [84,85]. Although reactive oxygen species (ROS) are the products of endogenous aerobic metabolism, RONS result from both endogenous (nicotinamide adenine dinucleotide phosphate oxidase, myeloperoxidase, lipoxygenase and angiotensin II) and exogenous sources (pollution, tobacco, alcohol, heavy metals) [86–88]. As in the case of ROS, RONS resulting from cellular metabolism due to the alteration of the balance between their generation and removal may aggravate the oxidative stress [84,85].

Experimental and observational studies have shown that an increase in both ROS and RONS levels is associated with various age-related diseases. For example, it is clear now that physiopathological alterations of the cardiovascular system may also occur due to a decreased tolerance to reactive oxygen species. Moreover, the aged organism carries a high risk of atherogenicity due to a significant increase in oxidized low-density lipoprotein (LDL) levels [89,90]. ROS also modulate the activation of transcription factors that further influence the release of proinflammatory biomolecules. Moreover, the transcription of nuclear factor kappa-light-chain-enhancer of activated B cells (NF-kB) activated by TNF-α and RONS stimulates the genes involved in cell proliferation and carcinogenesis [84,91]. Thus, oxidative stress may activate immune cells and further exacerbate inflammation [84,92]. Recent studies have also shown that oxidative stress has detrimental effects on the normal function of neuronal cells [93]. The presence of active redox metals such as copper and iron, together with high concentrations of polyunsaturated fatty acids (PUFA) that are prone to lipid peroxidation, as well as low levels of antioxidant glutathione (GSH) may represent the main mechanisms involved in the development of neurodegenerative diseases such as Alzheimer's, Parkinson's, and Huntington's disease [86].

Taken together, the telomers shortening, cellular senescence, and oxidative stress may represent the main mechanisms responsible for the development of aging-related diseases. Moreover, all these mechanisms are also capable of inducing various functional alterations of the immune system which further promote and maintain a prolonged status of chronic inflammation that aggravates the progression of aging-associated diseases.

2. Chronic Inflammation and Immunosenescence in Aging

It is now generally accepted that ECS dynamically regulates many aspects of mammalian physiology [94]. Recent evidence indicates that ECS may play a pivotal role in aging-related diseases such as neurodegenerative, inflammatory, and immune-related diseases, neoplasia, and cardiovascular disorders [95,96]. In contrast, the relationship between ECS, inflammatory and immune-related diseases, and aging is still under debate. Recently, a beneficial influence of the cannabinoids on the abovementioned relationship was described and ongoing studies are focusing on the hypothesis that cannabinoids may improve the pathophysiological mechanisms associated with inflammation and immune system dysfunction [97]. In the next paragraphs, we focused on the description of the ECS alterations and the therapeutic potential of the natural, synthetic and endogenous cannabinoids in all the before mentioned disorders.

2.1. Cannabinoids in Chronic Inflammation

Chronic inflammation and subsequent alterations of the immune system that occur with advancing age, i.e., immunosenescence, are strongly related [98,99]. The majority of the studies focusing on the concept of immunosenescence points toward the conclusion that this represents the leading cause of most biological changes related to aging and associated pathologies. Although many features of immunosenescence may be considered harmful, there are also adaptive or remodeling characteristics which are necessary to ensure survival and longevity, as long as they are kept within normal limits [98]. We will further describe the harmful consequences of the immunosenescence-induced inflammation and also the potential beneficial role of cannabinoid use to improve this relationship.

As mentioned above, aging involves a nonspecific state of chronic inflammation, a particular condition that is usually characterized by increased levels of multiple inflammatory biomarkers such as C-reactive protein (CRP), TNF-α, IL-6, and interleukin 8 (IL-8) [100,101]. Experimental studies have shown that cannabinoids may have anti-inflammatory effects since their administration in various age-related diseases led to positive outcomes on various subpopulations of inflammatory cells. For example, in an in vivo experiment, Kaplan et collaborators have demonstrated in an animal model of inflammation that CBD has a significant anti-inflammatory effect since it was able to decrease the circulating levels of IL-6 [102]. In another in vitro experimental study focusing on allergic contact dermatitis, CBD was shown to suppress the inflammatory state by the inhibition of synthesis of proinflammatory cytokines such as IL-6, IL-8, and TNF-α [103]. Furthermore, in an animal model of myocardial ischemia, CBD demonstrated notable cardioprotective effects due to its ability to significantly reduce IL-6 levels [104]. In all these experimental studies, the anti-inflammatory effects of CBD were mediated through the cannabinoid receptors CB1 and CB2 [102]. In addition, activation of G protein coupled receptor 55 (GPR55), inhibition of FAAH, activation of TRPV1 receptors, and gamma receptor activated by PPAR-γ peroxisome proliferator, as well as CB2/5HT1A heterodimerization represents additional pathways through which CBD exerts its anti-inflammatory effects [105,106].

Another component of the cannabinoid system is Δ9-THC which also showed various anti-inflammatory effects in both in vivo and in vitro studies. Interestingly, unlike CBD, Δ9-THC exerts its anti-inflammatory action by inhibiting T-helper (Th)-1 lymphocytes and promoting the activity of Th-2 lymphocytes [106]. Moreover, THC plays an important role in modulating the inflammatory response by suppressing proliferation, chemotaxis, phagocytosis and cytokine production. In a study on human monocytes and astrocytes, Δ9-THC was shown to suppresses inflammatory responses through the suppression of the IL-1b monocyte synthesis and subsequent IL-6 astrocytes production [107]. Thus, like CBD, Δ9-THC is also able to reduce the pro-inflammatory state mediated by IL-6. This is of paramount importance given that the majority of experimental and clinical studies have shown that an increased concentration of IL-6 is strongly correlated with high morbidity and mortality in the elderly [108]. Moreover, the inflammatory pathways encompassing proinflammatory cytokines such as IL-6, IL-8, and IL-1α have also been shown to play a critical role in the expression of cardiovascular risk factors such as hypertension, atherosclerosis, diabetes, and obesity which increases the risk for cardiovascular disease with age [84,109]. Taken together, these experimental results suggest that the modulation of pro-inflammatory cytokines such as IL-6 by ECS may have beneficial effects on aging-related diseases.

Experimental studies have shown that ECS is also involved in the modulation of TNF-α levels, a cytokine which is known to play a key role in the proinflammatory status associated with aging [101,110]. Interestingly, in an in vitro study on the wild murine glial cells, abnormal cannabidiol (an atypical synthetic cannabinoid) developed anti-inflammatory effects by reducing lipopolysaccharide (LPS)-induced TNF-α production. Furthermore, abnormal cannabidiol significantly attenuated lipopolysaccharide-induced TNF-α expression in astrocytes [111]. In addition, in a murine model of chronic liver failure due to excessive alcohol consumption, CBD suppressed the expression of several proinflammatory cytokines including TNF-α [112]. In another murine study on a model of anti-CD40 colitis, THC was also able to reduce the circulating levels of TNF-α, interleukin 17A (IL-17A), interleukin 22 (IL-22), and interferon-γ (IFN-γ), leading to a significant reduction in both systemic and local inflammation [113]. Granja et al. have shown in an in vitro study on murine neuronal cultures that a synthetic cannabinoid (VCE-003) is able to significantly reduce the secretion of pro-inflammatory cytokines such as TNF-α, IL-6, and IL-1β. Interestingly, the mechanism of action is mediated by the activation of PPAR-γ receptors and the anti-inflammatory effect may be enhanced by various phytocannabinoids with high affinity for this receptors [114]. Taken together, the abovementioned results suggest that the inhibition of pro-inflammatory pathways through ECS may be a promising approach to ameliorate various aging-related pathologies and to improve thus the prognostic and quality of life of these patients.

It Is well known that the inflammation plays a key role not only in the onset, but also in the progression of age-related diseases. CRP is an inflammatory marker which has predictive roles in morbidity and mortality in the elderlies since its increased circulating level is usually associated with the development and progression of various cardiovascular, metabolic and neurodegenerative diseases [100,115,116]. Although the cannabinoids-induced anti-inflammatory effects have also been studied in the CRP-mediated inflammatory pathways, their role still remains controversial. For example, the results from a study on 1115 recently active cannabis smokers and 8041 non-smokers showed that recent and active cannabis smokers have lower serum CRP levels when compared to non-smokers [117]. Although this effect may be explained by gender differences, body mass index (BMI) disparities, and anti-inflammatory medication use, a retrospective analysis from Population Assessment of Tobacco Health (PATH) study found that recent cannabis use is associated with reduced levels of systemic inflammation biomarkers, including CRP [115,118]. Taken together, the abovementioned results indicate that cannabinoids present anti-inflammatory effects that may have additional benefits to classical drugs in reducing the progression of chronic inflammation associated with aging.

2.2. Immunosenescence and Cannabinoid System

It is clear now that a pro-inflammatory state is a hallmark of aging. The elderly population is characterized by an inability to develop a proper anti-inflammatory response to various exogenous and/or endogenous aggressors due to a particular state of immunosenescence [101]. Immunosenescence emerges due to a reduction in both qualitative and quantitative response of naive peripheral T and B lymphocytes as we age. Since elderly individuals have a reduced ability to respond to non-self structures and an increased susceptibility to infections, they have a higher probability to develop a chronic inflammatory state which further promote the development of various age-related diseases [119]. For example, longitudinal studies have shown that severe reduction in B cell count, reversal of CD4/CD8 T cell ratio, and reduced proliferative response lead to a decreased survival rates among the octogenarians and nonagenarians [120]. Recent studies in human and rodents have shown that both T and B lymphocytes express cannabinoid receptors on the surface of their membranes [121]. Although CBD demonstrated immunosuppressive and immunomodulatory effects in some experimental studies, there are still controversies among authors regarding the ability of this cannabinoid to reduce the pro-inflammatory status. Methodological conditions such as the concentration of the CBD used, cell culture parameters, the presence or the absence of the serum, and the modality of the immune system stimulation may explain in part these differences [102]. Although many of these conflicting results may be explained in part by the differences of methodological approaches, there is a continuous need for further studies focusing on the involvement of ECS on inflammatory state in general and on immunosenescence in particular [121].

The influence of cannabinoids on B lymphocytes has also been extensively studied. For example, in a study on mice investigating the role of 2-AG on B lymphocytes, the authors showed that this cannabinoid is able to induce the migration of B220 + CD19 + B cells through the chemoattraction of I B cells mediated by CB2 receptors [122]. 2-AG appears to modulate the differentiation of B cell populations and promote their migration during the development of the immune response [121].

The changes that occur with age influence both the adaptive and innate immune cells. For example, an increase in the number of Natural Killer (NK) cells in healthy aging has been reported as physiological. NK cells are considered the main subgroup of lymphocytes involved not only in antimicrobial defense, but also in removal of senescent cells, modulation of inflammation, and initiation of the adaptive immune response [119,123]. Additionally, both NK cell subpopulations express rCB1 and rCB2 and release considerable amounts of endocannabinoids [121]. Interestingly, the ECS is also involved in the modulation of the activity of this cell sub-population. In a study of $CB^{-/-}$ deficient mice, the authors showed that endocannabinoids with affinity for rCB2 play a key role in suppressing cytokine production by lung NK cells. Moreover, these endocannabinoids were able to decrease the inflammation associated with allergic asthma [124].

Other components of the immune system that undergo functional changes with aging are neutrophils and macrophages. It is known that the alteration of the functions of these cells will alter the phagocytic response to a bacterial invasion. Moreover, macrophages are characterized by a reduced chemotaxis in the elderly [119]. Interestingly, both macrophages and neutrophils express rCB1 and rCB2, and the activation of CB2 receptors in neutrophils reduce the release of metalloproteases which reduce the vulnerability of atherosclerotic plaque [56,125]. In addition, in vivo studies have shown that 2-AG is a potent regulator of the host defense and is involved in activating human neutrophils by stimulating the release of kinases, myeloperoxidases, B4 leukotrienes, and by mobilizing cellular calcium [121].

Macrophages are mainly involved in the clearance of apoptotic cells and pathogens and interactions with other immune cells. Studies on murine macrophages have shown that 2-AG inhibits TNF-α and IL-6 production and promotes the anti-inflammatory effects of macrophages. Conversely, in the same study, 2-AG increased inducible nitric oxide synthase-dependent nitric oxide production based on arachidonic acid pathway [121]. Moreover, studies involving cancer patients have shown that targeting cannabinoid receptors from macrophages membrane may be helpful in reducing disease progression [126].

It is clear now that the ECS is involved in the regulation of the immune system at many levels. The cannabinoid system–immunosenescence–aging relationship remains provocative. However, encouraging results from experimental studies support the use of cannabinoids in various immune disorders which are associated with various aging-related neurodegenerative, autoimmune, cardiovascular, and cancer diseases [56].

Changes of Cannabinoid System in Immune Dysregulation Associated with an Increased Risk of Infections in Elderly Patients

Observational studies have reported that elderly patients present an overall higher risk of infection usually associated with an increased severity and poor prognosis. Immunosenescence, define as the state of dysregulated immune function that occurs as people age, is among of the main risk factors which increase the susceptibility of the elderly to infection [127]. It is well known that the immune system cells undergoes age-related changes through both intrinsic and extrinsic aging pathways leading to immunosenescence [128]. Dysregulated immune cell production and altered peripheral selection processes related to precursor cell's differentiation are related to intrinsic aging pathways. In contrast, the immune cells' lifelong exposure to antigenic and other stressors from the internal and external environment are usually related to extrinsic aging pathways [128]. Interestingly, recent evidence has reported that the ECS is involved in the modulation of the immune homeostasis as it may play the role of a gate-keeper for different immune cells [121,129–131]. As shown in Figure 2, all the immune cells also present cannabinoid receptors and perform various roles such as inhibition, modulation, or promotion of different inflammatory pathways [132]. For example, different immune cells interactions which contribute to the host defense mechanisms are also signaled through cannabinoid receptors [127]. Among a variety of alterations of physiological systems, aging is also linked to the immune system dysregulation which is known to be associated with an increased susceptibility to infectious diseases. Despite the increased number of studies focusing on CS, the knowledge regarding the age-related-changes of cannabinoid system and how immune dysregulation are linked to the ECS cannabinoid receptors in elderly patients is still fragmented, missing, or reduced to a few organs. Therefore, additional studies are required in order to achieve promising therapeutic benefits of the cannabinoids in aging therapy.

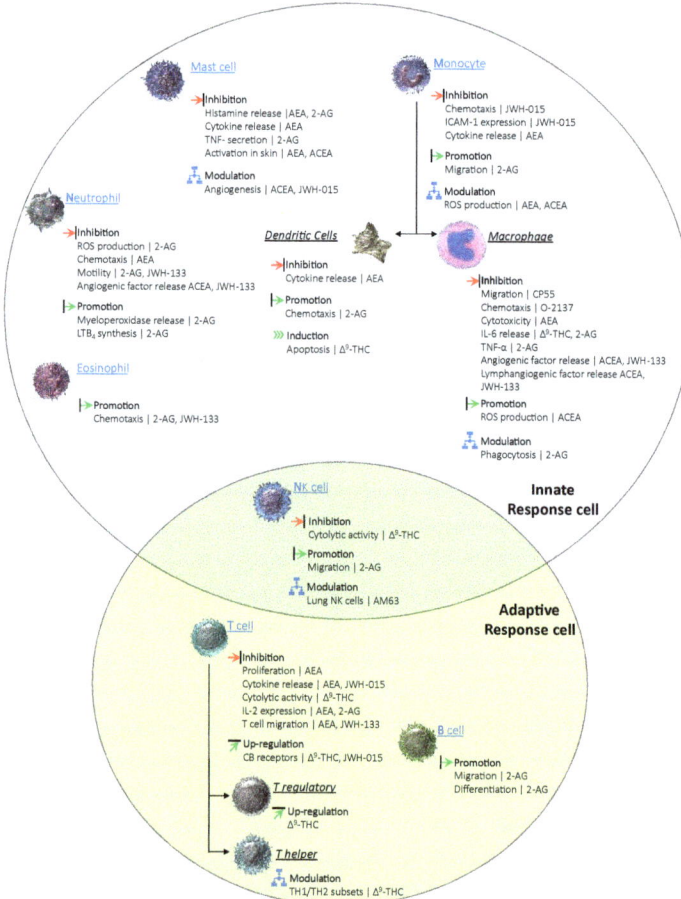

Figure 2. Schematic representation of main effects of the cannabinoid receptors on cells of innate and adaptive immune system; ⇥ = inhibition of; ⇥ = promotion of; ⋙ = induction of; ⋔ = modulation of.

3. The Interplay between Cannabinoid System and Age-Related Diseases

3.1. Cannabinoids Potential in Age-Related Neurodegenerative Diseases: Alzheimer's Disease

Alzheimer's disease (AD) is a neurodegenerative condition characterized by a gradual cognitive decline and behavioral impairment that interfere with professional and social functioning [133]. According to the Alzheimer's Association, the disease accounts for around 60 to 80% of dementia in elderly individuals, with advancing age being the strongest risk factor [134]. Currently, it is estimated that 50 million people worldwide suffer from AD and the prevalence is expected to double every two decades due to the increase of life expectancy and the rapidly aging population [134,135].

The continuous discovery of new signaling pathways in AD reflects the multifactorial pathophysiology of the disease, which is not yet fully understood [136]. Neuropathological hallmarks of AD include deposition of amyloid-β (Aβ) plaques and the presence of neurofibrillary tangles. These are strongly correlated with neuronal loss and neurodegeneration [137]. In the progression of the disease, it is believed that different physiological pathways play major roles, such as apolipoprotein E-mediated metabolism and cholesterol transportation, energy utilization, neuroinflammatory response, and vascular burden [138].

Despite the efforts made in the field of pharmacological research, acetylcholinesterase inhibitors remain the mainstay treatment option which provide only symptomatic relief without reducing the progression of the disease [133,139]. A plethora of factors contribute to the difficulty of developing effective therapies for AD such as gaps in knowledge regarding the molecular alterations and biological mechanisms in the brain that lead to the development of the disease. Furthermore, an inadequate number of patients enrolled into clinical trials and a prolonged time required to complete interventional studies represent additional factors which contribute to the inability to develop effective therapies [140]. For example, in the last 20 years, only Aducanumab, which represents a significant milestone for the treatment of AD, was approved for use in humans by the US Food and Drug Administration (FDA) in June 2021—on the condition of further successful trials [141]. The drug is an antibody that targets Aβ which decrease the number of Aβ plaques present in the brain and has the theoretical potential to ameliorate the cognitive deterioration typical for AD. Because the only target of aducanumab is Aβ plaques, the other features of the disease such as brain cell death or neuroinflammation remain unaddressed. Thus, the concept "one molecule–one target–one disease" fails to provide a comprehensive solution for AD treatment due to the complex and multilayered nature of the disease [142]. As a result, the ideal treatment for AD should be able to modulate the disease through multiple mechanisms rather than targeting a single dysregulated pathway. In this context, exogenous and endogenous cannabinoids are an attractive and promising target against this condition, supported by growing evidence of improved Alzheimer's symptoms in various disease models after exposure to these compounds. This improvement may result from the modulation of the endocannabinoid system, as well from their positive effects on neuroinflammation, Aβ and tau processing, microglial activation, oxidative stress, mitochondrial dysfunction, glucose uptake in the brain, and excitotoxicity [143–145].

The Link between the Cannabinoid Systems and Alzheimer's Disease through Its Effects on Inflammation, on the Immune System and on Oxidative Stress

Early scientific evidence that cannabinoid compounds may be effective therapeutic tools for treating AD was obtained from the study of the ECS [44]. As mentioned before, the ECS contains at least two well-described receptors (rCB1 and rCB2). CB1 receptors are widely expressed in the central nervous system where they are involved in the regulation of the main functions of the brain [146]. In addition, CB1 receptors play a significant role in protecting against neurotoxicity and promoting repair mechanisms in response to neuronal injury [147,148]. Although CB2 receptors are mainly expressed in the immune system with relatively low expression in neuronal cells, specific CB2 receptor agonists have gained major attention in AD due to their lack of psychoactive properties [44,149]. Interestingly, it has been shown that CB2 receptors are selectively overexpressed in cells associated with Aβ enriched neuritic plaques in AD samples from postmortem human brains [150]. The growing interest in cannabinoids as a promising neuroprotective therapy in AD is based on their ability to decrease neuroinflammation through the activation of the CB1 and CB2 receptors. Moreover, they are also able to reduce the pathological action of Aβ and promote brain repair mechanisms [151–154]. In this regard, recent studies have shown that CB1 receptor activation maintains the viability of neurons by suppressing pro-apoptotic signaling pathways and by decreasing Aβ-mediated lysosomal membrane permeabilization [155,156]. CB2 receptors, expressed mainly in microglia, may suppress the AD neuroinflammatory processes by their immunomodulatory effect. Thus, in vitro studies have suggested that the release of pro-inflammatory cytokines in microglial cell cultures exposed to Aβ peptide can by reduced by selective agonists JWH-133, JWH-015, HU-308, and CB1 + CB2 agonists HU-210 and WIN55,212-2 [151,157]. These results were confirmed in animal models of AD, in which chronic administration of these compounds resulted in reduced microglial reactivity and decreased levels of various proinflammatory cytokines [151,153]. Moreover, in transgenic mice models of AD an improved cognitive performance was obtained after CB1 and CB2 targeting, as summarized in Figure 3 [158,159].

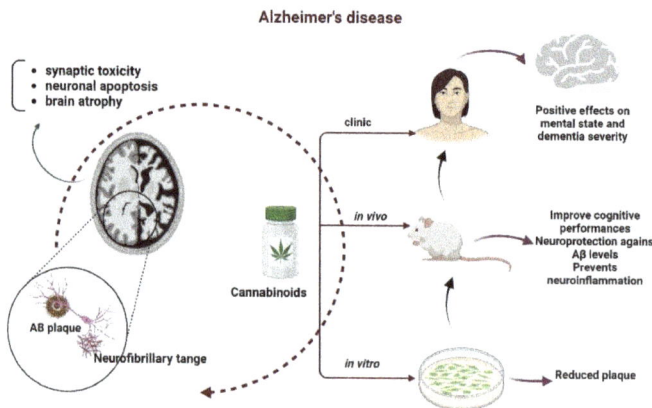

Figure 3. Schematic representation of the involvement of cannabinoids therapy in Alzheimer's disease.

Another significant effect of the CS in AD is on oxidative stress. Two studies have shown that CB2 agonists may decrease the production of free radical nitric oxide induced by exposure to Aβ in microglial cell culture [151,157]. However, these results could not be replicated in a glioma cell line [160]. A series of in vivo studies have also shown that activation of CB2 receptors decreases oxidative stress injury and stimulates anti-oxidative stress responses; long-term treatment with low-dose of JWH-133 reduces the expression of hydroxynonenal adducts and increases the levels of both superoxide dismutase 1 and 2 around plaques in APP/PS1 transgenic mice [159]. The underlying mechanisms by which CB2 receptors mediate these antioxidant effects are not completely elucidated. Although it has been suggested that the CB1–CB2 agonist THC improves mitochondrial function leading thus to a reduction in free radicals, additional studies are needed to support this hypothesis [161].

Cannabinoids can also modulate both peripheral and cerebral immune system by influencing the expression of cytokine and T cell subpopulations, ameliorating thus the balance between neurodegeneration and neuroinflammation [162]. Interestingly, immune cells may produce endocannabinoids and may be influenced by cannabinoid analogues [163]. The use of cell and animal models that reproduce some of the cerebral abnormalities that occur in AD has led to the discovery of the therapeutic potential of cannabinoids (Table 3). It is particularly noteworthy that the few clinical trials to date also support the use of these compounds to alleviate some of the behavioral alterations associated with AD.

Table 3. Preclinical and clinical findings in cannabinoids use in Alzheimer's disease.

Compound and Endocannabinoid System Targets	Experimental Model	Main Findings
Cannabidiol mixed rCB1 and CB2 agonist	→ treatment of PC12 cells with cannabidiol (10^{-7}–10^{-4} m) prior to Aβ- peptide exposure	→ increased cell survival while it reduced lipid peroxidation, ROS production, caspase 3 levels, DNA fragmentation, and intracellular calcium [164]
	→ neuronal (SH-SY5Y) and microglial (BV-2) cell culture, 10 μM compound	→ neuroprotection against $Aβ_{1-42}$ [165]

Table 3. Cont.

Compound and Endocannabinoid System Targets	Experimental Model	Main Findings
Cannabidiol mixed rCB1 and CB2 agonist	→ primary mixed glial cells treated with 100 nM compound and 20 mg/kg of cannabidiol for 3 weeks delivered to Aβ-inoculated C57/Bl6 mice	→ reduce microglial activation and prevent Aβ-induced cognitive impairment and cytokine gene expression [151]
	→ 10 mg/kg of compound administered ip every other day for 2 weeks in 5xFAD mice	→ ameliorates cognitive function [166]
	→ daily administration of 0.75 mg/kg, ip compound for 5 weeks in AβPP/PS1 mice	→ improves cognitive performance, reduce Aβ deposition-related astrogliosis, and cytokine expression [167]
ACEA rCB1 agonist	→ a non-amnesic dose (1.5 mg/kg) of the compound for 5 weeks, administered ip to AβPP/PS1 transgenic mice	→ reduces the cognitive impairment [147]
THC mixed rCB1 and CB2 agonist	→ N2a/AβPPswe cells treated with 100 μL THC	→ decrease Aβ levels [161]
	→ neuronal (SH-SY5Y) and microglial (BV-2) cell culture, 10 μM compound	→ neuroprotection against Aβ$_{1-42}$ [165]
	→ THC was administered ip in 3 different doses (0.75, 1.5 and 3.0 mg/kg) for 7 days (acute therapy) and 21 days (chronic treatment) in Sprague–Dawley rats	→ induce neurogenesis and improve cognitive performances of animals [168]
	→ 1.5 mg/kg/day of compound in ip delivery for 7 days in Sprague–Dawley rats	→ increases the expression, at both protein levels of BDNF and mRNA [27]
	→ daily administration of 0.75 mg/kg, ip compound for 5 weeks in AβPP/PS1 mice	→ reduces Aβ deposition-related astrogliosis and cytokine expression, improves cognitive performance [167]
	→ double-blind, randomized, placebo-controlled, crossover trial (10 old individuals with dementia), 12 weeks oral THC therapy (weeks 1–6, 0.75 mg; weeks 7–12, 1.5 mg)	→ encourages amyloidogenesis [169]
	→ an-open label 4 weeks pilot study in ten AD patients treated with different doses of THC (2.5 mg, 5 mg or 7.5 mg twice a day)	→ positive effects on mental state, dementia severity; and behavioral symptoms such as irritability, delusions, sleep [170]
	→ a double-blind study in mixed dementia and vascular patients and the administered dose was low (1.5 mg three times daily)	→ no improvement in neuropsychiatric symptoms score [171]
WIN 55,212-2 mixed rCB1 and CB2 agonist	→ 0.2 mg/kg/day of WIN 55,212-2 in the drinking water during 4 months in Tg APP 2576 mice	→ prevents neuroinflammation, increase Aβ clearance [158]
	→ human fetal astrocytes treated with 10 μM of compound for 72 h	→ inhibition of the production of inflammatory mediators (nitric oxide, cytokines, and chemokines) [172]
HU210 mixed rCB1 and CB2 agonist	→ 25 or 100 μg/kg of HU210 in ip administration for 10 days in Long-Evans, Wistar, and Fischer 344 rats	→ promote hippocampal neurogenesis and improves cognitive performance [173]

Table 3. Cont.

Compound and Endocannabinoid System Targets	Experimental Model	Main Findings
JWH-133 selective rCB2 agonist	→ 0.2 mg/kg/day of JWH-133 in the drinking water during 4 months in Tg APP 2576 mice →	improves cognitive performance and lowers β-amyloid levels [158]
	→ acute JWH133 injection of 0.2 mg/kg in Tg APP 2576 mice →	enhances glucose uptake [174]

CB1 agonist ACEA, cannabinoid receptor type 1 (CB1) agonist arachidonyl-2-chloroethylamide (ACEA); ip, intraperitoneally; ROS, reactive oxygen species; 5xFAD mice, expressing human APP and PSEN1 transgenes with a total of five AD-linked mutations; THC, Δ9-tetrahydrocannabinol; N2a/AβPPswe cells, N2a cells stably expressing 184 human AβPP carrying the K670N/M671L Swedish 185 mutation (APPswe); BDNF, brain-derived neurotrophic factor.

Although a plethora of scientific advances on the functional relevance of cannabinoids in AD were achieved in the past decades, a series of outstanding research questions still remain. For example, the beneficial effects of cannabinoids in neurodegenerative diseases such as dementia is still controversial as reported by Krishnan et al. [175]. Thus, a more detailed knowledge of the mechanisms of action of these cannabinoid compounds on animal models of Alzheimer's and other neurodegenerative diseases is required for a better optimization of future therapies.

3.2. Cannabinoids Potential in Age-Related Neurodegenerative Diseases: Parkinson's Disease

Parkinson's disease (PD) is a neurodegenerative disorder characterized by basal ganglia (BG) dysfunction due to the loss of dopaminergic neurons in substantia nigra pars compacta (SNc) [176]. Growing evidence supports the hypothesis that neuroinflammation and oxidative stress are the main contributors to the neurodegenerative processes in PD [177]. It has also been suggested that the alteration in α-synuclein proteostasis may be an epiphenomenon mediated by inflammation [178]. There are also theories regarding the ability of extracellular α-synuclein to activate glial cells and induce neuroinflammation [179]. Higher concentrations of proapoptotic proteins have been found in the BG and the cerebrospinal fluid of PD patients. Striatal activated microglia that synthetize proinflammatory cytokines, such as transforming growth factor-β (TGF-β), interleukin 1β (IL-1β), IL-6, IFN-γ, and IL-1, have been detected as well [180,181]. Activated glial cells also seem to produce ROS and RONS in the substantia nigra (SN) [182,183].

Several alterations of the ECS in PD have been described [45,184]. Whether these modifications are compensatory and meant to limit the effects of dopamine loss in the BG or whether they contribute to the development of the motor symptoms in PD is still a matter of extensive debate, but the use of cannabinoids as a therapeutic option for this condition has become of interest [45,185].

The cannabinoid receptors expressed in the BG are rCB1, rCB2, GPR55, and TRPV1. Their presence is indicative for their role in the modulation of various signaling pathways present at this level [186–188]. rCB1 is found in gamma-aminobutyric acid (GABA)ergic and glutamatergic neurons projecting to globus pallidus pars interna (GPi), globus pallidus pars externa (GPe) and substantia nigra pars reticulata (SNr). Even though this receptor has not been discovered in dopaminergic neurons, it seems to modulate dopamine release through the GABAergic and glutamatergic neurons nearby and the formation of heteromers with the D1 and D2 dopamine receptors [45,188,189]. rCB1 seems to have different effects depending on where it is expressed [188]. The activation of this receptor in the GPi and SNr inhibits glutamate release from the afferent neurons of the subthalamic nucleus and seems to alleviate the symptoms and signs of PD. Conversely, enhanced transmission in the GPe may exacerbate the disease by reducing GABA reuptake at this level [188,190,191]. rCB2 is expressed in the striatum, globus pallidus, dopaminergic neurons in the ventral tegmental area, SNr, and basal thalamus [192–196]. Several studies have demonstrated the presence of this receptor in the cytosol and axon terminals of nigrostriatal dopaminergic neurons. However, rCB2 is mainly found in astrocytes and microglia and involved in the regulation of neuroinflammation [197,198]. TRPV1 is expressed by glial cells, nigrostriatal dopaminergic neurons in the BG, and the tyrosine hydroxylase-positive neurons of SNc. Through their presence in dopaminergic neurons, TRPV1 and rCB2 seem to be directly involved in the regulation of dopamine release [188,199–201].

In idiopathic and experimental PD, the ECS seems to reorganize at the level of the BG. An increase in the activity of rCB1 and AEA levels and a decrease in cannabinoid clearance have been described [45]. Another important finding is that rCB2 expression is upregulated in 1-methyl-4-phenyl-1,2,3,6-tetrahydropyridine (MPTP) treated mice and this seems to be a part of a neuroprotective mechanism which prevents the activation of microglia, the expression of astroglial myeloperoxidase and the disruption of the blood-brain barrier [182,183].

Because of the modifications in the ECS that have been identified in PD patients and PD models and the involvement of the cannabinoid receptors in the regulation of circuits within the BG, rCB1 and rCB2 have become new potential therapeutic targets. Most rCB1 agonists that have been tested had an inhibitory effect on dopamine release in the BG and therefore they are not expected to show any improvement in PD patients [45]. However, rCB1 agonists may prove useful in the attenuation of tremor and L-3,4-dihydroxyphenylalanine (L-DOPA)-induced dyskinesia [202–204]. A study by Song et al. also revealed that the chronic use of WIN 55,212-2, a rCB1 agonist, reduced the abnormal behavioral changes caused by L-DOPA in rat models of 6-hydroxydopamine (6-OHDA)-induced PD [205]. WIN 55,212-2 had been shown to inhibit the accumulation of α-synuclein and parkin as well [206]. A study on rats with 6-OHDA-induced lesions compared the effects of L-DOPA with those of an rCB1 antagonist called rimonabant and demonstrated that both L-DOPA and rimonabant improved stepping and the combined administration of L-DOPA and rimonabant had a better effect than either drug alone [207]. Moghaddam et al. conducted a study using both an rCB1 antagonist, AM251, and an agonist, ACPA, and measured the catalepsy in PD models of reserpinized rats and normal controls. AM251 alleviated the catalepsy in a dose dependent manner. In contrast, the administration of ACPA increased the catalepsy [208]. Such studies prove that rCB1 antagonist could be the next step as drug of choice in the alleviation of motor symptoms in PD. Cannabinoids may also improve non-motor symptoms in PD. An experimental study on rodents has shown that the systemic administration of CBD led to an increase in total sleep time by increasing AEA levels and having a modulatory effect in regions expressing rCB1 and involved in the sleep–wake cycle [209,210].

In regard to rCB2, preclinical trials have shown that the activation of this receptor suppresses microglial activation, therefore reducing neuroinflammation [211]. JWH-015, an rCB2 agonist, had a protective effect against MPTP-induced degeneration in mice by reducing the activation of microglia by MPTP. The same study also demonstrated that there was an exacerbation in MPTP toxicity following the genetic ablation of rCB2 [183]. The fact that rCB2 stimulation is involved in neuroprotection was also suggested in a study on tetrahydrocannabivarin (Δ9-THCV). Both the acute and chronic administration of Δ9-THCV led to a preservation of tyrosine hydroxylase-positive neurons in the SN of rats with 6-OHDA-induced lesions [212]. In support of these findings, another study using the same animal model showed that rats treated with GW842166x, a selective rCB2 agonist, scored better in balance beam walking, pole, grip strength, rotarod, and amphetamine-induced rotation tests [213]. In rotenone-induced animal models of PD, there is clear evidence of oxidative stress, loss of antioxidant enzymes, and enhanced production of proinflammatory cytokines, such as IL-1β, IL-6, and TNF-α. Treatment with the selective rCB2 agonist β-caryophyllene reduced the levels of these cytokines, prevented glutathione depletion, decreased lipid peroxidation, and increased the concentration of antioxidant enzymes [214].

Data on the neuroprotective effect of Δ9-THC and CBD were also provided by several studies [31,215–217]. Δ9-THC provided direct neuroprotection in PD-induced SH-SY5Y cell cultures and marmoset models of PD which were treated with Δ9-THC had a major improvement in locomotion. It has been hypothesized that rCB1 stimulation by THC in the striatum is able to overrule the inhibitory effects upon movement determined by the activation of rCB1 in the GPe [218–220]. Regarding CBD, its administration led to a downregulation of glycogen synthase kinase-3, which seems to be a major inhibitor of the WNT/β-catenin pathway. The WNT/β-catenin pathway is a signaling system that amplifies oxidative stress and inflammation and has been shown to be part of the metabolic reprogramming that characterizes PD [216]. CBD also seems to upregulate Cu/Zn-superoxide dismutase and, therefore, increases the endogenous mechanisms of defense against oxidative stress [215]. Through a preferential action on the astrocytes and the stimulation of the TRPV1 receptor, CBD also enhances the endogenous neuroprotection provided by the ciliary neurotrophic factor and, thus, maintains the viability of dopaminergic neurons [31].

Given the growing evidence for the benefits of administering cannabinoids in PD animal models, interest for studying their effects in PD patients has risen [221]. A survey of 339 patients showed that 25% had taken cannabis and 45.9% of these reported some benefit in regard to general improvement, tremor, bradykinesia, rigidity, and L-DOPA induced dyskinesia [222]. The improvement of motor symptoms was also described in a smaller study on 22 patients. In addition, some patients reported an improvement in the quality of sleep and a decrease in the visual analog scale of pain score could also be identified [223]. Several other uncontrolled trials have found improvement in the motor symptoms and also non-motor symptoms, such as pain, mood, and sleep [224–226]. An open-label study focusing on CBD administration in 6 PD patients described lower Unified Parkinson's Disease Rating Scale (UPDRS) score with CBD use. The psychotic symptoms were also significantly decreased in these patients [227].

Only a few randomized controlled trials (RCTs) testing the use of cannabinoids in PD have been conducted and they provided contradictory results [221]. Two RCTs, one studying the effects of rimonabant, and the other Cannador®, a plant extract with a Δ9-THC to CBD ratio of 2:1 and standardized Δ9-THC content, failed to show significant improvement of the UPDRS scores [220,228]. In contrast, a RCT evaluating the effects of nabilone, a rCB1 and rCB2 agonist, on the L-DOPA induced dyskinesia showed significant improvement at a total dose of 0.03 mg/kg body weight when half of the dose was administered 12 h before and the rest 1 h before an acute L-DOPA challenge [229]. A dose of 75 mg/day or 300 mg/day of CBD did not provide a statistically significant improvement in the UPDRS, but it increased the quality of life [210]. An acute dose of 300 mg of CBD also provided a significant anxiolytic effect and a decrease in tremor amplitude [230].

The involvement of the ECS in the regulation of movement and the complex alterations within this system that become apparent in PD are far from being deciphered. Preclinical data show promising results regarding the use of cannabinoids in PD. Nevertheless, the clinical data is very lacking. More evidence is needed before cannabinoids become a viable option in the treatment of PD.

3.3. Cannabinoids Potential in Age-Related Neurodegenerative Diseases: Multiple Sclerosis

Multiple sclerosis (MS) is a chronic inflammatory autoimmune disease which involves complex interactions and underlying mechanisms which are not yet fully understood. Although many clinical and experimental studies focus on discovering new treatment strategies to improve the symptoms, quality of life, and overall prognosis of MS, no significant progress was achieved in the past decade. Thus, the cannabinoid approach in MS has evolved as a promising alternative not only for the improvement of symptomatology, but also for their potential to increase the efficacy of existing drugs since recent clinical evidence has shown that cannabinoids may ameliorate the symptomatology of pain, fatigue, depression, tremor, or sleep disorders [231]. For example, approval of Nabiximols

(Sativex®), a 1:1 mixture Δ9-THC and CBD for MS related spasticity was a real progress for the management of this disease. From the first studies of Collin et al., it was recognizable that the improvement was significantly higher in subjective patient-reported measures than in objective parameters [232]. A plethora of further observational and randomized studies have confirmed the efficacy of Nabiximols, cannabis, and other cannabinoids to control spasticity, pain, sfincterian problems, and sleep disturbances in MS patients [64,233–238].

In patients with an advanced stage of MS, pain is a common symptom and may have various forms such as neuropathic pain, headache, trigeminal neuralgia, joint and muscle pain due to motor deficits, and walk abnormalities or spasticity. The antalgic effect induced by cannabinoids may be partially explained by a central mechanism which involves the restoration of cortical pain gating mechanisms, most likely through the modulation of sensory–motor cortical integration [239]. In a systematic review published by Longoria et al., pain reduction was found at −3.42 points after cannabinoids administration when compared to a control group [240]. In another paper focusing on the effects of cannabinoids on MS neuropathic pain, Jones and collaborators identified a clinically relevant difference between placebo and treatment groups but without reaching statistical significance [241]. Although modest evidence for the use of cannabinoids in MS for alleviating pain was reported by Jones et al., the aforementioned results pave the way for further experimental studies focusing on finding promising cannabinoids compounds which may have a more pronounced antalgic effects.

Although case reports and nonrandomized trials found evidence that cannabinoids may provide some benefits in MS-related tremor, none of the placebo-controlled trials reviewed by Pourmohamaddi and collaborators found any significant differences [242]. In a recent survey, cannabis consumption in the past 3 months in MS patients was associated with an improvement of bladder symptoms such as urinary frequency, urinary urgency, bladder leakage and wetness, pad use, and bladder emptying [243]. The same results were reported in a systematic review focusing on efficacy and tolerability of cannabinoids in MS which showed that bladder symptoms are significantly improved by the use of cannabis or cannabinoids [43].

Data from experimental studies using animal models of MS show a favorable effect of cannabinoids on clinical and biological parameters. For example, significant improvement in disability and behavior was described in experimental autoimmune encephalomyelitis (EAE) after administration of cannabinoid oil extract formulations. These results were based on complex biological mechanisms and included the reduction of TNF-α production and the enhancement of brain-derived neurotrophic factor (BDNF) synthesis [244].

Cannabinoids may play an important role in modulating the complex physiopathology of MS and may be used as immune modulators, neuroprotectors, or remyelination promoters. Although current MS treatment approaches are focused on the modulation of the immune system by using substances such as cladribine, alemtuzumab, or even bone marrow transplant, significant results were not yet obtained. Recent evidence has suggested that endocannabinoid system dysregulation contributes to the progression of inflammatory and degenerative processes associated with MS. For example, in MS patients, the ECS's components were found altered not only in cerebrospinal fluid (CSF), but also in plasma and peripheral lymphocytes in different patterns depending on MS type and severity class [245–248]. Moreover, the involvement of cannabinoid systems in various MS related pathological mechanisms was confirmed not only by pharmacological modulation of receptors and enzymes, but also by their genetic deletion [249]. Interestingly, both neuroprotective (usually obtained through the activation of CB1 receptors) and anti-inflammatory (usually linked to CB2 activation) cannabinoids-induced effects are abolished by specific receptor blockade. Additionally, experimental studies have shown that neuroprotection is at least in part explained by the modulation of glutamate release which is dependent on CB1 receptors [250,251].

Other pathways may also contribute to the neuroprotective and anti-inflammatory cannabinoids dependent effects. VCE-004.8, a derivative of CBD, has a dual PPAR-γ and CB2 agonist action and also activates the HIF pathway in oligodendrocytes and microglia cells. In EAE and Theiler's virus-induced encephalopathy (TMEV), VCE-004.8 enhanced migration of oligodendrocytes, prevented demyelination, axonal damage, immune cells infiltration, and downregulated the expression of several genes associated with MS physiopathology [252]. Hydroxy CBD enantiomers (HU-446, Hu465) prevented myelin oligodendrocyte glycoprotein (MOG) stimulated T cells to produce interleukin 17 (IL-17) via a CB1/CB2 independent mechanism [253].

Autoimmunity was postulated as another mechanism involved in the physiopathology of MS. Briefly, autoimmunity in MS comprises persistent activation of local astrocytes, microglial cells, recurrent and persistent infiltration of both peripheral leukocytes, and soluble inflammatory mediators. The immune aggression involves mainly cells of adaptive immunity such as CD8 and CD4 Th1 and Th17 lymphocytes. B-cells function as APCs and also produce autoantibodies that have been shown to contribute to neurodegeneration and cortical demyelination, particularly in the case of meningeal ectopic B cell follicles [254]. Intriguingly, in Theiler's murine encephalomyelitis virus-induced demyelinating disease (TMEV-IDD), activation of PPAR-γ nuclear receptors by a CB agonist (WIN55,212-2) led to downregulation of intercellular adhesion molecule-1 (ICAM-1) and vascular cell adhesion molecule-1 (VCAM-1) in brain endothelium. Moreover, a reduced infiltration of CD4 T lymphocytes and microglial activation was also reported [255]. Similarly, anandamide-reduced VCAM-1 expression in brain endothelial cell cultures through a CB1-dependent mechanism and possibly A2A receptors [256,257].

The complex action of cannabinoids in MS is also demonstrated in a study focused on the effect of THC+CBD combination in murine EAE. The improvement of clinical manifestations in this model was based on the reduction of neuroinflammatory processes mediated by CB1 and CB2 activation. Authors found reduced levels of Th1 and Th17 cells, decreased CD4+ T infiltrative cells into the brain, decreased pro-inflammatory molecules (IL-17, INF-γ, TNF-α, IL-1β, IL-6, and TBX21), and increased FoxP3, STAT5b, interleukin 4 (IL-4), interleukin 10 (IL-10), and TGF-β, and apoptosis. The effects were also mirrored by changes in miRNA profile in brain-infiltrating cells [258].

Growing evidence indicates that epigenetic regulation is involved in CBD immune modulation. In MOG-sensitized lymphocytes, different histone methylation levels in binding sites of certain transcription factors suggest that these may play important roles in CBD-mediated immune modulation. Abnormal expression patterns of various miRNAs with pro- and anti-inflammatory properties was counteracted by CBD. In transcriptome expression analysis, CBD suppressed 876 MOG-induced transcripts and induced 396 MOG-suppressed transcripts. These changes are known to be involved in cell cycle and immune response and are in line with previous results showing that CBD inhibits T cell proliferation [259].

Recent data from experimental studies focusing on innate immunity might provide new insights into MS physiopathology and may reveal new evidence of a potential causal relationship between MS and viral infection [260]. O'Brien and collaborators postulated that this relationship may represent the pillar of the progression of MS [261]. Furthermore, experimental studies have shown that signaling pathways involving the family of the toll-like receptors (TLR) may influence the progression of MS in animal models [262]. For example, the expression of the TLR3 and TLR 4 receptors is increased in active lesions [263]. A study in MS patients focused on the effects of cannabidiol and Δ9-THC on TLR3 and TLR4 from peripheral blood mononuclear cells revealed anti-inflammatory responses since reduced expression of IFN-β was documented in both groups. Additionally, a pronounced favorable effect was reported if cells were pretreated with a 1:1 association of THC:CBD compared to the effect of each of them alone [264].

Microglia fulfill the role of resident mononuclear phagocytes in the brain parenchyma. They are essential players in local homeostasis and defense. Microglia is maintained in a stable surveillant phenotype by various signals from healthy neurons and astrocytes [265]. Once stimulated, microglia switch to either the M1 proinflammatory state producing pro-inflammatory cytokines such as IL-1β, IL-12, IL-18, IL-6, TNF-α, or to an alternative M2 state which is associated with regeneration and repairing (subtype M2a), immunoregulation (M2b) or an acquired-deactivating phenotype (M2c) [266]. M2 state microglia release anti-inflammatory factors such as IL-10 and IL-4 and express higher levels of receptors associated with phagocytosis [265]. Activated M1 microglia produce endocannabinoids [267] which promote the M2 phenotypes mainly through CB2 receptors [266]. In human brain samples from MS patients, CB2 receptors were present in T-lymphocytes, astrocytes, and perivascular and reactive microglia while CB1 receptors were found mostly on cortical neurons, oligodendrocytes, oligodendrocyte precursor cells, macrophages, and infiltrated T-lymphocytes. Interestingly, CB2-positive microglial cells were found into active plaques while in the case of chronic plaques, they were identified at the periphery [268].

In vitro studies have shown that cannabinoids activate the phosphoinositide 3 kinase/protein kinase B/mechanistic target of rapamycine (PI3K/Akt/mTOR) pathway which is known to play a central role in the regulation of inflammation, cell survival and differentiation. This is mainly achieved through CB1 receptors leading to a protective effect on astrocytes [269] and oligodendrocyte progenitor cells [270]. Interestingly, in EAE mice study, cannabidiol was able to restore PI3K/Akt/mTOR function. Moreover, a reduction of pro-inflammatory cytokines such as IFN-γ and IL-17, an increased level of BNDF together with up-regulation of PPAR-γ and inhibition of c-Jun N-terminal kinase (JNK) and p38 mitogen-activated protein kinase (MAP) kinases were reported in the same study [271].

The dysfunction of the oligodendrocyte plays a major role in the physiopathology of MS and pharmacological interventions that specifically target their protection or regeneration may provide a promising approach towards their remyelination. It is clear now that oligodendrogenesis is not restricted only to developmental periods. In contrast, recent evidence showed that this process is a permanent part of brain activity [272,273]. Oligodendrocyte progenitor cells (OPC) differentiate into oligodendrocytes under the influence of a plethora of intrinsic and extrinsic factors [274]. Among them, the cannabinoid system may play an essential role in the modulation of this process. Both CB1 and CB2 receptors are found on oligodendrocytes and their precursors and cannabinoids have been shown to exert a protective effect that involves the activation of the PI3K/Akt signaling pathway [270]. Additionally, other endocannabinoid-dependent protective mechanisms are stimulated during inflammation such as the reduction of endoplasmic reticulum stress pathways-related apoptosis and the inhibition of LPS/IFN-γ induced phosphorylation of eiF2α and protein kinase R (PKR) [275]. Intriguingly, a dose-dependent relationship was documented since different doses of a cannabinoid drug may induce opposite effects. For example, exposure of cuprizone fed mice to CB1 agonist WIN-55,212-2 at a dose of 1 mg/kg aggravated demyelination and prevented OPC proliferation while a lower dose of 0.5 mg/kg had a protective and anti-inflammatory effect [276].

Unfortunately, the promising results from in vitro and in vivo studies are not yet fully paralleled by the results from observational studies or clinical trials and controversies still exist. For example, in a sub-study of CAMS (Cannabinoids in MS), no evidence for a benefic cannabinoid influence on serum levels of IFN-γ, IL-10, IL-12, or C-reactive protein was found. Moreover, mitogenic stimulation experiments also failed to demonstrate any significant reduction of CD3+ and IFN-γ production [277]. In contrast, a recent prospective case control study showed that the levels of pro-inflammatory cytokines such as IL-1, IL-2, IL-6, IL-17, IL-22, TNF-α, and IFN-γ were significantly increased in the MS group when compared to the MS/cannabis and control groups. Moreover, the same study showed that in the MS population, anti-inflammatory cytokines such as IL-4, IL-10, and interferon-β1 (IFN-β1) had significantly lower values [278].

Although MS is still challenging and is not completely understood in terms of causality and pathogeny, the ECS may represent a promising approach not only for the treatment, but also for the alleviation of MS-associated symptoms and/or for increasing the efficacy of existing drugs. Recent and growing evidence has shown that CS may have the potential to modulate virtually all the major processes in MS involving genetic expression, inflammatory reactions, cell survival and interaction. Moreover, the beneficial effects of cannabinoids in neurodegenerative diseases such as multiple sclerosis may result from their antioxidant properties, as well as their regulatory functions in the inflammatory responses mediated by ECS [279]. Though promising, further studies involving the ECS in MS are necessary to overcome the potential adverse effects, lack of specificity, and/or methodological issues.

4. The Endocannabinoid System and Aging-Related Musculoskeletal Changes

Aging is a physiological process associated with changes in bone density, decreased muscle mass and function, and joint degradation [280–282]. Whereas various risk factors and pathological mechanisms have been identified and described with respect to aging-related musculoskeletal changes, the potential role of endocannabinoid signaling is yet to be fully understood. Nevertheless, recent studies highlight the active involvement of ECS in bone metabolism, sarcopenia, and degenerative joint disease [283–285].

4.1. The Endocannabinoid System and Bone Changes

Older adults experience a marked decrease in bone density mainly due to a disruption in bone metabolism. In this respect, the imbalance between bone formation and resorption favoring the latter in aging individuals has been linked to endocrine factors, comorbidities, inflammaging, medications, low physical activity or bedrest, sarcopenia, increased bone marrow adipogenesis, and poor diet [286–289]. While osteopenia and osteoporosis are more frequently found in postmenopausal women, a notable aging-related decrease in bone density has also been described in men and some authors suggest that this is a largely underestimated issue in the older male population [290].

Studies have indicated that bone metabolism is significantly impacted by the activity of the ECS. The connection between ECS activity and bone mass is supported by recent findings describing the presence in bone tissue of ECS-related molecules such as the receptors CB1 and CB2, together with AEA, 2-AG, as well as the enzymatic equipment involved in endogenous cannabinoid metabolism. Moreover, the cannabinoid receptors CB1 and CB2 have been described as potential future therapeutic targets for osteoporosis [289,291].

The release of norepinephrine by sympathetic fibers leads to an enhancement in bone resorption and a decrease in bone formation. Through its effect on the sympathetic nervous system which includes the interruption of noradrenaline release, rCB1 stimulation by 2-AG has been shown to decelerate the process of bone resorption in mice [291]. The deterring effect of skeletal rCB1 on norepinephrine release followed by temporary stimulation of bone formation has been previously demonstrated in acute conditions. However, Deis et al. aimed to examine the potential feedback loop between sympathetic nerve fiber activity and bone-forming osteoblasts in chronic conditions. The evaluation included bone mass changes at the level of the distal femoral metaphysis and vertebrae of young rCB1 deficient (12 weeks old) and older male mice (35 weeks old) compared to age-matched controls. Although in young rCB1 null mice, there was no difference in bone mass compared to wild-type controls, in the aging CB1r-deficient animals, the authors noted an unexpected increase in bone mass. rCB1 deficiency at the level of sympathetic neurons was linked to an upregulation of bone formation and a decreased osteoclast genesis, indicating that rCB1 deletion interfere with the feedback circuit between ECS and sympathetic nerve activity with regard to bone formation [292]. The relationship between endocannabinoid system and bone changes is summarized in Figure 4.

The activity of renal proximal tubule cells (RPTC) impacts bone metabolism. These cells express rCB1 (RPTC-CB1r), the latter influencing the regulation of bone mass. Baraghithy et al. found that rRPTC-CB1 deficient mice led to an increased bone mass phenotype (higher trabecular bone volume ratio in the distal femoral metaphysis—BV/TV, with an augmented trabecular thickness and number) and greater bone mineral density compared to the control group. In rRPTC-CB1-/- mice, the authors noted an enhancement of osteoblast activity linked to an increased bone formation. Interestingly, a higher number of osteoclasts per trabecular perimeter was also identified in null mice, yet without a corresponding augmentation of osteoclast activity [293].

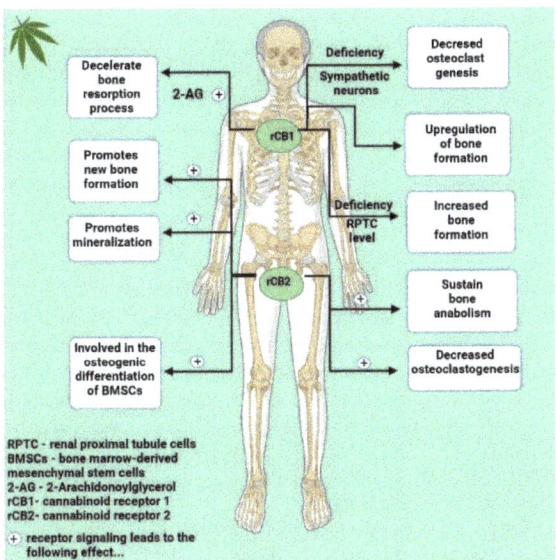

Figure 4. Schematic representation of the relationship between endocannabinoid system and bone changes.

According to a number of animal studies, rCB2 signaling has the ability to sustain bone anabolism. rCB2-deficient mice may exhibit age-related trabecular and cortical bone changes similar to postmenopausal osteoporosis. Additionally, decreased bone strength and lower bone mineral density were linked to polymorphisms in the coding region of rCB2 in human subjects, suggesting that ECS-related genetic factors may contribute to the risk of osteopenia or osteoporosis [291].

rCB2 signaling was shown to either promote new bone formation and mineralization or decrease osteoclastogenesis [294]. However, in cultured murine macrophages, Li and Sun found that the rCB2-selective agonist AM1241 boosted receptor activator of nuclear factor kappa-B ligand (RANKL) dependent osteoclast differentiation, whereas the selective antagonist AM630 hampered this process [295].

Bone marrow-derived mesenchymal stem cells (BMSCs) are multipotent cells which have the ability to differentiate into osteoblasts. Moreover, these cells express rCB2 [296]. rCB2 is believed to be involved in the osteogenic differentiation of BMSCs. Cultured BMSCs isolated from the bone marrow samples of healthy donors and patients with osteoporosis revealed a decreased expression of CB2r in osteoporotic subjects compared to the control group. The study conducted by Wang et al. focused on analyzing the potential role of rCB2 signaling in the restoration of osteogenic differentiation of BMSCs sampled from human subjects with osteoporosis. The overexpression of rCB2 in human osteoporotic BMSCs boosted alkaline phosphatase (ALP) activity, favored osteogenic gene expression and increased mineralized extracellular matrix deposition [297].

Sophocleous et al. examined the effects of double rCB deficiency (rCB1 and rCB2) on bone development (from birth to aging mice) and studied its impact on ovariectomy-induced bone loss in female mice. rCB1/CB2 deficiency in mice led to an osteoclast defect and a subsequent protective effect on ovariectomy-induced and age-related bone loss in experimental animals. Moreover, the positive effect of reduced osteoclast number surpassed the negative impact of the observed reduction in bone formation leading thus to the preservation of bone mass. These findings were not paralleled by those obtained from the distinct inactivation of rCB1 and rCB2, suggesting that the two receptors have coinciding (but not redundant) effects on bone mass in aging experimental animals and ovariectomized female mice [298].

AEA and 2-AG may be produced at the level of trabecular bone, as shown in animal studies. Additionally, AEA and 2-AG were found to be produced by human osteoclasts. Moreover, experimental studies have shown that 2-AG treatment of rodent BMSCs resulted in an increase of ALP which is known as a marker of osteoblast differentiation. However, other research studies did not report an increase of ALP in murine osteoblast cell lines [294]. Smith et al. examined the effects of endocannabinoids AEA and 2-AG on cultured human osteoblast activity. At four days, AEA and 2-AG prevent osteoblast differentiation with a concentration-related augmentation of ALP levels. Overall, AEA was linked to early osteoblast differentiation, while 2-AG was associated with an early increase and a late decrease in the levels of osteoblast differentiation biomarkers [299].

Two endocannabinoid-like molecules, palmitoylethanolamide (PEA) and oleoylethanolamide (OEA), were studied with respect to a variety of processes including endocannabinoid tone during osteoblastic differentiation. Kostrzewa et al. analyzed this relationship in a murine osteoblast cell line MC3T3-E1 and found that during osteoblastic differentiation, the levels of OEA increased while AEA and 2-AG declined in maturing and mineralized cells. In the femurs of male mice, there was a notable age-related reduction in PEA, OEA and 2-AG expression [294].

Monoacylglycerol lipase, a lipolytic enzyme which is known to degrade the endogenous cannabinoid 2-AG, has been described as a potential therapeutic target for osteoporosis due to its presumed impact on osteoclast differentiation. Interestingly, during osteoclast differentiation the monoacylglycerol lipase protein expression may be augmented. Moreover, Liu et al. found that monoacylglycerol lipase deletion in bone marrow-derived macrophages was linked with the inhibition of both bone resorption and osteoclast genesis [300].

4.2. The Endocannabinoid System and Osteoarthritis

Osteoarthritis (OA) is the most prevalent joint disease in aging individuals and is mainly characterized by a progressive degeneration of articular structures. Whereas other changes such as bone remodeling and synovial inflammation have also been described in osteoarthritic joints, cartilage degradation plays a central role in the pathogenic process [301].

A large number of studies focusing on analgesia have described the pain as the most prominent symptom of the disease and also the ability of the ECS to modulate pain in OA [302]. Mlost et al. found that β-caryophyllene (a natural low-efficacy agonist of CB2r that is present in human diet) had both antinociceptive and chondroprotective effects in animals with experimentally induced osteoarthritis. Additionally, chronic administration of β-caryophyllene reduced cartilage degradation without inducing tolerance to its analgesic properties [303].

In wild-type mice, the selective rCB2 agonist HU308 developed beneficial effects on knee osteoarthritis secondary to a surgically-induced destabilization of the medial meniscus [304]. The examination of cultured chondrocytes from rCB2-deficient experimental animals revealed that these cells produced lower amounts of proteoglycans compared to chondrocytes obtained from wild-type mice, indicating a role for rCB2 signaling in the development and progression of OA in mice [305].

Bryk et al. conducted a study on rodents with monoiodoacetate-induced knee OA and investigated the gene expression of ECS constituents at the level of the spine and knees of the experimental animals during the early and late stages of osteoarthritis development. The authors found an enhancement of AEA synthesis and degradation enzymes in the early phases of OA. There was no upregulation of rCB1 and rCB2 gene expression in the rats' cartilage. Also, the transcript levels of AEA synthesis and degradation enzymes did not vary significantly in the animals' cartilage. However, in the synovial membrane samples, Cnr2 gene expression started to increase from day 2 after monoiodoacetate injection and was significantly upregulated after 2 weeks up to the end of the study (14 to 28 days after injection). N-arachidonoyl phosphatidylethanolamine phospholipase D (Nape-plD) gene expression was augmented from the second day of the experiment. Both the cartilage and synovial membrane samples exhibited modifications in the transcript levels of the AEA alternative synthesis and degradation pathways. Nonetheless, more changes were seen in the synovial membrane [306].

Gaisberger et al. recruited elderly patients with knee OA who underwent spa treatment with or without low-dose radon therapy for 2 weeks. Plasma AEA levels were measured at baseline and after 2 weeks. AEA values were significantly decreased post-treatment and were paralleled by pain reduction in both study groups. No relationship between AEA and the tested potential serum and urinary markers of cartilage degradation was described [307].

4.3. The Endocannabinoid System and Skeletal Muscle Changes

Aging-related sarcopenia includes a marked decrease in both muscle mass and function compared to young adults and is frequently accompanied by different degrees of disability [308]. Whereas particular ECS constituents have been associated with age-dependent muscle changes, the impact of endocannabinoids on muscle mass and function over time requires further investigations.

Le Bacquer et al. aimed to describe the relationship between endocannabinoids and muscle-related parameters in young adult versus older male Wistar rats. The authors evaluated the levels of endocannabinoids AEA and 2-AG, and endocannabinoid-related N-acylethanolamines PEA and OEA in the animals' plasma, skeletal muscles (oxidative and glycolytic), and adipose tissue. While the subjects' weight did not differ, the body composition of the older rats revealed a higher fat mass and a lower lean mass. Sarcopenic animals demonstrated impaired motor activity and significantly lower plasma levels of PEA and AEA. In rats with sarcopenia, the authors found a marked augmentation of 2-AG levels in the soleus muscle (oxidative) and a low OEA expression in the extensor digitorum longus muscle (glycolytic). Elevated levels of AEA, PEA, and OEA were described in the sarcopenic animals' subcutaneous fat. Moreover, the abovementioned changes were accompanied by altered ECS-linked gene expression in both the skeletal muscles and the adipose tissue of older rats compared to young adults [284].

Dalle and Koppo examined the expression of cannabinoid receptors in young men (20–27 years of age) versus old non-sarcopenic males (65–84 years of age) and found that rCB1 expression in the vastus lateralis muscle was bigger in aging individuals while rCB2 expression did not significantly differ. In healthy older adults (physically active, non-sarcopenic participants over 65 years of age, males and females), a 12-week resistance exercise program increased both rCB1 and rCB2 expression at the level of the vastus lateralis muscle but without statistical significance. Intriguingly, in older participants of both sexes, the authors identified statistically significant correlations between the difference in rCB2 expression post- versus pre-resistance training and the levels of muscle maintenance markers (FOXO3a and the myogenic markers MyoD and Pax7) [309].

In the past decade, a growing body of evidence has paved the way for ascertaining a relationship between ECS constituents and endocannabinoid-like molecules in various aging-associated musculoskeletal changes [301,303,306,309]. Most scientific evidence pertaining to this relationship derives from in vitro and in vivo studies and the potential applicability of these findings to the management of osteoporosis, osteoarthritis or sarcopenia in human subjects require further studies. Nevertheless, recent and encouraging studies provide valuable insight into the involvement of ECS in the musculo-skeletal changes associated with aging.

5. Cannabinoid Implications in Age-Related Oncological Diseases

Since the median age of cancer diagnosis is around 66 years, this disorder is now considered the disease of aging [310]. The advances in oncological disease prevention strategies together with the improvements in healthcare systems will shift towards a greater incidence and prevalence the neoplasic conditions in the elderly. According to the

World Health Organization (WHO), in the majority of developed countries in which life expectancy is now exceeding 80 years, the prevalence of cancer is projected to increase by 45% until 2030 [311,312]. Thus, various strategies of the healthcare systems focusing on the improvement of the prevention and treatment effectiveness to cure or ameliorate the quality of life of oncological patients are mandatory.

Among many molecular pathological pathways involved in the development of cancer disease, recent evidence has shown that the cellular senescence may play an important role. As mentioned before, senescent cells have the ability to secrete pro-inflammatory cytokines and growth factors (the SASP phenotype) which are known to induce and maintain a chronic inflammatory state. Together with their ability to provide a supportive environment for the development and progression of cancer cells, senescent cell targeting may be a promising approach to improve the management of cancer conditions [313,314].

Recent experimental and clinical studies focusing on identifying novel and promising therapeutic approaches addressed to both oncological conditions and cancer-related disorders have described a potential benefit of the endocannabinoid system. It is already known that cannabinoids are indicated to ameliorate cancer related pain, chemotherapy-induced nausea and vomiting, cachexia, or anorexia [315]. However, recent studies suggested that dysregulation of the ECS may also promote cancer development by fostering physiological conditions which allow cancer cells to proliferate and migrate. Clearly, targeting this mechanism with various natural or synthetic compounds may have the theoretical potential of an improved control of cancer progression. Moreover, in the past years many authors proposed the hypothesis that the endocannabinoid system may be used not only as a prognosis marker, but also as a marker of carcinogenesis.

5.1. The Relationship between the Endocannabinoid System, Carcinogenesis, and Tumor Progression

Experimental studies have shown that both rCB1 and rCB2 agonists induce antiproliferative and pro-apoptotic effects most likely through the downregulation of gene transcription and the increase of intracellular ceramide [316]. The mechanisms responsible for cannabinoid-induced autophagy are still under debate, some authors proposing the inhibition of protein kinase B/the target of rapamycin kinase complex 1 (Akt/mTORC1) axis [317], while others suggest that upregulation of cyclooxygenase 2 (Cox-2) and prostaglandin E-2 (PGE2) are more probably involved [318].

Several studies have focused on evaluating the antineoplastic effects of cannabinoids in geriatric patients. For example, in vitro studies using prostatic cancer cells sampled from patients, cannabinoids administration in various concentrations caused a decrease of the tumoral volume by the induction of apoptosis, decrease in cell viability or interfering with different cell signaling pathways which counteract oncogenesis [319–324]. Interestingly, further in vivo studies have confirmed the antitumoral effect of cannabinoids since encouraging results such as reduction in the rate of growth and size of the tumors were reported [321,322]. The same antiproliferative effects were also reported in breast cancer together with the reduction of cell viability, alteration of signaling pathways and impeding cell cycle and promoting apoptosis [325–330]. Reduction of both tumoral volume and metastases have been also reported in in vivo studies [330]. Moreover, in a recent paper aiming to evaluate the cancer risk in cannabis users, Clark et al. reported that several types of head and neck cancer occur less frequently in this population suggesting that the ECS may represent a promising approach for the management of cancer [331]. The main effects of cannabinoids in prostatic and breast cancer are summarized in Figure 5.

The ECS has also been linked to essential events in the cascade of cancer progression such as invasion, metastasis and angiogenesis [318]. For example, in various types of solid tumors such as glioblastoma, prostate cancer, endometrial sarcoma, and colon cancer, increased concentrations of AEA and 2-AG have been reported when compared to non-cancerous tissues suggesting thus a possible endocannabinoid control mechanism of cancer growth [332]. Furthermore, in animal models of breast cancer, peritumoral administration of CBD induced a decrease in the recruitment of tumor-associated M2 pro-tumorigenic macrophages type [333]. This suggests that cannabinoids may have the ability to modulate tumoral microenvironment by lowering the CC chemokine ligand 3 (CCL3) levels reducing, and thus the macrophage chemotactic activity and metastasis induction [334–336].

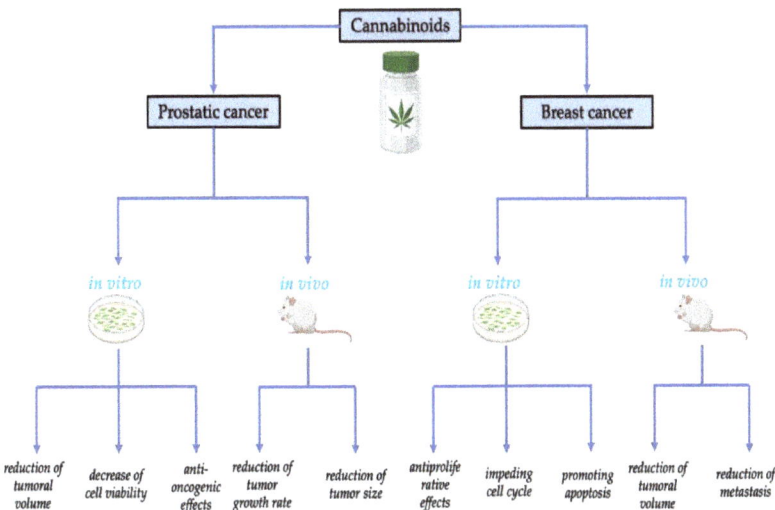

Figure 5. Schematic representation of the effects of cannabinoids in prostatic and breast cancer.

Recent evidence has shown that the variance of CB1 and CB2 receptors expression may impact the prognosis of the disease, as summarized in Table 4. For example, in tissular hepatocarcinoma samples, overexpression of both CB1 and CB2 receptors was correlated with a decreased likelihood of portal vein invasion and a subsequent improvement in disease-free survival rate [337]. An inverse correlation between rCB2 expression and tumor aggressiveness was also reported for gliomas [338]. Moreover, in non-small cell lung cancer patients, a statistically significant positive correlation was described between an increased CB1 and CB2 receptor expression and survival rate [339]. The association between rCB1 and disease severity and outcome has been also documented in prostatic cancer. Specifically, a higher expression of the cannabinoid receptor in tumoral tissue was correlated with an increased Gleason score and the presence of metastases at diagnosis [340]. Furthermore, patients with a high CB1-immunoreactivity (CB1-IR) score had shorter disease-specific survival rate [341]. In another study focusing on malignant and non-malignant thyroid cells, an increased rCB2 expression was correlated with a high recurrence rate, lymphatic and vascular invasion, and lymph node metastasis [342]. Similarly, a study on human pancreatic ductal carcinoma samples suggested that there is an inverse correlation between rCB1 levels and survival rate [343]. The impact of cannabinoids receptor expression on cancer development and their implication on the disease prognosis is summarized in Table 4.

Table 4. The impact of cannabinoids receptor expression on cancer development and their implication on the disease prognosis.

Cancer Type	Receptor Expression	Effects	Ref.
Colorectal cancer	↑ CB2 ↑ CB1	↓ disease-free survival, ↓ overall survival, ↑ tumor growth ↓ disease outcome	[344,345]
Prostate cancer	↑ CB1	↑ Gleason score, ↑ incidence of metastases at diagnosis, ↑ tumor size, ↑ rate of proliferation, ↓ disease-specific survival	[340,341]
Pancreatic cancer	↓ CB1	↓ survival	[343]
Head and neck squamos cell carcinoma	↑ CB2	↓ survival	[346]
Hepatocellular carcinoma	↑ CB1 ↑ CB2	↑ disease-free survival	[337]
Glioma	↑ CB2	↑ tumor aggressivity	[338]
Glioblastoma	↑ CB2	↑ histologic grade	[347]
Non-small cell lung cancer	↑ CB1, ↑ CB2	↑ survival	[339]

↑ = increase of; ↓ = decrease of.

5.2. Cannabinoid Usage for the Management of Pain-Associated Cancer

Various aging-associated comorbidities such as dementia, arthritis, and osteoporosis may challenge the proper management of pain in the elderly oncological population and often such patients may receive an inadequate antalgic treatment [348,349]. Recent evidence has shown that ECS may be considered a promising approach since encouraging results from clinical and experimental studies were reported. Several molecular mechanisms for the analgesic effect of CBD have been proposed and studied in animal models. For example, in neuropathic and taxol-induced pain animal models, CBD showed favorable analgesic effects [350]. Although some experimental studies stated exciting results, clinical trials still report conflicting effects. In a randomized, double-blind study focusing on the effects of topical CBD on neuropathic pain, the authors reported more beneficial effects when compared to placebo [351]. Moreover, two randomized, placebo-controlled trials have shown that in patients with an inadequate analgesia control despite the use of opioids, Nabiximols significantly reduces cancer-related pain when compared to placebo [352,353]. On the other hand, a randomized study investigating the potential antalgic effect of Nabiximols for chemotherapy-induced neuropathic pain reported no significant benefits when compared to placebo [354]. Clearly, further experimental and clinical studies are required to find novel ECS-related molecules which may interact with various pathways involved in cancer-associated pain to improve the quality of life of oncological patients.

5.3. Cannabinoid Usage to Ameliorate Chemotherapy-Induced Nausea and Vomiting

In the cancer population, observational studies have reported an increased frailty index which is a predictor of mortality and morbidity related to chemotoxicity [355,356]. Additionally, in such patients, an increased incidence of chemotherapy-induced organ toxicity was also described which frequently requires the lowering of the chemotherapeutic doses to ameliorate this undesirable effect.

Chemotherapy-induced emesis significantly influences the quality of life leading usually to anorexia and metabolic disorders which may negatively impact the administration of anticancer drugs. Currently, two cannabinoid drugs are approved for the usage in clinical practice, while dronabinol is indicated as a first line drug for the treatment of chemotherapy-induced emesis, nabilone is recommended in patients who have failed to respond to conventional antiemetic treatments [357]. Interestingly, cannabinoid administration in such patients reduced the emetic reflex by inhibiting the release of excitatory neurotransmitters, mainly through rCB1 dependent mechanisms [358]. Furthermore, in a large multicenter randomized placebo-controlled trial, oral THC:CBD cannabis extract successfully ameliorated symptoms induced-chemotherapy such as nausea and vomiting when compared to standard antiemetic therapy, although more side effects were reported in THC:CBD group [359]. Moreover, in a phase II clinical trial including 16 patients, 4.8 sprays of Nabiximols were more effective than placebo in further reducing chemotherapy-induced nausea and vomiting in patients on standard antiemetics [360].

5.4. Cannabinoid Usage to Ameliorate Cancer—Associated Cachexia and Anorexia

As before mentioned, a common feature of aging is sarcopenia, which represents the physiological loss of both muscle mass and function [361]. In cancer patients, the muscle loss is usually accelerated leading to cachexia which is associated with a functional impairment, reduced physical performance and a decreased survival rate. Particularly, if cachexia occurs in patients that are already sarcopenic, an increase of the risk of malnutrition and deleterious side effects is commonly reported [362]. The ECS may have an important role to ameliorate cancer associated cachexia since cannabinoids are known to modulate eating behavior. Early reports showed a benefit of Dronabinol on the appetite and weight stability of HIV/AIDS patients [363]. However, the data supporting cannabinoids for cancer cachexia are limited. In a clinical study, Jatoi et al. showed that Megestrol acetate provided superior anorexia palliation among advanced cancer patients when compared to dronabinol alone (75% versus 49% for appetite and 11% versus 10% for baseline weight gain). Unfortunately, the administration of both drugs did not show additional benefits [364]. Although cannabinoids must be used with caution in the geriatric population due to the risk of delirium, growing evidence supports the hypothesis that these drugs may be considered for use in daily clinical practice to ameliorate cachexia-associated cancer in patients with life expectancy of days to months.

5.5. Cannabinoid Usage to Ameliorate Cancer—Associated Anxiety and Depression

Observational studies have reported poorer treatment outcomes, decreased compliance, prolonged hospitalization, and suicide in cancer patients in which the rate of both anxiety and depression is up to 23% and 26%, respectively [365–369]. It is clear now that the treatment against anxiety and depression is mandatory in such patients to improve not only the quality of life but also the overall prognosis. Although the role of CBD as an anxiolytic agent has been intensively studied in a variety of diseases such as generalized anxiety disorder, social phobia, and schizophrenia, a limited number of studies assessed the effects of cannabinoids on cancer associated anxiety or depression. Good et al. investigated the effects of cannabinoids in palliative care and reported a significant reduction of anxiety and depression. Moreover, the same study reported a decrease in the median depression, anxiety, and stress scale (DASS 21) scores, with the biggest reduction of depression and stress [370].

The modulation of the ECS which may counteract the processes involved in cancer development such as the promotion of cell autophagy and apoptosis, antiproliferative effects, or reduction of metastasis outgrowth is an attractive and promising pharmacological intervention. Although encouraging results are reported from both experimental and clinical studies, further investigations are required to confirm all these benefits of cannabinoids on ameliorating or even cure cancer associated various symptoms such as nausea, vomiting, anxiety, or depression.

6. Cardiovascular Aging and Cannabinoid System

Cardiovascular diseases (CVDs) represent the leading cause of mortality globally with recent epidemiological studies showing an increasing trend of prevalence and incidence. Since in the next decade it is estimated that one-fifth of the world's population will be over 65 years and giving that aging has the greatest impact on cardiovascular homeostasis, it is a certainty that the global burden of cardiovascular diseases will increase [371,372]. Thus, emerging non-pharmacological and pharmacological therapies are mandatory to reduce the burden of CVDs.

Growing evidence suggests that ECS may play an important role in the modulation of cardiovascular parameters such as blood pressure, vasomotor tone, cardiac contractility, vascular inflammation, and angiogenesis [373]. Interestingly, in various aging associated cardiovascular diseases such as obesity, diabetes, and hypertension, dysregulation of the ECS signaling was shown to play pivotal roles. Moreover, a decreased plasma levels of 2-AG and AEA is associated with the alteration of cannabinoid receptor expression in the vasculature, suggesting that the ECS may represent a promising complementary therapeutic approach for the treatment of aging associated cardiovascular diseases [374–378]. We will further focus on describing the relationship between the ECS modulation and the physiopathology of the two most prevalent risk factor for CVDs associated with aging: arterial hypertension and atherosclerosis.

6.1. The Endocannabinoid System and Aging—Associated Hypertension

Among the risk factors for CVDs, arterial hypertension has the highest prevalence and is the major cause for heart failure, atrial fibrillation, coronary heart disease, stroke, chronic kidney disease, and dementia. Since aging is strongly correlated with an increase in arterial blood pressure values, it is expected that the prevention of age-related increase in blood pressure would decrease the vascular consequences commonly attributed to aging [379].

Although a plethora of antihypertensive drugs are currently available, a proper management of arterial hypertension is still challenging to be achieved. For example, observational studies reported a prevalence of resistant hypertension between 10 and 25% in the general population and up to 12% in elderly patients [380]. Interestingly, the ECS may play a major role in the physiopathology of arterial hypertension since significant antihypertensive effects of cannabinoids, their endogenous and synthetic analogs were reported. Among the mechanisms of action, NO-related pathways, CB1, and TRPV1 receptors were postulated to be involved [381,382]. Moreover, one of the endogenous cannabinoids' metabolism is arachidonic acid which is further converted in vasoactive products and modulate the regulation of vascular tone, local blood flow, and blood pressure [383].

Experimental studies have suggested that AEA may play a pivotal role in the physiopathology of arterial hypertension since AEA treatment has been shown to induce various antihypertensive effects in in vivo [382,384,385]. For example, AEA administration led to a transient decrease of blood pressure and heart rate due to the activation of the vanilloid TRPV1 receptors from sensory vagal neurons in the heart. Moreover, through rCB1 found in heart and blood vessels which are involved in counteracting the production of noradrenaline, AEA is able to reduce the cardiac contractility and peripheral resistance [386]. Intriguingly, AEA is also able to modulate vascular tone through the release of nitric oxide (NO) and endothelium-derived hyperpolarizing factor (EDHF) from the vascular endothelium [387]. Furthermore, ECS is also postulated to be involved in the long-term control of blood pressure since antihypertensive effects were linked to AEA and COX-2 metabolites from renal medulla. For example, AEA infusion into renal medulla promotes diuresis and natriuresis due to NO generation and inhibition of Na^+/H^+ and $Na^+/K^+/2Cl^-$ cotransporters through the rCB1 [388–390]. These findings suggest that an increased AEA concentration at various levels which may be achieved by the inhibition of the enzymatic breakdown or cellular uptake may represent a promising therapeutic approach for the treatment of arterial hypertension. Thus, the development of active drugs targeting AEA pathways may complement the traditional lowering blood pressure therapy.

6.2. The ECS and Aging—Associated Atherosclerosis

Atherosclerosis is a chronic arterial disease and represent the leading cause of vascular death globally due to cardiovascular and neurological complications such as ischemic heart and peripheral disease and stroke [391]. Recent evidence has shown that atherosclerosis is a systemic inflammatory disease in which the accumulation of lipids into arterial wall is mirrored by a pro-inflammatory state driven by chemokines and leukocytes leading to the formation of atherosclerotic plaque [392]. Atherosclerosis is also known as a disease of aging and the interplay between increasing age and atherosclerosis is still under research. It is clear now that aging is an independent risk factor for the development of atherosclerosis and the cellular senescence is the main factor which promote atherosclerosis [393].

Clinical and experimental evidence has reported high levels of both local and systemic endocannabinoid levels paralleling local atherogenic lesions or systemic atherosclerosis. For example, in patients with coronary artery disease, increased levels of systemic endocannabinoids were reported [394]. Montecucco et al. also found high levels of endocannabinoids and an increased expression of both rCB1 and rCB2 in human carotid plaque samples [125]. Moreover, in an animal model of atherosclerosis, Steffens et al. have reported lower dimensions of atherosclerotic plaques and reduced local inflammation in mice treated with THC. Interestingly, these favorable effects were mitigated by the administration of rCB2-selective antagonists, suggesting that the anti-atherosclerotic effects induced by THC are modulated through rCB2 pathways [395]. These findings are in line with another experimental study on LDL receptor knockout mice ($LDLr^{-/-}$) which demonstrated that rCB2-deletion increased macrophage infiltration in atherosclerotic lesions [396]. Furthermore, Chiurchiu et al. demonstrated that the treatment of human-derived foam cells with rCB2 agonist have anti-inflammatory effects since it was able to significantly lower TNF-α, IL-10, and IL-12 levels. They also reported a reduced expression of the CD36 scavenger receptor which is known to be involved in the uptake of oxidized LDL during foam cell production [397]. Although the CB2 receptor pathway clearly has favorable effects in the physiopathology of atherosclerosis, rCB1 seems to have opposite mechanisms of action since their activation led to ROS generation and induction of apoptosis in primary human coronary artery endothelial cells [398]. Interestingly, an increased expression of rCB1 was also reported in vulnerable atherosclerotic plaques in which a high level of activated immune cells is usually found, suggesting that CB1 pathway may be involved in the modulation of inflammatory processes during plaque development [399]. This hypothesis is supported by the experimental results showing that CB1 pathway inhibition improved endothelial dysfunction, prevented cell proliferation, and foam-cells development and induced arterial vasodilatation [399,400]. The main effects of cannabinoids in hypertension and atherosclerosis are summarized in Figure 6.

Taken together, these findings suggest that selective rCB2 activation and rCB1 inhibition may have promising anti-atherosclerotic effects. Additionally, these encouraging results pave the way for further experimental and clinical studies to develop novel therapeutic agents which may have additional benefits to those of classical therapy currently used for the treatment of atherosclerosis.

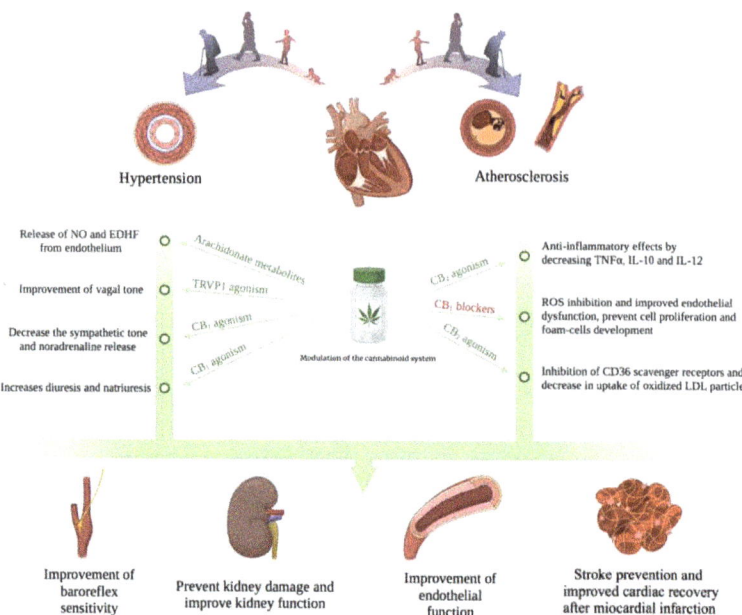

Figure 6. Schematic representation of the main effects of cannabinoids in hypertension and atherosclerosis (NO—Nitric Oxide; EDHF—endothelium-derived hyperpolarizing factor; TRVP1—transient receptor potential vanilloid 1; CB1—cannabinoids receptor 1; CB2—cannabinoids receptor 2; TNF-α—Tumor Necrosis Factor Alpha; IL-10—Interleukin 10; IL-12—Interleukin12; ROS—Reactive Oxygen Species; CD-36—Cluster of Differentiation 36; LDL—Low Density Lipoproteins).

7. Study Limitations

Although we have tried to emphasize the beneficial effects of ECS on various pathological mechanisms involved in multiple aging-related diseases, a series of limitations of this comprehensive review must be also discussed. For example, the contribution of genetic factors, as well as various influences from living environment which definitely influence the physiology of aging were not sufficiently take into account in this review [401,402]. In addition, various drug formulation and dosage as well as multiple adverse psychiatric reactions may also be considered as limitations of this study [403,404]. Therefore, from a pharmacokinetic point of view, cannabinoids are difficult to be managed in both animal and human studies since their absorption may vary. Furthermore, during chronic administration, cannabinoids may lead to drug tolerance which usually requires the increase of daily dosage with subsequent rise of psychiatric secondary effects [405]. These limitations hamper the translation of the results from experimental studies to daily clinical practice.

8. Conclusions and Perspectives

The cannabinoid system has the potential to ameliorate different underlying mechanism involved in the progression of aging-related diseases. Additionally, ECS may represent a promising approach not only for the treatment, but also for the alleviation of age-related disorder-associated symptoms and/or for increasing the efficacy of existing drugs. Moreover, our findings show that cannabinoids may be able to modulate various mechanisms rather than targeting a single dysregulated pathway in age-related diseases. Natural as well as synthetic cannabinoids ameliorate the balance between neurodegeneration and neuroinflammation in neurodegenerative diseases. In addition, they may play an important role in modulating the complex physio-pathology of MS and may be used as immune modulators, neuroprotectors, or remyelination promoters. The modulation of pro-inflammatory cytokines through the endogenous cannabinoid system may have beneficial effects on MS, AD, PD, aging-related musculoskeletal changes, and CVDs. On the other hand, it is clearly now that targeting the ECS with various natural or synthetic compounds may have the theoretical potential of an improved control of cancer progression.

Although a plethora of scientific advances on the functional relevance of cannabinoids in age-related diseases was recently achieved, a series of outstanding research questions still remain. We strongly believe that further experimental studies are mandatory to encourage the translational approach to clinical trials assessing the therapeutic potential of cannabinoids in various aging-related diseases.

Author Contributions: Conceptualization: I.M.T. and B.I.T.; methodology: I.M.T., B.I.T. and I.T.; writing—original draft preparation: I.M.T., G.D.S., C.C., M.C., A.S., B.I., A.B., E.R., T.A.-S., I.C. and I.T.; writing—review and editing: I.M.T., I.T. and B.I.T.; visualization: I.M.T., G.D.S., C.C., M.C., A.S., B.I., A.B., E.R., T.A.-S., I.C. and I.T.; project administration: I.M.T. and B.I.T. All authors have read and agreed to the published version of the manuscript.

Funding: This work was supported by a grant of the Romanian Ministry of Education and Research, CNCS–UEFISCDI, project number PN-III-P4-ID-PCE-2020-1247, within PNCDI III.

Institutional Review Board Statement: Not applicable.

Informed Consent Statement: Not applicable.

Data Availability Statement: Not applicable.

Conflicts of Interest: The authors declare no conflict of interest.

References

1. Battista, N.; Di Tommaso, M.; Bari, M.; Maccarrone, M. The endocannabinoid system: An overview. *Front. Behav. Neurosci.* **2012**, *6*, 9. [CrossRef] [PubMed]
2. Aizpurua-Olaizola, O.; Elezgarai, I.; Rico-Barrio, I.; Zarandona, I.; Etxebarria, N.; Usobiaga, A. Targeting the endocannabinoid system: Future therapeutic strategies. *Drug Discov. Today* **2017**, *22*, 105–110. [CrossRef] [PubMed]
3. Lowe, H.; Toyang, N.; Steele, B.; Bryant, J.; Ngwa, W. The endocannabinoid system: A potential target for the treatment of various diseases. *Int. J. Mol. Sci.* **2021**, *22*, 9372. [CrossRef] [PubMed]
4. Śledziński, P.; Nowak-Terpiłowska, A.; Zeyland, J. Cannabinoids in medicine: Cancer, immunity, and microbial diseases. *Int. J. Mol. Sci.* **2020**, *22*, 263. [CrossRef]
5. Donvito, G.; Nass, S.R.; Wilkerson, J.L.; Curry, Z.A.; Schurman, L.D.; Kinsey, S.G.; Lichtman, A.H. The endogenous cannabinoid system: A budding source of targets for treating inflammatory and neuropathic pain. *Neuropsychopharmacology* **2018**, *43*, 52–79. [CrossRef] [PubMed]
6. Mücke, M.; Weier, M.; Carter, C.; Copeland, J.; Degenhardt, L.; Cuhls, H.; Radbruch, L.; Häuser, W.; Conrad, R. Systematic review and meta-analysis of cannabinoids in palliative medicine. *J. Cachexia Sarcopenia Muscle* **2018**, *9*, 220–234. [CrossRef]
7. Lu, H.-C.; Mackie, K. Review of the endocannabinoid system. *Biol. Psychiatry Cogn. Neurosci. Neuroimaging* **2021**, *6*, 607–615. [CrossRef] [PubMed]
8. Glass, M.; Dragunow, M.; Faull, R.L. Cannabinoid receptors in the human brain: A detailed anatomical and quantitative autoradiographic study in the fetal, neonatal and adult human brain. *Neuroscience* **1997**, *77*, 299–318. [CrossRef]
9. Devane, W.A.; Dysarz, F.A.; Johnson, M.R.; Melvin, L.S.; Howlett, A.C. Determination and characterization of a cannabinoid receptor in rat brain. *Mol. Pharmacol.* **1988**, *34*, 605–613.
10. Munro, S.; Thomas, K.L.; Abu-Shaar, M. Molecular characterization of a peripheral receptor for cannabinoids. *Nature* **1993**, *365*, 61–65. [CrossRef]
11. Hua, T.; Vemuri, K.; Nikas, S.P.; Laprairie, R.B.; Wu, Y.; Qu, L.; Pu, M.; Korde, A.; Jiang, S.; Ho, J.-H.; et al. Crystal structures of agonist-bound human cannabinoid receptor CB1. *Nature* **2017**, *547*, 468–471. [CrossRef] [PubMed]
12. Congreve, M.; de Graaf, C.; Swain, N.A.; Tate, C.G. Impact of GPCR structures on drug discovery. *Cell* **2020**, *181*, 81–91. [CrossRef]
13. Hryhorowicz, S.; Kaczmarek-Ryś, M.; Andrzejewska, A.; Staszak, K.; Hryhorowicz, M.; Korcz, A.; Słomski, R. Allosteric Modulation of Cannabinoid Receptor 1-Current Challenges and Future Opportunities. *Int. J. Mol. Sci.* **2019**, *20*, 5874. [CrossRef] [PubMed]
14. Deng, L.; Cornett, B.L.; Mackie, K.; Hohmann, A.G. CB1 Knockout Mice Unveil Sustained CB2-Mediated Antiallodynic Effects of the Mixed CB1/CB2 Agonist CP55,940 in a Mouse Model of Paclitaxel-Induced Neuropathic Pain. *Mol. Pharmacol.* **2015**, *88*, 64–74. [CrossRef]

15. Tham, S.M.; Angus, J.A.; Tudor, E.M.; Wright, C.E. Synergistic and additive interactions of the cannabinoid agonist CP55,940 with mu opioid receptor and alpha2-adrenoceptor agonists in acute pain models in mice. *Br. J. Pharmacol.* **2005**, *144*, 875–884. [CrossRef] [PubMed]
16. Colombo, G.; Agabio, R.; Diaz, G.; Lobina, C.; Reali, R.; Gessa, G.L. Appetite suppression and weight loss after the cannabinoid antagonist SR 141716. *Life Sci.* **1998**, *63*, PL113–PL117. [CrossRef]
17. Bensaid, M.; Gary-Bobo, M.; Esclangon, A.; Maffrand, J.P.; Le Fur, G.; Oury-Donat, F.; Soubrié, P. The cannabinoid CB1 receptor antagonist SR141716 increases Acrp30 mRNA expression in adipose tissue of obese fa/fa rats and in cultured adipocyte cells. *Mol. Pharmacol.* **2003**, *63*, 908–914. [CrossRef]
18. Shearman, L.P.; Rosko, K.M.; Fleischer, R.; Wang, J.; Xu, S.; Tong, X.S.; Rocha, B.A. Antidepressant-like and anorectic effects of the cannabinoid CB1 receptor inverse agonist AM251 in mice. *Behav. Pharmacol.* **2003**, *14*, 573–582. [CrossRef]
19. Zamberletti, E.; Viganò, D.; Guidali, C.; Rubino, T.; Parolaro, D. Long-lasting recovery of psychotic-like symptoms in isolation-reared rats after chronic but not acute treatment with the cannabinoid antagonist AM251. *Int. J. Neuropsychopharmacol.* **2012**, *15*, 267–280. [CrossRef] [PubMed]
20. Ostadhadi, S.; Haj-Mirzaian, A.; Nikoui, V.; Kordjazy, N.; Dehpour, A.-R. Involvement of opioid system in antidepressant-like effect of the cannabinoid CB1 receptor inverse agonist AM-251 after physical stress in mice. *Clin. Exp. Pharmacol. Physiol.* **2016**, *43*, 203–212. [CrossRef]
21. Vimalanathan, A.; Gidyk, D.C.; Diwan, M.; Gouveia, F.V.; Lipsman, N.; Giacobbe, P.; Nobrega, J.N.; Hamani, C. Endocannabinoid modulating drugs improve anxiety but not the expression of conditioned fear in a rodent model of post-traumatic stress disorder. *Neuropharmacology* **2020**, *166*, 107965. [CrossRef]
22. Morena, M.; Berardi, A.; Colucci, P.; Palmery, M.; Trezza, V.; Hill, M.N.; Campolongo, P. Enhancing Endocannabinoid Neurotransmission Augments the Efficacy of Extinction Training and Ameliorates Traumatic Stress-Induced Behavioral Alterations in Rats. *Neuropsychopharmacology* **2018**, *43*, 1284–1296. [CrossRef]
23. Ni, X.; Geller, E.B.; Eppihimer, M.J.; Eisenstein, T.K.; Adler, M.W.; Tuma, R.F. Win 55212-2, a cannabinoid receptor agonist, attenuates leukocyte/endothelial interactions in an experimental autoimmune encephalomyelitis model. *Mult. Scler.* **2004**, *10*, 158–164. [CrossRef] [PubMed]
24. Herzberg, U.; Eliav, E.; Bennett, G.J.; Kopin, I.J. The analgesic effects of R(+)-WIN 55,212-2 mesylate, a high affinity cannabinoid agonist, in a rat model of neuropathic pain. *Neurosci. Lett.* **1997**, *221*, 157–160. [CrossRef]
25. Alonso-Alconada, D.; Álvarez, F.J.; Goñi-de-Cerio, F.; Hilario, E.; Álvarez, A. Cannabinoid-mediated Modulation of Oxidative Stress and Early Inflammatory Response after Hypoxia-Ischemia. *Int. J. Mol. Sci.* **2020**, *21*, 1283. [CrossRef] [PubMed]
26. Paronis, C.A.; Nikas, S.P.; Shukla, V.G.; Makriyannis, A. $\Delta(9)$-Tetrahydrocannabinol acts as a partial agonist/antagonist in mice. *Behav. Pharmacol.* **2012**, *23*, 802–805. [CrossRef] [PubMed]
27. Butovsky, E.; Juknat, A.; Goncharov, I.; Elbaz, J.; Eilam, R.; Zangen, A.; Vogel, Z. In vivo up-regulation of brain-derived neurotrophic factor in specific brain areas by chronic exposure to Delta-tetrahydrocannabinol. *J. Neurochem.* **2005**, *93*, 802–811. [CrossRef]
28. Patra, P.H.; Barker-Haliski, M.; White, H.S.; Whalley, B.J.; Glyn, S.; Sandhu, H.; Jones, N.; Bazelot, M.; Williams, C.M.; McNeish, A.J. Cannabidiol reduces seizures and associated behavioral comorbidities in a range of animal seizure and epilepsy models. *Epilepsia* **2019**, *60*, 303–314. [CrossRef]
29. Malvestio, R.B.; Medeiros, P.; Negrini-Ferrari, S.E.; Oliveira-Silva, M.; Medeiros, A.C.; Padovan, C.M.; Luongo, L.; Maione, S.; Coimbra, N.; de Freitas, R. Cannabidiol in the prelimbic cortex modulates the comorbid condition between the chronic neuropathic pain and depression-like behaviour in rats: The role of medial prefrontal cortex 5-HT1A and CB1 receptors. *Brain Res. Bull.* **2021**, *174*, 323–338. [CrossRef]
30. McAllister, S.D.; Christian, R.T.; Horowitz, M.P.; Garcia, A.; Desprez, P.-Y. Cannabidiol as a novel inhibitor of Id-1 gene expression in aggressive breast cancer cells. *Mol. Cancer Ther.* **2007**, *6*, 2921–2927. [CrossRef] [PubMed]
31. Giuliano, C.; Francavilla, M.; Ongari, G.; Petese, A.; Ghezzi, C.; Rossini, N.; Blandini, F.; Cerri, S. Neuroprotective and symptomatic effects of cannabidiol in an animal model of parkinson's disease. *Int. J. Mol. Sci.* **2021**, *22*, 8920. [CrossRef]
32. Craft, R.M.; Greene, N.Z.; Wakley, A.A. Antinociceptive effects of JWH015 in female and male rats. *Behav. Pharmacol.* **2018**, *29*, 280–289. [CrossRef]
33. Fechtner, S.; Singh, A.K.; Srivastava, I.; Szlenk, C.T.; Muench, T.R.; Natesan, S.; Ahmed, S. Cannabinoid Receptor 2 Agonist JWH-015 Inhibits Interleukin-1β-Induced Inflammation in Rheumatoid Arthritis Synovial Fibroblasts and in Adjuvant Induced Arthritis Rat via Glucocorticoid Receptor. *Front. Immunol.* **2019**, *10*, 1027. [CrossRef] [PubMed]
34. Sheng, W.S.; Chauhan, P.; Hu, S.; Prasad, S.; Lokensgard, J.R. Antiallodynic Effects of Cannabinoid Receptor 2 (CB2R) Agonists on Retrovirus Infection-Induced Neuropathic Pain. *Pain Res. Manag.* **2019**, *2019*, 1260353. [CrossRef]
35. Cabañero, D.; Ramírez-López, A.; Drews, E.; Schmöle, A.; Otte, D.M.; Wawrzczak-Bargiela, A.; Encabo, H.H.; Kummer, S.; Ferrer-Montiel, A.; Przewlocki, R.; et al. Protective role of neuronal and lymphoid cannabinoid CB_2 receptors in neuropathic pain. *eLife* **2020**, *9*, e55582. [CrossRef]
36. Jing, N.; Fang, B.; Li, Z.; Tian, A. Exogenous activation of cannabinoid-2 receptor modulates TLR4/MMP9 expression in a spinal cord ischemia reperfusion rat model. *J. Neuroinflammation* **2020**, *17*, 101. [CrossRef] [PubMed]
37. Ilyasov, A.A.; Milligan, C.E.; Pharr, E.P.; Howlett, A.C. The endocannabinoid system and oligodendrocytes in health and disease. *Front. Neurosci.* **2018**, *12*, 733. [CrossRef]

38. Araujo, D.J.; Tjoa, K.; Saijo, K. The endocannabinoid system as a window into microglial biology and its relationship to autism. *Front. Cell Neurosci.* **2019**, *13*, 424. [CrossRef]
39. Komorowska-Müller, J.A.; Schmöle, A.-C. CB2 Receptor in Microglia: The Guardian of Self-Control. *Int. J. Mol. Sci.* **2020**, *22*, 19. [CrossRef] [PubMed]
40. Schurman, L.D.; Lu, D.; Kendall, D.A.; Howlett, A.C.; Lichtman, A.H. Molecular mechanism and cannabinoid pharmacology. *Handb. Exp. Pharmacol.* **2020**, *258*, 323–353. [CrossRef]
41. Jordà, M.A.; Verbakel, S.E.; Valk, P.J.M.; Vankan-Berkhoudt, Y.V.; Maccarrone, M.; Finazzi-Agrò, A.; Löwenberg, B.; Delwel, R. Hematopoietic cells expressing the peripheral cannabinoid receptor migrate in response to the endocannabinoid 2-arachidonoylglycerol. *Blood* **2002**, *99*, 2786–2793. [CrossRef] [PubMed]
42. Spigelman, I. Therapeutic targeting of peripheral cannabinoid receptors in inflammatory and neuropathic pain states. In *Translational Pain Research: From Mouse to Man*; Kruger, L., Light, A.R., Eds.; CRC Press; Taylor & Francis: Boca Raton, FL, USA, 2010.
43. Torres-Moreno, M.C.; Papaseit, E.; Torrens, M.; Farré, M. Assessment of Efficacy and Tolerability of Medicinal Cannabinoids in Patients with Multiple Sclerosis: A Systematic Review and Meta-analysis. *JAMA Netw. Open* **2018**, *1*, e183485. [CrossRef]
44. Abate, G.; Uberti, D.; Tambaro, S. Potential and limits of cannabinoids in alzheimer's disease therapy. *Biology* **2021**, *10*, 542. [CrossRef]
45. Stampanoni Bassi, M.; Sancesario, A.; Morace, R.; Centonze, D.; Iezzi, E. Cannabinoids in parkinson's disease. *Cannabis Cannabinoid Res.* **2017**, *2*, 21–29. [CrossRef] [PubMed]
46. Gómez-Ruiz, M.; Hernández, M.; de Miguel, R.; Ramos, J.A. An overview on the biochemistry of the cannabinoid system. *Mol. Neurobiol.* **2007**, *36*, 3–14. [CrossRef]
47. Zuardi, A.W. History of cannabis as a medicine: A review. *Rev. Bras. Psiquiatr.* **2006**, *28*, 153–157. [CrossRef]
48. Zou, S.; Kumar, U. Cannabinoid receptors and the endocannabinoid system: Signaling and function in the central nervous system. *Int. J. Mol. Sci.* **2018**, *19*, 833. [CrossRef]
49. Fagundo, A.B.; de la Torre, R.; Jiménez-Murcia, S.; Agüera, Z.; Pastor, A.; Casanueva, F.F.; Granero, R.; Baños, R.; Botella, C.; Del Pino-Gutierrez, A.; et al. Modulation of the Endocannabinoids N-Arachidonoylethanolamine (AEA) and 2-Arachidonoylglycerol (2-AG) on Executive Functions in Humans. *PLoS ONE* **2013**, *8*, e66387. [CrossRef]
50. Di Marzo, V. Endocannabinoids: Synthesis and degradation. In *Reviews of Physiology, Biochemistry and Pharmacology*; Springer: Berlin/Heidelberg, Germany, 2008; Volume 160, pp. 1–24. [CrossRef]
51. Finn, D.P.; Haroutounian, S.; Hohmann, A.G.; Krane, E.; Soliman, N.; Rice, A.S.C. Cannabinoids, the endocannabinoid system, and pain: A review of preclinical studies. *Pain* **2021**, *162*, S5–S25. [CrossRef]
52. de Lago, E.; Petrosino, S.; Valenti, M.; Morera, E.; Ortega-Gutierrez, S.; Fernandez-Ruiz, J.; Di Marzo, V. Effect of repeated systemic administration of selective inhibitors of endocannabinoid inactivation on rat brain endocannabinoid levels. *Biochem. Pharmacol.* **2005**, *70*, 446–452. [CrossRef]
53. Goparaju, S.K.; Ueda, N.; Yamaguchi, H.; Yamamoto, S. Anandamide amidohydrolase reacting with 2-arachidonoylglycerol, another cannabinoid receptor ligand. *FEBS Lett.* **1998**, *422*, 69–73. [CrossRef]
54. Kohnz, R.A.; Nomura, D.K. Chemical approaches to therapeutically target the metabolism and signaling of the endocannabinoid 2-AG and eicosanoids. *Chem. Soc. Rev.* **2014**, *43*, 6859–6869. [CrossRef]
55. Marrs, W.R.; Blankman, J.L.; Horne, E.A.; Thomazeau, A.; Lin, Y.H.; Coy, J.; Bodor, A.L.; Muccioli, G.; Hu, S.S.-J.; Woodruff, G.; et al. The serine hydrolase ABHD6 controls the accumulation and efficacy of 2-AG at cannabinoid receptors. *Nat. Neurosci.* **2010**, *13*, 951–957. [CrossRef] [PubMed]
56. Almogi-Hazan, O.; Or, R. Cannabis, the Endocannabinoid System and Immunity-the Journey from the Bedside to the Bench and Back. *Int. J. Mol. Sci.* **2020**, *21*, 4448. [CrossRef]
57. Sholler, D.J.; Huestis, M.A.; Amendolara, B.; Vandrey, R.; Cooper, Z.D. Therapeutic potential and safety considerations for the clinical use of synthetic cannabinoids. *Pharmacol. Biochem. Behav.* **2020**, *199*, 173059. [CrossRef]
58. Chand, M.; Tung, R.L. The Aging of the World's Population and Its Effects on Global Business. JSTOR. Available online: https://www.jstor.org/stable/43822378 (accessed on 12 August 2022).
59. López-Otín, C.; Blasco, M.A.; Partridge, L.; Serrano, M.; Kroemer, G. The hallmarks of aging. *Cell* **2013**, *153*, 1194–1217. [CrossRef]
60. Li, Z.; Zhang, Z.; Ren, Y.; Wang, Y.; Fang, J.; Yue, H.; Ma, S.; Guan, F. Aging and age-related diseases: From mechanisms to therapeutic strategies. *Biogerontology* **2021**, *22*, 165–187. [CrossRef]
61. McDonald, W.I.; Compston, A.; Edan, G.; Goodkin, D.; Hartung, H.P.; Lublin, F.D.; McFarland, H.F.; Paty, D.W.; Polman, C.H.; Reingold, S.C.; et al. Recommended diagnostic criteria for multiple sclerosis: Guidelines from the International Panel on the diagnosis of multiple sclerosis. *Ann. Neurol.* **2001**, *50*, 121–127. [CrossRef]
62. Schimrigk, S.; Marziniak, M.; Neubauer, C.; Kugler, E.M.; Werner, G.; Abramov-Sommariva, D. Dronabinol Is a Safe Long-Term Treatment Option for Neuropathic Pain Patients. *Eur. Neurol.* **2017**, *78*, 320–329. [CrossRef]
63. van Amerongen, G.; Kanhai, K.; Baakman, A.C.; Heuberger, J.; Klaassen, E.; Beumer, T.L.; Strijers, R.L.; Killestein, J.; Van Gerven, J.; Cohen, A.; et al. Effects on Spasticity and Neuropathic Pain of an Oral Formulation of Δ9-tetrahydrocannabinol in Patients WithProgressive Multiple Sclerosis. *Clin. Ther.* **2018**, *40*, 1467–1482. [CrossRef]
64. Markovà, J.; Essner, U.; Akmaz, B.; Marinelli, M.; Trompke, C.; Lentschat, A.; Vila, C. Sativex®as add-on therapy vs. further optimized first-line ANTispastics (SAVANT) in resistant multiple sclerosis spasticity: A double-blind, placebo-controlled randomised clinical trial. *Int. J. Neurosci.* **2019**, *129*, 119–128. [CrossRef]

65. Hunter, D.; Oldfield, G.; Tich, N.; Messenheimer, J.; Sebree, T. Synthetic transdermal cannabidiol for the treatment of knee pain due to osteoarthritis. *Osteoarthr. Cartil.* **2018**, *26*, S26. [CrossRef]
66. Herrmann, N.; Ruthirakuhan, M.; Gallagher, D.; Verhoeff, N.P.L.G.; Kiss, A.; Black, S.E.; Lanctôt, K.L. Randomized Placebo-Controlled Trial of Nabilone for Agitation in Alzheimer's Disease. *Am. J. Geriatr. Psychiatry* **2019**, *27*, 1161–1173. [CrossRef]
67. Eisenstein, M. Does the human lifespan have a limit? *Nature* **2022**, *601*, S2–S4. [CrossRef]
68. Partridge, L.; Deelen, J.; Slagboom, P.E. Facing up to the global challenges of ageing. *Nature* **2018**, *561*, 45–56. [CrossRef]
69. DiLoreto, R.; Murphy, C.T. The cell biology of aging. *Mol. Biol. Cell* **2015**, *26*, 4524–4531. [CrossRef]
70. Campisi, J. Aging, cellular senescence, and cancer. *Annu. Rev. Physiol.* **2013**, *75*, 685–705. [CrossRef]
71. da Costa, J.P.; Vitorino, R.; Silva, G.M.; Vogel, C.; Duarte, A.C.; Rocha-Santos, T. A synopsis on aging-Theories, mechanisms and future prospects. *Ageing Res. Rev.* **2016**, *29*, 90–112. [CrossRef]
72. Harley, C.B. Telomere loss: Mitotic clock or genetic time bomb? *Mutat. Res.* **1991**, *256*, 271–282. [CrossRef]
73. Chakravarti, D.; LaBella, K.A.; DePinho, R.A. Telomeres: History, health, and hallmarks of aging. *Cell* **2021**, *184*, 306–322. [CrossRef]
74. Harley, C.B.; Vaziri, H.; Counter, C.M.; Allsopp, R.C. The telomere hypothesis of cellular aging. *Exp. Gerontol.* **1992**, *27*, 375–382. [CrossRef]
75. Calado, R.T.; Young, N.S. Telomere diseases. *N. Engl. J. Med.* **2009**, *361*, 2353–2365. [CrossRef]
76. Nault, J.-C.; Ningarhari, M.; Rebouissou, S.; Zucman-Rossi, J. The role of telomeres and telomerase in cirrhosis and liver cancer. *Nat. Rev. Gastroenterol. Hepatol.* **2019**, *16*, 544–558. [CrossRef]
77. Calcinotto, A.; Kohli, J.; Zagato, E.; Pellegrini, L.; Demaria, M.; Alimonti, A. Cellular senescence: Aging, cancer, and injury. *Physiol. Rev.* **2019**, *99*, 1047–1078. [CrossRef]
78. Zou, Y.; Sfeir, A.; Gryaznov, S.M.; Shay, J.W.; Wright, W.E. Does a sentinel or a subset of short telomeres determine replicative senescence? *Mol. Biol. Cell* **2004**, *15*, 3709–3718. [CrossRef] [PubMed]
79. Itahana, K.; Campisi, J.; Dimri, G.P. Mechanisms of cellular senescence in human and mouse cells. *Biogerontology* **2004**, *5*, 1–10. [CrossRef]
80. Gomes, N.M.V.; Ryder, O.A.; Houck, M.L.; Charter, S.J.; Walker, W.; Forsyth, N.R.; Austad, S.N.; Venditti, C.; Pagel, M.; Shay, J.W.; et al. Comparative biology of mammalian telomeres: Hypotheses on ancestral states and the roles of telomeres in longevity determination. *Aging Cell* **2011**, *10*, 761–768. [CrossRef]
81. Pignolo, R.J.; Passos, J.F.; Khosla, S.; Tchkonia, T.; Kirkland, J.L. Reducing senescent cell burden in aging and disease. *Trends Mol. Med.* **2020**, *26*, 630–638. [CrossRef]
82. van Deursen, J.M. The role of senescent cells in ageing. *Nature* **2014**, *509*, 439–446. [CrossRef]
83. Kowald, A.; Passos, J.F.; Kirkwood, T.B.L. On the evolution of cellular senescence. *Aging Cell* **2020**, *19*, e13270. [CrossRef]
84. Liguori, I.; Russo, G.; Curcio, F.; Bulli, G.; Aran, L.; Della-Morte, D.; Gargiulo, G.; Testa, G.; Cacciatore, F.; Bonaduce, D.; et al. Oxidative stress, aging, and diseases. *Clin. Interv. Aging* **2018**, *13*, 757–772. [CrossRef] [PubMed]
85. Pomatto, L.C.D.; Davies, K.J.A. Adaptive homeostasis and the free radical theory of ageing. *Free Radic. Biol. Med.* **2018**, *124*, 420–430. [CrossRef]
86. Singh, A.; Kukreti, R.; Saso, L.; Kukreti, S. Oxidative stress: A key modulator in neurodegenerative diseases. *Molecules* **2019**, *24*, 1583. [CrossRef]
87. Salisbury, D.; Bronas, U. Reactive oxygen and nitrogen species: Impact on endothelial dysfunction. *Nurs. Res.* **2015**, *64*, 53–66. [CrossRef]
88. Phaniendra, A.; Jestadi, D.B.; Periyasamy, L. Free radicals: Properties, sources, targets, and their implication in various diseases. *Indian J. Clin. Biochem.* **2015**, *30*, 11–26. [CrossRef]
89. Gradinaru, D.; Borsa, C.; Ionescu, C.; Prada, G.I. Oxidized LDL and NO synthesis–Biomarkers of endothelial dysfunction and ageing. *Mech. Ageing Dev.* **2015**, *151*, 101–113. [CrossRef] [PubMed]
90. Brinkley, T.E.; Nicklas, B.J.; Kanaya, A.M.; Satterfield, S.; Lakatta, E.G.; Simonsick, E.M.; Sutton-Tyrrell, K.; Kritchevsky, S. Plasma oxidized low-density lipoprotein levels and arterial stiffness in older adults: The health, aging, and body composition study. *Hypertension* **2009**, *53*, 846–852. [CrossRef] [PubMed]
91. Arfin, S.; Jha, N.K.; Jha, S.K.; Kesari, K.K.; Ruokolainen, J.; Roychoudhury, S.; Rathi, B.; Kumar, D. Oxidative stress in cancer cell metabolism. *Antioxidants* **2021**, *10*, 642. [CrossRef]
92. Wójcik, P.; Gęgotek, A.; Žarković, N.; Skrzydlewska, E. Oxidative stress and lipid mediators modulate immune cell functions in autoimmune diseases. *Int. J. Mol. Sci.* **2021**, *22*, 723. [CrossRef] [PubMed]
93. Paloczi, J.; Varga, Z.V.; Hasko, G.; Pacher, P. Neuroprotection in Oxidative Stress-Related Neurodegenerative Diseases: Role of Endocannabinoid System Modulation. *Antioxid. Redox Signal.* **2018**, *29*, 75–108. [CrossRef]
94. Hodges, E.L.; Marshall, J.P.; Ashpole, N.M. Age-dependent hormesis-like effects of the synthetic cannabinoid CP55940 in C57BL/6 mice. *npj Aging Mech. Dis.* **2020**, *6*, 7. [CrossRef] [PubMed]
95. Khan, M.I.; Sobocińska, A.A.; Czarnecka, A.M.; Król, M.; Botta, B.; Szczylik, C. The Therapeutic Aspects of the Endocannabinoid System (ECS) for Cancer and their Development: From Nature to Laboratory. *Curr. Pharm. Des.* **2016**, *22*, 1756–1766. [CrossRef] [PubMed]
96. Maurya, N.; Velmurugan, B.K. Therapeutic applications of cannabinoids. *Chem. Biol. Interact.* **2018**, *293*, 77–88. [CrossRef]

97. Baban, B.; Khodadadi, H.; Salles, É.L.; Costigliola, V.; Morgan, J.C.; Hess, D.C.; Vaibhav, K.; Dhandapani, K.M.; Yu, J.C. Inflammaging and Cannabinoids. *Ageing Res. Rev.* **2021**, *72*, 101487. [CrossRef] [PubMed]
98. Fulop, T.; Larbi, A.; Dupuis, G.; Le Page, A.; Frost, E.H.; Cohen, A.A.; Witkowski, J.M.; Franceschi, C. Immunosenescence and Inflamm-Aging as Two Sides of the Same Coin: Friends or Foes? *Front. Immunol.* **2017**, *8*, 1960. [CrossRef] [PubMed]
99. Franceschi, C.; Garagnani, P.; Parini, P.; Giuliani, C.; Santoro, A. Inflammaging: A new immune-metabolic viewpoint for age-related diseases. *Nat. Rev. Endocrinol.* **2018**, *14*, 576–590. [CrossRef]
100. Tang, Y.; Fung, E.; Xu, A.; Lan, H.-Y. C-reactive protein and ageing. *Clin. Exp. Pharmacol. Physiol.* **2017**, *44* (Suppl. S1), 9–14. [CrossRef]
101. Bektas, A.; Schurman, S.H.; Sen, R.; Ferrucci, L. Human T cell immunosenescence and inflammation in aging. *J. Leukoc. Biol.* **2017**, *102*, 977–988. [CrossRef]
102. Nichols, J.M.; Kaplan, B.L.F. Immune responses regulated by cannabidiol. *Cannabis Cannabinoid Res.* **2020**, *5*, 12–31. [CrossRef] [PubMed]
103. Petrosino, S.; Verde, R.; Vaia, M.; Allarà, M.; Iuvone, T.; Di Marzo, V. Anti-inflammatory Properties of Cannabidiol, a Nonpsychotropic Cannabinoid, in Experimental Allergic Contact Dermatitis. *J. Pharmacol. Exp. Ther.* **2018**, *365*, 652–663. [CrossRef] [PubMed]
104. Durst, R.; Danenberg, H.; Gallily, R.; Mechoulam, R.; Meir, K.; Grad, E.; Beeri, R.; Pugatsch, T.; Tarsish, E.; Lotan, C. Cannabidiol, a nonpsychoactive Cannabis constituent, protects against myocardial ischemic reperfusion injury. *Am. J. Physiol. Heart Circ. Physiol.* **2007**, *293*, H3602–H3607. [CrossRef] [PubMed]
105. Hegde, V.L.; Singh, U.P.; Nagarkatti, P.S.; Nagarkatti, M. Critical Role of Mast Cells and Peroxisome Proliferator-Activated Receptor γ in the Induction of Myeloid-Derived Suppressor Cells by Marijuana Cannabidiol In Vivo. *J. Immunol.* **2015**, *194*, 5211–5222. [CrossRef] [PubMed]
106. Suryavanshi, S.V.; Kovalchuk, I.; Kovalchuk, O. Cannabinoids as key regulators of inflammasome signaling: A current perspective. *Front. Immunol.* **2020**, *11*, 613613. [CrossRef] [PubMed]
107. Rizzo, M.D.; Crawford, R.B.; Bach, A.; Sermet, S.; Amalfitano, A.; Kaminski, N.E. ∆9-Tetrahydrocannabinol Suppresses Monocyte-Mediated Astrocyte Production of Monocyte Chemoattractant Protein 1 and Interleukin-6 in a Toll-Like Receptor 7-Stimulated Human Coculture. *J. Pharmacol. Exp. Ther.* **2019**, *371*, 191–201. [CrossRef]
108. Franceschi, C.; Garagnani, P.; Vitale, G.; Capri, M.; Salvioli, S. Inflammaging and "Garb-aging". *Trends Endocrinol. Metab.* **2017**, *28*, 199–212. [CrossRef]
109. Rodgers, J.L.; Jones, J.; Bolleddu, S.I.; Vanthenapalli, S.; Rodgers, L.E.; Shah, K.; Karia, K.; Panguluri, S.K. Cardiovascular Risks Associated with Gender and Aging. *J. Cardiovasc. Dev. Dis.* **2019**, *6*, 19. [CrossRef]
110. Jang, D.-I.; Lee, A.-H.; Shin, H.-Y.; Song, H.-R.; Park, J.-H.; Kang, T.-B.; Lee, S.R.; Yang, S.H. The Role of Tumor Necrosis Factor Alpha (TNF-α) in Autoimmune Disease and Current TNF-α Inhibitors in Therapeutics. *Int. J. Mol. Sci.* **2021**, *22*, 2719. [CrossRef]
111. Cardinal von Widdern, J.; Hohmann, T.; Dehghani, F. Abnormal Cannabidiol Affects Production of Pro-Inflammatory Mediators and Astrocyte Wound Closure in Primary Astrocytic-Microglial Cocultures. *Molecules* **2020**, *25*, 496. [CrossRef]
112. Wang, Y.; Mukhopadhyay, P.; Cao, Z.; Wang, H.; Feng, D.; Haskó, G.; Mechoulam, R.; Gao, B.; Pacher, P. Cannabidiol attenuates alcohol-induced liver steatosis, metabolic dysregulation, inflammation and neutrophil-mediated injury. *Sci. Rep.* **2017**, *7*, 12064. [CrossRef]
113. Becker, W.; Alrafas, H.R.; Wilson, K.; Miranda, K.; Culpepper, C.; Chatzistamou, I.; Cai, G.; Nagarkatti, M.; Nagarkatti, P.S. Activation of Cannabinoid Receptor 2 Prevents Colitis-Associated Colon Cancer through Myeloid Cell De-activation Upstream of IL-22 Production. *iScience* **2020**, *23*, 101504. [CrossRef]
114. Granja, A.G.; Carrillo-Salinas, F.; Pagani, A.; Gómez-Cañas, M.; Negri, R.; Navarrete, C.; Mecha, M.; Mestre, L.; Fiebich, B.L.; Cantarero, I.; et al. A cannabigerol quinone alleviates neuroinflammation in a chronic model of multiple sclerosis. *J. Neuroimmune Pharmacol.* **2012**, *7*, 1002–1016. [CrossRef] [PubMed]
115. Ferguson, E.G.; Mannes, Z.L.; Ennis, N. Is marijuana use associated with lower inflammation? Results from waves III and IV of the national longitudinal study of adolescent to adult health. *Drug Alcohol Depend.* **2019**, *198*, 162–167. [CrossRef]
116. Puzianowska-Kuźnicka, M.; Owczarz, M.; Wieczorowska-Tobis, K.; Nadrowski, P.; Chudek, J.; Slusarczyk, P.; Skalska, A.; Jonas, M.; Franek, E.; Mossakowska, M. Interleukin-6 and C-reactive protein, successful aging, and mortality: The PolSenior study. *Immun. Ageing* **2016**, *13*, 21. [CrossRef] [PubMed]
117. Alshaarawy, O.; Anthony, J.C. Cannabis smoking and serum C-reactive protein: A quantile regressions approach based on NHANES 2005-2010. *Drug Alcohol Depend.* **2015**, *147*, 203–207. [CrossRef] [PubMed]
118. Okafor, C.N.; Li, M.; Paltzer, J. Self-reported cannabis use and biomarkers of inflammation among adults in the United States. *Brain Behav. Immun. Health* **2020**, *7*, 100109. [CrossRef] [PubMed]
119. Aiello, A.; Farzaneh, F.; Candore, G.; Caruso, C.; Davinelli, S.; Gambino, C.M.; Ligotti, M.E.; Zareian, N.; Accardi, G. Immunosenescence and its hallmarks: How to oppose aging strategically? A review of potential options for therapeutic intervention. *Front. Immunol.* **2019**, *10*, 2247. [CrossRef]
120. Wikby, A.; Månsson, I.A.; Johansson, B.; Strindhall, J.; Nilsson, S.E. The immune risk profile is associated with age and gender: Findings from three Swedish population studies of individuals 20-100 years of age. *Biogerontology* **2008**, *9*, 299–308. [CrossRef]
121. Chiurchiù, V.; Battistini, L.; Maccarrone, M. Endocannabinoid signalling in innate and adaptive immunity. *Immunology* **2015**, *144*, 352–364. [CrossRef] [PubMed]

122. Tanikawa, T.; Kurohane, K.; Imai, Y. Induction of preferential chemotaxis of unstimulated B-lymphocytes by 2-arachidonoylglycerol in immunized mice. *Microbiol. Immunol.* **2007**, *51*, 1013–1019. [CrossRef] [PubMed]
123. Gounder, S.S.; Abdullah, B.J.J.; Radzuanb, N.E.I.B.M.; Zain, F.D.B.M.; Sait, N.B.M.; Chua, C.; Subramani, B. Effect of aging on NK cell population and their proliferation at ex vivo culture condition. *Anal. Cell Pathol.* **2018**, *2018*, 7871814. [CrossRef]
124. Ferrini, M.E.; Hong, S.; Stierle, A.; Stierle, D.; Stella, N.; Roberts, K.; Jaffar, Z. CB2 receptors regulate natural killer cells that limit allergic airway inflammation in a murine model of asthma. *Allergy* **2017**, *72*, 937–947. [CrossRef] [PubMed]
125. Montecucco, F.; Di Marzo, V.; da Silva, R.F.; Vuilleumier, N.; Capettini, L.; Lenglet, S.; Pagano, S.; Piscitelli, F.; Quintao, S.; Bertolotto, M.; et al. The activation of the cannabinoid receptor type 2 reduces neutrophilic protease-mediated vulnerability in atherosclerotic plaques. *Eur. Heart J.* **2012**, *33*, 846–856. [CrossRef]
126. Xiang, W.; Shi, R.; Kang, X.; Zhang, X.; Chen, P.; Zhang, L.; Hou, A.; Wang, R.; Zhao, Y.; Zhao, K.; et al. Monoacylglycerol lipase regulates cannabinoid receptor 2-dependent macrophage activation and cancer progression. *Nat. Commun.* **2018**, *9*, 2574. [CrossRef]
127. Castle, S.C. Impact of age-related immune dysfunction on risk of infections. *Z. Gerontol. Geriatr.* **2000**, *33*, 341–349. [CrossRef]
128. Müller, L.; Di Benedetto, S.; Pawelec, G. The Immune System and Its Dysregulation with Aging. In *Biochemistry and Cell Biology of Ageing: Part II Clinical Science*; Subcellular Biochemistry; Springer: Singapore, 2019; Volume 91, pp. 21–43. [CrossRef]
129. Chiurchiù, V. Endocannabinoids and Immunity. *Cannabis Cannabinoid Res.* **2016**, *1*, 59–66. [CrossRef]
130. Lu, Y.; Anderson, H.D. Cannabinoid signaling in health and disease. *Can. J. Physiol. Pharmacol.* **2017**, *95*, 311–327. [CrossRef] [PubMed]
131. Maccarrone, M.; Valverde, O.; Barbaccia, M.L.; Castañé, A.; Maldonado, R.; Ledent, C.; Parmentier, M.; Finazzi-Agrò, A. Age-related changes of anandamide metabolism in CB1 cannabinoid receptor knockout mice: Correlation with behaviour. *Eur. J. Neurosci.* **2002**, *15*, 1178–1186. [CrossRef] [PubMed]
132. Braile, M.; Marcella, S.; Marone, G.; Galdiero, M.R.; Varricchi, G.; Loffredo, S. The Interplay between the Immune and the Endocannabinoid Systems in Cancer. *Cells* **2021**, *10*, 1282. [CrossRef]
133. Stanciu, G.D.; Luca, A.; Rusu, R.N.; Bild, V.; Beschea Chiriac, S.I.; Solcan, C.; Bild, W.; Ababei, D.C. Alzheimer's disease pharmacotherapy in relation to cholinergic system involvement. *Biomolecules* **2019**, *10*, 40. [CrossRef] [PubMed]
134. Alzheimer's Association. 2020 Alzheimer's disease facts and figures. *Alzheimers Dement.* **2020**, *16*, 391–460. [CrossRef]
135. Alzheimer's Association. 2021 Alzheimer's disease facts and figures. *Alzheimers Dement.* **2021**, *17*, 327–406. [CrossRef]
136. Fan, L.; Mao, C.; Hu, X.; Zhang, S.; Yang, Z.; Hu, Z.; Sun, H.; Fan, Y.; Dong, Y.; Yang, J.; et al. New insights into the pathogenesis of alzheimer's disease. *Front. Neurol.* **2019**, *10*, 1312. [CrossRef]
137. Abubakar, M.B.; Sanusi, K.O.; Ugusman, A.; Mohamed, W.; Kamal, H.; Ibrahim, N.H.; Khoo, C.S.; Kumar, J. Alzheimer's disease: An update and insights into pathophysiology. *Front. Aging Neurosci.* **2022**, *14*, 742408. [CrossRef]
138. Kim, C.K.; Lee, Y.R.; Ong, L.; Gold, M.; Kalali, A.; Sarkar, J. Alzheimer's Disease: Key Insights from Two Decades of Clinical Trial Failures. *J. Alzheimers Dis.* **2022**, *87*, 83–100. [CrossRef]
139. Stanciu, G.D.; Bild, V.; Ababei, D.C.; Rusu, R.N.; Cobzaru, A.; Paduraru, L.; Bulea, D. Link Between Diabetes and Alzheimer's Disease due to the Shared Amyloid Aggregation and Deposition Involving both Neurodegenerative Changes and Neurovascular Damages. *J. Clin. Med.* **2020**, *9*, 1713. [CrossRef]
140. DeTure, M.A.; Dickson, D.W. The neuropathological diagnosis of Alzheimer's disease. *Mol. Neurodegener.* **2019**, *14*, 32. [CrossRef] [PubMed]
141. FDA's Decision to Approve New Treatment for Alzheimer's Disease. FDA. n.d. Available online: https://www.fda.gov/drugs/news-events-human-drugs/fdas-decision-approve-new-treatment-alzheimers-disease (accessed on 14 August 2022).
142. Knez, D.; Coquelle, N.; Pišlar, A.; Žakelj, S.; Jukič, M.; Sova, M.; Mravljak, J.; Nachon, F.; Brazzolotto, X.; Kos, J.; et al. Multi-target-directed ligands for treating Alzheimer's disease: Butyrylcholinesterase inhibitors displaying antioxidant and neuroprotective activities. *Eur. J. Med. Chem.* **2018**, *156*, 598–617. [CrossRef]
143. Smith, T.H.; Sim-Selley, L.J.; Selley, D.E. Cannabinoid CB1 receptor-interacting proteins: Novel targets for central nervous system drug discovery? *Br. J. Pharmacol.* **2010**, *160*, 454–466. [CrossRef]
144. Lange, J.H.M.; Coolen, H.K.A.C.; van der Neut, M.A.W.; Borst, A.J.M.; Stork, B.; Verveer, P.C.; Kruse, C.G. Design, synthesis, biological properties, and molecular modeling investigations of novel tacrine derivatives with a combination of acetylcholinesterase inhibition and cannabinoid CB1 receptor antagonism. *J. Med. Chem.* **2010**, *53*, 1338–1346. [CrossRef]
145. Oliveira, C.; Cagide, F.; Teixeira, J.; Amorim, R.; Sequeira, L.; Mesiti, F.; Silva, T.; Garrido, J.; Remião, F.; Vilar, S.; et al. Hydroxybenzoic Acid Derivatives as Dual-Target Ligands: Mitochondriotropic Antioxidants and Cholinesterase Inhibitors. *Front. Chem.* **2018**, *6*, 126. [CrossRef] [PubMed]
146. Wilson, R.I.; Nicoll, R.A. Endocannabinoid signaling in the brain. *Science* **2002**, *296*, 678–682. [CrossRef] [PubMed]
147. Aso, E.; Palomer, E.; Juvés, S.; Maldonado, R.; Muñoz, F.J.; Ferrer, I. CB1 agonist ACEA protects neurons and reduces the cognitive impairment of AβPP/PS1 mice. *J. Alzheimers Dis.* **2012**, *30*, 439–459. [CrossRef] [PubMed]
148. Aguado, T.; Romero, E.; Monory, K.; Palazuelos, J.; Sendtner, M.; Marsicano, G.; Lutz, B.; Guzmán, M.; Galve-Roperh, I. The CB1 cannabinoid receptor mediates excitotoxicity-induced neural progenitor proliferation and neurogenesis. *J. Biol. Chem.* **2007**, *282*, 23892–23898. [CrossRef] [PubMed]

149. Callén, L.; Moreno, E.; Barroso-Chinea, P.; Moreno-Delgado, D.; Cortés, A.; Mallol, J.; Casadó, V.; Lanciego, J.L.; Franco, R.; Lluis, C.; et al. Cannabinoid receptors CB1 and CB2 form functional heteromers in brain. *J. Biol. Chem.* **2012**, *287*, 20851–20865. [CrossRef]
150. Bedse, G.; Romano, A.; Lavecchia, A.M.; Cassano, T.; Gaetani, S. The role of endocannabinoid signaling in the molecular mechanisms of neurodegeneration in Alzheimer's disease. *J. Alzheimers Dis.* **2015**, *43*, 1115–1136. [CrossRef]
151. Martín-Moreno, A.M.; Reigada, D.; Ramírez, B.G.; Mechoulam, R.; Innamorato, N.; Cuadrado, A.; de Ceballos, M.L. Cannabidiol and other cannabinoids reduce microglial activation in vitro and in vivo: Relevance to Alzheimer's disease. *Mol. Pharmacol.* **2011**, *79*, 964–973. [CrossRef]
152. Campbell, V.A.; Gowran, A. Alzheimer's disease; taking the edge off with cannabinoids? *Br. J. Pharmacol.* **2007**, *152*, 655–662. [CrossRef]
153. Esposito, G.; Scuderi, C.; Valenza, M.; Togna, G.I.; Latina, V.; De Filippis, D.; Cipriano, M.; Carratù, M.R.; Iuvone, T.; Steardo, L. Cannabidiol reduces Aβ-induced neuroinflammation and promotes hippocampal neurogenesis through PPARγ involvement. *PLoS ONE* **2011**, *6*, e28668. [CrossRef]
154. Esposito, G.; Scuderi, C.; Savani, C.; Steardo, L.; De Filippis, D.; Cottone, P.; Iuvone, T.; Cuomo, V.; Steardo, L. Cannabidiol in vivo blunts beta-amyloid induced neuroinflammation by suppressing IL-1beta and iNOS expression. *Br. J. Pharmacol.* **2007**, *151*, 1272–1279. [CrossRef]
155. Chen, X.; Zhang, J.; Chen, C. Endocannabinoid 2-arachidonoylglycerol protects neurons against β-amyloid insults. *Neuroscience* **2011**, *178*, 159–168. [CrossRef]
156. Noonan, J.; Tanveer, R.; Klompas, A.; Gowran, A.; McKiernan, J.; Campbell, V.A. Endocannabinoids prevent β-amyloid-mediated lysosomal destabilization in cultured neurons. *J. Biol. Chem.* **2010**, *285*, 38543–38554. [CrossRef] [PubMed]
157. Ehrhart, J.; Obregon, D.; Mori, T.; Hou, H.; Sun, N.; Bai, Y.; Klein, T.; Fernandez, F.; Tan, J.; Shytle, R.D. Stimulation of cannabinoid receptor 2 (CB2) suppresses microglial activation. *J. Neuroinflammation* **2005**, *2*, 29. [CrossRef] [PubMed]
158. Martín-Moreno, A.M.; Brera, B.; Spuch, C.; Carro, E.; García-García, L.; Delgado, M.; Pozo, M.A.; Innamorato, N.G.; Cuadrado, A.; De Ceballos, M.L. Prolonged oral cannabinoid administration prevents neuroinflammation, lowers β-amyloid levels and improves cognitive performance in Tg APP 2576 mice. *J. Neuroinflamm.* **2012**, *9*, 8. [CrossRef]
159. Aso, E.; Juvés, S.; Maldonado, R.; Ferrer, I. CB2 cannabinoid receptor agonist ameliorates Alzheimer-like phenotype in AβPP/PS1 mice. *J. Alzheimers Dis.* **2013**, *35*, 847–858. [CrossRef]
160. Esposito, G.; De Filippis, D.; Steardo, L.; Scuderi, C.; Savani, C.; Cuomo, V.; Iuvone, T. CB1 receptor selective activation inhibits beta-amyloid-induced iNOS protein expression in C6 cells and subsequently blunts tau protein hyperphosphorylation in co-cultured neurons. *Neurosci. Lett.* **2006**, *404*, 342–346. [CrossRef] [PubMed]
161. Cao, C.; Li, Y.; Liu, H.; Bai, G.; Mayl, J.; Lin, X.; Sutherland, K.; Nabar, N.; Cai, J. The potential therapeutic effects of THC on Alzheimer's disease. *J. Alzheimers Dis.* **2014**, *42*, 973–984. [CrossRef] [PubMed]
162. Tanasescu, R.; Constantinescu, C.S. Cannabinoids and the immune system: An overview. *Immunobiology* **2010**, *215*, 588–597. [CrossRef]
163. Cabral, G.A.; Dove Pettit, D.A. Drugs and immunity: Cannabinoids and their role in decreased resistance to infectious disease. *J. Neuroimmunol.* **1998**, *83*, 116–123. [CrossRef]
164. Iuvone, T.; Esposito, G.; Esposito, R.; Santamaria, R.; Di Rosa, M.; Izzo, A.A. Neuroprotective effect of cannabidiol, a non-psychoactive component from *Cannabis sativa*, on beta-amyloid-induced toxicity in PC12 cells. *J. Neurochem.* **2004**, *89*, 134–141. [CrossRef]
165. Janefjord, E.; Mååg, J.L.V.; Harvey, B.S.; Smid, S.D. Cannabinoid effects on β amyloid fibril and aggregate formation, neuronal and microglial-activated neurotoxicity in vitro. *Cell Mol. Neurobiol.* **2014**, *34*, 31–42. [CrossRef]
166. Khodadadi, H.; Salles, É.L.; Jarrahi, A.; Costigliola, V.; Khan, M.B.; Yu, J.C.; Morgan, J.C.; Hess, D.C.; Vaibhav, K.; Dhandapani, K.M.; et al. Cannabidiol Ameliorates Cognitive Function via Regulation of IL-33 and TREM2 Upregulation in a Murine Model of Alzheimer's Disease. *J. Alzheimers Dis.* **2021**, *80*, 973–977. [CrossRef] [PubMed]
167. Aso, E.; Sánchez-Pla, A.; Vegas-Lozano, E.; Maldonado, R.; Ferrer, I. Cannabis-based medicine reduces multiple pathological processes in AβPP/PS1 mice. *J. Alzheimers Dis.* **2015**, *43*, 977–991. [CrossRef]
168. Suliman, N.A.; Taib, C.N.M.; Moklas, M.A.M.; Basir, R. Delta-9-Tetrahydrocannabinol (Δ9-THC) Induce Neurogenesis and Improve Cognitive Performances of Male Sprague Dawley Rats. *Neurotox. Res.* **2018**, *33*, 402–411. [CrossRef] [PubMed]
169. Ahmed, A.I.A.; van den Elsen, G.A.H.; Colbers, A.; Kramers, C.; Burger, D.M.; van der Marck, M.A.; Rikkert, M.G.M.O. Safety, pharmacodynamics, and pharmacokinetics of multiple oral doses of delta-9-tetrahydrocannabinol in older persons with dementia. *Psychopharmacology* **2015**, *232*, 2587–2595. [CrossRef] [PubMed]
170. Shelef, A.; Barak, Y.; Berger, U.; Paleacu, D.; Tadger, S.; Plopsky, I.; Baruch, Y. Safety and Efficacy of Medical Cannabis Oil for Behavioral and Psychological Symptoms of Dementia: An-Open Label, Add-On, Pilot Study. *J. Alzheimers Dis.* **2016**, *51*, 15–19. [CrossRef] [PubMed]
171. van den Elsen, G.A.H.; Ahmed, A.I.A.; Verkes, R.-J.; Kramers, C.; Feuth, T.; Rosenberg, P.B.; Van Der Marck, M.A.; Rikkert, M.G.O. Tetrahydrocannabinol for neuropsychiatric symptoms in dementia: A randomized controlled trial. *Neurology* **2015**, *84*, 2338–2346. [CrossRef]
172. Sheng, W.S.; Hu, S.; Min, X.; Cabral, G.A.; Lokensgard, J.R.; Peterson, P.K. Synthetic cannabinoid WIN55,212-2 inhibits generation of inflammatory mediators by IL-1beta-stimulated human astrocytes. *Glia* **2005**, *49*, 211–219. [CrossRef]

173. Jiang, W.; Zhang, Y.; Xiao, L.; Van Cleemput, J.; Ji, S.-P.; Bai, G.; Zhang, X. Cannabinoids promote embryonic and adult hippocampus neurogenesis and produce anxiolytic- and antidepressant-like effects. *J. Clin. Investig.* **2005**, *115*, 3104–3116. [CrossRef]
174. Köfalvi, A.; Lemos, C.; Martín-Moreno, A.M.; Pinheiro, B.S.; García-García, L.; Pozo, M.A.; Valério-Fernandes, Â.; Beleza, R.O.; Agostinho, P.; Rodrigues, R.J.; et al. Stimulation of brain glucose uptake by cannabinoid CB2 receptors and its therapeutic potential in Alzheimer's disease. *Neuropharmacology* **2016**, *110*, 519–529. [CrossRef]
175. Krishnan, S.; Cairns, R.; Howard, R. Cannabinoids for the treatment of dementia. *Cochrane Database Syst. Rev.* **2009**, CD007204. [CrossRef]
176. Meoni, S.; Cury, R.G.; Moro, E. New players in basal ganglia dysfunction in Parkinson's disease. *Prog. Brain Res.* **2020**, *252*, 307–327. [CrossRef] [PubMed]
177. Little, J.P.; Villanueva, E.B.; Klegeris, A. Therapeutic potential of cannabinoids in the treatment of neuroinflammation associated with Parkinson's disease. *Mini Rev. Med. Chem.* **2011**, *11*, 582–590. [CrossRef]
178. Hirsch, E.C.; Vyas, S.; Hunot, S. Neuroinflammation in Parkinson's disease. *Parkinsonism Relat. Disord.* **2012**, *18* (Suppl. S1), S210–S212. [CrossRef]
179. Caggiu, E.; Arru, G.; Hosseini, S.; Niegowska, M.; Sechi, G.; Zarbo, I.R.; Sechi, L.A. Inflammation, infectious triggers, and parkinson's disease. *Front. Neurol.* **2019**, *10*, 122. [CrossRef]
180. Nagatsu, T.; Mogi, M.; Ichinose, H.; Togari, A. Cytokines in Parkinson's disease. *J. Neural. Transm. Suppl.* **2000**, *10*, 143–151.
181. McGeer, P.L.; McGeer, E.G. Inflammation and neurodegeneration in Parkinson's disease. *Parkinsonism Relat. Disord.* **2004**, *10* (Suppl. S1), S3–S7. [CrossRef]
182. Chung, Y.C.; Shin, W.-H.; Baek, J.Y.; Cho, E.J.; Baik, H.H.; Kim, S.R.; Won, S.-Y.; Jin, B.K. CB2 receptor activation prevents glial-derived neurotoxic mediator production, BBB leakage and peripheral immune cell infiltration and rescues dopamine neurons in the MPTP model of Parkinson's disease. *Exp. Mol. Med.* **2016**, *48*, e205. [CrossRef] [PubMed]
183. Price, D.A.; Martinez, A.A.; Seillier, A.; Koek, W.; Acosta, Y.; Fernandez, E.; Strong, J.R.; Lutz, B.; Marsicano, G.; Roberts, J.L.; et al. WIN55,212-2, a cannabinoid receptor agonist, protects against nigrostriatal cell loss in the 1-methyl-4-phenyl-1,2,3,6-tetrahydropyridine mouse model of Parkinson's disease. *Eur. J. Neurosci.* **2009**, *29*, 2177–2186. [CrossRef]
184. Soti, M.; Ranjbar, H.; Kohlmeier, K.A.; Shabani, M. Parkinson's disease related alterations in cannabinoid transmission. *Brain Res. Bull.* **2022**, *178*, 82–96. [CrossRef]
185. Figura, M.; Koziorowski, D.; Sławek, J. Cannabis in Parkinson's Disease—The patient's perspective versus clinical trials: A systematic literature review. *Neurol. Neurochir. Pol.* **2022**, *56*, 21–27. [CrossRef]
186. Di Marzo, V.; Hill, M.P.; Bisogno, T.; Crossman, A.R.; Brotchie, J.M. Enhanced levels of endogenous cannabinoids in the globus pallidus are associated with a reduction in movement in an animal model of Parkinson's disease. *FASEB J.* **2000**, *14*, 1432–1438. [CrossRef]
187. Herkenham, M.; Lynn, A.B.; Little, M.D.; Johnson, M.R.; Melvin, L.S.; de Costa, B.R.; Rice, K.C. Cannabinoid receptor localization in brain. *Proc. Natl. Acad. Sci. USA* **1990**, *87*, 1932–1936. [CrossRef]
188. Wang, M.; Liu, H.; Ma, Z. Roles of the cannabinoid system in the basal ganglia in parkinson's disease. *Front. Cell. Neurosci.* **2022**, *16*, 832854. [CrossRef] [PubMed]
189. Covey, D.P.; Mateo, Y.; Sulzer, D.; Cheer, J.F.; Lovinger, D.M. Endocannabinoid modulation of dopamine neurotransmission. *Neuropharmacology* **2017**, *124*, 52–61. [CrossRef] [PubMed]
190. Brotchie, J. CB cannabinoid receptor signalling in Parkinson's disease. *Curr. Opin. Pharmacol.* **2003**, *3*, 54–61. [CrossRef]
191. van der Stelt, M.; Di Marzo, V. The endocannabinoid system in the basal ganglia and in the mesolimbic reward system: Implications for neurological and psychiatric disorders. *Eur. J. Pharmacol.* **2003**, *480*, 133–150. [CrossRef] [PubMed]
192. Sierra, S.; Luquin, N.; Rico, A.J.; Gómez-Bautista, V.; Roda, E.; Dopeso-Reyes, I.G.; Vázquez, A.; Martínez-Pinilla, E.; Labandeira-García, J.L.; Franco, R.; et al. Detection of cannabinoid receptors CB1 and CB2 within basal ganglia output neurons in macaques: Changes following experimental parkinsonism. *Brain Struct. Funct.* **2015**, *220*, 2721–2738. [CrossRef] [PubMed]
193. Jordan, C.J.; Xi, Z.-X. Progress in brain cannabinoid CB2 receptor research: From genes to behavior. *Neurosci. Biobehav. Rev.* **2019**, *98*, 208–220. [CrossRef]
194. Canseco-Alba, A.; Schanz, N.; Sanabria, B.; Zhao, J.; Lin, Z.; Liu, Q.-R.; Onaivi, E.S. Behavioral effects of psychostimulants in mutant mice with cell-type specific deletion of CB2 cannabinoid receptors in dopamine neurons. *Behav. Brain Res.* **2019**, *360*, 286–297. [CrossRef]
195. Gómez-Gálvez, Y.; Palomo-Garo, C.; Fernández-Ruiz, J.; García, C. Potential of the cannabinoid CB(2) receptor as a pharmacological target against inflammation in Parkinson's disease. *Prog. Neuropsychopharmacol. Biol. Psychiatry* **2016**, *64*, 200–208. [CrossRef]
196. Amenta, P.S.; Jallo, J.I.; Tuma, R.F.; Elliott, M.B. A cannabinoid type 2 receptor agonist attenuates blood-brain barrier damage and neurodegeneration in a murine model of traumatic brain injury. *J. Neurosci. Res.* **2012**, *90*, 2293–2305. [CrossRef]
197. López-Ramírez, G.; Sánchez-Zavaleta, R.; Ávalos-Fuentes, A.; José Sierra, J.; Paz-Bermúdez, F.; Leyva-Gómez, G.; Vila, J.S.; Cortés, H.; Florán, B. D2 autoreceptor switches CB2 receptor effects on [3 H]-dopamine release in the striatum. *Synapse* **2020**, *74*, e22139. [CrossRef] [PubMed]

198. Suárez, J.; Llorente, R.; Romero-Zerbo, S.Y.; Mateos, B.; Bermúdez-Silva, F.J.; de Fonseca, F.R.; Viveros, M.-P. Early maternal deprivation induces gender-dependent changes on the expression of hippocampal CB(1) and CB(2) cannabinoid receptors of neonatal rats. *Hippocampus* **2009**, *19*, 623–632. [CrossRef] [PubMed]
199. Marinelli, S.; Di Marzo, V.; Berretta, N.; Matias, I.; Maccarrone, M.; Bernardi, G.; Mercuri, N.B. Presynaptic facilitation of glutamatergic synapses to dopaminergic neurons of the rat substantia nigra by endogenous stimulation of vanilloid receptors. *J. Neurosci.* **2003**, *23*, 3136–3144. [CrossRef]
200. Cristino, L.; de Petrocellis, L.; Pryce, G.; Baker, D.; Guglielmotti, V.; Di Marzo, V. Immunohistochemical localization of cannabinoid type 1 and vanilloid transient receptor potential vanilloid type 1 receptors in the mouse brain. *Neuroscience* **2006**, *139*, 1405–1415. [CrossRef] [PubMed]
201. Calabresi, P.; Picconi, B.; Tozzi, A.; Ghiglieri, V.; Di Filippo, M. Direct and indirect pathways of basal ganglia: A critical reappraisal. *Nat. Neurosci.* **2014**, *17*, 1022–1030. [CrossRef]
202. Mohanty, D.; Lippmann, S. Marijuana for parkinson's disease? *Innov. Clin. Neurosci.* **2019**, *16*, 33–34.
203. Gilgun-Sherki, Y.; Melamed, E.; Mechoulam, R.; Offen, D. The CB1 cannabinoid receptor agonist, HU-210, reduces levodopa-induced rotations in 6-hydroxydopamine-lesioned rats. *Pharmacol. Toxicol.* **2003**, *93*, 66–70. [CrossRef]
204. Fox, S.H.; Henry, B.; Hill, M.; Crossman, A.; Brotchie, J. Stimulation of cannabinoid receptors reduces levodopa-induced dyskinesia in the MPTP-lesioned nonhuman primate model of Parkinson's disease. *Mov. Disord.* **2002**, *17*, 1180–1187. [CrossRef]
205. Song, L.; Yang, X.; Ma, Y.; Wu, N.; Liu, Z. The CB1 cannabinoid receptor agonist reduces L-DOPA-induced motor fluctuation and ERK1/2 phosphorylation in 6-OHDA-lesioned rats. *Drug Des. Devel. Ther.* **2014**, *8*, 2173–2179. [CrossRef] [PubMed]
206. Jeon, P.; Yang, S.; Jeong, H.; Kim, H. Cannabinoid receptor agonist protects cultured dopaminergic neurons from the death by the proteasomal dysfunction. *Anat. Cell. Biol.* **2011**, *44*, 135–142. [CrossRef]
207. Kelsey, J.E.; Harris, O.; Cassin, J. The CB(1) antagonist rimonabant is adjunctively therapeutic as well as monotherapeutic in an animal model of Parkinson's disease. *Behav. Brain Res.* **2009**, *203*, 304–307. [CrossRef]
208. Moghaddam, H.F.; Khodayar, M.J.; Abarghouei, S.M.Z.; Ardestani, M.S. Evaluation of the role of striatal cannabinoid CB1 receptors on movement activity of parkinsonian rats induced by reserpine. *Saudi Pharm. J.* **2010**, *18*, 207–215. [CrossRef]
209. Han, Q.-W.; Yuan, Y.-H.; Chen, N.-H. The therapeutic role of cannabinoid receptors and its agonists or antagonists in Parkinson's disease. *Prog. Neuropsychopharmacol. Biol. Psychiatry* **2020**, *96*, 109745. [CrossRef]
210. Chagas, M.H.N.; Zuardi, A.W.; Tumas, V.; Pena-Pereira, M.A.; Sobreira, E.T.; Bergamaschi, M.M.; Dos Santos, A.C.; Teixeira, A.L.; Hallak, J.E.C.; Crippa, J.A.S. Effects of cannabidiol in the treatment of patients with Parkinson's disease: An exploratory double-blind trial. *J. Psychopharmacol.* **2014**, *28*, 1088–1098. [CrossRef]
211. Kibret, B.G.; Ishiguro, H.; Horiuchi, Y.; Onaivi, E.S. New insights and potential therapeutic targeting of CB2 cannabinoid receptors in CNS disorders. *Int. J. Mol. Sci.* **2022**, *23*, 975. [CrossRef]
212. García, C.; Palomo-Garo, C.; García-Arencibia, M.; Ramos, J.; Pertwee, R.; Fernández-Ruiz, J. Symptom-relieving and neuroprotective effects of the phytocannabinoid Δ^9-THCV in animal models of Parkinson's disease. *Br. J. Pharmacol.* **2011**, *163*, 1495–1506. [CrossRef]
213. Yu, H.; Liu, X.; Chen, B.; Vickstrom, C.R.; Friedman, V.; Kelly, T.J.; Bai, X.; Zhao, L.; Hillard, C.J.; Liu, Q.-S. The Neuroprotective Effects of the CB2 Agonist GW842166x in the 6-OHDA Mouse Model of Parkinson's Disease. *Cells* **2021**, *10*, 3548. [CrossRef]
214. Javed, H.; Azimullah, S.; Haque, M.E.; Ojha, S.K. Cannabinoid Type 2 (CB2) Receptors Activation Protects against Oxidative Stress and Neuroinflammation Associated Dopaminergic Neurodegeneration in Rotenone Model of Parkinson's Disease. *Front. Neurosci.* **2016**, *10*, 321. [CrossRef]
215. García-Arencibia, M.; González, S.; de Lago, E.; Ramos, J.A.; Mechoulam, R.; Fernández-Ruiz, J. Evaluation of the neuroprotective effect of cannabinoids in a rat model of Parkinson's disease: Importance of antioxidant and cannabinoid receptor-independent properties. *Brain Res.* **2007**, *1134*, 162–170. [CrossRef]
216. Vallée, A.; Vallée, J.-N.; Lecarpentier, Y. Potential role of cannabidiol in Parkinson's disease by targeting the WNT/β-catenin pathway, oxidative stress and inflammation. *Aging* **2021**, *13*, 10796–10813. [CrossRef]
217. Lastres-Becker, I.; Molina-Holgado, F.; Ramos, J.A.; Mechoulam, R.; Fernández-Ruiz, J. Cannabinoids provide neuroprotection against 6-hydroxydopamine toxicity in vivo and in vitro: Relevance to Parkinson's disease. *Neurobiol. Dis.* **2005**, *19*, 96–107. [CrossRef]
218. Cooray, R.; Gupta, V.; Suphioglu, C. Current aspects of the endocannabinoid system and targeted THC and CBD phytocannabinoids as potential therapeutics for parkinson's and alzheimer's diseases: A review. *Mol. Neurobiol.* **2020**, *57*, 4878. [CrossRef] [PubMed]
219. van Vliet, S.A.M.; Vanwersch, R.A.P.; Jongsma, M.J.; Olivier, B.; Philippens, I.H.C.H.M. Therapeutic effects of Delta9-THC and modafinil in a marmoset Parkinson model. *Eur. Neuropsychopharmacol.* **2008**, *18*, 383–389. [CrossRef]
220. Carroll, C.B.; Zeissler, M.L.; Hanemann, C.O.; Zajicek, J.P. Δ^9-tetrahydrocannabinol (Δ^9-THC) exerts a direct neuroprotective effect in a human cell culture model of Parkinson's disease. *Neuropathol. Appl. Neurobiol.* **2012**, *38*, 535–547. [CrossRef]
221. Bougea, A.; Koros, C.; Simitsi, A.-M.; Chrysovitsanou, C.; Leonardos, A.; Stefanis, L. Medical cannabis as an alternative therapeutics for Parkinsons' disease: Systematic review. *Complement. Ther. Clin. Pract.* **2020**, *39*, 101154. [CrossRef]
222. Venderová, K.; Růzicka, E.; Vorísek, V.; Visnovský, P. Survey on cannabis use in Parkinson's disease: Subjective improvement of motor symptoms. *Mov. Disord.* **2004**, *19*, 1102–1106. [CrossRef]

223. Lotan, I.; Treves, T.A.; Roditi, Y.; Djaldetti, R. Cannabis (medical marijuana) treatment for motor and non-motor symptoms of Parkinson disease: An open-label observational study. *Clin. Neuropharmacol.* **2014**, *37*, 41–44. [CrossRef]
224. Balash, Y.; Bar-Lev Schleider, L.; Korczyn, A.D.; Shabtai, H.; Knaani, J.; Rosenberg, A.; Baruch, Y.; Djaldetti, R.; Giladi, N.; Gurevich, T. Medical Cannabis in Parkinson Disease: Real-Life Patients' Experience. *Clin. Neuropharmacol.* **2017**, *40*, 268–272. [CrossRef]
225. Shohet, A.; Khlebtovsky, A.; Roizen, N.; Roditi, Y.; Djaldetti, R. Effect of medical cannabis on thermal quantitative measurements of pain in patients with Parkinson's disease. *Eur. J. Pain* **2017**, *21*, 486–493. [CrossRef]
226. Finseth, T.A.; Hedeman, J.L.; Brown, R.P.; Johnson, K.I.; Binder, M.S.; Kluger, B.M. Self-reported efficacy of cannabis and other complementary medicine modalities by Parkinson's disease patients in colorado. *Evid.-Based Complement. Alternat. Med.* **2015**, *2015*, 874849. [CrossRef]
227. Zuardi, A.W.; Crippa, J.A.S.; Hallak, J.E.C.; Pinto, J.P.; Chagas, M.H.N.; Rodrigues, G.G.R.; Dursun, S.M.; Tumas, V. Cannabidiol for the treatment of psychosis in Parkinson's disease. *J. Psychopharmacol.* **2009**, *23*, 979–983. [CrossRef] [PubMed]
228. Mesnage, V.; Houeto, J.L.; Bonnet, A.M.; Clavier, I.; Arnulf, I.; Cattelin, F.; Le Fur, G.; Damier, P.; Welter, M.L.; Agid, Y. Neurokinin B, Neurotensin, and cannabinoid receptor antagonists and Parkinson disease. *Clin. Neuropharmacol.* **2004**, *27*, 108–110. [CrossRef] [PubMed]
229. Sieradzan, K.A.; Fox, S.H.; Hill, M.; Dick, J.P.; Crossman, A.R.; Brotchie, J.M. Cannabinoids reduce levodopa-induced dyskinesia in Parkinson's disease: A pilot study. *Neurology* **2001**, *57*, 2108–2111. [CrossRef] [PubMed]
230. de Faria, S.M.; de Morais Fabrício, D.; Tumas, V.; Castro, P.C.; Ponti, M.A.; Hallak, J.E.; Zuardi, A.W.; Crippa, J.A.S.; Chagas, M.H.N. Effects of acute cannabidiol administration on anxiety and tremors induced by a Simulated Public Speaking Test in patients with Parkinson's disease. *J. Psychopharmacol.* **2020**, *34*, 189–196. [CrossRef]
231. Lassmann, H. Multiple Sclerosis Pathology. *Cold Spring Harb. Perspect. Med.* **2018**, *8*, a028936. [CrossRef]
232. Collin, C.; Davies, P.; Mutiboko, I.K.; Ratcliffe, S.; Sativex Spasticity in MS Study Group. Randomized controlled trial of cannabis-based medicine in spasticity caused by multiple sclerosis. *Eur. J. Neurol.* **2007**, *14*, 290–296. [CrossRef]
233. D'hooghe, M.; Willekens, B.; Delvaux, V.; D'haeseleer, M.; Guillaume, D.; Laureys, G.; Nagels, G.; Vanderdonckt, P.; Van Pesch, V.; Popescu, V. Sativex®(nabiximols) cannabinoid oromucosal spray in patients with resistant multiple sclerosis spasticity: The Belgian experience. *BMC Neurol.* **2021**, *21*, 227. [CrossRef] [PubMed]
234. Patti, F.; Messina, S.; Solaro, C.; Amato, M.P.; Bergamaschi, R.; Bonavita, S.; Bossio, R.B.; Morra, V.B.; Costantino, G.F.; Cavalla, P.; et al. Efficacy and safety of cannabinoid oromucosal spray for multiple sclerosis spasticity. *J. Neurol. Neurosurg. Psychiatry* **2016**, *87*, 944–951. [CrossRef] [PubMed]
235. Turri, M.; Teatini, F.; Donato, F.; Zanette, G.; Tugnoli, V.; Deotto, L.; Bonetti, B.; Squintani, G. Pain Modulation after Oromucosal Cannabinoid Spray (SATIVEX®) in Patients with Multiple Sclerosis: A Study with Quantitative Sensory Testing and Laser-Evoked Potentials. *Medicines* **2018**, *5*, 59. [CrossRef]
236. Flachenecker, P.; Henze, T.; Zettl, U.K. Nabiximols (THC/CBD oromucosal spray, Sativex®) in clinical practice–results of a multicenter, non-interventional study (MOVE 2) in patients with multiple sclerosis spasticity. *Eur. Neurol.* **2014**, *71*, 271–279. [CrossRef]
237. Meuth, S.G.; Henze, T.; Essner, U.; Trompke, C.; Vila Silván, C. Tetrahydrocannabinol and cannabidiol oromucosal spray in resistant multiple sclerosis spasticity: Consistency of response across subgroups from the SAVANT randomized clinical trial. *Int. J. Neurosci.* **2020**, *130*, 1199–1205. [CrossRef] [PubMed]
238. Paolicelli, D.; Direnzo, V.; Manni, A.; D'Onghia, M.; Tortorella, C.; Zoccolella, S.; Di Lecce, V.; Iaffaldano, A.; Trojano, M. Long-Term Data of Efficacy, Safety, and Tolerability in a Real-Life Setting of THC/CBD Oromucosal Spray-Treated Multiple Sclerosis Patients. *J. Clin. Pharmacol.* **2016**, *56*, 845–851. [CrossRef]
239. Russo, M.; Naro, A.; Leo, A.; Sessa, E.; D'Aleo, G.; Bramanti, P.; Calabrò, R.S. Evaluating sativex®in neuropathic pain management: A clinical and neurophysiological assessment in multiple sclerosis. *Pain Med.* **2016**, *17*, 1145–1154. [CrossRef] [PubMed]
240. Longoria, V.; Parcel, H.; Toma, B.; Minhas, A.; Zeine, R. Neurological benefits, clinical challenges, and neuropathologic promise of medical marijuana: A systematic review of cannabinoid effects in multiple sclerosis and experimental models of demyelination. *Biomedicines* **2022**, *10*, 539. [CrossRef]
241. Jones, É.; Vlachou, S. A Critical Review of the Role of the Cannabinoid Compounds Δ9-Tetrahydrocannabinol (Δ9-THC) and Cannabidiol (CBD) and their Combination in Multiple Sclerosis Treatment. *Molecules* **2020**, *25*, 4930. [CrossRef]
242. Pourmohammadi, A.; Riahi, R.; Hosseini, S.M.; Adibi, I. Pharmacological treatment of tremor in multiple sclerosis; a systematic review. *Mult. Scler. Relat. Disord.* **2022**, *60*, 103722. [CrossRef]
243. Kim-Fine, S.; Greenfield, J.; Chaput, K.H.; Robert, M.; Metz, L.M. Cannabinoids and bladder symptoms in multiple sclerosis. *Mult. Scler. Relat. Disord.* **2021**, *54*, 103105. [CrossRef]
244. Dopkins, N.; Miranda, K.; Wilson, K.; Holloman, B.L.; Nagarkatti, P.; Nagarkatti, M. Effects of orally administered cannabidiol on neuroinflammation and intestinal inflammation in the attenuation of experimental autoimmune encephalomyelitis. *J. Neuroimmune Pharmacol.* **2021**; *online ahead of print*. [CrossRef]
245. Centonze, D.; Bari, M.; Rossi, S.; Prosperetti, C.; Furlan, R.; Fezza, F.; De Chiara, V.; Battistini, L.; Bernardi, G.; Bernardini, S.; et al. The endocannabinoid system is dysregulated in multiple sclerosis and in experimental autoimmune encephalomyelitis. *Brain* **2007**, *130*, 2543–2553. [CrossRef]

246. Sánchez López, A.J.; Román-Vega, L.; Ramil Tojeiro, E.; Giuffrida, A.; García-Merino, A. Regulation of cannabinoid receptor gene expression and endocannabinoid levels in lymphocyte subsets by interferon-β: A longitudinal study in multiple sclerosis patients. *Clin. Exp. Immunol.* **2015**, *179*, 119–127. [CrossRef]
247. Jean-Gilles, L.; Feng, S.; Tench, C.R.; Chapman, V.; Kendall, D.A.; Barrett, D.A.; Constantinescu, C. Plasma endocannabinoid levels in multiple sclerosis. *J. Neurol. Sci.* **2009**, *287*, 212–215. [CrossRef]
248. Di Filippo, M.; Pini, L.A.; Pellicciolo, G.P.; Calabresi, P.; Sarchielli, P. Abnormalities in the cerebrospinal fluid levels of endocannabinoids in multiple sclerosis. *J. Neurol. Neurosurg. Psychiatry* **2008**, *79*, 1224–1229. [CrossRef]
249. Rodrigues, R.S.; Lourenço, D.M.; Paulo, S.L.; Mateus, J.M.; Ferreira, M.F.; Mouro, F.M.; Moreira, J.B.; Ribeiro, F.F.; Sebastião, A.M.; Xapelli, S. Cannabinoid actions on neural stem cells: Implications for pathophysiology. *Molecules* **2019**, *24*, 1350. [CrossRef] [PubMed]
250. Marsicano, G.; Goodenough, S.; Monory, K.; Hermann, H.; Eder, M.; Cannich, A.; Azad, S.C.; Cascio, M.G.; Gutiérrez, S.O.; van der Stelt, M.; et al. CB1 cannabinoid receptors and on-demand defense against excitotoxicity. *Science* **2003**, *302*, 84–88. [CrossRef]
251. Musella, A.; Sepman, H.; Mandolesi, G.; Gentile, A.; Fresegna, D.; Haji, N.; Conrad, A.; Lutz, B.; Maccarrone, M.; Centonze, D. Pre- and postsynaptic type-1 cannabinoid receptors control the alterations of glutamate transmission in experimental autoimmune encephalomyelitis. *Neuropharmacology* **2014**, *79*, 567–572. [CrossRef] [PubMed]
252. Navarrete, C.; Carrillo-Salinas, F.; Palomares, B.; Mecha, M.; Jiménez-Jiménez, C.; Mestre, L.; Feliú, A.; Bellido, M.L.; Fiebich, B.L.; Appendino, G.; et al. Hypoxia mimetic activity of VCE-004.8, a cannabidiol quinone derivative: Implications for multiple sclerosis therapy. *J. Neuroinflammation* **2018**, *15*, 64. [CrossRef] [PubMed]
253. Kozela, E.; Haj, L.; Hanuš, L.; Chourasia, M.; Shurki, A.; Juknat, A.; Kaushansky, N.; Mechoulam, R.; Vogel, Z. HU-446 and HU-465, Derivatives of the Non-psychoactive Cannabinoid Cannabidiol, Decrease the Activation of Encephalitogenic T Cells. *Chem. Biol. Drug Des.* **2016**, *87*, 143–153. [CrossRef] [PubMed]
254. Fraussen, J.; de Bock, L.; Somers, V. B cells and antibodies in progressive multiple sclerosis: Contribution to neurodegeneration and progression. *Autoimmun. Rev.* **2016**, *15*, 896–899. [CrossRef]
255. Mestre, L.; Docagne, F.; Correa, F.; Loría, F.; Hernangómez, M.; Borrell, J.; Guaza, C. A cannabinoid agonist interferes with the progression of a chronic model of multiple sclerosis by downregulating adhesion molecules. *Mol. Cell Neurosci.* **2009**, *40*, 258–266. [CrossRef] [PubMed]
256. Mestre, L.; Iñigo, P.M.; Mecha, M.; Correa, F.G.; Hernangómez-Herrero, M.; Loría, F.; Docagne, F.; Borrell, J.; Guaza, C. Anandamide inhibits Theiler's virus induced VCAM-1 in brain endothelial cells and reduces leukocyte transmigration in a model of blood brain barrier by activation of CB(1) receptors. *J. Neuroinflamm.* **2011**, *8*, 102. [CrossRef]
257. Mecha, M.; Feliú, A.; Iñigo, P.M.; Mestre, L.; Carrillo-Salinas, F.J.; Guaza, C. Cannabidiol provides long-lasting protection against the deleterious effects of inflammation in a viral model of multiple sclerosis: A role for A2A receptors. *Neurobiol. Dis.* **2013**, *59*, 141–150. [CrossRef] [PubMed]
258. Al-Ghezi, Z.Z.; Miranda, K.; Nagarkatti, M.; Nagarkatti, P.S. Combination of Cannabinoids, Δ9- Tetrahydrocannabinol and Cannabidiol, Ameliorates Experimental Multiple Sclerosis by Suppressing Neuroinflammation Through Regulation of miRNA-Mediated Signaling Pathways. *Front. Immunol.* **2019**, *10*, 1921. [CrossRef]
259. Yang, X.; Bam, M.; Nagarkatti, P.S.; Nagarkatti, M. Cannabidiol Regulates Gene Expression in Encephalitogenic T cells Using Histone Methylation and noncoding RNA during Experimental Autoimmune Encephalomyelitis. *Sci. Rep.* **2019**, *9*, 15780. [CrossRef]
260. Bjornevik, K.; Cortese, M.; Healy, B.C.; Kuhle, J.; Mina, M.J.; Leng, Y.; Elledge, S.J.; Niebuhr, D.W.; Scher, A.I.; Munger, K.L.; et al. Longitudinal analysis reveals high prevalence of Epstein-Barr virus associated with multiple sclerosis. *Science* **2022**, *375*, 296–301. [CrossRef] [PubMed]
261. O'Brien, K.; Fitzgerald, D.C.; Naiken, K.; Alugupalli, K.R.; Rostami, A.M.; Gran, B. Role of the innate immune system in autoimmune inflammatory demyelination. *Curr. Med. Chem.* **2008**, *15*, 1105–1115. [CrossRef]
262. Prinz, M.; Garbe, F.; Schmidt, H.; Mildner, A.; Gutcher, I.; Wolter, K.; Piesche, M.; Schroers, R.; Weiss, E.; Kirschning, C.J.; et al. Innate immunity mediated by TLR9 modulates pathogenicity in an animal model of multiple sclerosis. *J. Clin. Investig.* **2006**, *116*, 456–464. [CrossRef]
263. Bsibsi, M.; Ravid, R.; Gveric, D.; van Noort, J.M. Broad expression of Toll-like receptors in the human central nervous system. *J. Neuropathol. Exp. Neurol.* **2002**, *61*, 1013–1021. [CrossRef]
264. Fitzpatrick, J.-M.; Hackett, B.; Costelloe, L.; Hind, W.; Downer, E.J. Botanically-Derived Δ9-Tetrahydrocannabinol and Cannabidiol, and Their 1:1 Combination, Modulate Toll-like Receptor 3 and 4 Signalling in Immune Cells from People with Multiple Sclerosis. *Molecules* **2022**, *27*, 1763. [CrossRef]
265. Orihuela, R.; McPherson, C.A.; Harry, G.J. Microglial M1/M2 polarization and metabolic states. *Br. J. Pharmacol.* **2016**, *173*, 649–665. [CrossRef]
266. Mecha, M.; Carrillo-Salinas, F.J.; Feliú, A.; Mestre, L.; Guaza, C. Microglia activation states and cannabinoid system: Therapeutic implications. *Pharmacol. Ther.* **2016**, *166*, 40–55. [CrossRef]
267. Stella, N. Endocannabinoid signaling in microglial cells. *Neuropharmacology* **2009**, *56* (Suppl. S1), 244–253. [CrossRef]
268. Benito, C.; Romero, J.P.; Tolón, R.M.; Clemente, D.; Docagne, F.; Hillard, C.J.; Guaza, C. Cannabinoid CB1 and CB2 receptors and fatty acid amide hydrolase are specific markers of plaque cell subtypes in human multiple sclerosis. *J. Neurosci.* **2007**, *27*, 2396–2402. [CrossRef] [PubMed]

269. Gómez Del Pulgar, T.; De Ceballos, M.L.; Guzmán, M.; Velasco, G. Cannabinoids protect astrocytes from ceramide-induced apoptosis through the phosphatidylinositol 3-kinase/protein kinase B pathway. *J. Biol. Chem.* **2002**, *277*, 36527–36533. [CrossRef]
270. Molina-Holgado, E.; Vela, J.M.; Arévalo-Martín, A.; Almazán, G.; Molina-Holgado, F.; Borrell, J.; Guaza, C. Cannabinoids promote oligodendrocyte progenitor survival: Involvement of cannabinoid receptors and phosphatidylinositol-3 kinase/Akt signaling. *J. Neurosci.* **2002**, *22*, 9742–9753. [CrossRef] [PubMed]
271. Giacoppo, S.; Pollastro, F.; Grassi, G.; Bramanti, P.; Mazzon, E. Target regulation of PI3K/Akt/mTOR pathway by cannabidiol in treatment of experimental multiple sclerosis. *Fitoterapia* **2017**, *116*, 77–84. [CrossRef] [PubMed]
272. Hughes, E.G.; Orthmann-Murphy, J.L.; Langseth, A.J.; Bergles, D.E. Myelin remodeling through experience-dependent oligodendrogenesis in the adult somatosensory cortex. *Nat. Neurosci.* **2018**, *21*, 696–706. [CrossRef] [PubMed]
273. Xiao, L.; Ohayon, D.; McKenzie, I.A.; Sinclair-Wilson, A.; Wright, J.L.; Fudge, A.D.; Emery, B.; Li, H.; Richardson, W.D. Rapid production of new oligodendrocytes is required in the earliest stages of motor-skill learning. *Nat. Neurosci.* **2016**, *19*, 1210–1217. [CrossRef]
274. Elbaz, B.; Popko, B. Molecular control of oligodendrocyte development. *Trends Neurosci.* **2019**, *42*, 263–277. [CrossRef]
275. Mecha, M.; Torrao, A.S.; Mestre, L.; Carrillo-Salinas, F.J.; Mechoulam, R.; Guaza, C. Cannabidiol protects oligodendrocyte progenitor cells from inflammation-induced apoptosis by attenuating endoplasmic reticulum stress. *Cell Death Dis.* **2012**, *3*, e331. [CrossRef]
276. Tomas-Roig, J.; Agbemenyah, H.Y.; Celarain, N.; Quintana, E.; Ramió-Torrentà, L.; Havemann-Reinecke, U. Dose-dependent effect of cannabinoid WIN-55,212-2 on myelin repair following a demyelinating insult. *Sci. Rep.* **2020**, *10*, 590. [CrossRef]
277. Katona, S.; Kaminski, E.; Sanders, H.; Zajicek, J. Cannabinoid influence on cytokine profile in multiple sclerosis. *Clin. Exp. Immunol.* **2005**, *140*, 580–585. [CrossRef]
278. Mustafa, W.; Elgendy, N.; Salama, S.; Jawad, M.; Eltoukhy, K. The Effect of Cannabis on the Clinical and Cytokine Profiles in Patients with Multiple Sclerosis. *Mult. Scler. Int.* **2021**, *2021*, 6611897. [CrossRef] [PubMed]
279. Walter, L.; Stella, N. Cannabinoids and neuroinflammation. *Br. J. Pharmacol.* **2004**, *141*, 775–785. [CrossRef]
280. Chandra, A.; Rajawat, J. Skeletal aging and osteoporosis: Mechanisms and therapeutics. *Int. J. Mol. Sci.* **2021**, *22*, 3553. [CrossRef]
281. Qaisar, R.; Karim, A.; Muhammad, T.; Shah, I.; Khan, J. Prediction of sarcopenia using a battery of circulating biomarkers. *Sci. Rep.* **2021**, *11*, 8632. [CrossRef] [PubMed]
282. Moon, P.M.; Shao, Z.Y.; Wambiekele, G.; Appleton, C.; Laird, D.W.; Penuela, S.; Beier, F. Global Deletion of Pannexin 3 Accelerates Development of Aging-induced Osteoarthritis in Mice. *Arthritis Rheumatol.* **2021**, *73*, 1178–1188. [CrossRef] [PubMed]
283. Rankin, L.; Fowler, C.J. The basal pharmacology of palmitoylethanolamide. *Int. J. Mol. Sci.* **2020**, *21*, 7942. [CrossRef] [PubMed]
284. Le Bacquer, O.; Salles, J.; Piscitelli, F.; Sanchez, P.; Martin, V.; Montaurier, C.; Di Marzo, V.; Walrand, S. Alterations of the endocannabinoid system and circulating and peripheral tissue levels of endocannabinoids in sarcopenic rats. *J. Cachexia Sarcopenia Muscle* **2022**, *13*, 662–676. [CrossRef] [PubMed]
285. Raphael-Mizrahi, B.; Gabet, Y. The cannabinoids effect on bone formation and bone healing. *Curr. Osteoporos. Rep.* **2020**, *18*, 433–438. [CrossRef]
286. Li, J.; Ayoub, A.; Xiu, Y.; Yin, X.; Sanders, J.O.; Mesfin, A.; Xing, L.; Yao, Z.; Boyce, B.F. TGFβ-induced degradation of TRAF3 in mesenchymal progenitor cells causes age-related osteoporosis. *Nat. Commun.* **2019**, *10*, 2795. [CrossRef]
287. Serna, J.; Bergwitz, C. Importance of dietary phosphorus for bone metabolism and healthy aging. *Nutrients* **2020**, *12*, 3001. [CrossRef] [PubMed]
288. Bettis, T.; Kim, B.J.; Hamrick, M.W. Impact of muscle atrophy on bone metabolism and bone strength: Implications for muscle-bone crosstalk with aging and disuse. *Osteoporos. Int.* **2018**, *29*, 1713–1720. [CrossRef]
289. Noh, J.-Y.; Yang, Y.; Jung, H. Molecular mechanisms and emerging therapeutics for osteoporosis. *Int. J. Mol. Sci.* **2020**, *21*, 7623. [CrossRef]
290. Rinonapoli, G.; Ruggiero, C.; Meccariello, L.; Bisaccia, M.; Ceccarini, P.; Caraffa, A. Osteoporosis in men: A review of an underestimated bone condition. *Int. J. Mol. Sci.* **2021**, *22*, 2105. [CrossRef]
291. Tam, J.; Hinden, L.; Drori, A.; Udi, S.; Azar, S.; Baraghithy, S. The therapeutic potential of targeting the peripheral endocannabinoid/CB1 receptor system. *Eur. J. Intern. Med.* **2018**, *49*, 23–29. [CrossRef]
292. Deis, S.; Srivastava, R.K.; de Azua, I.R.; Bindila, L.; Baraghithy, S.; Lutz, B.; Bab, I.; Tam, J. Age-related regulation of bone formation by the sympathetic cannabinoid CB1 receptor. *Bone* **2017**, *108*, 34–42. [CrossRef]
293. Baraghithy, S.; Soae, Y.; Assaf, D.; Hinden, L.; Udi, S.; Drori, A.; Gabet, Y.; Tam, J. Renal Proximal Tubule Cell Cannabinoid-1 Receptor Regulates Bone Remodeling and Mass via a Kidney-to-Bone Axis. *Cells* **2021**, *10*, 414. [CrossRef]
294. Kostrzewa, M.; Mahmoud, A.M.; Verde, R.; Scotto di Carlo, F.; Gianfrancesco, F.; Piscitelli, F.; Ligresti, A. Modulation of Endocannabinoid Tone in Osteoblastic Differentiation of MC3T3-E1 Cells and in Mouse Bone Tissue over Time. *Cells* **2021**, *10*, 1199. [CrossRef]
295. Li, W.; Sun, Y. Nrf2 is required for suppressing osteoclast RANKL-induced differentiation in RAW 264.7 cells via inactivating cannabinoid receptor type 2 with AM630. *Regen. Ther.* **2020**, *14*, 191–195. [CrossRef]
296. López-González, I.; Zamora-Ledezma, C.; Sanchez-Lorencio, M.I.; Tristante Barrenechea, E.; Gabaldón-Hernández, J.A.; Meseguer-Olmo, L. Modifications in Gene Expression in the Process of Osteoblastic Differentiation of Multipotent Bone Marrow-Derived Human Mesenchymal Stem Cells Induced by a Novel Osteoinductive Porous Medical-Grade 3D-Printed Poly(ε-caprolactone)/β-tricalcium Phosphate Composite. *Int. J. Mol. Sci.* **2021**, *22*, 11216. [CrossRef] [PubMed]

297. Wang, B.; Lian, K.; Li, J.; Mei, G. Restoration of osteogenic differentiation by overexpression of cannabinoid receptor 2 in bone marrow mesenchymal stem cells isolated from osteoporotic patients. *Exp. Ther. Med.* **2018**, *15*, 357–364. [CrossRef]
298. Sophocleous, A.; Marino, S.; Kabir, D.; Ralston, S.H.; Idris, A.I. Combined deficiency of the Cnr1 and Cnr2 receptors protects against age-related bone loss by osteoclast inhibition. *Aging Cell* **2017**, *16*, 1051–1061. [CrossRef]
299. Smith, M.; Wilson, R.; O'Brien, S.; Tufarelli, C.; Anderson, S.I.; O'Sullivan, S.E. The Effects of the Endocannabinoids Anandamide and 2-Arachidonoylglycerol on Human Osteoblast Proliferation and Differentiation. *PLoS ONE* **2015**, *10*, e0136546. [CrossRef]
300. Liu, H.; Zhou, C.; Qi, D.; Gao, Y.; Zhu, M.; Tao, T.; Sun, X.; Xiao, J. Inhibiting Monoacylglycerol Lipase Suppresses RANKL-Induced Osteoclastogenesis and Alleviates Ovariectomy-Induced Bone Loss. *Front. Cell Dev. Biol.* **2021**, *9*, 640867. [CrossRef]
301. Rezuş, E.; Burlui, A.; Cardoneanu, A.; Macovei, L.A.; Tamba, B.I.; Rezuş, C. From Pathogenesis to Therapy in Knee Osteoarthritis: Bench-to-Bedside. *Int. J. Mol. Sci.* **2021**, *22*, 2697. [CrossRef] [PubMed]
302. Valdes, A.M. Metabolic syndrome and osteoarthritis pain: Common molecular mechanisms and potential therapeutic implications. *Osteoarth. Cartil.* **2019**, *28*, 7–9. [CrossRef]
303. Mlost, J.; Kac, P.; Kędziora, M.; Starowicz, K. Antinociceptive and chondroprotective effects of prolonged β-caryophyllene treatment in the animal model of osteoarthritis: Focus on tolerance development. *Neuropharmacology* **2021**, *204*, 108908. [CrossRef]
304. Sophocleous, A.; Börjesson, A.E.; Salter, D.M.; Ralston, S.H. The type 2 cannabinoid receptor regulates susceptibility to osteoarthritis in mice. *Osteoarth. Cartil.* **2015**, *23*, 1586–1594. [CrossRef]
305. Xin, Y.; Tang, A.; Pan, S.; Zhang, J. Components of the Endocannabinoid System and Effects of Cannabinoids Against Bone Diseases: A Mini-Review. *Front. Pharmacol.* **2021**, *12*, 793750. [CrossRef] [PubMed]
306. Bryk, M.; Chwastek, J.; Kostrzewa, M.; Mlost, J.; Pędracka, A.; Starowicz, K. Alterations in Anandamide Synthesis and Degradation during Osteoarthritis Progression in an Animal Model. *Int. J. Mol. Sci.* **2020**, *21*, 7381. [CrossRef]
307. Gaisberger, M.; Fuchs, J.; Riedl, M.; Edtinger, S.; Reischl, R.; Grasmann, G.; Hölzl, B.; Landauer, F.; Dobias, H.; Eckstein, F.; et al. Endogenous anandamide and self-reported pain are significantly reduced after a 2-week multimodal treatment with and without radon therapy in patients with knee osteoarthritis: A pilot study. *Int. J. Biometeorol.* **2021**, *65*, 1151–1160. [CrossRef]
308. Rezuş, E.; Burlui, A.; Cardoneanu, A.; Rezuş, C.; Codreanu, C.; Pârvu, M.; Zota, G.R.; Tamba, B.I. Inactivity and skeletal muscle metabolism: A vicious cycle in old age. *Int. J. Mol. Sci.* **2020**, *21*, 592. [CrossRef] [PubMed]
309. Dalle, S.; Koppo, K. Cannabinoid receptor 1 expression is higher in muscle of old vs. young males, and increases upon resistance exercise in older adults. *Sci. Rep.* **2021**, *11*, 18349. [CrossRef]
310. SEER Incidence Data, 1975–2019. n.d. Available online: https://seer.cancer.gov/data/ (accessed on 14 August 2022).
311. Smith, B.D.; Smith, G.L.; Hurria, A.; Hortobagyi, G.N.; Buchholz, T.A. Future of cancer incidence in the United States: Burdens upon an aging, changing nation. *J. Clin. Oncol.* **2009**, *27*, 2758–2765. [CrossRef]
312. Sung, H.; Ferlay, J.; Siegel, R.L.; Laversanne, M.; Soerjomataram, I.; Jemal, A.; Bray, F. Global cancer statistics 2020: GLOBOCAN estimates of incidence and mortality worldwide for 36 cancers in 185 countries. *CA Cancer J. Clin.* **2021**, *71*, 209–249. [CrossRef]
313. Krtolica, A.; Parrinello, S.; Lockett, S.; Desprez, P.Y.; Campisi, J. Senescent fibroblasts promote epithelial cell growth and tumorigenesis: A link between cancer and aging. *Proc. Natl. Acad. Sci. USA* **2001**, *98*, 12072–12077. [CrossRef] [PubMed]
314. Falandry, C.; Bonnefoy, M.; Freyer, G.; Gilson, E. Biology of cancer and aging: A complex association with cellular senescence. *J. Clin. Oncol.* **2014**, *32*, 2604–2610. [CrossRef]
315. Jugl, S.; Keshwani, S.; Adkins, L.; Heldermon, C.D.; Winterstein, A.; Goodin, A. A systematic review of evidence for cannabis and cannabinoids as adjuvant therapy in palliative and supportive oncology care. *J. Clin. Oncol.* **2020**, *38*, 12091. [CrossRef]
316. Laezza, C.; Pagano, C.; Navarra, G.; Pastorino, O.; Proto, M.C.; Fiore, D.; Piscopo, C.; Gazzerro, P.; Bifulco, M. The endocannabinoid system: A target for cancer treatment. *Int. J. Mol. Sci.* **2020**, *21*, 747. [CrossRef]
317. Ramer, R.; Schwarz, R.; Hinz, B. Modulation of the endocannabinoid system as a potential anticancer strategy. *Front. Pharmacol.* **2019**, *10*, 430. [CrossRef]
318. Hinz, B.; Ramer, R. Anti-tumour actions of cannabinoids. *Br. J. Pharmacol.* **2019**, *176*, 1384–1394. [CrossRef]
319. Ruiz, L.; Miguel, A.; Díaz-Laviada, I. Delta9-tetrahydrocannabinol induces apoptosis in human prostate PC-3 cells via a receptor-independent mechanism. *FEBS Lett.* **1999**, *458*, 400–404. [CrossRef]
320. Orellana-Serradell, O.; Poblete, C.E.; Sanchez, C.; Castellón, E.A.; Gallegos, I.; Huidobro, C.; Llanos, M.N.; Contreras, H.R. Proapoptotic effect of endocannabinoids in prostate cancer cells. *Oncol. Rep.* **2015**, *33*, 1599–1608. [CrossRef] [PubMed]
321. De Petrocellis, L.; Ligresti, A.; Schiano Moriello, A.; Iappelli, M.; Verde, R.; Stott, C.G.; Cristino, L.; Orlando, P.; Di Marzo, V. Non-THC cannabinoids inhibit prostate carcinoma growth in vitro and in vivo: Pro-apoptotic effects and underlying mechanisms. *Br. J. Pharmacol.* **2013**, *168*, 79–102. [CrossRef]
322. Morell, C.; Bort, A.; Vara, D.; Ramos-Torres, A.; Rodríguez-Henche, N.; Díaz-Laviada, I. The cannabinoid WIN 55,212-2 prevents neuroendocrine differentiation of LNCaP prostate cancer cells. *Prostate Cancer Prostatic Dis.* **2016**, *19*, 248–257. [CrossRef] [PubMed]
323. Sarfaraz, S.; Afaq, F.; Adhami, V.M.; Malik, A.; Mukhtar, H. Cannabinoid receptor agonist-induced apoptosis of human prostate cancer cells LNCaP proceeds through sustained activation of ERK1/2 leading to G1 cell cycle arrest. *J. Biol. Chem.* **2006**, *281*, 39480–39491. [CrossRef]
324. Sánchez, M.G.; Sánchez, A.M.; Ruiz-Llorente, L.; Díaz-Laviada, I. Enhancement of androgen receptor expression induced by (R)-methanandamide in prostate LNCaP cells. *FEBS Lett.* **2003**, *555*, 561–566. [CrossRef]

325. Santoro, A.; Pisanti, S.; Grimaldi, C.; Izzo, A.A.; Borrelli, F.; Proto, M.C.; Malfitano, A.M.; Gazzerro, P.; Laezza, C.; Bifulco, M. Rimonabant inhibits human colon cancer cell growth and reduces the formation of precancerous lesions in the mouse colon. *Int. J. Cancer* **2009**, *125*, 996–1003. [CrossRef]
326. Lin, Y.; Xu, J.; Lan, H. Tumor-associated macrophages in tumor metastasis: Biological roles and clinical therapeutic applications. *J. Hematol. Oncol.* **2019**, *12*, 76. [CrossRef]
327. Nallathambi, R.; Mazuz, M.; Namdar, D.; Shik, M.; Namintzer, D.; Vinayaka, A.C.; Ion, A.; Faigenboim, A.; Nasser, A.; Laish, I.; et al. Identification of Synergistic Interaction Between Cannabis-Derived Compounds for Cytotoxic Activity in Colorectal Cancer Cell Lines and Colon Polyps That Induces Apoptosis-Related Cell Death and Distinct Gene Expression. *Cannabis Cannabinoid Res.* **2018**, *3*, 120–135. [CrossRef] [PubMed]
328. Proto, M.C.; Gazzerro, P.; Di Croce, L.; Santoro, A.; Malfitano, A.M.; Pisanti, S.; Laezza, C.; Bifulco, M. Interaction of endocannabinoid system and steroid hormones in the control of colon cancer cell growth. *J. Cell Physiol.* **2012**, *227*, 250–258. [CrossRef] [PubMed]
329. McAllister, S.D.; Murase, R.; Christian, R.T.; Lau, D.; Zielinski, A.J.; Allison, J.; Almanza, C.; Pakdel, A.; Lee, J.; Limbad, C.; et al. Pathways mediating the effects of cannabidiol on the reduction of breast cancer cell proliferation, invasion, and metastasis. *Breast Cancer Res. Treat.* **2011**, *129*, 37–47. [CrossRef]
330. Hirao-Suzuki, M.; Takeda, S.; Koga, T.; Takiguchi, M.; Toda, A. Cannabidiolic acid dampens the expression of cyclooxygenase-2 in MDA-MB-231 breast cancer cells: Possible implication of the peroxisome proliferator-activated receptor β/δ abrogation. *J. Toxicol. Sci.* **2020**, *45*, 227–236. [CrossRef]
331. Clark, T.M. Scoping Review and Meta-Analysis Suggests that Cannabis Use May Reduce Cancer Risk in the United States. *Cannabis Cannabinoid Res.* **2021**, *6*, 413–434. [CrossRef] [PubMed]
332. Hermanson, D.J.; Marnett, L.J. Cannabinoids, endocannabinoids, and cancer. *Cancer Metastasis Rev.* **2011**, *30*, 599–612. [CrossRef]
333. Elbaz, M.; Nasser, M.W.; Ravi, J.; Wani, N.A.; Ahirwar, D.K.; Zhao, H.; Oghumu, S.; Satoskar, A.R.; Shilo, K.; Carson, W.E.; et al. Modulation of the tumor microenvironment and inhibition of EGF/EGFR pathway: Novel anti-tumor mechanisms of Cannabidiol in breast cancer. *Mol. Oncol.* **2015**, *9*, 906–919. [CrossRef] [PubMed]
334. Wu, Y.; Li, Y.-Y.; Matsushima, K.; Baba, T.; Mukaida, N. CCL3-CCR5 axis regulates intratumoral accumulation of leukocytes and fibroblasts and promotes angiogenesis in murine lung metastasis process. *J. Immunol.* **2008**, *181*, 6384–6393. [CrossRef] [PubMed]
335. Su, S.; Liu, Q.; Chen, J.; Chen, J.; Chen, F.; He, C.; Huang, D.; Wu, W.; Lin, L.; Huang, W.; et al. A positive feedback loop between mesenchymal-like cancer cells and macrophages is essential to breast cancer metastasis. *Cancer Cell* **2014**, *25*, 605–620. [CrossRef]
336. Hsu, C.-J.; Wu, M.-H.; Chen, C.-Y.; Tsai, C.-H.; Hsu, H.-C.; Tang, C.-H. AMP-activated protein kinase activation mediates CCL3-induced cell migration and matrix metalloproteinase-2 expression in human chondrosarcoma. *Cell Commun. Signal.* **2013**, *11*, 68. [CrossRef]
337. Xu, X.; Liu, Y.; Huang, S.; Liu, G.; Xie, C.; Zhou, J.; Fan, W.; Li, Q.; Wang, Q.; Zhong, D.; et al. Overexpression of cannabinoid receptors CB1 and CB2 correlates with improved prognosis of patients with hepatocellular carcinoma. *Cancer Genet. Cytogenet.* **2006**, *171*, 31–38. [CrossRef]
338. Sánchez, C.; de Ceballos, M.L.; Gomez del Pulgar, T.; Rueda, D.; Corbacho, C.; Velasco, G.; Galve-Roperh, I.; Huffman, J.W.; Ramón y Cajal, S.; Guzmán, M. Inhibition of glioma growth in vivo by selective activation of the CB(2) cannabinoid receptor. *Cancer Res.* **2001**, *61*, 5784–5789.
339. Milian, L.; Mata, M.; Alcacer, J.; Oliver, M.; Sancho-Tello, M.; Martín de Llano, J.J.; Camps, C.; Galbis, J.; Carretero, J.; Carda, C. Cannabinoid receptor expression in non-small cell lung cancer. Effectiveness of tetrahydrocannabinol and cannabidiol inhibiting cell proliferation and epithelial-mesenchymal transition in vitro. *PLoS ONE* **2020**, *15*, e0228909. [CrossRef] [PubMed]
340. Cipriano, M.; Häggström, J.; Hammarsten, P.; Fowler, C.J. Association between cannabinoid CB_1 receptor expression and Akt signalling in prostate cancer. *PLoS ONE* **2013**, *8*, e65798. [CrossRef]
341. Chung, S.C.; Hammarsten, P.; Josefsson, A.; Stattin, P.; Granfors, T.; Egevad, L.; Mancini, G.; Lutz, B.; Bergh, A.; Fowler, C.J. A high cannabinoid CB(1) receptor immunoreactivity is associated with disease severity and outcome in prostate cancer. *Eur. J. Cancer* **2009**, *45*, 174–182. [CrossRef]
342. Lakiotaki, E.; Giaginis, C.; Tolia, M.; Alexandrou, P.; Delladetsima, I.; Giannopoulou, I.; Kyrgias, G.; Patsouris, E.; Theocharis, S. Clinical significance of cannabinoid receptors CB1 and CB2 expression in human malignant and benign thyroid lesions. *Biomed. Res. Int.* **2015**, *2015*, 839403. [CrossRef] [PubMed]
343. Michalski, C.W.; Oti, F.E.; Erkan, M.; Sauliunaite, D.; Bergmann, F.; Pacher, P.; Batkai, S.; Müller, M.W.; Giese, N.A.; Friess, H.; et al. Cannabinoids in pancreatic cancer: Correlation with survival and pain. *Int. J. Cancer* **2008**, *122*, 742–750. [CrossRef] [PubMed]
344. Martínez-Martínez, E.; Martín-Ruiz, A.; Martín, P.; Calvo, V.; Provencio, M.; García, J.M. CB2 cannabinoid receptor activation promotes colon cancer progression via AKT/GSK3β signaling pathway. *Oncotarget* **2016**, *7*, 68781–68791. [CrossRef]
345. Jung, C.K.; Kang, W.K.; Park, J.M.; Ahn, H.J.; Kim, S.W.; Taek Oh, S.; Choi, K.Y. Expression of the cannabinoid type I receptor and prognosis following surgery in colorectal cancer. *Oncol. Lett.* **2013**, *5*, 870–876. [CrossRef]
346. Klein Nulent, T.J.W.; Van Diest, P.J.; van der Groep, P.; Leusink, F.K.J.; Kruitwagen, C.L.J.J.; Koole, R.; Van Cann, E.M. Cannabinoid receptor-2 immunoreactivity is associated with survival in squamous cell carcinoma of the head and neck. *Br. J. Oral. Maxillofac. Surg.* **2013**, *51*, 604–609. [CrossRef]
347. Ellert-Miklaszewska, A.; Grajkowska, W.; Gabrusiewicz, K.; Kaminska, B.; Konarska, L. Distinctive pattern of cannabinoid receptor type II (CB2) expression in adult and pediatric brain tumors. *Brain Res.* **2007**, *1137*, 161–169. [CrossRef] [PubMed]

348. Urban, D.; Cherny, N.; Catane, R. The management of cancer pain in the elderly. *Crit. Rev. Oncol. Hematol.* **2010**, *73*, 176–183. [CrossRef]
349. Herr, K.; Coyne, P.J.; McCaffery, M.; Manworren, R.; Merkel, S. Pain assessment in the patient unable to self-report: Position statement with clinical practice recommendations. *Pain Manag. Nurs.* **2011**, *12*, 230–250. [CrossRef] [PubMed]
350. Mlost, J.; Bryk, M.; Starowicz, K. Cannabidiol for pain treatment: Focus on pharmacology and mechanism of action. *Int. J. Mol. Sci.* **2020**, *21*, 8870. [CrossRef]
351. Xu, D.H.; Cullen, B.D.; Tang, M.; Fang, Y. The effectiveness of topical cannabidiol oil in symptomatic relief of peripheral neuropathy of the lower extremities. *Curr. Pharm. Biotechnol.* **2020**, *21*, 390–402. [CrossRef]
352. Portenoy, R.K.; Ganae-Motan, E.D.; Allende, S.; Yanagihara, R.; Shaiova, L.; Weinstein, S.; McQuade, R.; Wright, S.; Fallon, M.T. Nabiximols for opioid-treated cancer patients with poorly-controlled chronic pain: A randomized, placebo-controlled, graded-dose trial. *J. Pain* **2012**, *13*, 438–449. [CrossRef]
353. Johnson, J.R.; Burnell-Nugent, M.; Lossignol, D.; Ganae-Motan, E.D.; Potts, R.; Fallon, M.T. Multicenter, double-blind, randomized, placebo-controlled, parallel-group study of the efficacy, safety, and tolerability of THC:CBD extract and THC extract in patients with intractable cancer-related pain. *J. Pain Symptom Manag.* **2010**, *39*, 167–179. [CrossRef]
354. Lynch, M.E.; Cesar-Rittenberg, P.; Hohmann, A.G. A double-blind, placebo-controlled, crossover pilot trial with extension using an oral mucosal cannabinoid extract for treatment of chemotherapy-induced neuropathic pain. *J. Pain Symptom Manag.* **2014**, *47*, 166–173. [CrossRef]
355. Hamaker, M.E.; Prins, M.C.; Stauder, R. The relevance of a geriatric assessment for elderly patients with a haematological malignancy–a systematic review. *Leuk. Res.* **2014**, *38*, 275–283. [CrossRef]
356. Pérez-Zepeda, M.U.; Cárdenas-Cárdenas, E.; Cesari, M.; Navarrete-Reyes, A.P.; Gutiérrez-Robledo, L.M. Cancer and frailty in older adults: A nested case-control study of the Mexican Health and Aging Study. *J. Cancer Surviv.* **2016**, *10*, 736–742. [CrossRef] [PubMed]
357. Pagano, C.; Navarra, G.; Coppola, L.; Avilia, G.; Bifulco, M.; Laezza, C. Cannabinoids: Therapeutic use in clinical practice. *Int. J. Mol. Sci.* **2022**, *23*, 3344. [CrossRef] [PubMed]
358. Sharkey, K.A.; Wiley, J.W. The Role of the Endocannabinoid System in the Brain-Gut Axis. *Gastroenterology* **2016**, *151*, 252–266. [CrossRef] [PubMed]
359. Grimison, P.; Mersiades, A.; Kirby, A.; Lintzeris, N.; Morton, R.; Haber, P.; Olver, I.; Walsh, A.; McGregor, I.; Cheung, Y.; et al. Oral THC:CBD cannabis extract for refractory chemotherapy-induced nausea and vomiting: A randomised, placebo-controlled, phase II crossover trial. *Ann. Oncol.* **2020**, *31*, 1553–1560. [CrossRef] [PubMed]
360. Duran, M.; Pérez, E.; Abanades, S.; Vidal, X.; Saura, C.; Majem, M.; Arriola, E.; Rabanal, M.; Pastor, A.; Farré, M.; et al. Preliminary efficacy and safety of an oromucosal standardized cannabis extract in chemotherapy-induced nausea and vomiting. *Br. J. Clin. Pharmacol.* **2010**, *70*, 656–663. [CrossRef] [PubMed]
361. Williams, G.R.; Rier, H.N.; McDonald, A.; Shachar, S.S. Sarcopenia & aging in cancer. *J. Geriatr. Oncol.* **2019**, *10*, 374–377. [CrossRef]
362. Fearon, K.; Strasser, F.; Anker, S.D.; Bosaeus, I.; Bruera, E.; Fainsinger, R.L.; Jatoi, A.; Loprinzi, C.; MacDonald, N.; Mantovani, G.; et al. Definition and classification of cancer cachexia: An international consensus. *Lancet Oncol.* **2011**, *12*, 489–495. [CrossRef]
363. Haney, M.; Gunderson, E.W.; Rabkin, J.; Hart, C.L.; Vosburg, S.K.; Comer, S.D.; Foltin, R.W. Dronabinol and marijuana in HIV-positive marijuana smokers. Caloric intake, mood, and sleep. *J. Acquir. Immune Defic. Syndr.* **2007**, *45*, 545–554. [CrossRef]
364. Jatoi, A.; Windschitl, H.E.; Loprinzi, C.L.; Sloan, J.A.; Dakhil, S.R.; Mailliard, J.A.; Pundaleeka, S.; Kardinal, C.G.; Fitch, T.R.; Krook, J.E.; et al. Dronabinol versus megestrol acetate versus combination therapy for cancer-associated anorexia: A North Central Cancer Treatment Group study. *J. Clin. Oncol.* **2002**, *20*, 567–573. [CrossRef]
365. Rao, A.; Cohen, H.J. Symptom management in the elderly cancer patient: Fatigue, pain, and depression. *J. Natl. Cancer Inst. Monogr.* **2004**, *2004*, 150–157. [CrossRef]
366. Katon, W.J.; Schoenbaum, M.; Fan, M.-Y.; Callahan, C.M.; Williams, J.; Hunkeler, E.; Harpole, L.; Zhou, X.-H.A.; Langston, C.; Unützer, J. Cost-effectiveness of improving primary care treatment of late-life depression. *Arch. Gen. Psychiatry* **2005**, *62*, 1313–1320. [CrossRef]
367. Roth, A.J.; Modi, R. Psychiatric issues in older cancer patients. *Crit. Rev. Oncol. Hematol.* **2003**, *48*, 185–197. [CrossRef]
368. Kurtz, M.E.; Kurtz, J.C.; Stommel, M.; Given, C.W.; Given, B. Predictors of depressive symptomatology of geriatric patients with colorectal cancer: A longitudinal view. *Support Care Cancer* **2002**, *10*, 494–501. [CrossRef] [PubMed]
369. Alici, Y.; Weiss, T.; Holland, J.C.; Nelson, C.; Roth, A. Common psychiatric problems in older patients with cancer: Report of one-year experience of a psychiatry outpatient clinic. *J. Geriatr. Oncol.* **2011**, *2*, 137–141. [CrossRef]
370. Good, P.D.; Greer, R.M.; Huggett, G.E.; Hardy, J.R. An Open-Label Pilot Study Testing the Feasibility of Assessing Total Symptom Burden in Trials of Cannabinoid Medications in Palliative Care. *J. Palliat. Med.* **2020**, *23*, 650–655. [CrossRef] [PubMed]
371. Heidenreich, P.A.; Trogdon, J.G.; Khavjou, O.A.; Butler, J.; Dracup, K.; Ezekowitz, M.D.; Finkelstein, E.A.; Hong, Y.; Johnston, S.C.; Khera, A.; et al. Forecasting the future of cardiovascular disease in the United States: A policy statement from the American Heart Association. *Circulation* **2011**, *123*, 933–944. [CrossRef] [PubMed]
372. Costantino, S.; Paneni, F.; Cosentino, F. Ageing, metabolism and cardiovascular disease. *J. Physiol.* **2016**, *594*, 2061–2073. [CrossRef] [PubMed]
373. Bondarenko, A.I. Cannabinoids and cardiovascular system. *Adv. Exp. Med. Biol.* **2019**, *1162*, 63–87. [CrossRef]

374. Bondarenko, A.I.; Panasiuk, O.; Okhai, I.; Montecucco, F.; Brandt, K.J.; Mach, F. Ca^{2+}-dependent potassium channels and cannabinoid signaling in the endothelium of apolipoprotein E knockout mice before plaque formation. *J. Mol. Cell. Cardiol.* **2018**, *115*, 54–63. [CrossRef]
375. Khan, R.N.; Maner-Smith, K.; Owens, J.A.; Barbian, M.E.; Jones, R.M.; Naudin, C.R. At the heart of microbial conversations: Endocannabinoids and the microbiome in cardiometabolic risk. *Gut Microbes* **2021**, *13*, 1911572. [CrossRef]
376. Bátkai, S.; Pacher, P.; Osei-Hyiaman, D.; Radaeva, S.; Liu, J.; Harvey-White, J.; Offertáler, L.; Mackie, K.; Rudd, M.A.; Bukoski, R.D.; et al. Endocannabinoids acting at cannabinoid-1 receptors regulate cardiovascular function in hypertension. *Circulation* **2004**, *110*, 1996–2002. [CrossRef]
377. Pacher, P.; Steffens, S. The emerging role of the endocannabinoid system in cardiovascular disease. *Semin. Immunopathol.* **2009**, *31*, 63–77. [CrossRef]
378. Haspula, D.; Clark, M.A. Cannabinoid receptors: An update on cell signaling, pathophysiological roles and therapeutic opportunities in neurological, cardiovascular, and inflammatory diseases. *Int. J. Mol. Sci.* **2020**, *21*, 7693. [CrossRef] [PubMed]
379. Fuchs, F.D.; Whelton, P.K. High blood pressure and cardiovascular disease. *Hypertension* **2020**, *75*, 285–292. [CrossRef] [PubMed]
380. Noubiap, J.J.; Nansseu, J.R.; Nyaga, U.F.; Sime, P.S.; Francis, I.; Bigna, J.J. Global prevalence of resistant hypertension: A meta-analysis of data from 3.2 million patients. *Heart* **2019**, *105*, 98–105. [CrossRef] [PubMed]
381. Pacher, P.; Bátkai, S.; Kunos, G. The endocannabinoid system as an emerging target of pharmacotherapy. *Pharmacol. Rev.* **2006**, *58*, 389–462. [CrossRef]
382. Martín Giménez, V.M.; Noriega, S.E.; Kassuha, D.E.; Fuentes, L.B.; Manucha, W. Anandamide and endocannabinoid system: An attractive therapeutic approach for cardiovascular disease. *Ther. Adv. Cardiovasc. Dis.* **2018**, *12*, 177–190. [CrossRef] [PubMed]
383. Chawengsub, Y.; Gauthier, K.M.; Campbell, W.B. Role of arachidonic acid lipoxygenase metabolites in the regulation of vascular tone. *Am. J. Physiol. Heart Circ. Physiol.* **2009**, *297*, H495–H507. [CrossRef]
384. Varga, K.; Lake, K.D.; Huangfu, D.; Guyenet, P.G.; Kunos, G. Mechanism of the hypotensive action of anandamide in anesthetized rats. *Hypertension* **1996**, *28*, 682–686. [CrossRef]
385. Pacher, P.; Bátkai, S.; Kunos, G. Blood pressure regulation by endocannabinoids and their receptors. *Neuropharmacology* **2005**, *48*, 1130–1138. [CrossRef]
386. Grzęda, E.; Schlicker, E.; Toczek, M.; Zalewska, I.; Baranowska-Kuczko, M.; Malinowska, B. CB1 receptor activation in the rat paraventricular nucleus induces bi-directional cardiovascular effects via modification of glutamatergic and GABAergic neurotransmission. *Naunyn-Schmiedebergs Arch. Pharmacol.* **2017**, *390*, 25–35. [CrossRef]
387. Pratt, P.F.; Hillard, C.J.; Edgemond, W.S.; Campbell, W.B. N-arachidonylethanolamide relaxation of bovine coronary artery is not mediated by CB1 cannabinoid receptor. *Am. J. Physiol.* **1998**, *274*, H375–H381. [CrossRef]
388. Ritter, J.K.; Li, G.; Xia, M.; Boini, K. Anandamide and its metabolites: What are their roles in the kidney? *Front. Biosci.* **2016**, *8*, 264–277. [CrossRef]
389. Kudalkar, S.N.; Kingsley, P.J.; Marnett, L.J. Assay of Endocannabinoid Oxidation by Cyclooxygenase-2. *Methods Mol. Biol.* **2016**, *1412*, 205–215. [CrossRef]
390. Ritter, J.K.; Li, C.; Xia, M.; Poklis, J.L.; Lichtman, A.H.; Abdullah, R.A.; Dewey, W.L.; Li, P.-L. Production and actions of the anandamide metabolite prostamide E2 in the renal medulla. *J. Pharmacol. Exp. Ther.* **2012**, *342*, 770–779. [CrossRef] [PubMed]
391. Herrington, W.; Lacey, B.; Sherliker, P.; Armitage, J.; Lewington, S. Epidemiology of atherosclerosis and the potential to reduce the global burden of atherothrombotic disease. *Circ. Res.* **2016**, *118*, 535–546. [CrossRef] [PubMed]
392. Haba, M.Ș.C.; Șerban, D.N.; Șerban, L.; Tudorancea, I.M.; Haba, R.M.; Mitu, O.; Iliescu, R.; Tudorancea, I. Nanomaterial-Based Drug Targeted Therapy for Cardiovascular Diseases: Ischemic Heart Failure and Atherosclerosis. *Crystals* **2021**, *11*, 1172. [CrossRef]
393. Wang, J.C.; Bennett, M. Aging and atherosclerosis: Mechanisms, functional consequences, and potential therapeutics for cellular senescence. *Circ. Res.* **2012**, *111*, 245–259. [CrossRef] [PubMed]
394. Sugamura, K.; Sugiyama, S.; Nozaki, T.; Matsuzawa, Y.; Izumiya, Y.; Miyata, K.; Nakayama, M.; Kaikita, K.; Obata, T.; Takeya, M.; et al. Activated endocannabinoid system in coronary artery disease and antiinflammatory effects of cannabinoid 1 receptor blockade on macrophages. *Circulation* **2009**, *119*, 28–36. [CrossRef]
395. Steffens, M.; Zentner, J.; Honegger, J.; Feuerstein, T.J. Binding affinity and agonist activity of putative endogenous cannabinoids at the human neocortical CB1 receptor. *Biochem. Pharmacol.* **2005**, *69*, 169–178. [CrossRef]
396. Netherland, C.D.; Pickle, T.G.; Bales, A.; Thewke, D.P. Cannabinoid receptor type 2 (CB2) deficiency alters atherosclerotic lesion formation in hyperlipidemic Ldlr-null mice. *Atherosclerosis* **2010**, *213*, 102–108. [CrossRef] [PubMed]
397. Chiurchiù, V.; Lanuti, M.; Catanzaro, G.; Fezza, F.; Rapino, C.; Maccarrone, M. Detailed characterization of the endocannabinoid system in human macrophages and foam cells, and anti-inflammatory role of type-2 cannabinoid receptor. *Atherosclerosis* **2014**, *233*, 55–63. [CrossRef] [PubMed]
398. Pacher, P.; Steffens, S.; Haskó, G.; Schindler, T.H.; Kunos, G. Cardiovascular effects of marijuana and synthetic cannabinoids: The good, the bad, and the ugly. *Nat. Rev. Cardiol.* **2018**, *15*, 151–166. [CrossRef] [PubMed]
399. Alfulaij, N.; Meiners, F.; Michalek, J.; Small-Howard, A.L.; Turner, H.C.; Stokes, A.J. Cannabinoids, the heart of the matter. *J. Am. Heart Assoc.* **2018**, *7*, e009099. [CrossRef]

400. Rajesh, M.; Mukhopadhyay, P.; Bátkai, S.; Haskó, G.; Liaudet, L.; Huffman, J.W.; Csiszar, A.; Ungvari, Z.; Mackie, K.; Chatterjee, S.; et al. CB2-receptor stimulation attenuates TNF-alpha-induced human endothelial cell activation, transendothelial migration of monocytes, and monocyte-endothelial adhesion. *Am. J. Physiol. Heart Circ. Physiol.* **2007**, *293*, H2210–H2218. [CrossRef] [PubMed]
401. Dato, S.; Bellizzi, D.; Rose, G.; Passarino, G. The impact of nutrients on the aging rate: A complex interaction of demographic, environmental and genetic factors. *Mech. Ageing Dev.* **2016**, *154*, 49–61. [CrossRef]
402. Morris, B.J.; Willcox, B.J.; Donlon, T.A. Genetic and epigenetic regulation of human aging and longevity. *Biochim. Biophys. Acta Mol. Basis Dis.* **2019**, *1865*, 1718–1744. [CrossRef] [PubMed]
403. Bridgeman, M.B.; Abazia, D.T. Medicinal cannabis: History, pharmacology, and implications for the acute care setting. *Pharm. Ther.* **2017**, *42*, 180–188.
404. MacCallum, C.A.; Russo, E.B. Practical considerations in medical cannabis administration and dosing. *Eur. J. Intern. Med.* **2018**, *49*, 12–19. [CrossRef]
405. Colizzi, M.; Bhattacharyya, S. Cannabis use and the development of tolerance: A systematic review of human evidence. *Neurosci. Biobehav. Rev.* **2018**, *93*, 1–25. [CrossRef]

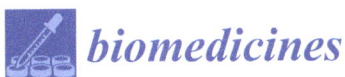

Review

Anti-Microbial Activity of Phytocannabinoids and Endocannabinoids in the Light of Their Physiological and Pathophysiological Roles

Ronit Vogt Sionov * and Doron Steinberg

The Biofilm Laboratory, The Institute of Biomedical and Oral Sciences, The Faculty of Dentistry, The Hebrew University—Hadassah Medical School, Jerusalem 9112102, Israel; dorons@ekmd.huji.ac.il
* Correspondence: ronit.sionov@mail.huji.ac.il

Abstract: Antibiotic resistance has become an increasing challenge in the treatment of various infectious diseases, especially those associated with biofilm formation on biotic and abiotic materials. There is an urgent need for new treatment protocols that can also target biofilm-embedded bacteria. Many secondary metabolites of plants possess anti-bacterial activities, and especially the phytocannabinoids of the *Cannabis sativa* L. varieties have reached a renaissance and attracted much attention for their anti-microbial and anti-biofilm activities at concentrations below the cytotoxic threshold on normal mammalian cells. Accordingly, many synthetic cannabinoids have been designed with the intention to increase the specificity and selectivity of the compounds. The structurally unrelated endocannabinoids have also been found to have anti-microbial and anti-biofilm activities. Recent data suggest for a mutual communication between the endocannabinoid system and the gut microbiota. The present review focuses on the anti-microbial activities of phytocannabinoids and endocannabinoids integrated with some selected issues of their many physiological and pharmacological activities.

Keywords: anti-microbial activity; anti-biofilm activity; *Cannabis sativa* L.; endocannabinoids; gut microbiota; pathogens; phytocannabinoids

Citation: Sionov, R.V.; Steinberg, D. Anti-Microbial Activity of Phytocannabinoids and Endocannabinoids in the Light of Their Physiological and Pathophysiological Roles. *Biomedicines* **2022**, *10*, 631. https://doi.org/10.3390/biomedicines10030631

Academic Editor: Wesley M. Raup-Konsavage

Received: 17 February 2022
Accepted: 8 March 2022
Published: 9 March 2022

Publisher's Note: MDPI stays neutral with regard to jurisdictional claims in published maps and institutional affiliations.

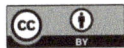

Copyright: © 2022 by the authors. Licensee MDPI, Basel, Switzerland. This article is an open access article distributed under the terms and conditions of the Creative Commons Attribution (CC BY) license (https://creativecommons.org/licenses/by/4.0/).

1. Introduction

Plant medicine has often been used for the treatment of diverse diseases, including bacterial and fungal infections [1–8]. The plants produce a series of secondary metabolites, many of which have pharmacological as well as anti-microbial activities [4–6,9–11]. Evolutionarily, plants have developed various anti-microbial mechanisms to protect them from infectious diseases [11]. Usually, these include the production of compounds that have anti-biofilm and bacteriostatic activities rather than biocidal effect [11]. Compounds with anti-biofilm activities are believed not to induce resistance mechanisms in the microbes, since they target processes not essential for their survival. In contrast, compounds with bactericidal activity might lead to the development of resistance mechanisms in the microbe as part of the bacterial fitness adaptation process with increased probability of developing microbial plant infections.

Cannabis sativa L. subspecies are plants that contain a large variety of secondary metabolites, including phytocannabinoids, terpenoids and flavonoids, which have profound anti-microbial activities, in addition to possessing anti-inflammatory, anti-oxidative and neuromodulatory properties [12–14]. In mammalians, the phytocannabinoids interact with the same receptors (e.g., cannabinoid receptors CB1 and CB2) as the endocannabinoids [15], which are endogenous substances with anti-microbial, anti-inflammatory and neuromodulatory activities [16–24]. While much is known about the cannabinoid targets in mammalians, so far, little is known about the microbial targets of these compounds. It is likely that these compounds also interact with specific targets in the microbes. The present review focuses on the anti-microbial activities of phytocannabinoids and endocannabinoids interwoven with selected aspects of their many physiological and pathophysiological activities.

2. Cannabis sativa L.

The hemp plant (*Cannabis sativa* L.; L = Linnaeus) belonging to the family *Cannabaceae*, originates in central-northeast Asia where it has been cultivated for more than 5000 years [15,25,26]. The Han Chinese dynasty used *Cannabis* to treat inflammatory disorders and malaria [27,28]. The Chinese pharmacopoeia of the Emperor Shen Nung, who lived approximately around 2700 BCE and is considered "The Father of Chinese Medicine", indicated *Cannabis* plant usage for the treatment of rheumatic pain, constipation, malaria, and gynecological disorders [26]. In modern times, this plant has been used for different medical conditions, including alleviating chronic pain (e.g., in cancer patients and in rheumatic diseases), muscle spasms (e.g., in multiple sclerosis), epileptic convulsion (e.g., Dravet syndrome and Lennox–Gastaut syndrome in children), nausea (e.g., following chemotherapy), intestinal inflammation (e.g., colitis, inflammatory bowel disease (IBD)), and for stimulating appetite (e.g., in devastating AIDS syndrome, anorexia, and cancer patients) [26,29,30]. It has also been used as a treatment remedy for cancer patients, since the phytocannabinoids can inhibit cell growth of certain tumor cells and enhance the efficacy of certain cancer therapeutics [31].

The phenotypes of *Cannabis* plants are highly variable and can be classified into three major subspecies: *Cannabis sativa* subsp. *sativa*, *Cannabis sativa* subsp. *indica*, and *Cannabis sativa* subsp. *ruderalis* [32]. The different subspecies have all been classified to the *Cannabis sativa* L. species [32]. There are also several chemovariants, chemotypes, or cultivars of this plant harboring different composition of chemical compounds [33–36]. Different *Cannabis* cultivars or chemotypes have been developed that contain various ratios of cannabidiol (CBD) and Δ^9-tetrahydrocannabinol (Δ^9-THC), and even those containing high CBD and low Δ^9-THC content, which is favorable for avoiding the psychomimetic effects of Δ^9-THC [33,37]. The cannabinoids are found in most parts of the plant, with the highest concentrations in glandular trichomes on the surfaces of leaves and flowers [38–42].

The chemical composition of *Cannabis* is affected by the ripeness and maturation state of the plant, growth conditions, the sowing and the harvest times, as well as the storage conditions [34,38–41,43]. The plant composition of phytocannabinoids is affected by light, temperature, water supply, nutrition, heavy metals, phytohormones, soil bacteria, insects and microbial pathogens, among others [44–47]. Cannabidiolic acid (CBDA), the precursor of cannabinols, predominates in the unripen plant, while it is converted to CBD, Δ^9-THC and cannabinol (CBN) upon ripening of the resin [48]. In the intermediate ripening state, CBD is predominant, then Δ^9-THC dominates in the ripened state, while CBN, the final conversion product, is the major compound in the overripened resin [48]. High anti-microbial activity was found especially in unripen *Cannabis* harvested from regions with unfavorable climate for this plant, whereas ripened *Cannabis* taken from tropical areas had a more hashish-active composition [48]. For the optimal production of essential oil, the recommended stage for harvest is one to three weeks before seed maturity [43].

The difference between industrial hemp and the high Δ^9-THC hemp breed type marijuana is that the industrial hemp contains minute amounts of Δ^9-THC (less than 0.2% (w/v)), while marijuana flowers and leaves may contain as much as 17–28% Δ^9-THC [49]. Even concentrated THC products, such as oil, shatter, and dab, have been produced with a concentration of up to 95% Δ^9-THC [49]. The use of marijuana is associated with hallucinations due to the high Δ^9-THC content and may lead to addiction, lack of judgement, and reduced cognition, especially during adolescence when the brain is undergoing significant development [49]. Smoking hemp may lead to decreased immune function with a consequent increase in opportunistic infections [50–53]. *Cannabis* users have a higher probability to get fungal infections than non-*Cannabis* users, which might in part be due to fungal contamination of the *Cannabis* product [54].

2.1. Anti-Microbial Activity of Cannabis sativa L. Extracts

Z. Krejčí, in the 1950s, observed that *Cannabis* has antibiotic activity and introduced it to the clinics in Czechoslovakia [55], a practice that was discontinued in 1990 [33]. The first compound identified by Krejčí with antibiotic activity was named cannabidiolic acid (CBDA) [56,57]. From then on, several other *Cannabis* components with antibiotic activities have been isolated and characterized [48,58–63], which will be further discussed below. In 1956, L. Ferenczy published a paper documenting that plant seeds from various plant species, including those from *Cannabis sativa*, exhibited antibacterial activity, especially against Gram-positive bacteria [64]. Wasim et al. [65] documented that both ethanolic and petroleum ether extracts of *Cannabis sativa* leaves showed anti-microbial activity against *Bacillus subtilis*, *Staphylococcus aureus*, *Micrococcus flavus*, *Bordetella bronchiseptica*, *Proteus vulgaris*, *Aspergillus niger*, and *Candida albicans*. Ali et al. [66] observed that the oil of the seeds of *Cannabis sativa* exerted pronounced anti-bacterial activity against *Bacillus subtilis* and *Staphylococcus aureus*, with moderate activity against *Escherichia coli* and *Pseudomonas aeruginosa*, without any activity against *Aspergillus niger* and *Candida albicans*. The petroleum ether extract of the whole plant showed high anti-bacterial activity against *Bacillus subtilis* and *Staphylococcus aureus*, moderate activity against *Escherichia coli*, while no activity against *Pseudomonas aeruginosa* or the tested fungi [66]. Thus, the extraction method and the source affect the composition of the anti-microbial content and the spectrum of responding microbes.

2.2. Anti-Microbial Activity of Essential Oils from Cannabis sativa L.

Novak et al. [67] analyzed the anti-bacterial effect of essential oils prepared from five different cultivars of *Cannabis sativa* L. These essential oils contained, among others, α-pinene, myrcene, trans-β-ocimene, α-terpinolene, trans-caryophyllene, and α-humulene, but undetectable levels of Δ^9-THC and very poor levels of other cannabinoids [67]. They observed differences in the anti-bacterial activity between the various cultivars. All five essential oils showed anti-bacterial activity against *Acinetobacter calcoaceticus*, *Beneckea natriegens*, *Brochothrix thermosphacta* and *Staphylococcus aureus* [67]. Only one of the five essential oils had an anti-bacterial effect on *Escherichia coli*, while none affected *Enterobacter aerogenes*, *Klebsiella pneumoniae*, *Proteus vulgaris*, *Salmonella pullorum*, *Serratia marcescens*, or *Streptococcus faecalis* [67].

Nissen et al. [34] observed that essential oils of *Cannabis sativa* L., prepared from 50–70% of seed maturity, showed anti-bacterial activity against the Gram-positive bacteria *Enterococcus faecium* and *Streptococcus salivarius* at less than 1% (v/v) but were unable to inhibit the growth of the yeast *Saccharomyces cerevisiae*. Zengin et al. [68] found that essential oils distilled from leaves, inflorescences, and thinner stems of the hemp plant showed anti-oxidative properties and had significant anti-bacterial activity against clinical *Helicobacter pylori* strains (MIC = 16–64 µg/mL), with lower activity against clinical *Staphylococcus aureus* isolates (MIC = 8 mg/mL) and no significant activity against *Candida* spp. and *Malassezia* spp. The minimum bacterial biofilm inhibitory concentration (MBIC) of the hemp essential oil against *Helicobacter pyroli* was similar to the MIC [68]. The hemp essential oil showed cytotoxicity against human breast cancer, cholangiocarcinoma, and colon carcinoma cell lines at 50–75 µg/mL, while 250 µg/mL was required to inhibit the cell proliferation of a nonmalignant cholangiocyte cell line [68]. The LD_{50} of hemp essential oil against larvae of *Galleria mellonella* was found to be 1.56 mg/mL, which is much higher than the anti-bacterial activity against *Helicobacter pyroli*, but lower than that found to be active against *Staphylococcus aureus* strains [68].

Pellegrini et al. [69] observed that essential oil prepared from *Cannabis sativa* L. cultivar Futura 75 inflorescences with low Δ^9-THC content (<0.2%) cultivated in the Abruzzo territory showed anti-bacterial activity against *Staphylococcus aureus* and *Listeria monocytogenes* with a MIC of 1.25–5 µL/mL, while being ineffective against *Salmonella enterica*. They also showed that the essential oil possessed anti-oxidative properties [69]. The essential oils produced from the *Cannabis sativa* L. cultivar Futura 75 inflorescences was also found to have insecticidal activity with LD_{50} values of 65.8 µg/larva on *Spodoptera littoralis*, 122.1 µg/adult on *Musca domestica*, and LC_{50} of 124.5 µL/L on *Culex quinquefasciatus* larvae [70]. The insecticidal effect might in part be due to an inhibition of the enzyme acetylcholinesterase (AChE) [70]. Thomas et al. [71] found that essential oil of *Cannabis sativa* could induce 100% mortality in the mosquito larvae of *Culex tritaeniorhynchus*, *Anopheles stephensi*, *Aedes aegypti*, and *Culex quinquefasciatus* at concentrations of 0.06, 0.1, 0.12, and 0.2 µL/mL, respectively.

Palmieri et al. [72] studied the variability of *Cannabis* essential oils from various origins and observed that the time of distillation affected the chemical composition of terpenic components, sesquiterpenes, and CBD with consequent variations in the anti-microbial activities against *Staphylococcus aureus*, *Listeria monocytogenes*, and *Enterococcus faecium*. Zheljazkov et al. [73] compared the anti-microbial activity of nine wild hemp (*Cannabis sativa* spp. *spontanea* Vavilov) accessions sampled from agricultural fields in northeastern Serbia with 13 EU registered cultivars, eight breeding lines, and one cannabidiol (CBD) hemp strain, which showed variations in the secondary metabolites β-caryophyllene, α-humulene, caryophyllene oxide, and humulene epoxide. The CBD concentration in the essential oils of wild hemp varied from 6.9 to 52.4%, while the CBD content in the essential oils of the registered cultivars, breeding lines, and the CBD strain varied from 7.1 to 25%; 6.4 to 25%; and 7.4 to 8.8%, respectively [73]. The Δ^9-THC concentration showed high variability between the different strains, with the highest concentration being 3.5% [73]. The essential oils of the wild hemp had greater anti-microbial activity compared with the essential oil of registered cultivars [73]. In general, with variations between the different essential oils, anti-microbial activity was observed toward *Staphylococcus aureus*, *Enterococcus faecalis*, *Streptococcus pneumoniae*, *Pseudomonas aeruginosa*, *Yersenia enterocolitica*, *Salmonella enterica*, *Candida albicans*, *Candida krusei*, and *Candida tropicalis* using the disc diffusion method [73]. Altogether, the data presented above show that there is high variability of the composition of hemp essential oils, which might explain the many contradictory publications of the anti-microbial activities toward the same microbial species. In general, a good anti-bacterial response is achieved on Gram-positive bacteria, with less or no effect on Gram-negative bacteria, and variable effect on fungi.

2.3. Anti-Microbial Activity of Terpenoids in Cannabis Essential Oils

Several terpenoids in the *Cannabis* essential oils have been demonstrated to have anti-microbial effect, which include the monoterpenes α-pinene, linalool, and limonene, and the bitter-tasting sesquiterpenes nerolidol, β-caryophyllene, and caryophyllene oxide [33,74–76]. α-Pinene inhibited the growth of both Gram-positive bacteria (e.g., various *Clostridium* species, *Enterococcus faecium*, *Streptococcus salivarius*, *Staphylococcus aureus*, *Staphylococcus epidermidis*, *Streptococcus pyogenes*, *Streptococcus pneumoniae*) and Gram-negative bacteria (e.g., various *Pseudomonas* species), as well as the fungus *Candida albicans* [34,77–79]. Myrcene, which is also found in tea tree oil, inhibited the growth of *Staphylococcus aureus* that was associated with the leakage of K^+ ions from the bacterial cells and damage to the cell membrane [80]. Linalool, a monoterpenoid alcohol, and α-terpineol, a fragrant terpene, showed anti-bacterial activity against *Propionibacterium acne* and *Staphylococcus epidermidis* with a minimum inhibitory concentration (MIC) of 0.625–1.25 µg/mL [77]. Linalool is also effective against the yeast and hyphal forms of *Candida albicans*, where it alters the membrane integrity and induces cell cycle arrest [81]. Limonene showed anti-bacterial activity against *Staphylococcus epidermidis* [77] and *Listeria monocytogenes* [82], and exerted anti-biofilm activity against *Streptococcus pyogenes*, *Streptococcus mutans*, and *Streptococcus mitis* [83]. α-Humulene showed potent anti-fungal activity against *Cryptococcus neoformans*, *Candida glabrata*, and *Candida krusei* with MIC values of 5.0, 1.45, and 10.0 µg/mL, respectively, without any effect on methicillin-sensitive *Staphylococcus aureus* (MSSA) 29213, methicillin-resistant *Staphylococcus aureus* (MRSA) 33591, or *Mycobacterium intracellulare* [84]. Nerolidol is a sesquiterpene with sedative properties and inhibits the growth of *Leishmania amazonensis*, *Leishmania braziliensis*, and *Leishmania chagasi* promastigotes, and *Leishmania amazonensis* amastigotes [85], as well as the growth of *Plasmodium falciparum* at the trophozoite and schizont stages [86,87]. The anti-oxidative β-caryophyllene possesses anti-microbial activity against *Staphylococcus aureus* (MIC 2–4 µM), *Bacillus subtilis* (MIC 6–10 µM), *Escherichia coli* (MIC 7–11 µM), *Pseudomonas aeruginosa* (6–8 µM), *Aspergillus niger* (MIC 5–7 µM), and *Trichoderma reesei* (MIC 3–5 µM) without any significant cytotoxic effect on normal mammalian cell lines [88]. The anti-inflammatory oxygenated sesquiterpene caryophyllene oxide exhibited anti-fungal activities against the dermatophytes *Trichophyton mentagrophytes* var. *mentagrophytes*, *Trichophyton mentagrophytes* var. *interdigitale*, and *Trichophyton rubrum* [89].

3. Phytocannabinoids

The *Cannabis sativa* L. plants produce more than 560 chemicals, including at least 144 cannabinoids and 200 terpenoids, as well as flavonoids and polyunsaturated fatty acids [15,33,34,42,63,67,72,73,90–107]. The most common phytocannabinoids are Δ^9-tetrahydrocannabinol (Δ^9-THC) and cannabidiol (CBD), which are the neutral homologs of tetrahydrocannabinolic acid (THCA) and cannabidiol acid (CBDA), respectively [108]. The phytocannabinoids are terpenophenolic compounds containing a resorcinyl core with a para-positioned isoprenyl, alkyl, or aralkyl side chain [39,40] (Figure 1). The tetrahydrobenzochromen ring is quite unique to the genus *Cannabis*, although a related compound has been found in the liverwort *Radula marginata* [109], and cannabigerol (CBG) and its corresponding acid have been isolated from *Helichrysum umbraculigerum* [110].

Apart from exerting anti-microbial activities, which will be discussed in more detail below (Section 3.3), phytocannabinoids modulate several physiological and pathophysiological processes in humans and other mammalians, making them potential therapeutic drugs in various settings [12–14,31,111–115]. Among others, these compounds have been shown to have anti-inflammatory, anti-oxidative, anti-nausea, anti-nociceptive, anti-convulsant, anti-neoplastic, anxiolytic, and neuroprotective properties [14,111,112,114–117]. Cannabinoids also affect cognition, such as learning and memory, consciousness, and emotion, including anxiety and depression [118,119].

Some cannabinoid-based drugs (e.g., Marinol, Syndros, Cesamet, Sativex, and Epidiolex) have been approved by the U.S. Food and Drug Administration (FDA) for the treatment of epilepsy, Dravet syndrome, Lennox–Gastaut syndrome, Parkinson's disease, spasticity associated with multiple sclerosis, neuropathic pain, mental illnesses, chemotherapy-induced nausea, and AIDS wasting syndrome [117,120–122]. Marinol and Syndros contain the (-)-trans-Δ^9-THC dronabinol; Cesamet contains the synthetic cannabinoid nabilone that shows structural similarities to Δ^9-THC; and Epidiolex contains CBD. Sativex is produced from a *Cannabis*-derived extract that is composed of approximately equal quantities of Δ^9-THC and CBD. A major concern is the production of many psychotropic synthetic cannabinoids distributed on the illicit market, which poses a potential health treat due to their high potency and toxicity [123].

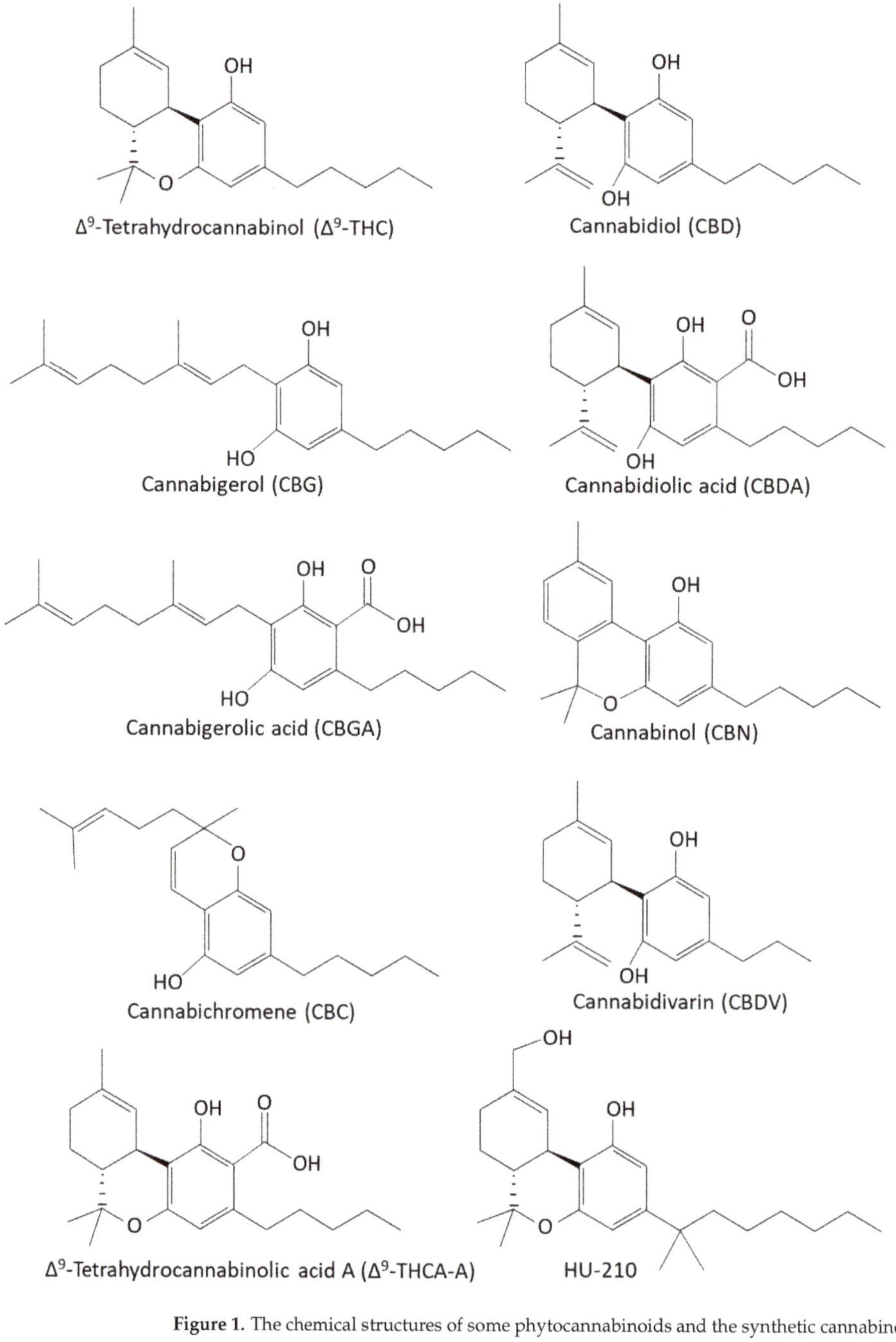

Figure 1. The chemical structures of some phytocannabinoids and the synthetic cannabinoid HU-210.

3.1. Cannabinoid Receptors

The effects of phytocannabinoids on humans and other mammalians are partly mediated by the $G_{i/o}$ protein-coupled CB1 (encoded by the CNR1 gene) and CB2 (encoded by the CNR2 gene) cannabinoid receptors that consist of seven transmembrane domains [124–126].

The stimulation of these receptors leads to the inhibition of adenylyl cyclase with consequent reduction in the intracellular cAMP levels, activation of potassium channels, activation of mitogen-activated protein kinases (MAPKs) such as the extracellular signal-regulated kinase (ERK) and c-Jun N-terminal kinase (JNK), as well as activation of the phosphoinositide-3 kinase (PI3K)/Akt signaling pathways and the mammalian target of rapamycin (mTOR) [126–134].

The CB1 and CB2 receptors also recognize the endogenous arachidonic acid-derived endocannabinoids, such as N-Arachidonoylethanolamine (anandamide; AEA) and 2-arachidonoylglycerol (2-AG) [134–136]. Both CB1 and CB2 are expressed in various cells in the brain and in peripheral tissues [137]. CB1 is especially expressed at high levels in the neocortex, hippocampus, basal ganglia, cerebellum, and brainstem, but it is also found in peripheral nerve terminals and some tissues, such as the vascular endothelium, spleen, testis, and eye [137]. CB2 is predominantly found in cells of the immune system, and in the central nervous system, it is primarily localized to microglia and tissue macrophages [137].

The CB1 receptor regulates the balance between excitatory and inhibitory neuronal activity. The psychoactive effect is believed to be mediated through the CB1 receptor in the brain, whereas the immunomodulatory effects are anticipated to be mediated via the CB2 receptor expressed on immune cells [138,139]. In addition, CB1 signaling affects metabolism and is involved in maintaining whole body energy homeostasis by increasing appetite and stimulating feeding [140]. Many efforts have been made to develop CB2 specific agonists at an attempt to achieve anti-inflammatory actions without psychotropic adverse effects [13,141–143]. The sesquiterpene (E)-β-caryophyllene produced by *Cannabis* as well as other plants, including oregano (*Origanum vulgare* L.), cinnamon (*Cinnamomum* spp.), and black pepper (*Piper nigrum* L.), was found to bind selectively to the CB2 receptor and exert anti-inflammatory activities [144–147].

Other cannabinoid receptors include transient receptor potential vanilloid 1 (TRPV1), the G-protein-coupled receptors GPR18 and GPR55, and peroxisome proliferator activated receptors (PPARs) [126,134,148–152]. The anti-nociceptive effect of *Cannabis sativa* extracts was found to be mediated by the binding of CBD to TRPV1 [153]. A study by Ibrahim et al. [154] showed that activation of the CB2 receptor by its agonist AM1241 stimulated the release of beta-endorphin from keratinocytes, which, in turn, acted on neuronal μ-opioid receptors to inhibit nociception. The *Cannabis sativa* extract containing multiple cannabinoids, terpenes, and flavonoids had stronger anti-nociceptive effect than a single cannabinoid given alone [153], suggesting an "entourage" effect of the various *Cannabis*-containing compounds [74].

The CB1 and CB2 can form receptor heteromers [155]. The activity of the receptor heteromer is affected by the agonists and antagonists that bind to each of them. A CB1 antagonist can block the effect of a CB2 agonist and vice versa; a CB2 antagonist can block the effect of a CB1 receptor agonist [155]. CB1 has also been shown to form heteromers with dopamine and adenosine receptors [156–158], AT1 angiotensin receptor [159], μ_1-opioid receptor [160,161], and OX1 orexin A receptor [162]. The many interacting partners put CB1 signaling under strict regulation.

3.2. Pharmacological Effects of Selected Phytocannabinoids

3.2.1. Δ^9-Tetrahydrocannibinol (Δ^9-THC)

Δ^9-THC binds to CB1 and CB2 receptors at a more or less equal affinity [138,163,164]. It also acts on CB1-CB2 receptor heterodimers [165]. Δ^9-THC is well known for its psychomimetic activities that are exerted by its binding to CB1 receptor in the brain, resulting in a calm and sedated mental state [49]. Besides euphoria, Δ^9-THC is an appetite stimulator [166]. Oral Δ^9-THC (Dronabinol, Marinol) and its synthetic nabilone (Cesamet) have been used for the treatment of nausea and appetite stimulation for people undergoing chemotherapy and for AIDS wasting syndrome [167,168]. The activation of CB1 by Δ^9-THC is believed to mediate its anti-nausea and anti-emetic effects [169]. Sativex, which contains a combination of Δ^9-THC and CBD, has been used for relief of neuropathic pain in multiple sclerosis [170].

3.2.2. Cannabidiol (CBD)

The non-psychotropic cannabidiol (CBD) shows low affinity to the CB1 and CB2 receptors [135] and can exert antagonistic modulatory actions on these receptors [138,171]. CBD can also activate the TRPV1 channel, serotonin 1A (5-HT$_{1A}$) receptors, and opioid receptors [24,172]. CBD has anti-inflammatory, anti-oxidative, anti-epileptic, analgesic, anti-neoplastic, sedative, neuroprotective, and anti-anxiety activities [173–188]. Moreover, CBD inhibits sebocyte lipogenesis by activating the TRPV4 ion channel that interferes with the pro-lipogenic ERK1/2 MAPK pathway [189].

The neuroprotective activity of CBD has been attributed in part to its anti-oxidative activity [190,191]. Based on its immunomodulatory activities, CBD has been implicated in the treatment of various autoimmune diseases [14,21], and its anti-nociceptive activity was found to be beneficial in relieving chronic pain [192]. In addition, CBD has potential uses in psychiatry due to its neuromodulatory activities in the brain that control recognition, emotional and behavioral responses [111,193,194]. CBD has especially been reported to have therapeutic effect for psychopathological conditions, such as substance use disorders, chronic psychosis, and anxiety [193]. CBD has been shown to be well tolerated in humans at concentrations as high as 3500–6000 mg/day [195–197], and the FDA-approved CBD (marketed as Epidiolex) is indicated for preventing epileptic seizures in Lennox–Gastaut syndrome and Dravet syndrome in children [198].

In experimental mice and rat models, CBD has been shown to have immunosuppressive activities [181], which are partly due to inhibition of TNFα production [199,200] and induction of myeloid-derived suppressor cells (MDSCs) [201]. CBD alleviated the symptoms of experimental autoimmune encephalomyelitis (EAE) and collagen-induced arthritis and prevented the onset of autoimmune diabetes in experimental murine models [199,200,202]. In mice, the anti-inflammatory activity of CBD was found to have a bell-shaped dose–response with an optimal dose of 5 mg/kg [203]. The use of a standardized extract from a CBD-rich, Δ^9-THC^{low} *Cannabis indica* cultivar overcame this bell-shaped dose–response, suggesting a synergistic effect among the different compounds of the *Cannabis* extract [199].

3.2.3. Cannabigerol (CBG)

CBG is another non-psychoactive *Cannabis* component that is produced at elevated levels in some industrial hemps [204–206]. It binds to both CB1 and CB2 receptors and modulates the signaling through these receptors, as well as the CB1-CB2 receptor heteromer, at concentrations as low as 0.1–1 µM [207]. CBG competes with the binding of [^{3}H]-WIN-55,212-2 to CB2, but not to CB1 [207]. Further studies suggest that CBG is a partial agonist of CB1 and CB2 [207–209]. CBG activates TRPV1, TRPV2, TRPV3, TRPV4, TRPA1, 5-HT$_{1a}$ receptor, α2-adrenergic receptor, and PPARγ, while being a TRPM8 antagonist [210–215]. CBG has anti-inflammatory, anti-oxidative, and anti-nociceptive activities [117,209,213,216]. The anti-inflammatory property is thought to be achieved by modulating the CB2 receptor, TRP channels, and PPARγ, and by inhibiting cyclooxygenase 1 and 2 (COX-1/2) [210,211,217], while the analgesic effect of CBG is thought to be mediated through the α2-adrenergic receptor [211]. CBG has been shown to have potential beneficial effects in treating inflammatory bowel disease and neurological disorders, such as Huntington's disease, Parkinson's disease, and multiple sclerosis [213,215,216,218,219].

3.2.4. Cannabichromene (CBC)

CBC is a non-psychoactive phytocannabinoid that activates the CB1 and CB2 receptors, resulting in decreased intracellular levels of cAMP [209]. CBC also activates the TRPA1, TRPV3, and TRPV4 channels [210]. CBC has anti-inflammatory, anti-nociceptive, and neuroprotective activities [220–225]. CBC reduces the activity of both the ON and OFF neurons in the rostral ventromedial medulla (RVM) and elevates the endocannabinoid levels in the ventrolateral periaqueductal gray matter [221]. The anti-nociceptive activity of CBC is mediated by the adenosine A1 and TRPA1 receptors [221]. CBC increases the viability of neural stem progenitor cells through activation of the adenosine A1 receptor [224]. Moreover, it has been shown to suppress reactive astrocytes, thus offering a protective effect against neuro-inflammation and Alzheimer's disease [225]. CBC had anti-convulsant properties in a mouse model of Dravet syndrome [226], and it exhibited cytotoxic activity against some carcinoma cells [227,228].

3.2.5. Cannabidiolic Acid (CBDA)

CBDA has low affinity for both CB1 and CB2 receptors, with moderate inhibition of adenylyl cyclase activity [209,229], and functions as an allosteric regulator on the 5-HT$_{1A}$ receptor, resulting in anti-emetic effects [230–233]. In addition, it activates PPARα and PPARγ [212]. CBDA shows anti-nociceptive and anti-inflammatory effects that are in part mediated by COX-2 inhibition and activation of the TRPV1 channel [217,234,235]. CBDA has anxiolytic and anti-convulsant effects in animal models [236–238].

3.2.6. Cannabigerolic Acid (CBGA)

CBGA displays low affinity for both CB1 and CB2 receptors but causes a similar decrease in intracellular cAMP levels as Δ^9-THC [229]. Since CBGA can activate PPARs [212], it is expected to affect lipid metabolism [117]. A *Cannabis sativa* cultivar containing high levels of CBG and CBGA inhibited the activity of the aldose reductase enzyme, which catalyzes the reduction of glucose to sorbitol [239]. Since the aldose reductase level is increased at high glucose levels and has been implicated in the development of neuropathy, nephropathy, retinopathy, and cataract in diabetes, CBGA has been suggested as a potential drug in preventing diabetic complications [239]. In the Scn1a$^{+/-}$ mouse model of Dravet syndrome, CBGA was found to have an anti-convulsant effect that was mediated by its interaction with the GPR55, TRPV1, and GABA$_A$ receptors [240].

3.2.7. Cannabinol (CBN)

CBN is formed during the degradation of Δ^9-THC and has a lower binding affinity to CB1 and CB2 receptors than Δ^9-THC [117]. CBN is an agonist of the TRPV1, TRPV2, TRPV3, TRPV4, and TRPA1 cation channels [210]. CBN is a non-psychotropic phytocannabinoid with analgesic and anti-inflammatory properties and acts as an appetite stimulant [117]. CBN has neuroprotective activity that is associated with its anti-oxidative actions, trophic support, and elimination of intraneuronal β-amyloid in neuronal cells [241]. CBN preserves mitochondrial functions, such as redox regulation, calcium uptake, mitochondrial membrane potential, and bioenergetics [242]. CBN promotes endogenous antioxidant defense mechanisms and triggers AMP-activated protein kinase (AMPK) signaling pathways [242].

3.3. Anti-Microbial Effects of Phytocannabinoids

Several phytocannabinoids have been shown to have anti-bacterial activities, especially on Gram-positive bacteria, including various antibiotic-resistant strains [58,59,62,63,101,220,243–247] (Table 1). Phytocannabinoids have been shown to exert both bactericidal and bacteriostatic effects [61,62,244,247]. Most of the studies have analyzed the half maximal inhibitory concentration (IC$_{50}$) or minimum inhibitory concentration (MIC) for each of the compounds against different bacterial species, fungi, and protozoa, while only a few studies have looked at the underlying mechanisms [61,243,244,247–250] (Figure 2).

Table 1. Examples of *Cannabis sativa* constituents that have been documented to possess anti-bacterial, anti-fungal, and/or anti-protozoal activities *.

Phytocannabinoids	Anti-Microbial Activity	Reference
Δ⁹-Tetrahydrocannabinol (Δ⁹-THC)	MIC: 2–5 µg/mL against *Staphylococcus aureus* ATCC 6538 MIC: 1 µg/mL against *Staphylococcus aureus* ATCC 25923 MIC: 2 µg/mL against *Staphylococcus aureus* SA-1199B (NorA overexpression) MIC: 2 µg/mL against *Staphylococcus aureus* EMRSA-15 MIC: 0.5 µg/mL against *Staphylococcus aureus* EMRSA-16 MIC: 2 µg/mL against MRSA USA300 MIC: 4–8 µg/mL against MRSA ATCC 43300 MIC: 5 µg/mL against *Streptococcus pyogenes* MIC: 2 µg/mL against *Streptococcus milleri* MIC: 5 µg/mL against *Streptococcus faecalis* MIC: 4–8 µg/mL against *Neisseria gonorrhoeae* ATCC 19424 IC_{50}: 4.8 µM against *Staphylococcus aureus* ATCC 29213 IC_{50}: 6.9 µM against *Bacillus cereus* IIIM 25 IC_{50}: 2.8 µM against *Lactococcus lactis* MTCC 440 IC_{50}: 3.5 µM against *Shigella boydii* NC-09357 IC_{50}: 6.4 µM against *Staphylococcus warneri* MTCC 4436 No effect against *Escherichia coli*, *Salmonella typhi* or *Proteus vulgaris*	[58,61,245–247]
Cannabidiol (CBD)	MIC: 1–5 µg/mL against *S. aureus* ATCC 6538 MIC: 0.5–1 µg/mL against *Staphylococcus aureus* ATCC 25923 MIC: 1 µg/mL against *Staphylococcus aureus* SA-1199B (NorA overexpression) MIC: 1 µg/mL against *Staphylococcus aureus* EMRSA-15 MIC: 1 µg/mL against *Staphylococcus aureus* EMRSA-16 MIC: 1–4 µg/mL against MRSA USA300 MIC: 1–2 µg/mL against various *Staphylococcus aureus* isolates. MIC: 1–2 µg/mL against *Staphylococcus epidermidis*. MIC: 4 µg/mL against methicillin-resistant *Staphylococcus epidermidis*. MIC: 2 µg/mL against *Streptococcus pyogenes* MIC: 1 µg/mL against *Streptococcus milleri* MIC: 5 µg/mL against *Streptococcus faecalis* MIC: 1–4 µg/mL against various *Streptococcus pneumoniae* species MIC: 0.5–4 µg/mL against various *Enterococcus faecalis* species MIC: 4 µg/mL against *Listereria monocytogenes* MIC: 1–2 µg/mL against *Cutibacterium (Propionibacterium) acnes* ATCC 6919 MIC: 2–4 µg/mL against *Clostridioides (Clostridium) difficile* M7404 human ribotype 027 MIC: 1–2 µg/mL against various *Neisseria gonorrhoeae* isolates. MIC: 0.25 µg/mL against various *Neisseria meningitidis* ATCC 13090 MIC: 1 µg/mL against *Moraxella catarrhalis* MMX 3782 MIC: 1 µg/mL against *Legionella pneumophila* MMX 7515 IC_{50}: 3.8 µM against *Staphylococcus aureus* ATCC 29213 IC_{50}: 9.5–11.1 µM against *Staphylococcus aureus* ATCC 6538 IC_{50}: 9.8 µM against *Bacillus cereus* IIIM 25 IC_{50}: 2.9 µM against *Lactococcus lactis* MTCC 440 IC_{50}: 4.3 µM against *Shigella boydii* NC-09357 IC_{50}: 4.1 µM against *Pseudomonas fluorescens* MTCC 103 IC_{50}: 5.7 µM against *Staphylococcus warneri* MTCC 4436 Moderate effect against *Mycobacterium smegmatis* (MIC 16 µg/mL) and marginal activity against *Mycobacterium tuberculosis* H37Rv, *Candida albicans*, and *Cryptococcus neoformans* with a MIC > 64 µg/mL. No effect against *Escherichia coli*, *Salmonella typhimurium*, *Shigella dysenteriae*, *Proteus vulgaris*, *Proteus mirabilis*, *Klebsiella pneumoniae*, *Pseudomonas aeruginosa*, *Acinetobacter baumannii*, *Serratia marcescens*, *Burkholderia cepacian*, and *Haemophilus influenzae*. *Anti-biofilm effect*: MBEC: 1–4 µg/mL against MSSA and MRSA biofilms. BIC_{50}: 12.5 µg/mL against *Candida albicans* SC5314 MBIC: 100 µg/mL against *Candida albicans* SC5314	[58,61,62,245–247,251–253]

Table 1. *Cont.*

Phytocannabinoids	Anti-Microbial Activity	Reference
Cannabigerol (CBG)	MIC: 0.5 µg/mL against *Staphylococcus aureus* ATCC 25923 MIC: 1 µg/mL against *Staphylococcus aureus* SA-1199B (NorA overexpression) MIC: 2 µg/mL against *Staphylococcus aureus* EMRSA-15 MIC: 1 µg/mL against *Staphylococcus aureus* EMRSA-16 MIC: 2 µg/mL against MRSA USA300 MIC: 2–4 µg/mL against various MRSA clinical isolates, with some requiring > 8 µg/mL MIC: 4–8 µg/mL against MRSA ATCC 43300 MIC: 2.5 µg/mL against *Streptococcus mutans* UA159 ATCC 700610 MIC: 1 µg/mL against *Streptococcus sanguis* ATCC 10556 MIC: 5 µg/mL against *Streptococcus sobrinus* ATCC 27351 MIC: 5 µg/mL against *Streptococcus salivarius* ATCC 25975 MIC: 1–2 µg/mL against *Neisseria gonorrhoeae* ATCC 19424 IC_{50}: 15 µg/mL against *Mycobacterium intracellulare* Anti-biofilm effect: MBIC: 2–4 µg/mL against biofilm formation by MRSA 4 µg/mL eradicated preformed biofilms of MRSA MBIC: 2.5 µg/mL against biofilm formation by *Streptococcus mutans* UA159 ATCC 70061 Anti-quorum sensing effect 1 µg/mL CBG inhibited quorum sensing in *Vibrio harveyi* BB120.	[58,61,100,243,244,247,248]
Cannabidiolic acid (CBDA)	MIC: 1–2 µg/mL against *Neisseria gonorrhoeae* ATCC 19424 MIC: 2 µg/mL against *Staphylococcus aureus* ATCC 25923 MIC: 4 µg/mL against *Staphylococcus aureus* USA300 MIC: 4 µg/mL against *Staphylococcus epidermidis* CA#71 and ATCC 51625 MIC: 16–32 µg/mL against MRSA ATCC 43300 No effect on *Escherichia coli* ATCC 25922 or *Pseudomonas aeruginosa* PA01 with a MIC > 64 µg/mL.	[62,247]
Cannabigerolic acid (CBGA)	IC_{50}: 12 µg/mL against *Leishmania donovani* MIC: 4 µg/mL against MRSA USA300 MIC: 2–4 µg/mL against MRSA ATCC 43300 MIC: 1–2 µg/mL against *Neisseria gonorrhoeae* ATCC 19424	[61,100,247]
Cannabichromene (CBC)	MIC: 1.56 µg/mL against *Staphylococcus aureus* ATCC 6538 MIC: 2 µg/mL against *Staphylococcus aureus* ATCC 25923 MIC: 2 µg/mL against *Staphylococcus aureus* SA-1199B (NorA overexpression) MIC: 2 µg/mL against *Staphylococcus aureus* EMRSA-15 MIC: 2 µg/mL against *Staphylococcus aureus* EMRSA-16 MIC: 8 µg/mL against MRSA USA300 MIC: 0.39 µg/mL against *Bacillus subtilis* ATCC 6633 MIC 12.5 µg/mL against *Mycobacterium smegmatis* ATCC 607 IC_{50}: 5.9 µM against *Staphylococcus aureus* ATCC 29213 IC_{50}: 9.2 µM against *Bacillus cereus* IIIM 25 IC_{50}: 2.6 µM against *Lactococcus lactis* MTCC 440 IC_{50}: 3.4 µM against *Shigella boydii* NC-09357 IC_{50}: 5.6 µM against *Staphylococcus warneri* MTCC 4436	[58,61,220,246]
Cannabichromenic acid (CBCA)	MIC: 2 µg/mL against MRSA USA300 MIC: 7.8 µM against *Staphylococcus aureus* MSSA 34397 MIC: 3.9 µM against a clinical MRSA isolate MIC: 7.8 µM against vancomycin-resistance *Enterococcus faecalis* (VRE)	[61,254]

Table 1. Cont.

Phytocannabinoids	Anti-Microbial Activity	Reference
Cannabinol (CBN)	MIC: 1 µg/mL against *Staphylococcus aureus* ATCC 25923 MIC: 1 µg/mL against *Staphylococcus aureus* SA-1199B (NorA overexpression) MIC: 1 µg/mL against *Staphylococcus aureus* EMRSA-15 MIC: 2 µg/mL against MRSA USA300 IC_{50}: 7.9 µM against *Staphylococcus aureus* ATCC 29213 IC_{50}: 3.2 µM against *Bacillus cereus* IIIM 25 IC_{50}: 5.8 µM against *Lactococcus lactis* MTCC 440 IC_{50}: 11.7 µM against *Shigella boydii* NC-09357 IC_{50}: 8.3 µM against *Pseudomonas fluorescens* MTCC 103 IC_{50}: 9.2 µM against *Staphylococcus warneri* MTCC 4436	[58,61,246]
Cannabidivarin (CBDV)	MIC: 2–4 µg/mL against MRSA ATCC 43300 MIC: 0.03–0.5 µg/mL against *Neisseria gonorrhoeae* ATCC 19424 IC_{50}: 7.8 µM against *Staphylococcus aureus* ATCC 29213 IC_{50}: 3.1 µM against *Bacillus cereus* IIIM 25 IC_{50}: 3.2 µM against *Lactococcus lactis* MTCC 440 IC_{50}: 10.4 µM against *Shigella boydii* NC-09357 IC_{50}: 5.9 µM against *Pseudomonas fluorescens* MTCC 103 IC_{50}: 7.9 µM against *Staphylococcus warneri* MTCC 4436 IC_{50}: 11.9 µM against *Candida albicans* MTCC 4748	[61,246,247]
(-)Δ^8-Tetrahydrocannabinol (Δ^8-THC)	MIC: 8 µg/mL against MRSA USA300 MIC: 2 µg/mL against MRSA USA300 MIC: 4–8 µg/mL against MRSA ATCC 43300 MIC: 2–4 µg/mL against *Neisseria gonorrhoeae* ATCC 19424	[61,247]
Exo-tetrahydrocannabinol (exo-THC)	MIC: 2 µg/mL against MRSA USA300	[61]
Δ^9-Tetrahydrocannabinolic acid A (THCA-A)	MIC: 4 µg/mL against MRSA USA300	[61]
Δ^9-Tetrahydrocannabivarin (THCV)	MIC: 4 µg/mL against MRSA USA300 MIC: 64 µg/mL against MRSA ATCC 43300 MIC: 16 µg/mL against *Neisseria gonorrhoeae* ATCC 19424	[61,247]
Δ^1-Tetrahydrocannabidivarol	IC_{50}: 6.9 µM against *Staphylococcus aureus* ATCC 29213 IC_{50}: 6.9 µM against *Bacillus cereus* IIIM 25 IC_{50}: 5.1 µM against *Lactococcus lactis* MTCC 440 IC_{50}: 3.9 µM against *Shigella boydii* NC-09357 IC_{50}: 7.8 µM against *Pseudomonas fluorescens* MTCC 103 IC_{50}: 7.6 µM against *Staphylococcus warneri* MTCC 4436	[246]
($\pm$)-4-Acetoxycannabichromene	IC_{50}: 40.3 µM against *Leishmania donovani* IC_{50}: 4–7.2 µM against *Plasmodium falciparum*	[63]
($\pm$)-3″-Hydroxy-$\Delta^{(4'',5'')}$ cannabichromene	IC_{50}: 24.4 µM against MRSA ATCC 33591 IC_{50}: 29.6 µM against *Staphylococcus aureus* ATCC 29213 IC_{50}: 60.5 µM against *Candida albicans* ATCC 90028 IC_{50}: 60.5 µM against *Candida krusei* ATCC 6258 IC_{50}: 57.5 µM against *Leishmania donovani* Not active against *Escherichia coli*, *Mycobacterium intracellulare*, or *Plasmodium falciparum*.	[63]
5-Acetyl-4-hydroxycannabigerol	IC_{50}: 53.4 µM against MRSA ATCC 33591 IC_{50}: 10.7 µM against *Leishmania donovani* IC_{50}: 6.7–7.2 µM against *Plasmodium falciparum* Not active against *Staphylococcus aureus*, *Escherichia coli*, *Mycobacterium intracellulare*, or *Candida albicans*.	[63]

Table 1. Cont.

Phytocannabinoids	Anti-Microbial Activity	Reference
4-Acetoxy-2-geranyl-5-hydroxy-3-n-pentylphenol	IC_{50}: 6.7 µM against MRSA ATCC 33591 IC_{50}: 12.2 µM against *Staphylococcus aureus* ATCC 29213 IC_{50}: 53.4 µM against *Candida krusei* ATCC 6258 IC_{50}: 42.7 µM against *Leishmania donovani* Not active against *Escherichia coli, Mycobacterium intracellulare, Candida albicans*, or *Plasmodium falciparum*.	[63]
8-Hydroxycannabinol	IC_{50}: 4.6 µM against *Candida albicans* ATCC 90028 IC_{50}: 30.6 µM against *Mycobacterium intracellulare* Not active against *Escherichia coli*.	[63]
8-Hydroxycannabinolic acid A	IC_{50}: 54 µM against *Candida krusei* ATCC 6258 IC_{50}: 3.5 µM against *Staphylococcus aureus* ATCC 29213 IC_{50}: 54 µM against *Escherichia coli* Not active against *Mycobacterium intracellulare*.	[63]
Non-Cannabinoid constituents of *Cannabis sativa* L.		
5-Acetoxy-6-geranyl-3-n-pentyl-1,4-benzoquinone	IC_{50}: 15 µg/mL against MRSA ATCC 43300 IC_{50}: 13 µg/mL against *Leishmania donovani* IC_{50}: 2.6–2.8 µg/mL against *Plasmodium falciparum*	[101]
Cannflavin A	IC_{50}: 4.5 µg/mL against *Leishmania donovani*	[101]
Cannflavin B	IC_{50}: 5 µg/mL against *Leishmania donovani*	[100]
Cannflavin C	IC_{50}: 17 µg/mL against *Leishmania donovani*	[101]
6-Prenylapigenin	IC_{50}: 6.5 µg/mL against MRSA ATCC 43300 IC_{50}: 20 µg/mL against *Candida albicans* IC_{50}: 2.0–2.8 µg/mL against *Plasmodium falciparum*	[101]
Prenylspirodinone	IC_{50}: 49.6 µM against *Bacillus thuringiensis* MTCC 809	[246]

* BIC_{50} = The test concentration that prevents 50% biofilm formation compared to control cells. IC_{50} = The test concentration that causes 50% growth inhibition in comparison to control cells. MBEC = Minimum biofilm eradication concentration is the lowest concentration that completely eradicates preformed biofilm. MBIC = Minimum biofilm inhibitory concentration is the lowest concentration that is required to completely prevent any biofilm formation. MIC = Minimum inhibitory concentration is the lowest concentration that completely inhibits bacterial growth (when no turbidity is observed).

3.3.1. Bacterial Growth Inhibitory Effects of Phytocannabinoids

The minimum inhibitory concentration (MIC) of Δ^9-THC and CBD on various *Staphylococcus aureus* strains, including MRSA and *Streptococci* species (e.g., *Streptococcus pyogenes* and *Streptococcus. faecalis*) was found to be in the range of 1–5 µg/mL [58,62,245,246]. There was no significant difference between the anti-bacterial effect of Δ^9-THC and CBD [58,245,246]. The anti-microbial effect was attenuated by the presence of either serum or blood, suggesting that serum components can bind the compounds and prevent them from acting on the microorganisms [245]. CBG shows anti-bacterial activity against Gram-positive bacteria, including MSSA, MRSA, and the oral cariogenic *Streptococcus mutans* at low concentrations similar to CBD [58,61,244,247]. CBC and CBDA showed a MIC of 1–2 µg/mL against *Staphylococcus aureus* and *Staphylococcus epidermidis* [62,220]. In these studies, CBDA was less active than CBD [62]. Cannabichromenic acid (CBCA) caused a rapid reduction in the colony-forming units (CFUs) of a clinical MRSA isolate both during the exponential and stationary growth phase, suggesting a bactericidal activity that is independent of the metabolic state of the bacteria [254]. None of the phytocannabinoids had any significant anti-bacterial activity against Gram-negative bacteria, such as *Escherichia coli*, *Salmonella typhi*, *Pseudomonas aeruginosa*, and *Proteus vulgaris* [61,62,220,245,247]. This might be due to the inability of these compounds to penetrate the outer membrane of the Gram-negative bacteria [61], or the outer membrane protects the bacteria from cell death caused by damage to the inner membrane.

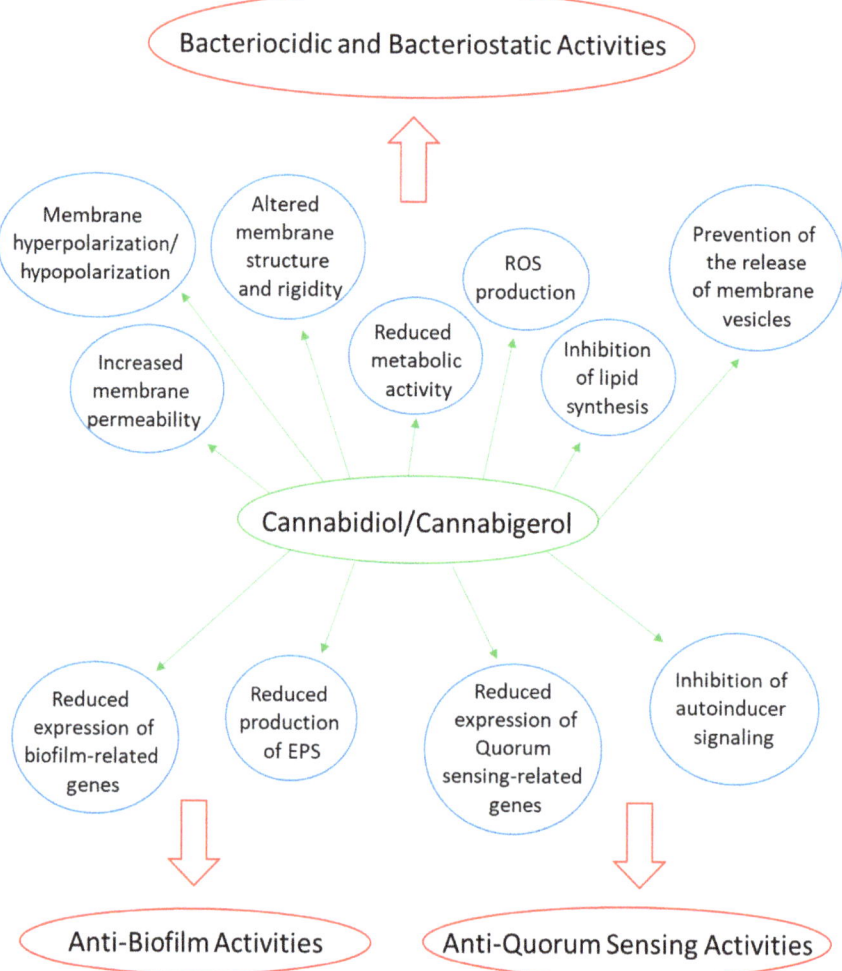

Figure 2. The anti-bacterial activities of phytocannabinoids.

3.3.2. Outer Membrane Permeabilization of Gram-Negative Bacteria Sensitizes Them to Phytocannabinoids

Interestingly, CBD and CBG could act on some Gram-negative bacteria (e.g., *Escherichia coli, Acinetobacter baumannii, Klebsiella pneumoniae, Pseudomonas aeruginosa*) if the outer membrane was permeabilized with the LPS-binding antibiotic polymyxin B [61,247]. It was shown that an *Escherichia coli* ΔbamBΔtolC deletion strain that renders the bacteria hyperpermeable to many small molecules was sensitive to CBG with a MIC of 4 μg/mL, which is in contrast to the parental *Escherichia coli* wild-type strain that showed a MIC above 128 μg/mL [61]. Similarly, a lipo-oligosaccharide-deficient *Acinetobacter baumannii* strain became sensitive to CBG with a MIC of 0.5 μg/mL compared to the parental strain showing a MIC of 64 μg/mL [61].

3.3.3. Combined Treatment of Phytocannabinoids with Antibiotics

No synergistic or antagonistic effects of CBD were observed on MRSA strain USA300 when combined with different conventional antibiotics, such as clindamycin, ofloxacin, meropenem, tobramycin, methicillin, teicoplanin, and vancomycin [62]. These authors concluded that the membrane-perturbing effect of CBD was not sufficient to enhance the uptake of conventional antibiotics [62]. However, Wassmann et al. [251] observed that CBD could reduce the MIC value of bacitracin against several Gram-positive bacteria, including *Staphylococcus* species, *Listeria monocytogenes*, and *Enterococcus faecalis*. The simultaneous use of CBD and bacitracin on MRSA USA300 resulted in the formation of multiple septa during cell division, appearance of membrane irregularities, reduced autolysis, and decreased membrane potential [251]. The combined CBD/bacitracin treatment did not affect the growth of the Gram-negative bacteria *Pseudomonas aeruginosa*, *Salmonella typhimurium*, *Klebsiella pneumoniae*, and *Escherichia coli* [251].

3.3.4. Phytocannabinoids Also Act on Persister Cells and Do Not Induce Drug Resistance

CBG was found to be active against MRSA persister cells, which are dormant, non-dividing bacteria [61]. This trait is therapeutically important, since many antibiotics require cell division to be effective, and they are frequently unable to eradicate persister cells that usually recover after antibiotic withdrawal [255–257]. Another obstacle of antibiotic therapy is the development of drug resistance, a frequent reason for treatment failure [258]. Farha et al. [61] attempted to develop CBG-resistant bacteria in the hopes of finding the target molecules. Despite rechallenging the MRSA with 2x and 16x MIC concentration of CBG, they were unable to get any spontaneously CBG-resistant mutants [61]. Similarly, MRSA that had been daily exposed to sub-lethal concentration of CBD for 20 days were still sensitive to CBD [247]. The authors of these two studies [61,247] concluded that CBD and CBG do not induce drug resistance. However, it should be noted that following exposure to CBD or CBG, the surviving growth-arrested bacteria could regain growth after withdrawal of the drug.

3.3.5. Therapeutic Anti-Microbial Potential of Phytocannabinoids

The hemolytic activity of CBD and CBG was found to be 256 µg/mL and 32 µg/mL, respectively, which is far above the MIC of 1–4 µg/mL for MRSA [61,247]. Additionally, the hemolytic activity of CBDA was found to be above 32 µg/mL [62]. This makes phytocannabinoids potential drugs that can act within a reasonable therapeutic window.

Farha et al. [61] observed that treating MRSA-infected mice with a high dose of 100 mg/kg CBG could reduce the bacterial burden in the spleen by a 2.8 $\log_{10}$ of CFU. Blaskovich et al. [247] tried various CBD-containing ointment formulations that could reduce a 2–3 $\log_{10}$ of CFU of MRSA inoculated on porcine skin after 1 h and a reduction of more than 5 $\log_{10}$ of CFU after a 24 h incubation. CBD, however, failed to significantly reduce the bacterial load of MRSA ATCC 43300 in a thigh infection mouse model [247].

3.3.6. Anti-Biofilm Activities of Phytocannabinoids

Biofilms are communities of bacteria embedded in an extracellular matrix that have attached to a biotic surface (e.g., lung tissue, gastrointestinal tract, nasal mucosa, inner ear) or an abiotic surface (e.g., medical devices, such as catheters, heart valves, stents, prostheses) [259]. The majority of infectious diseases involve bacterial biofilms that are usually difficult to eradicate due to reduced antibiotic sensitivity [259,260]. Several studies show that CBD and CBG can prevent biofilm formation of various Gram-positive bacteria (e.g., MSSA, MRSA, *Streptococcus mutans*) [61,243,247]. The extent of anti-biofilm activity of CBD and CBG against these bacteria correlated with their anti-bacterial activity [61,243,244,247]. In most cases, a similar concentration of these compounds was required to achieve both effects, suggesting that some of the anti-biofilm effect is caused by the anti-bacterial activity [61,243,244]. Moreover, CBD was found to be able to eradicate preformed MSSA and MRSA biofilms with a minimum biofilm eradication concentration (MBEC) of 1–4 µg/mL, indicating that CBD can penetrate the biofilms and act on the biofilm-embedded bacteria [247]. Some cannabinoids (e.g., CBD, CBG, CBC, and CBN) were shown to reduce the bacterial content of dental plaques in an in vitro assay where dental plaques were spread on agar plates coated with the cannabinoids [261]. The anti-biofilm activity of the cannabinoids has significant clinical importance, since the bacteria-embedded bacteria frequently show antibiotic resistance, and some antibiotics are unable to penetrate through the extracellular matrix of the biofilms [259,262,263].

3.3.7. Anti-Fungal Biofilm Activities of Phytocannabinoids

CBD barely affects the viability of *Candida albicans* with a MIC above 50–100 µg/mL [247,253], but it reduces biofilm formation with a biofilm inhibitory concentration 50 (BIC_{50}) at 12.5 µg/mL and a $MBIC_{90}$ of 100 µg/mL [253]. CBD reduced the metabolic activity of preformed *Candida albicans* biofilms by 50–60% at 6.25 µg/mL with no further reduction at higher concentrations, even at 100 µg/mL [253]. The morphology of the *Candida albicans* biofilm becomes altered in the presence of CBD. While the hyphal form was predominant in control biofilms, the CBD (25 µg/mL)-treated biofilms appeared in clusters mostly in yeast and pseudohyphal forms [253]. CBD caused a dose-dependent reduction in the cell wall chitin content and the intracellular ATP level, while increasing the intracellular reactive oxygen species (ROS) levels [253]. Gene expression studies showed that after a 24 h incubation with 25 µg/mL CBD, there is a significant downregulation of: *ADH5* (Alcohol dehydrogenase 5), involved in extracellular matrix production; *BIG1*, required for synthesis of the extracellular matrix component β-1,6-glucan; *ECE1* (extent of cell elongation protein 1), involved in biofilm formation; *EED1*, involved in filamentous growth; *CHT1* and *CHT3* chitinases, involved in the remodeling of chitin in the fungal cell wall; and *TRR1* (thioredoxin reductase) with anti-oxidant properties. On the other hand, a significant upregulation of *YWP1* (yeast-form wall protein 1) which is expressed predominantly in the yeast form, was observed [253]. These changes in gene expression might explain, at least in part, the reduced biofilm mass of *Candida albicans* in the presence of CBD and the increase in oxidative stress [253].

3.3.8. Anti-Viral Activities of Phytocannabinoids

There are some lines of evidence for an anti-viral activity of phytocannabinoids [60,264]. Some phytocannabinoids, especially Δ^9-THC and CBD, bind to the M^{pro} protease of SARS-CoV-2, which plays a role in viral replication [60,264]. CBGA and CBDA were found to be allosteric and orthosteric ligands for the spike protein of SARS-CoV-2 and prevented infection of human epithelial cells by a pseudovirus expressing the SARS-CoV-2 spike protein [265]. Phytocannabinoids might indirectly relieve the disease progress of COVID-19 patients through their anti-inflammatory properties [266]. However, CBD failed to alter the clinical disease development of COVID-19 when given at a daily dose of 300 mg for 14 days [267]. Additionally, caution should be taken into account due to the immunosuppressive activities of phytocannabinoids that can prevent proper anti-viral immune responses [268]. Notably, the use of *Cannabis* was increased in U.S. and Canada by 6–8% during the COVID-19 pandemic in comparison to the pre-pandemic period [269], with a special increase among people with mental health [270]. Vulnerability to COVID-19 was correlated with genetic liability to *Cannabis* use disorder (CUD) [271].

3.4. Some Mechanistic Insight into the Anti-Bacterial Activity of Phytocannabinoids

The ability of phytocannabinoids such as CBD and CBG, to kill MRSA, NorA-overexpressing *Staphylococcus aureus*, vancomycin-resistant *Staphylococcus aureus* (VRSA), vancomycin-resistant *enterococci* (VRE) to a similar extent as the respective antibiotic-sensitive strains [58,245,247], suggests that its action mechanism is not hindered by the common antibiotic-resistance mechanisms. Thus, phytocannabinoids can be used as an alternative drug or an antibiotic adjuvant for infectious diseases caused by drug-resistant Gram-positive bacteria.

3.4.1. CBD and CBG Target the Cytoplasmic Membrane, Increase Membrane Permeability, and Reduce Metabolic Activity

There is evidence that CBD and CBG act by targeting the cytoplasmic membrane of the Gram-positive bacteria [61,247]. Exposure of MSSA and MRSA to CBD or CBG caused a dose-dependent increase in the fluorescence of the potentiometric probe 3,3′-dipropylthiadicarbocyanine iodide [DiSC3(5)], suggesting a CBG-induced membrane depolarization [61,247]. CBD inhibited protein, DNA, RNA, and peptidoglycan synthesis in a *Staphylococcus aureus strain* when using concentrations close to the MIC [247]. At sub-MIC levels, CBD inhibited lipid synthesis [247]. CBG was found to inhibit the enzyme enoyl acyl carrier protein reductase (InhA) [272], which is involved in type II fatty acid biosynthesis in *Mycobacterium tuberculosis*. The rapid uptake of the SYTOX green dye into *Staphylococcus aureus* and *Bacillus subtilis* by CBD at MIC, suggests that CBD causes an increase in membrane permeability [247].

CBG prevents the growth of oral cariogenic *Streptococcus mutans* in a concentration and bacterial cell density manner [243]. At a MIC of 2.5 µg/mL, CBG exhibited a bacteriostatic effect on *Streptococcus mutans*, while at 2x MIC and 4x MIC, a bactericidal activity was observed [243]. CBG treatment was found to alter the morphology of *Streptococcus mutans* and cause intracellular accumulation of membrane-like structures [243]. CBG induced an immediate membrane hyperpolarization, followed by increased uptake of propidium iodide, suggesting increased membrane permeabilization [243]. At the same time, Laurdan incorporation into the membranes was reduced in a dose-dependent manner [243], indicative of a more rigid membrane structure. The metabolic activity was decreased in a dose-dependent manner, which might contribute to the growth inhibitory effect [243].

3.4.2. CBD Inhibits the Release of Membrane Vesicles from *Escherichia coli*

Kosgodage et al. [250] observed that CBD inhibits the release of membrane vesicles from the Gram-negative *Escherichia coli* VCS257, while having negligible effect on the membrane vesicle release from the Gram-positive *Staphylococcus aureus* subsp. *aureus* Rosenbach. Membrane vesicles participate in inter-bacterial communication by the transfer of cargo molecules and virulence factors [273]. CBD was found to enhance the anti-bacterial effect of erythromycin, rifampicin, and vancomycin against the tested *Escherichia coli* strain [250].

3.4.3. CBG Reduces the Expression of Biofilm and Quorum Sensing-Related Genes in *Streptococcus mutans*

CBG inhibited sucrose-induced biofilm formation by *Streptococcus mutans* with a minimum biofilm inhibitory concentration (MBIC) of 2.5 µg/mL [243]. Higher concentrations (10 µg/mL) of CBG were required to reduce the metabolic activity of preformed *Streptococcus mutans* biofilms [243]. CBG reduced the expression of various biofilm-related genes (e.g., *gtfB*, *gtfC*, *gtfD*, *ftf*, *gbpA*, *gbpA*, *brpA*, *wapA*) with concomitant reduction in the production of extracellular polymeric substances (EPS) [243]. The quorum sensing-related genes *comE*, *comD*, and *luxS* were downregulated by CBG, while no effect was observed on the gene expression of the stress-associated chaperones *groEL* and *dnaK* [243]. Moreover, CBG induced reactive oxygen species (ROS) production in *Streptococcus mutans*, which might be related to the reduced expression of the oxidative stress defense genes, *sod* and *nox* [243]. Thus, CBG has specific anti-biofilm activity unrelated to its membrane-acting effect. This conclusion is further supported by the study of Aqawi et al. [248] showing that CBG inhibited quorum sensing, bacterial motility, and biofilm formation of the marine Gram-negative *Vibrio harveyi* without affecting the planktonic growth.

3.4.4. CBG and HU-210 Inhibit Quorum Sensing in *Vibrio harveyi*

Quorum sensing is an inter-bacterial communication system mediated by secreted autoinducers that interact with their respective receptors, resulting in the activation of a signal transduction cascade that alters the gene expression repertoire in a cell-density-dependent manner [274]. CBG prevented the bioluminescence induced by the master quorum sensing regulator LuxR of *Vibrio harveyi* at a concentration of 1 µg/mL [248]. Using a ΔluxM, ΔlusS *Vibrio harveyi* mutant that does not produce autoinducers AI-1 and AI-2, CBG was found to prevent the signals delivered by exogenously added autoinducers, with a more profound inhibitory effect on the AI-2-induced than on the AI-1-induced bioluminescence [248]. Further studies show that CBG prevented the expression of several quorum sensing genes in *Vibrio harveyi*, including *luxU*, *luxO*, *qrr1–5*, and *luxR*, which can explain the inhibitory effect of CBG on LuxR-mediated bioluminescence [248]. Altogether, these data demonstrate that CBG can interfere with bacterial quorum sensing.

The synthetic cannabinoid HU-210, which is a dimethylheptyl analog of Δ^8-THC (Figure 1) and acts as a high-affinity CB1 and CB2 agonist [275,276], has been shown to inhibit quorum sensing in the *Vibrio harveyi* AI-1$^-$, AI-2$^+$ BB152 mutant, but it had barely any effect on the wild-type bacteria or the AI-1$^+$, AI-2$^-$ MM30 mutant [249]. This suggests that HU-210 specifically antagonizes the AI-2 pathway [249]. The concentration of HU-210 required to achieve the anti-quorum sensing activity was relatively high (20–200 µg/mL) [249], which is 2–3 magnitudes higher than that of CBG [248]. HU-210 prevented biofilm formation of the AI-1$^-$, AI-2$^+$ BB152 mutant with a BIC_{50} of 2 µg/mL and $MBIC_{90}$ of 200 µg/mL, while no significant effect was seen on biofilm formation by the wild-type bacteria or the AI-1$^+$, AI-2$^-$ MM30 mutant [249]. However, the motility of *Vibrio harveyi* was reduced in all three strains at both 20 and 200 µg/mL HU-210 [249]. Gene expression studies showed that HU-210 at a concentration of 2 µg/mL reduced the expression of the master regulator *luxR* in both wild-type and AI-1$^-$, AI-2$^+$ BB152 strain, while it had no effect on the AI-1$^+$, AI-2$^-$ MM30 *Vibrio harveyi* mutant strain [249]. The *luxM* gene that encodes for AI-1 was upregulated by HU-210 [249].

4. Endocannabinoids

The endocannabinoid system (ECS) modulates many physiological processes, including the cardiovascular, gastrointestinal and immune systems, pain, learning, memory, perception, mood, appetite, metabolism, emotions, and sleep [22,112,113,277–285]. The bioactive endocannabinoid lipid mediators have potent anti-inflammatory activities [286–291]. In addition, they promote neural progenitor cell proliferation and differentiation, and have neuroprotective effects [20,292–294]. The effect on neural cell proliferation is mediated by both the CB1 and CB2 receptors [293,295,296].

4.1. The Endocannabinoid System

The endocannabinoid system is composed of: (1) the lipid active endogenous ligands N-Arachidonoylethanolamine (anandamide; AEA) and 2-arachidonoylglycerol (2-AG); (2) their biosynthetic enzymes (e.g., diacylglycerol lipases (DAGL), N-acyl-phosphatidylethanolamine phospholipase D-like esterase (NAPE-PLD), and Ca^{2+}-dependent and Ca^{2+}-independent N-acetyltransferases); (3) their degradative enzymes (e.g., fatty acyl amide hydrolase (FAAH) and monoacylglycerol lipase (MAGL)); and (4) the CB1 and CB2 cannabinoid receptors [15,297,298]. The precursors of endocannabinoids (e.g., N-acyl-phosphatidylethanolamine (NAPE) and phosphatidylinositol-4,5-bisphosphate (PIP2)) are present in the lipid membranes, and the endocannabinoids are produced upon demand, usually after activation of certain G-protein-coupled receptors (GPCRs) and in response to an increase in the intracellular calcium levels [299–302].

4.2. The Production of AEA and 2-AG

The production of endocannabinoids requires one or two enzymatic steps, followed by their release into the extracellular space. AEA is usually produced from N-arachidonoyl-phosphatidylethanolamine phospholipid, and 2-AG is produced primarily from membrane phospholipid 1-stearoyl-2-arachidonoyl-sn-glycerol [297]. The synthesis of 2-AG involves two steps: first, the hydrolysis of its precursor phospholipid by a phospholipase (PLCβ, PLCγ2, or PLCε), followed by further cleavage by diacylglycerol lipase (DAGL) [303–305].

The biosynthesis of these endocannabinoids occurs in areas of the brain functionally related to cognitive processes, motivation, and movement control [306,307]. 2-AG was found to be present at 170 times higher concentrations than AEA in brain lysate [308]. While AEA was initially detected in the brain [135] and 2-AG in the canine gut [309], today it is known that these host-derived endocannabinoid lipid hormones are found in various peripheral tissues (e.g., the intestine) and in the serum, and produced by certain immune cells [23,290,309–317]. For instance, lipopolysaccharides induced the production of AEA in adipose tissue macrophages [318]. T and B cells produce elevated levels of 2-AG upon activation [290]. Astrocytes were found to produce AEA, as well as homo-γ-linolenoylethanolamine (HEA), docosatetraenoylethanolamine (DEA), oleoylethanolamine (OAE), and palmitoylethanolamine (PEA) [319].

4.3. The Circulating Levels of AEA and 2-AG

The circulating endocannabinoid levels are affected by various factors, and under physiological conditions, the AEA serum level was found to be between 1 to 5 nM, and the 2-AG serum level between 10–500 nM [316,320]. Physical exercise mobilizes endocannabinoids, which could contribute to the analgesic and mood-elevating effects of exercise [316]. The circulating levels of 2-AG show a circadian rhythm that gets altered when sleep is disrupted [316,320]. CBD inhibits the degradation of AEA and 2-AG, which is associated with the anti-inflammatory and anti-oxidative activities [321].

4.4. Endogenous Receptors for AEA and 2-AG

AEA and 2-AG act as agonists of the CB1 and CB2 receptors [135,322–325]. While 2-AG binds with high affinity to CB1 and CB2 cannabinoid receptors, AEA binds with low affinity to these receptors [323,324]. Although phytocannabinoids and endocannabinoids bind to the same CB1 and CB2 receptors, their chemical structure is quite different [297] (Figures 1 and 3). Both AEA and 2-AG have an alkyl-amide (alkamide) chemical structure, while cannabinoids are terpenophenolic compounds.

In addition to acting on CB1 and CB2, AEA activates the ionotropic TRPV1 channel, resulting in the opening of the ion channel and Ca^{2+} influx [312,326–331], the G-protein-coupled receptor GPR55 [332,333], and the cation channel TRPA1 [334], while it inhibits the TRPM8 channel [334]. In addition, AEA activates PPARγ, and 2-AG activates PPARα [335]. The vasodilation action of AEA was found to be mediated via activation of TRPV1 [336]. Endocannabinoids activating TRPV1 have been included in the endovanilloid system [337–339]. Recent studies suggest that potassium channels are also the targets of endocannabinoids [340].

In the brain, endocannabinoids serve as retrograde synaptic messengers [299,341]. They are released from postsynaptic neurons and inhibit the release of presynaptic neurotransmitters, such as glutamate and gamma-aminobutyric acid (GABA) by binding to the CB1 receptor and TRPV1 expressed in the presynaptic terminals [299,342,343]. This has led to the hypothesis that endocannabinoids regulate over-excitability and promote synaptic homeostasis [344]. Endocannabinoids differ from the classical neurotransmitters in that they are not stored in vesicles but are released immediately after their production.

The solubility of endocannabinoids is low in water, raising the question of how AEA diffuses through the synaptic cleft [345]. There is evidence that AEA can interact with cholesterol and ceramide, which are required for their insertion into and transport through the membrane [345–347]. In the brain, the lipid-binding protein α-synuclein is involved in the transport of arachidonic acid [348]. Fatty acid binding proteins have been shown to be intracellular carriers of AEA [349].

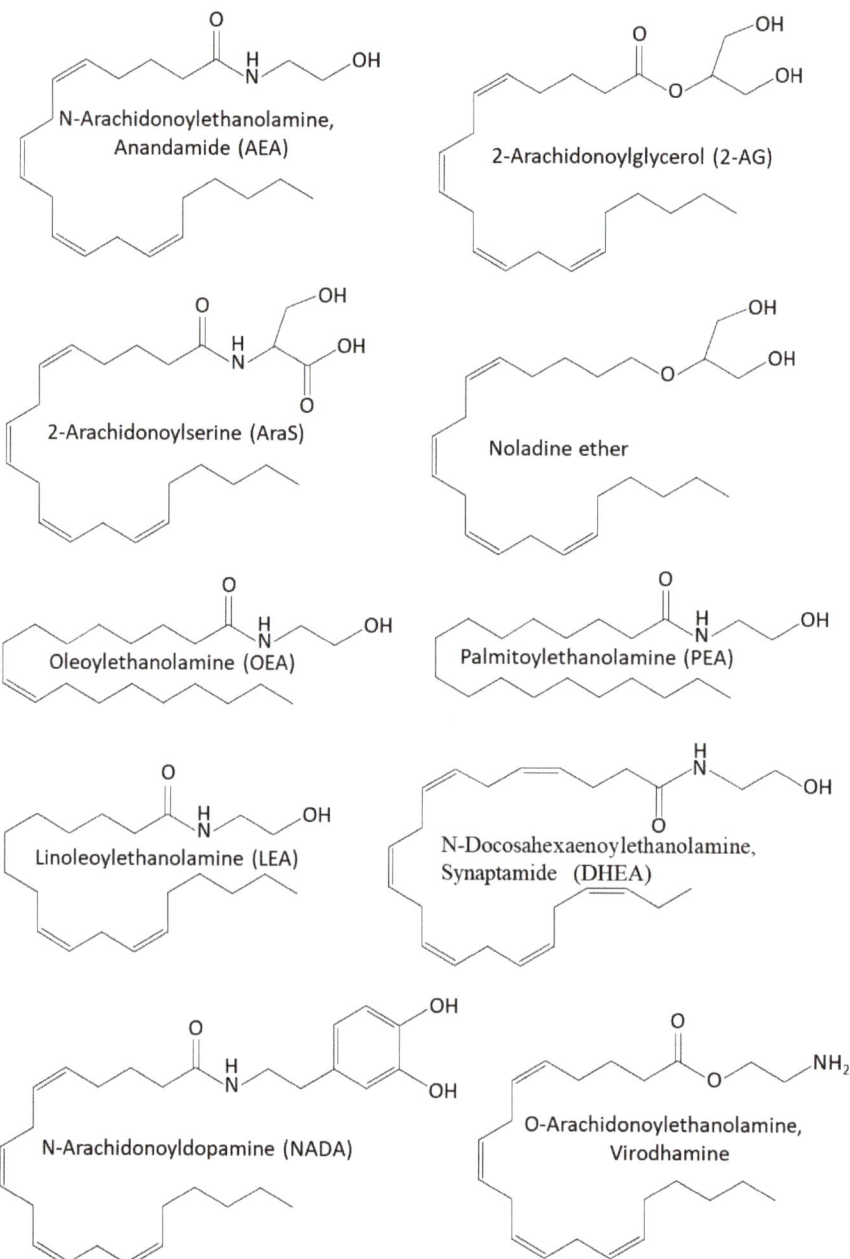

Figure 3. The chemical structures of some endocannabinoids.

Another communication system that exists between neurons is the release of lipid-based transport systems such as exosomes from neurons following a synaptic response, that are taken up by neighboring cells [350,351]. Gabrielli et al. [352] observed that endocannabinoids are secreted on extracellular membrane vesicles. In this study, extracellular vesicles secreted by microglial cells were found to carry AEA on their surface that was able to stimulate the CB1 receptor expressed on neurons and inhibit presynaptic transmission [352]. Microglial cells release endocannabinoids at much higher levels than neurons and astrocytes [319,353,354] and are thought to play a role in regulating the synaptic activity by a process termed gliotransmission, which functions to bridge the non-synaptic inter-neuronal communication [355].

4.5. Other Endocannabinoids and Endocannabinoid-like Compounds

Other endocannabinoids include the oleoyl- and palmitoyl-ethanolamines (OEA and PEA) that affect intestinal permeability by acting on TRPV-1 and PPARα [356,357], and 2-AG-ether and O-arachidonoylethanolamine (virodhamine) [22,358] (Figure 3). PEA is produced by neurons, microglia, and astrocytes in the central nervous system [359,360] where it plays an important role in neuroprotection [361,362]. Moreover, it was shown to have both anti-nociceptive and anti-inflammatory activities [363–366]. Immune cells release PEA that activates the CB2 receptor, resulting in downregulation of the inflammatory processes [367,368]. PEA, which is synthesized along with AEA, potentiates the action of AEA by increasing receptor affinity or reducing the degradation of AEA by FAAH [357,369–371]. The study of Lo Verme et al. [372] showed that PPARα was required for the anti-inflammatory effect of PEA. Borrelli et al. [365] observed that PEA alleviates the inflammation in a murine colitis model through acting on CB2, GPR55, and PPARα. OEA acts on PPARα and is secreted in the proximal intestine where it controls appetite, exhibits anti-inflammatory properties, and stimulates lipolysis and fatty acid oxidation [373–376].

The endocannabinoid noladin ether acts on CB2 and inhibits the intracellular effector adenylyl cyclase [377]. The endocannabinoid virodhamine, which is composed of arachidonic acid and ethanolamine joined by an ester linkage, is a partial agonist with an antagonist activity on CB1, while being a full agonist on CB2 [378]. At low concentrations, virodhamine activates GPR55, while at high concentrations it acts as an antagonist [379]. The endocannabinoid N-arachidonoyl-dopamine (NADA), which is highly expressed in the striatum, hippocampus, and cerebellum, activates TRPV1, induces the release of substance P and calcitonin gene-related peptide from dorsal spinal cord slices, and enhances hippocampal paired-pulse depression [380]. NADA and its epoxide metabolites also act as an agonist for the CB1 and CB2 receptors and show anti-inflammatory activities [337,381–383]. Other dopamine-related endocannabinoids include N-oleoyldopamine (OLDA), N-palmitoyldopamine (PALDA), and N-stearoyldopamine (STEARDA) [384]. OLDA is only a weak ligand of CB1, but it induced calcium influx, reduced the latency of paw withdrawal from a radiant heat source, and produced nocifensive behavior [384].

N-Arachidonoyl-L-serine (AraS) is an endogenous bioactive lipid found both in the central nervous system (CNS) and in the periphery, with a similar structure and physiological functions as AEA [385,386] (Figure 3). It possesses vasoactive, pro-angiogenic, pro-neurogenic, and neuroprotective properties [386–388]. Since AraS binds weakly to CB1 and CB2, it is not classified as an endocannabinoid, but rather has been coined as an "endocannabinoid-like" substance [386]. The pro-angiogenic activity of AraS is achieved by activation of GPR55 [387]. Moreover, AraS stimulates phosphorylation of MAPK and Akt protein kinases [385].

4.6. Anti-Microbial Activities of Endocannabinoids and Endocannabinoid-like Compounds

The anti-microbial effect of endocannabinoids depends on the strain studied and the endocannabinoid used [16–18,389,390] (Table 2). Among the tested organisms, *Streptococcus salivarius*, *Bacteroides fragilis*, and *Enterococcus faecalis* were the most susceptible bacteria to AEA and N-Linoleoylethanolamine (LEA) [390]. MSSA and MDRSA become immediately growth arrested by AEA, an effect that was transient and relieved upon time [16]. On the other hand, the growth of *Lactobacillus gasseri* species becomes enhanced by LEA and OEA [390].

Table 2. Anti-microbial activities of endocannabinoids and endocannabinoid-like compounds.

Endocannabinoids	Anti-Microbial Activity	References
Anandamide (AEA)	• MIC: 50 µM against *Streptococcus salivarius* RJX1086. • MIC > 256 µg/mL against MSSA ATCC 25923, MRSA ATCC 33592, MRSA ATCC 43300, a MRSA clinical isolate, and a MDRSA clinical isolate. • Transient bacteriostatic activity against drug-sensitive and drug-resistant *Staphylococcus aureus* species in a dose-dependent manner at concentration equal to an above 12.5 µg/mL AEA. • 50 and 100 µM AEA slightly inhibited the growth of *Alistipes shahii* RJX1084 and *Ruminococcus lactaris* RJX1085, and caused a delay in the log-phase growth of *Bacteriocides fragilis* ATCC 25285. 100 µM AEA retarded the growth of *Enterococcus faecalis* RJX1251. • 50 and 100 µM AEA slightly enhanced the growth of *Lactobacillus gasseri* DSM 20243, *Escherichia coli* RJX1083, and *Ruminococcus gnavus* RJX1118, while causing a small delay in the log-phase of *Ruminococcus gnavus* ATCC 29149. • 50 µM, but not 100 µM, AEA slightly increased the growth of *Lactobacillus gasseri* RJX1262. • 50 and 100 µM AEA had no effect on the growth of *Escherichia coli* AIEC NC101. • AEA sensitizes MRSA and MRDSA to antibiotics, including β-lactam antibiotics (ampicillin and methicillin), gentamicin, tetracycline, and norfloxacin. • MBIC: 12.5–35 µg/mL against MSSA ATCC 25923, MRSA ATCC 33592, MRSA ATCC 43300, a MRSA clinical isolate, and a MDRSA clinical isolate. • No anti-biofilm effect against *Candida albicans*. • Concentrations above 50 µg/mL prevented yeast-hyphal transition and hyphal extension of *Candida albicans* and inhibited their adhesion to cervical epithelial cells.	[16–18,389,390]
N-Arachidonoyl-L-serine (AraS)	• MIC: 16 µg/mL against MRSA ATCC 33592. • MIC: 128 µg/mL against MRSA ATCC 43300. • MIC > 256 µg/mL against a MRSA clinical isolate. • AraS sensitizes MRSA to antibiotics, including β-lactam antibiotics (ampicillin and methicillin), gentamicin, and tetracycline. • MBIC: 12.5–35 µg/mL against MRSA ATCC 33592, MRSA ATCC 43300, and a MRSA clinical isolate. • $MBIC_{50}$: 50 µg/mL against *Candida albicans*. • Concentrations above 50 µg/mL prevented yeast-hyphal transition and hyphal extension of *Candida albicans* and inhibited their adhesion to cervical epithelial cells.	[17,18,389]
2-Arachidonoylglycerol (2-AG)	• $MBIC_{50}$: 125 µg/mL against *Candida albicans*.	[389]
N-Linoleoylethanolamine (LEA)	• MIC: 50 µM against *Streptococcus salivarius* RJX1086. • MIC: 96 µM against *Bacteroides fragilis* ATCC 25285. A delayed log-phase growth was observed with 24 and 48 µM LEA on *Bacteroides fragilis* ATCC 25285. • MIC: 100 µM against *Enterococcus faecalis* RJX1251, with a strong growth retardation with 50 µM. • MIC: 100 µM against *Alistipes shahii* RJX1084. • 50 and 100 µM LEA reduced the growth of *Ruminococcus lactaris* RJX1085 by 24–40%. • 50 µM LEA strongly stimulated the growth of *Lactobacillus gasseri* DSM 20243 and *Lactobacillus gasseri* RJX1262. • 100 µM LEA strongly stimulated the growth of *Lactobacillus gasseri* DSM 20243 but slightly interfered with the growth of *Lactobacillus gasseri* RJX1262. • 50 and 100 µM LEA slightly increased the growth of *Escherichia coli* RJX1083. • It had no effect on the growth of *Ruminococcus gnavus* ATCC 29149 at 100 µM, with a small delay in the log-phase growth at 200 µM. • It had no effect on the growth of *Escherichia coli* AIEC NC101, even at 200 µM.	[390]

Table 2. Cont.

Endocannabinoids	Anti-Microbial Activity	References
Oleoylethanolamine (OEA)	• MIC: 50 µM against *Streptococcus salivarius* RJX1086. • 50 and 100 µM OEA had a slight growth inhibitory effect on *Ruminococcus lactaris* RJX1085 and caused a delay in the log-phase growth of *Alistipes shahii* RJX1084, *Bacteroides fragilis* ATCC 25285, and *Enterococcus faecalis* RJX1251. • 50 and 100 µM OEA strongly increased the growth of *Lactobacillus gasseri* RJX1262, while 100 µM was required to stimulate the growth of *Lactobacillus gasseri* DSM 20243 and *Ruminococcus gnavus* RJX1118. Both 50 and 100 µM had a slight growth-stimulating effect on *Escherichia coli* RJX1083, while no significant effect was observed on *Escherichia coli* AIEC NC101 and *Ruminococcus gnavus* ATCC 29149.	[390]
Palmitoylethanolamine (PEA)	• 50 and 100 µM PEA partly reduced the growth of *Ruminococcus lactaris* RJX1085 and *Streptococcus salivarius* RJX1086. The effect on *Alistipes shahii* RJX1084 was subtle. • 100 µM, but not 50 µM, PEA enhanced the growth of *Bacteroides fragilis* ATCC 25285 and *Enterococcus faecalis* RJX1251. • 50 and 100 µM PEA slightly increased the growth of *Lactobacillus gasseri* RJX1262 and DSM 20243, *Escherichia coli* RJX1083, *Ruminococcus gnavus* ATCC 29149 and RJX1118, while it had no significant effect on *Escherichia coli* AIEC NC101.	[390]

4.6.1. AEA and AraS Exert Bacteriostatic Activity on Both Drug-Sensitive and Drug-Resistant *Staphylococcus aureus*

Feldman et al. [18] observed that the MIC of AEA toward three MRSA species (MRSA ATCC 33592, MRSA ATCC 43300, and a MRSA clinical isolate) was above 256 µg/mL. AraS had a MIC of 16 and 128 µg/mL on MRSA ATCC 33592 and MRSA ATCC 43300, respectively, and a MIC above 256 µg/mL for the clinical MRSA isolate [18]. A kinetic study of AEA on a multidrug-resistant *Staphylococcus aureus* (MDRSA) clinical isolate and the MSSA ATCC 25923 strain showed that AEA caused a transient bacteriostatic effect that was overcome with time [16]. The bacteriostatic effect of AEA was independent of the drug-resistant phenotype [16]. Further analysis showed that AEA inhibited cell division just prior to daughter cell separation [16]. Gene expression studies showed that AEA reduced the expression of some autolysin genes, which might in part contribute to the growth arrest [16]. AEA altered the membrane structure of the MDRSA and caused an immediate membrane depolarization that recovered with time [16]. Both AEA and AraS reduced the hydrophobicity index of MRSA at a concentration of 16 µg/mL [18].

4.6.2. AEA and AraS Sensitize Drug-Resistant *Staphylococcus aureus* to Antibiotics

Importantly, it was observed that AEA and AraS sensitize MRSA and MDRSA strains to various antibiotics, including β-lactam antibiotics (ampicillin and methicillin), gentamicin, tetracycline, and norfloxacin [16,17]. For instance, the MIC of ampicillin against MRSA ATCC 33592 and 43300 was 128 and 256 µg/mL, respectively, but in the presence of 8–16 µg/mL AEA, it was reduced to 8 µg/mL [17]. The MIC of gentamicin against MRSA ATCC 33592 was 128 µg/mL, but in the presence of 8 µg/mL AEA, it was reduced to 4 µg/mL [17]. Treating a MDRSA clinical isolate with 50 µg/mL AEA reduced the MIC of methicillin from above 500 µg/mL to 50 µg/mL [16]. AEA was found to prevent drug efflux, resulting in intracellular drug accumulation, which might explain, at least in part, the sensitization of the bacteria to antibiotics [16]. Gene expression analysis shows that AEA reduces the expression of some efflux pump genes, including *norB*, *norC*, *mepA*, *kdpA*, and *opp1C* in MDRSA [16], but it is likely that the alterations in the membrane structure caused by AEA also contribute to intracellular drug retention.

It is notable that the sensitization of MRSA to methicillin takes place even when bacterial growth is inhibited by AEA [16], suggesting that the anti-bacterial effect of methicillin and other β-lactams does not require cell division as previously documented when used as a single agent [391,392]. Indeed, FtsZ inhibitors that arrest bacterial cell growth, also sensitize drug-resistant *Staphylococcus aureus* to β-lactam antibiotics, which was related to membrane relocalization of penicillin-binding proteins (PBPs) [393]. Further studies are required to fully understand the antibiotic-sensitization mechanisms of AEA and AraS.

4.6.3. AEA and AraS Exhibit Anti-Biofilm Activity against Drug-Sensitive and Drug-Resistant *Staphylococcus aureus*

AEA and AraS prevent biofilm formation of MRSA and MDRSA with a maximum effect at 12.5–35 µg/mL [16,18]. AEA and AraS had a rather weak effect on preformed biofilm of MRSA and MDRSA, where concentrations as high as 64 µg/mL were required to eradicate 50% of the biofilms after a 24 h incubation [16,18]. The simultaneous treatment of the MRSA and MDRSA strains with endocannabinoids and antibiotics significantly lowered the effective dose of the two compounds [16,17]. For instance, the MBICs of AEA and ampicillin on MRSA ATCC 33592 were, respectively, 33.8 and 128 µg/mL, while in combination, 8 µg/mL of each compound was required for inhibiting biofilm formation [17]. When combining the sub-MBIC concentration 3.125 µg/mL of AEA with 50 µg/mL norfloxacin, which, as a single agent, had no anti-biofilm effect, an 80% reduction in biofilm formation by MDRSA was observed [16]. A 90% reduction in preformed MDRSA biofilm was observed when 50 µg/mL of AEA was combined with 50 µg/mL methicillin, which is the synergistic condition required for killing the bacteria [16]. The latter observation shows that the combination of AEA with antibiotics is also effective against biofilm-embedded bacteria.

Gene expression studies showed that AEA reduced the expression of the regulatory *RNAIII* and the virulence gene α-helical phenol-soluble modulin (*psmα*) in MDRSA [16]. Additionally, the genes *fnbB*, *hla*, and *hld* encoding for the virulence factors fibronectin binding protein, α-hemolysin and δ-hemolysin (δ-toxin), respectively, were downregulated by AEA [16]. As Psmα plays a central role in *Staphylococcus aureus* biofilm formation by stabilizing the biofilms through amyloid formation [394–396], the inhibition of its expression might be one mechanism for the anti-biofilm effect of AEA (Figure 4).

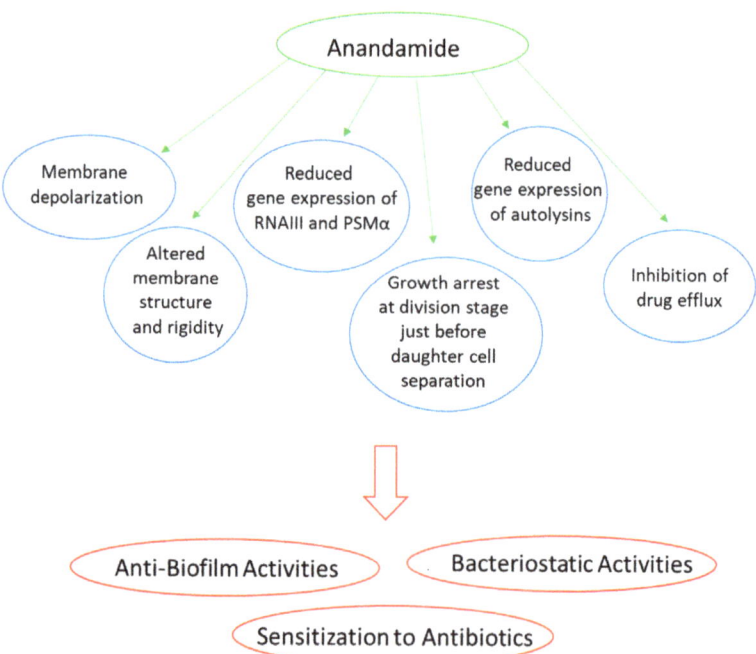

Figure 4. The anti-bacterial actions of anandamide on *Staphylococcus aureus*.

4.6.4. AEA and AraS Inhibit Yeast-Hypha Transition of *Candida albicans* and Prevent Adhesion of *Candida albicans* Hyphae to Epithelial Cells

AEA and AraS were found to inhibit yeast-hypha transition of *Candida albicans* at 125 and 250 µg/mL [389]. At 50 µg/mL, there was only a partial inhibition on the yeast-hypha transition, but this concentration was sufficient to prevent hyphal extension [389]. Importantly, *Candida albicans* hyphae that have been exposed to AEA at 50 µg/mL and higher concentrations showed strong reduction in their ability to adhere to the HeLa cervical epithelial carcinoma cells [389]. AraS-treated *Candida albicans* hyphae showed deficient adherence to HeLa cervical carcinoma cells similar to AEA-treated fungi, while 2-AG treatment had only a minor effect at the concentrations analyzed (up to 250 µg/mL) [389]. None of the endocannabinoids affected the adherence of the *Candida albicans* hyphae to polystyrene tissue culture plates within the first hour of incubation, while AraS and 2-AG, but not AEA, reduced the biofilm mass formed on the polystyrene tissue culture plates after a 24 h incubation [389].

Gene expression studies showed that AEA increased the expression of *NRG1*, which is a transcriptional repressor of filamentous growth, but reduced the expression of the hyphal cell wall protein 1 (*HWP1*), the Agglutinin-like protein 3 (*ALS3*), the Hypha-specific G1 cyclin-related protein 1 (*HGC1*), the Ras-like protein 1 (*RAS1*), the enhanced filamentous growth protein 1 (*EFG1*), the cell surface hydrophobicity-associated protein *CSH1*, and the extent of cell elongation protein 1 (*ECE1*). The combined effect of AEA on the expression of these genes might cumulate in the observed effects of AEA on *Candida albicans* adherence and hyphal growth (Figure 5).

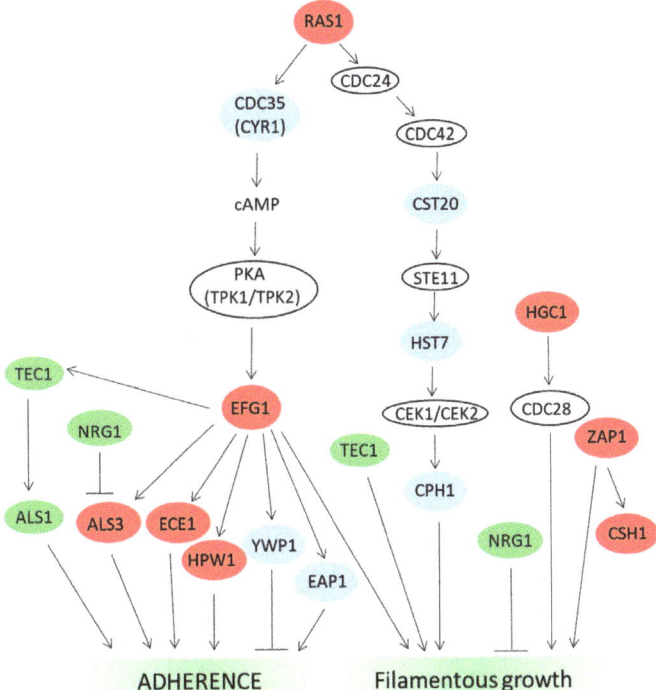

Figure 5. Effect of AEA on *Candida albicans* gene expression [381]. Genes in red are downregulated by AEA after a 2 h incubation. Genes in green are upregulated by AEA. Genes in light blue are unaffected by AEA. Open circles are genes that have not yet been analyzed. Ultimately, AEA prevents the adherence and hyphal extension of *Candida albicans*.

4.7. Dialog between the Gut Microbiota and the Endocannabinoid System

An intercommunication system has been found to exist between the gut microbiota and the endocannabinoid system [285,298,397–402]. The gut microbiota, representing more than 100 trillion microorganisms, including at least 1000 distinct species, lives in symbiosis with the host and assists in controlling the metabolic health of the host by degrading nutrients that the host is unable to digest and by providing a whole battery of small signaling molecules, metabolites, and nutrients beneficial for the host physiology [298,403]. The gut microbiome differs from individual to individual, and the composition of the microbiota is believed to affect various metabolic disorders, such as obesity, hyperglycemia, and dyslipidemia, which are risk factors for type 2 diabetes, hepatosteatosis, and arteriosclerosis [404]. Reduced diversity of gut microbiota has been linked with various pathophysiological conditions, such as depression, schizophrenia, neurological disorders, and chronic fatigue [405–409]. Microbiota can affect the endocannabinoid system and the nervous system, and vice versa; the nervous system and the endocannabinoids can influence the enteric microbiota composition [112,285,390,397,410,411].

4.7.1. The Relationship between Gut Microbiota, the Endocannabinoid System, and Depression

The effect of the gut microbiota on depressive-like behaviors in mice was found to be mediated by the endocannabinoid system [411]. These authors showed that the transfer of microbiota from stress-induced depressive mice to naïve unstressed hosts induced a depressive-like state in the recipients. This was accompanied by a reduced adult hippocampal neurogenesis that was related to decreased hippocampal 2-AG levels and deficient CB1-mediated activation of the mTOR signaling pathways [411]. The detrimental effects on hippocampal neurogenesis could be restored by a MAGL inhibitor that prevents 2-AG degradation, addition of the 2-AG precursor arachidonic acid to the diet, or by complementation with *Lactobacillus plantarum*^{WJL} [411]. The microbiota from the stress-induced depressive mice showed an increase in *Ruminococcaceae* and *Porphyromonodaceae* species, with a decrease in *Lactobacillaceae* [411]. The complementation with *Lactobacillus plantarum*^{WJL} restored hippocampal 2-AG to normal levels, as well as increased the levels of AEA, n-3, and n-6 polyunsaturated fatty acids (PUFAs) [411]. *Lactobacillus* species can regulate fatty acid metabolism, absorption, and fatty acid composition of the host [412,413], which in turn affects the endocannabinoid system [411]. Rousseaux et al. [414] observed that oral administration of *Lactobacillus acidophilus* induced the expression of both the μ_1 opioid receptor and CB2 receptor on colon epithelial cells, resulting in reduced abdominal pain in a rat colorectal distension model.

4.7.2. Association between Gut Microbiota, PEA, and Anhedonia/Amotivation

PEA was shown to mediate the association between gut microbial diversity and anhedonia/amotivation [410]. Increased serum levels of PEA were associated with antidepressive effects [357,415], while increased stool levels of PEA, indicative of increased excretion of PEA, were associated with alterations in synaptic plasticity, learning, and emotional responses [410,416,417]. The stool PEA levels were associated with gut microbial diversity, with implications on host mental health [285,357,410,418]. The relative abundance of microbes of the *Blautia* and *Dorea* taxa was particularly associated with fecal PEA and anhedonia/amotivation [410]. Reduced microbial diversity corresponded with increased excretion of PEA and more severe anhedonia/amotivation [410]. PEA was also found to counteract autistic-like behaviors in BTBR T$^+$ *tf*/J mice by dampening inflammation, reducing oxidative stress, reducing gut permeability, and altering the gut microbiota, besides its neuroprotection through induction of PPARα [419]. These authors found that PEA treatment increased the ratio of *Firmicutes/Bacteroidetes*, which was due to an increase in *Firmicutes* (e.g., *Clostridials*) and a decrease in *Bacteroidetes* [419].

4.7.3. The Relationship between Gut Microbiota, AEA, and Acute Respiratory Distress Syndrome

AEA was found to attenuate acute respiratory distress syndrome through modulating the gut microbiota [420]. In this study, the researchers investigated the effect of AEA on staphylococcal enterotoxin B (SEB)-mediated acute respiratory distress syndrome. SEB caused an increase in pathogenic bacteria in both the lungs and the gut [420]. AEA-treated mice showed increased level of anti-microbial peptides in the lung epithelial cells and prevented the increase in pathogenic bacteria induced by SEB [420]. AEA increased the level of several bacterial species (e.g., *Lachnospiraceae* and *Clostridia*) that produce elevated levels of SCFAs, such as butyrate and valerate, important for stabilizing the gut–lung microbial axis and suppressing inflammation [420]. In addition, AEA treatment increased the abundance of *Muribaculaceae* and reduced the abundance of *Pseudomonas* and *Enterobacteriaceae* [420].

4.7.4. The Relationship between Gut Microbiota, the Endocannabinoid System, and Obesity

Obesity is often characterized by low-grade inflammation, with increased levels of endocannabinoids in the plasma and adipose tissues and altered expression of CB1 [421]. Activation of CB1 and CB2 receptors reduces motility, limits secretion, and decreases hypersensitivity in the gut [422–424]. Impaired CB1 signaling protected against the development of obesity and steatosis [425–427]. Lipopolysaccharides from Gram-negative bacteria induce the production of endocannabinoids under inflammatory conditions that dampen the inflammatory response [318,428–430]. Vice versa, the activation of CB1 in mice increases circulating levels of lipopolysaccharides due to reduced expression of the tight junction proteins occludin and zonula occludens-1 (ZO-1), resulting in increased gut epithelial permeability [421,431].

The gut microbiota was found to modulate colon CB1 receptor expression in both normal and obese mice [421]. Obese mice fed with the prebiotic oligofructose showed reduced CB1 expression, lower AEA content, and increased expression of FAAH [421]. Obese mice treated with the CB1 antagonist SR141716A (Rimonabant) improved the gut barrier function and reduced body weight gain [421]. Mehrpouya-Bahrami et al. [432] observed that SR141716A attenuated diet-induced obesity and inflammation that was correlated with increased relative abundance of *Akkermansia muciniphila* and decreased abundance of *Lanchnospiraceae* and *Erysipelotrichaceae* in the gut. Interestingly, SR141716A prevented the intracellular replication of macrophage-phagocytosed *Brucella suis* by activating the macrophages, which was related to the inhibition of CB1 [433]. It would be interesting to study whether SR141716A also has a direct anti-microbial effect. In this context, it is worth mentioning that SR141716A could potentiate the anti-fungal activity of amphotericin B against *Candida albicans* and *Cryptococcus neoformans* by increasing cellular oxidative stress and cell membrane permeability [434].

Mice fed on high-fat, high-glucose diet showed altered microbiome with concomitant increase in AEA and 2-AG in the plasma [398]. The relative abundances of *Adlercreutzia*, *Barnesiella*, *Coprobacillus*, *Eubacterium*, and *Parasutterella* in the ileum were negatively associated with AEA levels [398]. The level of the AEA congener N-docosahexaenoylethanolamine (synaptamide, DHEA), which is required for normal brain development [435], was negatively associated with *Barnesiella*, *Enterococcus*, *Eubacterium*, *Flavonifractor*, and *Intestinimonas* in the ileum [398]. These authors also found a negative correlation between the *Delftia* genus and N-linoleoylethanolamine (LEA), while the *Lactobacillus* genus was associated with increased 2-docosahexaenoyl-glycerol (2-DHG) levels [398].

Repeated administration of OAE to mice fed on normal chow pellet diet for 11 days led to alteration in fecal microbial composition with an increase in *Bacteroidetes* (e.g., *Bacteroides* genus) and a decrease in *Firmicutes* (*Lactobacillus*), which is considered a "lean-like" phenotype [436]. OAE also reduced intestinal cytokines expression by immune cells isolated from Peyer's patches [436].

4.7.5. The Relationship between Gut Microbiota, the Endocannabinoid System, and Inflammatory Bowel Diseases

Both AEA and PEA have been observed to reduce inflammation in murine models of colitis and inflammatory bowel disease [437–439]. Elevating the levels of the endocannabinoids by inhibiting FAAH could relieve colitis and inflammatory bowel disease [440,441]. Butyrate that is produced by gut microbiota (e.g., bacteria of the *Ruminococcaceae* and *Lachnospiraceae* family) [442] reduces inflammation and pain in colitis animal models, which can in part be mediated through the endocannabinoid system [443]. Vijay et al. [443] studied the association of the endocannabinoids AEA, 2-AG, OEA, and PEA with gut microbiome composition upon exercise. Under resting condition, AEA and OEA were positively associated with alpha diversity and with SCFA producing bacteria such as *Bifidobacterium*, *Coprococcus 3*, and *Faecalibacterium*, while being negatively associated with *Collinsella* [443]. AEA, OEA, and PEA increased with exercise, and changes in AEA correlated with bacterial butyrate production [443]. The increases in AEA and PEA correlated with decreased expression of the inflammatory mediators TNFα and IL-6 and increased expression of the anti-inflammatory cytokine IL-10 [443].

PEA was found to increase the phagocytosis and intracellular killing of encapsulated *Escherichia coli* K1 by activated microglial cells and macrophages [444,445]. Pre-treatment with PEA significantly increased the survival of mice challenged with *Escherichia coli* K1 [445]. Similarly, Heide et al. [446] observed that prophylactic PEA attenuated inflammation and increased the survival of mice challenged with intracerebral *Escherichia coli* K1 infection. Lower bacterial loads were observed in the spleen, liver, and blood of the PEA pretreated animals [446]. This was related to the anti-inflammatory effect, since PEA at 1 µg/mL had no effect on *Escherichia coli* growth in vitro [446].

The gut microbiota of IBD patients differs from healthy individuals, with a decrease in butyrate- and indole-producing bacteria, decrease in bile salt-sensitive bacteria, while an enrichment in bile acid-metabolizing bacteria [390,447–449]. Among others, *Escherichia coli*, *Lactobacillus gasseri*, *Ruminococcus gnavus*, and *Blautia producta*, were more abundant in IBD, while *Bacteroides cellulosilyticus*, *Bacteroides fragilis*, and *Streptococcus salivarius* were depleted [390]. Fornelos et al. [390] observed that certain N-Acylethanolamines (NAEs), such as LEA, PEA, OEA and AEA, are elevated in the stool of IBD, Crohn's disease, and/or ulcerative colitis patients, and stimulate the growth of bacterial species overrepresented in IBD while inhibiting bacterial species lacking in IBD. N-acylethanolamine levels were highest in samples with most differences in the microbiome, suggesting a connection between N-Acylethanolamines and altered microbiota in IBD [390]. These researchers observed that LEA inhibited the growth of *Bacteroides fragilis*, *Bacteroides cellulosilyticus*, and *Enterococcus faecalis*, while slightly enhanced the growth of *Escherichia coli*, *Ruminococcus gnavus*, and *Blautia producta* [390]. AEA also transiently inhibited the growth of *Bacteroides fragilis* and *Enterococcus faecalis* that recovered with time [390]. The growth of *Lactobacillus gasseri*, which is enriched in IBD, was enhanced by OEA and LEA, and to a lesser extent by AEA [390]. LEA and AEA partly inhibited the growth of *Alistipes shahii* and *Ruminococcus lactaris* that are underrepresented in IBD subjects [390]. The growth of *Streptococcus salivarius* was completely prevented at a concentration of 50 µM LEA, AEA, or OEA, but only slightly inhibited by PEA [390].

4.7.6. Effect of N-Acylethanolamines on the Microbial Composition of Stool Chemostats

Fornelos et al. [390] also studied the effect of N-acylethanolamines, including endocannabinoids, on the composition of two different stool chemostats. In the control chemostat A, the *Enterobacteriaceae*, *Clostridiaceae*, and *Veillonellaceae* taxa dominated, while in the presence of AEA, the bacterial community was almost entirely overtaken by *Enterobacteriaceae* [390]. LEA-treated chemostat A was dominated by *Enterococcaceae*, *Veillonellaceae* and *Enterobacteriaceae* at the expense of *Streptococcaceae*, *Erysipelotrichaceae*, *Porphyromonadacea*, *Bacteroidaceae*, and *Rikenellaceae*, while OEA treatment did not impact *Enterobacteriaceae* abundance but increased the relative abundances of *Enterococcaceae* and *Streptococcaceae* and decreased those of *Bacteroidaceae* and *Rikenellaceae* [390]. AEA and LEA also reduced the abundance of *Barnesiella intestinihominis*, *Alistipes*, and *Bacteroides* species, while they increased the abundance of *Escherichia* species [390]. In Chemostat B, the abundance of *Blautia producta*, *Clostridium clostridioforme*, *Klebsiella pneumoniae*, and *Proteus mirabilis* was increased in the presence of AEA or LEA [390]. These data indicate that LEA, AEA, and other *N*-Acylethanolamines can shift the microbiome of a healthy individual into an IBD profile [390].

Transcriptional analysis showed that AEA upregulates both the anaerobic, reductive, and oxidative branches of the citrate cycle concomitant with increased energy metabolism and increased respiratory electron transport chain activity, especially in *Enterobacteriaceae* [390]. Metabolic changes occurring upon exposure to AEA, LEA, and other NAEs include the activation of bacterial processes involved in NAE metabolism [390].

Searching for an action mechanism of LEA and AEA on *Bacteroides fragilis*, the researchers found that the most upregulated genes are those encoding for membrane-associated efflux transport proteins, and the most downregulated gene was the long chain fatty acid (LCFA) importer *fadL* [390]. They further showed that two other genes involved in fatty acid metabolic processing were repressed: a *fadD* homolog that catalyzes esterification of incoming fatty acids into CoA thioesters and a *fadE* homolog involved in downstream fatty acid breakdown [390]. These data indicate that bacteria have developed mechanisms that can respond to endocannabinoids.

5. Conclusions

Both phytocannabinoids and endocannabinoids have diverse physiological activities that are, in part, mediated by common receptors in mammalians, each compound with its specificity and affinity, being agonists, partly agonists, inverse agonists, or antagonists. While these mechanisms have been widely investigated, the mechanisms leading to their anti-microbial effects are less understood. Despite the quite different structures of phytocannabinoids and endocannabinoids (Figures 1 and 3), there are some common dominators that characterize their anti-bacterial activities (Figures 2 and 4). For instance, they exert bacteriostatic activity, alter the membrane structure, induce either membrane hyperpolarization or depolarization, modulate gene expression including those involved in metabolism, affect virulence factors, and prevent biofilm formation (Figures 2 and 4). Additionally, the AEA-mediated inhibition of yeast-hypha transition of *Candida albicans* and the hyphal adherence to epithelial cells seem to be mediated by alterations in gene expression (Figure 5). The multiple actions of phytocannabinoids and endocannabinoids suggest that the compounds do much more than just affecting membrane permeability as previously thought.

The emergence of antibiotic-resistant microbes is a clinical problem worldwide, and novel treatment strategies are urged. The important observation that some of the phytocannabinoids and endocannabinoids act on both drug-sensitive and drug-resistant *Staphylococcus aureus* makes them potential antibiotic adjuvants in treating drug-resistant infections, for instance for topical infectious wound treatment. Especially important is the ability of AEA and AraS to sensitize drug-resistant *Staphylococcus aureus* to antibiotics in virtue of their ability to prevent drug efflux and induce growth arrest. The addition of these endocannabinoids to the treatment cocktail will revive the use of already existing antibiotics. The ability of both CBG and the synthetic cannabinoid HU-210 to antagonize quorum sensing may have implications in the new era where quorum sensing inhibitors or quorum quenchers have attracted attention for alternative antibiotic drugs for antibiotic-resistant bacteria [450]. To reach this goal, further studies should be performed to clarify the spectrum of bacteria whose quorum sensing pathways are affected by cannabinoids. The increasing recognition of the complex interplay between the gut microbiota and the endocannabinoid system with the accompanying implications for various physiological and pathophysiological conditions, places the therapeutic uses of cannabinoids into a new spotlight.

Author Contributions: Conceptualization, R.V.S. and D.S.; writing—original draft preparation, R.V.S.; writing—review and editing, R.V.S. and D.S. All authors have read and agreed to the published version of the manuscript.

Funding: This research received no external funding.

Institutional Review Board Statement: Not applicable.

Informed Consent Statement: Not applicable.

Data Availability Statement: Not applicable.

Acknowledgments: The authors want to thank Goldie Wolfson for her English editing of the manuscript.

Conflicts of Interest: The authors declare no conflict of interest.

Abbreviations

AEA	Anandamide, N-Arachidonoylethanolamine, N-Arachidonylethanolamide
2-AG	2-Arachidonoylglycerol
AraS	N-Arachidonoyl-L-serine
CBC	Cannabichromene
CBCA	Cannabichromenic acid
CBD	Cannabidiol
CBDA	Cannabidiolic acid
CBG	Cannabigerol
CBN	Cannabinol
CFU	Colony-forming unit
C. sativa L.	Cannabis sativa Linnaeus
DAGL	Diacylglycerol lipase
ECS	Endocannabinoid system
EPS	Extracellular polymeric substances
FAAH	Fatty acid amide hydrolase
GPCR	G-protein-coupled receptor
GPR18/GPR55	G-protein-coupled receptors 18/55
IBD	Inflammatory bowel disease
IC50	Half maximal inhibitory concentration
LD50	Half maximal lethal dose
LEA	N-Linoleoylethanolamine
MBEC	Minimum biofilm eradication concentration
MBIC	Minimum biofilm inhibitory concentration
MIC	Minimum inhibitory concentration
MDRSA	Multidrug resistant Staphylococcus aureus
MSSA	Methicillin sensitive Staphylococcus aureus
MRSA	Methicillin resistant Staphylococcus aureus
NAE	N-Acylethanolamine
NAPE	N-Acyl-phosphatidylethanolamine
OEA	Oleoylethanolamine
OLDA	N-Oleoyldopamine
PALDA	N-Palmitoyldopamine
PEA	Palmitoylethanolamine
PIP2	Phosphatidylinositol-4,5-bisphosphate
PPARα/γ	Peroxisome proliferator activated receptor α/γ
Psmα	α-Helical phenol-soluble modulin
SCFA	Small chain fatty acid
STEARDA	N-Stearoyldopamine
Δ^9-THC	Δ^9-Tetrahydrocannabinol
THCA	Tetrahydrocannabinolic acid
TRPA1	Ankyrin-type 1 transient receptor potential channel
TRPM8	Transient receptor potential cation channel subfamily M (melastatin) member 8
TRPV1	Transient receptor potential vanilloid-1

References

1. Sofowora, A.; Ogunbodede, E.; Onayade, A. The role and place of medicinal plants in the strategies for disease prevention. *Afr. J. Tradit. Complement. Altern. Med.* **2013**, *10*, 210–229. [CrossRef] [PubMed]
2. Bidlack, W.R.; Omaye, S.T.; Meskin, M.S.; Topham, D.K. *Phytochemicals as Bioactive Agents*; CRC Press: Boca Raton, FL, USA, 2000.
3. Ross, I.A. *Medicinal Plants of the World, Volumes 3: Chemical Constituents, Traditional and Modern Medicinal Uses*; Springer Science & Business Media: Berlin/Heidelberg, Germany, 2007; Volume 3.
4. Gorlenko, C.L.; Kiselev, H.Y.; Budanova, E.V.; Zamyatnin, A.A., Jr.; Ikryannikova, L.N. Plant secondary metabolites in the battle of drugs and drug-resistant bacteria: New heroes or worse clones of antibiotics? *Antibiotics* **2020**, *9*, 170. [CrossRef] [PubMed]
5. Radulović, N.S.; Blagojević, P.D.; Stojanović-Radić, Z.Z.; Stojanović, N.M. Antimicrobial plant metabolites: Structural diversity and mechanism of action. *Curr. Med. Chem.* **2013**, *20*, 932–952. [PubMed]
6. Vaou, N.; Stavropoulou, E.; Voidarou, C.; Tsigalou, C.; Bezirtzoglou, E. Towards advances in medicinal plant antimicrobial activity: A review study on challenges and future perspectives. *Microorganisms* **2021**, *9*, 2041. [CrossRef]
7. Lahiri, D.; Dash, S.; Dutta, R.; Nag, M. Elucidating the effect of anti-biofilm activity of bioactive compounds extracted from plants. *J. Biosci.* **2019**, *44*, 52. [CrossRef] [PubMed]
8. Ekor, M. The growing use of herbal medicines: Issues relating to adverse reactions and challenges in monitoring safety. *Front. Pharmacol.* **2014**, *4*, 177. [CrossRef]
9. Hussein, R.A.; El-Anssary, A.A. Chapter 2: Plants secondary metabolites: The key drivers of the pharmacological actions of medicinal plants. *Herb. Med.* **2019**, *1*, 13. [CrossRef]
10. Nunes, C.D.R.; Barreto Arantes, M.; Menezes de Faria Pereira, S.; Leandro da Cruz, L.; de Souza Passos, M.; Pereira de Moraes, L.; Vieira, I.J.C.; Barros de Oliveira, D. Plants as sources of anti-inflammatory agents. *Molecules* **2020**, *25*, 3726. [CrossRef]
11. Borges, A.; Abreu, A.C.; Dias, C.; Saavedra, M.J.; Borges, F.; Simões, M. New perspectives on the use of phytochemicals as an emergent strategy to control bacterial infections including biofilms. *Molecules* **2016**, *21*, 877. [CrossRef]
12. Kaur, S.; Sharma, N.; Roy, A. Role of cannabinoids in various diseases: A review. *Curr. Pharm. Biotechnol.* 2021; *in press*. [CrossRef]
13. Kogan, N.M.; Mechoulam, R. Cannabinoids in health and disease. *Dialogues Clin. Neurosci.* **2007**, *9*, 413–430. [CrossRef]
14. Rodríguez Mesa, X.M.; Moreno Vergara, A.F.; Contreras Bolaños, L.A.; Guevara Moriones, N.; Mejía Piñeros, A.L.; Santander González, S.P. Therapeutic prospects of cannabinoids in the immunomodulation of prevalent autoimmune diseases. *Cannabis Cannabinoid Res.* **2021**, *6*, 196–210. [CrossRef]
15. Mechoulam, R.; Hanuš, L.O.; Pertwee, R.; Howlett, A.C. Early phytocannabinoid chemistry to endocannabinoids and beyond. *Nat. Rev. Neurosci.* **2014**, *15*, 757–764. [CrossRef] [PubMed]
16. Banerjee, S.; Sionov, R.V.; Feldman, M.; Smoum, R.; Mechoulam, R.; Steinberg, D. Anandamide alters the membrane properties, halts the cell division and prevents drug efflux in multidrug resistant *Staphylococcus aureus*. *Sci. Rep.* **2021**, *11*, 8690. [CrossRef] [PubMed]
17. Feldman, M.; Smoum, R.; Mechoulam, R.; Steinberg, D. Potential combinations of endocannabinoid/endocannabinoid-like compounds and antibiotics against methicillin-resistant *Staphylococcus aureus*. *PLoS ONE* **2020**, *15*, e0231583. [CrossRef] [PubMed]
18. Feldman, M.; Smoum, R.; Mechoulam, R.; Steinberg, D. Antimicrobial potential of endocannabinoid and endocannabinoid-like compounds against methicillin-resistant *Staphylococcus aureus*. *Sci. Rep.* **2018**, *8*, 17696. [CrossRef] [PubMed]
19. Feldman, M.; Sionov, R.; Smoum, R.; Mechoulam, R.; Ginsburg, I.; Steinberg, D. Comparative evaluation of combinatory interaction between endocannabinoid system compounds and Poly-L-lysine against *Streptococcus mutans* growth and biofilm formation. *Biomed. Res. Int.* **2020**, *2020*, 7258380. [CrossRef] [PubMed]
20. Bilkei-Gorzo, A. The endocannabinoid system in normal and pathological brain ageing. *Philos. Trans. R. Soc. B Biol. Sci.* **2012**, *367*, 3326–3341. [CrossRef]
21. Cabral, G.A.; Rogers, T.J.; Lichtman, A.H. Turning Over a New Leaf: Cannabinoid and endocannabinoid modulation of immune function. *J. Neuroimmune Pharmacol.* **2015**, *10*, 193–203. [CrossRef]
22. Chiurchiù, V.; Battistini, L.; Maccarrone, M. Endocannabinoid signalling in innate and adaptive immunity. *Immunology* **2015**, *144*, 352–364. [CrossRef]
23. Maccarrone, M.; Bab, I.; Bíró, T.; Cabral, G.A.; Dey, S.K.; Di Marzo, V.; Konje, J.C.; Kunos, G.; Mechoulam, R.; Pacher, P.; et al. Endocannabinoid signaling at the periphery: 50 years after THC. *Trends Pharmacol. Sci.* **2015**, *36*, 277–296. [CrossRef]
24. Pacher, P.; Kogan, N.M.; Mechoulam, R. Beyond THC and endocannabinoids. *Annu. Rev. Pharmacol. Toxicol.* **2020**, *60*, 637–659. [CrossRef] [PubMed]
25. Li, H.L. The origin and use of *Cannabis* in eastern Asia linguistic-cultural implications. *J. Econ. Bot.* **1973**, *28*, 293–301. [CrossRef]
26. Pisanti, S.; Bifulco, M. Medical *Cannabis*: A plurimillennial history of an evergreen. *J. Cell. Physiol.* **2019**, *234*, 8342–8351. [CrossRef] [PubMed]
27. Jiang, H.E.; Li, X.; Zhao, Y.X.; Ferguson, D.K.; Hueber, F.; Bera, S.; Wang, Y.F.; Zhao, L.C.; Liu, C.J.; Li, C.S. A new insight into *Cannabis sativa* (Cannabaceae) utilization from 2500-year-old Yanghai Tombs, Xinjiang, China. *J. Ethnopharmacol.* **2006**, *108*, 414–422. [CrossRef]
28. Touw, M. The religious and medicinal uses of *Cannabis* in China, India and Tibet. *J. Psychoact. Drugs* **1981**, *13*, 23–34. [CrossRef] [PubMed]

29. Baron, E.P.; Lucas, P.; Eades, J.; Hogue, O. Patterns of medicinal cannabis use, strain analysis, and substitution effect among patients with migraine, headache, arthritis, and chronic pain in a medicinal cannabis cohort. *J. Headache Pain* **2018**, *19*, 37. [CrossRef]
30. Kantonen, T.; Karjalainen, T.; Pekkarinen, L.; Isojärvi, J.; Kalliokoski, K.; Kaasinen, V.; Hirvonen, J.; Nuutila, P.; Nummenmaa, L. Cerebral μ-opioid and CB_1 receptor systems have distinct roles in human feeding behavior. *Transl. Psychiatry* **2021**, *11*, 442. [CrossRef]
31. Lal, S.; Shekher, A.; Puneet; Narula, A.S.; Abrahamse, H.; Gupta, S.C. *Cannabis* and its constituents for cancer: History, biogenesis, chemistry and pharmacological activities. *Pharmacol. Res.* **2021**, *163*, 105302. [CrossRef]
32. Pollio, A. The Name of Cannabis: A short guide for nonbotanists. *Cannabis Cannabinoid Res.* **2016**, *1*, 234–238. [CrossRef]
33. Hanuš, L.O.; Hod, Y. Terpenes/terpenoids in *Cannabis*: Are They important? *Med. Cannabis Cannabinoids* **2020**, *3*, 25–60. [CrossRef]
34. Nissen, L.; Zatta, A.; Stefanini, I.; Grandi, S.; Sgorbati, B.; Biavati, B.; Monti, A. Characterization and antimicrobial activity of essential oils of industrial hemp varieties (*Cannabis sativa* L.). *Fitoterapia* **2010**, *81*, 413–419. [CrossRef] [PubMed]
35. Vergara, D.; Gaudino, R.; Blank, T.; Keegan, B. Modeling cannabinoids from a large-scale sample of *Cannabis sativa* chemotypes. *PLoS ONE* **2020**, *15*, e0236878. [CrossRef]
36. Borroto Fernandez, E.; Peterseil, V.; Hackl, G.; Menges, S.; de Meijer, E.; Staginnus, C. Distribution of chemical phenotypes (chemotypes) in European agricultural hemp (*Cannabis sativa* L.) cultivars. *J. Forensic Sci.* **2020**, *65*, 715–721. [CrossRef] [PubMed]
37. Casajuana Kögüel, C.; López-Pelayo, H.; Balcells-Olivero, M.M.; Colom, J.; Gual, A. Psychoactive constituents of *Cannabis* and their clinical implications: A systematic review. *Adicciones* **2018**, *30*, 140–151. [CrossRef] [PubMed]
38. Farag, S.; Kayser, O. Cultivation and breeding of *Cannabis sativa* L. for preparation of standardized extracts for medicinal purposes. In *Medicinal and Aromatic Plants of the World: Scientific, Production, Commercial and Utilization Aspects*; Máthé, Á., Ed.; Springer: Dordrecht, The Netherlands, 2015; pp. 165–186. [CrossRef]
39. Hanuš, L.O.; Meyer, S.M.; Muñoz, E.; Taglialatela-Scafati, O.; Appendino, G. Phytocannabinoids: A unified critical inventory. *Nat. Prod. Rep.* **2016**, *33*, 1357–1392. [CrossRef]
40. Gülck, T.; Møller, B.L. Phytocannabinoids: Origins and biosynthesis. *Trends Plant Sci.* **2020**, *25*, 985–1004. [CrossRef]
41. Livingston, S.J.; Quilichini, T.D.; Booth, J.K.; Wong, D.C.J.; Rensing, K.H.; Laflamme-Yonkman, J.; Castellarin, S.D.; Bohlmann, J.; Page, J.E.; Samuels, A.L. *Cannabis* glandular trichomes alter morphology and metabolite content during flower maturation. *Plant J.* **2020**, *101*, 37–56. [CrossRef]
42. Andre, C.M.; Hausman, J.F.; Guerriero, G. *Cannabis sativa*: The plant of the thousand and one molecules. *Front. Plant Sci.* **2016**, *7*, 19. [CrossRef]
43. Mediavilla, V.; Jonquera, M.; Schmid-Slembrouck, I.; Soldati, A. Decimal code for growth stages of hemp (*Cannabis sativa* L.). *J. Int. Hemp. Assoc.* **1998**, *5*, 68–74.
44. Eichhorn Bilodeau, S.; Wu, B.S.; Rufyikiri, A.S.; MacPherson, S.; Lefsrud, M. An update on plant photobiology and implications for Cannabis production. *Front. Plant Sci.* **2019**, *10*, 296. [CrossRef]
45. Magagnini, G.; Grassi, G.; Kotiranta, S. The effect of light spectrum on the morphology and cannabinoid content of *Cannabis sativa* L. *Med. Cannabis Cannabinoids* **2018**, *1*, 19–27. [CrossRef] [PubMed]
46. Bernstein, N.; Gorelick, J.; Zerahia, R.; Koch, S. Impact of N, P, K, and humic acid supplementation on the chemical profile of medical *Cannabis* (*Cannabis sativa* L.). *Front. Plant Sci.* **2019**, *10*, 736. [CrossRef] [PubMed]
47. Burgel, L.; Hartung, J.; Schibano, D.; Graeff-Hönninger, S. Impact of different phytohormones on morphology, yield and cannabinoid content of *Cannabis sativa* L. *Plants* **2020**, *9*, 725. [CrossRef]
48. Radoševič, A.; Kupinič, M.; Grlič, L. Antibiotic activity of various types of *Cannabis* resin. *Nature* **1962**, *195*, 1007–1009. [CrossRef] [PubMed]
49. Stuyt, E. The problem with the current high potency THC marijuana from the perspective of an addiction psychiatrist. *Mo. Med.* **2018**, *115*, 482–486. [PubMed]
50. Caiaffa, W.T.; Vlahov, D.; Graham, N.M.; Astemborski, J.; Solomon, L.; Nelson, K.E.; Muñoz, A. Drug smoking, *Pneumocystis carinii* pneumonia, and immunosuppression increase risk of bacterial pneumonia in human immunodeficiency virus-seropositive injection drug users. *Am. J. Respir. Crit. Care Med.* **1994**, *150*, 1493–1498. [CrossRef] [PubMed]
51. Roth, M.D.; Whittaker, K.; Salehi, K.; Tashkin, D.P.; Baldwin, G.C. Mechanisms for impaired effector function in alveolar macrophages from marijuana and cocaine smokers. *J. Neuroimmunol.* **2004**, *147*, 82–86. [CrossRef]
52. Cabral, G.A.; Dove Pettit, D.A. Drugs and immunity: Cannabinoids and their role in decreased resistance to infectious disease. *J. Neuroimmunol.* **1998**, *83*, 116–123. [CrossRef]
53. Maggirwar, S.B.; Khalsa, J.H. The link between *Cannabis* use, immune system, and viral infections. *Viruses* **2021**, *13*, 1099. [CrossRef]
54. Benedict, K.; Thompson, G.R., 3rd; Jackson, B.R. *Cannabis* use and fungal infections in a commercially insured population, United States, 2016. *Emerg. Infect. Dis.* **2020**, *26*, 1308–1310. [CrossRef]
55. Krejčí, Z. Antibacterial action of *Cannabis indica*. *Lek. Listy* **1952**, *7*, 500–503. [PubMed]
56. Krejčí, Z.; Horak, M.; Santavy, F. Hemp (*Cannabis sativa*)-an antibiotic drug. 3. Isolation and constitution of two acids from *Cannabis sativa*. *Die Pharmazie* **1959**, *14*, 349–355. [PubMed]
57. Krejčí, Z.; Šantavý, F. Isolace dalších látek z listí indického konopí *Cannabis sativa* L. *Acta Univ. Palacki. Olomuc.* **1955**, *6*, 59–66.

58. Appendino, G.; Gibbons, S.; Giana, A.; Pagani, A.; Grassi, G.; Stavri, M.; Smith, E.; Rahman, M.M. Antibacterial cannabinoids from *Cannabis sativa*: A structure-activity study. *J. Nat. Prod.* **2008**, *71*, 1427–1430. [CrossRef] [PubMed]
59. Mechoulam, R.; Gaoni, Y. Hashish. IV. The isolation and structure of cannabinolic cannabidiolic and cannabigerolic acids. *Tetrahedron* **1965**, *21*, 1223–1229. [CrossRef]
60. Mahmud, M.S.; Hossain, M.S.; Ahmed, A.; Islam, M.Z.; Sarker, M.E.; Islam, M.R. Antimicrobial and antiviral (SARS-CoV-2) potential of cannabinoids and *Cannabis sativa*: A comprehensive review. *Molecules* **2021**, *26*, 7216. [CrossRef]
61. Farha, M.A.; El-Halfawy, O.M.; Gale, R.T.; MacNair, C.R.; Carfrae, L.A.; Zhang, X.; Jentsch, N.G.; Magolan, J.; Brown, E.D. Uncovering the hidden antibiotic potential of *Cannabis*. *ACS Infect. Dis.* **2020**, *6*, 338–346. [CrossRef]
62. Martinenghi, L.D.; Jønsson, R.; Lund, T.; Jenssen, H. Isolation, purification, and antimicrobial characterization of cannabidiolic acid and cannabidiol from *Cannabis sativa* L. *Biomolecules* **2020**, *10*, 900. [CrossRef]
63. Radwan, M.M.; Elsohly, M.A.; Slade, D.; Ahmed, S.A.; Khan, I.A.; Ross, S.A. Biologically active cannabinoids from high-potency *Cannabis sativa*. *J. Nat. Prod.* **2009**, *72*, 906–911. [CrossRef]
64. Ferenczy, L. Antibacterial substances in seeds. *Nature* **1956**, *178*, 639–640. [CrossRef]
65. Wasim, K.; Haq, I.; Ashraf, M. Antimicrobial studies of the leaf of *Cannabis sativa* L. *Pak. J. Pharm. Sci.* **1995**, *8*, 29–38. [PubMed]
66. Ali, E.; Almagboul, A.; Khogali, S.; Gergeir, U. Antimicrobial activity of *Cannabis sativa* L. *Chin. Med.* **2012**, *3*, 61–64. [CrossRef]
67. Novak, J.; Zitterl-Eglseer, K.; Deans, S.G.; Franz, C.M. Essential oils of different cultivars of *Cannabis sativa* L. and their antimicrobial activity. *Flavour Fragance J.* **2001**, *16*, 259–262. [CrossRef]
68. Zengin, G.; Menghini, L.; Di Sotto, A.; Mancinelli, R.; Sisto, F.; Carradori, S.; Cesa, S.; Fraschetti, C.; Filippi, A.; Angiolella, L.; et al. Chromatographic analyses, In vitro biological activities, and cytotoxicity of *Cannabis sativa* L. essential oil: A multidisciplinary study. *Molecules* **2018**, *23*, 3266. [CrossRef]
69. Pellegrini, M.; Palmieri, S.; Ricci, A.; Serio, A.; Paparella, A.; Lo Sterzo, C. In vitro antioxidant and antimicrobial activity of *Cannabis sativa* L. cv 'Futura 75' essential oil. *Nat. Prod. Res.* **2021**, *35*, 6020–6024. [CrossRef]
70. Benelli, G.; Pavela, R.; Lupidi, G.; Nabissi, M.; Petrelli, R.; Ngahang Kamte, S.L.; Cappellacci, L.; Fiorini, D.; Sut, S.; Dall'Acqua, S.; et al. The crop-residue of fiber hemp cv. Futura 75: From a waste product to a source of botanical insecticides. *Environ. Sci. Pollut. Res. Int.* **2018**, *25*, 10515–10525. [CrossRef]
71. Thomas, T.G.; Sharma, S.K.; Prakash, A.; Sharma, B.R. Insecticidal properties of essential oil of *Cannabis sativa* Linn. against mosquito larvae. *Entomon* **2000**, *25*, 21–24.
72. Palmieri, S.; Maggio, F.; Pellegrini, M.; Ricci, A.; Serio, A.; Paparella, A.; Lo Sterzo, C. Effect of the distillation time on the chemical composition, antioxidant potential and antimicrobial activity of essential oils from different *Cannabis sativa* L. cultivars. *Molecules* **2021**, *26*, 4770. [CrossRef]
73. Zheljazkov, V.D.; Sikora, V.; Dincheva, I.; Kačániová, M.; Astatkie, T.; Semerdjieva, I.B.; Latkovic, D. Industrial, CBD, and wild hemp: How different are their essential oil profile and antimicrobial activity? *Molecules* **2020**, *25*, 4631. [CrossRef]
74. Russo, E.B. Taming THC: Potential cannabis synergy and phytocannabinoid-terpenoid entourage effects. *Br. J. Pharmacol.* **2011**, *163*, 1344–1364. [CrossRef]
75. Schofs, L.; Sparo, M.D.; Sánchez Bruni, S.F. The antimicrobial effect behind *Cannabis sativa*. *Pharmacol. Res. Perspect.* **2021**, *9*, e00761. [CrossRef]
76. Karas, J.A.; Wong, L.J.M.; Paulin, O.K.A.; Mazeh, A.C.; Hussein, M.H.; Li, J.; Velkov, T. The antimicrobial activity of cannabinoids. *Antibiotics* **2020**, *9*, 406. [CrossRef]
77. Kim, S.S.; Baik, J.S.; Oh, T.H.; Yoon, W.J.; Lee, N.H.; Hyun, C.G. Biological activities of Korean *Citrus obovoides* and *Citrus natsudaidai* essential oils against acne-inducing bacteria. *Biosci. Biotechnol. Biochem.* **2008**, *72*, 2507–2513. [CrossRef]
78. Rivas da Silva, A.C.; Lopes, P.M.; Barros de Azevedo, M.M.; Costa, D.C.; Alviano, C.S.; Alviano, D.S. Biological activities of α-pinene and β-pinene enantiomers. *Molecules* **2012**, *17*, 6305–6316. [CrossRef]
79. Leite, A.M.; Lima, E.O.; Souza, E.L.; Diniz, M.F.F.M.; Trajano, V.N.; Medeiros, I.A. Inhibitory effect of β-pinene, α-pinene and eugenol on the growth of potential infectious endocarditis causing Gram-positive bacteria. *Rev. Bras. De Ciências Farm.* **2007**, *43*, 121–126. [CrossRef]
80. Inoue, Y.; Shiraishi, A.; Hada, T.; Hamashima, H.; Shimada, J. The antibacterial effects of myrcene on *Staphylococcus aureus* and its role in the essential oil of the tea tree (*Melaleuca alternifolia*). *Nat. Med.* **2004**, *58*, 10–14.
81. Zore, G.B.; Thakre, A.D.; Jadhav, S.; Karuppayil, S.M. Terpenoids inhibit *Candida albicans* growth by affecting membrane integrity and arrest of cell cycle. *Phytomedicine* **2011**, *18*, 1181–1190. [CrossRef]
82. Han, Y.; Sun, Z.; Chen, W. Antimicrobial susceptibility and antibacterial mechanism of limonene against *Listeria monocytogenes*. *Molecules* **2019**, *25*, 33. [CrossRef]
83. Subramenium, G.A.; Vijayakumar, K.; Pandian, S.K. Limonene inhibits streptococcal biofilm formation by targeting surface-associated virulence factors. *J. Med. Microbiol.* **2015**, *64*, 879–890. [CrossRef]
84. Wanas, A.S.; Radwan, M.M.; Mehmedic, Z.; Jacob, M.; Khan, I.A.; Elsohly, M.A. Antifungal activity of the volatiles of high potency *Cannabis sativa* L. against *Cryptococcus neoformans*. *Rec. Nat. Prod.* **2016**, *10*, 214–220.
85. Arruda, D.C.; D'Alexandri, F.L.; Katzin, A.M.; Uliana, S.R. Antileishmanial activity of the terpene nerolidol. *Antimicrob. Agents Chemother.* **2005**, *49*, 1679–1687. [CrossRef]
86. Lopes, N.P.; Kato, M.J.; Andrade, E.H.; Maia, J.G.; Yoshida, M.; Planchart, A.R.; Katzin, A.M. Antimalarial use of volatile oil from leaves of *Virola surinamensis* (Rol.) Warb. by Waiãpi Amazon Indians. *J. Ethnopharmacol.* **1999**, *67*, 313–319. [CrossRef]

87. Rodrigues Goulart, H.; Kimura, E.A.; Peres, V.J.; Couto, A.S.; Aquino Duarte, F.A.; Katzin, A.M. Terpenes arrest parasite development and inhibit biosynthesis of isoprenoids in *Plasmodium falciparum*. *Antimicrob. Agents Chemother.* **2004**, *48*, 2502–2509. [CrossRef]
88. Dahham, S.S.; Tabana, Y.M.; Iqbal, M.A.; Ahamed, M.B.; Ezzat, M.O.; Majid, A.S.; Majid, A.M. The anticancer, antioxidant and antimicrobial properties of the sesquiterpene β-caryophyllene from the essential oil of *Aquilaria crassna*. *Molecules* **2015**, *20*, 11808–11829. [CrossRef]
89. Yang, D.; Michel, L.; Chaumont, J.P.; Millet-Clerc, J. Use of caryophyllene oxide as an antifungal agent in an in vitro experimental model of onychomycosis. *Mycopathologia* **1999**, *148*, 79–82. [CrossRef]
90. ElSohly, M.A.; Radwan, M.M.; Gul, W.; Chandra, S.; Galal, A. Phytochemistry of *Cannabis sativa* L. *Prog. Chem. Org. Nat. Prod.* **2017**, *103*, 1–36. [CrossRef]
91. Pourseyed Lazarjani, M.; Torres, S.; Hooker, T.; Fowlie, C.; Young, O.; Seyfoddin, A. Methods for quantification of cannabinoids: A narrative review. *J. Cannabis Res.* **2020**, *2*, 35. [CrossRef]
92. Hazekamp, A.; Choi, Y.H.; Verpoorte, R. Quantitative analysis of cannabinoids from *Cannabis sativa* using 1H-NMR. *Chem. Pharm. Bull.* **2004**, *52*, 718–721. [CrossRef]
93. Fischedick, J.; Van Der Kooy, F.; Verpoorte, R. Cannabinoid receptor 1 binding activity and quantitative analysis of *Cannabis sativa* L. smoke and vapor. *Chem. Pharm. Bull.* **2010**, *58*, 201–207. [CrossRef]
94. Ibrahim, E.A.; Gul, W.; Gul, S.W.; Stamper, B.J.; Hadad, G.M.; Abdel Salam, R.A.; Ibrahim, A.K.; Ahmed, S.A.; Chandra, S.; Lata, H.; et al. Determination of acid and neutral cannabinoids in extracts of different strains of *Cannabis sativa* using GC-FID. *Planta Med.* **2018**, *84*, 250–259. [CrossRef]
95. Russo, E.B.; Marcu, J. Cannabis Pharmacology: The usual suspects and a few promising leads. *Adv. Pharmacol.* **2017**, *80*, 67–134. [CrossRef]
96. Pellati, F.; Brighenti, V.; Sperlea, J.; Marchetti, L.; Bertelli, D.; Benvenuti, S. New methods for the comprehensive analysis of bioactive compounds in *Cannabis sativa* L. (hemp). *Molecules* **2018**, *23*, 2639. [CrossRef]
97. Iseppi, R.; Brighenti, V.; Licata, M.; Lambertini, A.; Sabia, C.; Messi, P.; Pellati, F.; Benvenuti, S. Chemical Characterization and evaluation of the antibacterial activity of essential oils from fibre-type *Cannabis sativa* L. (Hemp). *Molecules* **2019**, *24*, 2302. [CrossRef]
98. Mechoulam, R.; Gaoni, Y. Recent advances in the chemistry of hashish. *Fortschr. Chem. Org. Nat.* **1967**, *25*, 175–213. [CrossRef]
99. Elsohly, M.A.; Slade, D. Chemical constituents of marijuana: The complex mixture of natural cannabinoids. *Life Sci.* **2005**, *78*, 539–548. [CrossRef]
100. Radwan, M.M.; Ross, S.A.; Slade, D.; Ahmed, S.A.; Zulfiqar, F.; Elsohly, M.A. Isolation and characterization of new *Cannabis* constituents from a high potency variety. *Planta Med.* **2008**, *74*, 267–272. [CrossRef]
101. Radwan, M.M.; Elsohly, M.A.; Slade, D.; Ahmed, S.A.; Wilson, L.; El-Alfy, A.T.; Khan, I.A.; Ross, S.A. Non-cannabinoid constituents from a high potency *Cannabis sativa* variety. *Phytochemistry* **2008**, *69*, 2627–2633. [CrossRef]
102. Leizer, C.; Ribnicky, D.; Poulev, A.; Dushenkov, S.; Raskin, I. The composition of Hemp seed oil and its potential as an important source of nutrition. *J. Nutraceuticals Funct. Med. Foods* **2000**, *2*, 35–53. [CrossRef]
103. Radwan, M.M.; Chandra, S.; Gul, S.; ElSohly, M.A. Cannabinoids, phenolics, terpenes and alkaloids of *Cannabis*. *Molecules* **2021**, *26*, 2774. [CrossRef]
104. Turner, C.E.; Elsohly, M.A.; Boeren, E.G. Constituents of *Cannabis sativa* L. XVII. A review of the natural constituents. *J. Nat. Prod.* **1980**, *43*, 169–234. [CrossRef]
105. Appendino, G.; Chianese, G.; Taglialatela-Scafati, O. Cannabinoids: Occurrence and medicinal chemistry. *Curr. Med. Chem.* **2011**, *18*, 1085–1099. [CrossRef]
106. Yang, Y.; Vyawahare, R.; Lewis-Bakker, M.; Clarke, H.A.; Wong, A.H.C.; Kotra, L.P. Bioactive chemical composition of *Cannabis* extracts and cannabinoid receptors. *Molecules* **2020**, *25*, 3466. [CrossRef]
107. Rock, E.M.; Parker, L.A. Constituents of *Cannabis sativa*. *Adv. Exp. Med. Biol.* **2021**, *1264*, 1–13. [CrossRef]
108. Aizpurua-Olaizola, O.; Soydaner, U.; Öztürk, E.; Schibano, D.; Simsir, Y.; Navarro, P.; Etxebarria, N.; Usobiaga, A. Evolution of the cannabinoid and terpene content during the growth of *Cannabis sativa* plants from different chemotypes. *J. Nat. Prod.* **2016**, *79*, 324–331. [CrossRef]
109. Toyota, M.; Shimamura, T.; Ishii, H.; Renner, M.; Braggins, J.; Asakawa, Y. New bibenzyl cannabinoid from the New Zealand liverwort *Radula marginata*. *Chem. Pharm. Bull.* **2002**, *50*, 1390–1392. [CrossRef]
110. Bohlmann, F.; Hoffmann, E. Cannabigerol-ähnliche verbindungen aus *Helichrysum umbraculigerum*. *Phytochemistry* **1979**, *18*, 1371–1374. [CrossRef]
111. Kirkland, A.E.; Fadus, M.C.; Gruber, S.A.; Gray, K.M.; Wilens, T.E.; Squeglia, L.M. A scoping review of the use of cannabidiol in psychiatric disorders. *Psychiatry Res.* **2021**, *308*, 114347. [CrossRef]
112. Finn, D.P.; Haroutounian, S.; Hohmann, A.G.; Krane, E.; Soliman, N.; Rice, A.S.C. Cannabinoids, the endocannabinoid system, and pain: A review of preclinical studies. *Pain* **2021**, *162*, S5–S25. [CrossRef]
113. Lu, Y.; Anderson, H.D. Cannabinoid signaling in health and disease. *Can. J. Physiol. Pharmacol.* **2017**, *95*, 311–327. [CrossRef]
114. Slawek, D.E.; Curtis, S.A.; Arnsten, J.H.; Cunningham, C.O. Clinical approaches to Cannabis: A narrative review. *Med. Clin. N. Am.* **2022**, *106*, 131–152. [CrossRef]

115. Ligresti, A.; De Petrocellis, L.; Di Marzo, V. From phytocannabinoids to cannabinoid receptors and endocannabinoids: Pleiotropic physiological and pathological roles through complex pharmacology. *Physiol. Rev.* **2016**, *96*, 1593–1659. [CrossRef]
116. Atalay, S.; Jarocka-Karpowicz, I.; Skrzydlewska, E. Antioxidative and anti-inflammatory properties of cannabidiol. *Antioxidants* **2019**, *9*, 21. [CrossRef]
117. Walsh, K.B.; McKinney, A.E.; Holmes, A.E. Minor cannabinoids: Biosynthesis, molecular pharmacology and potential therapeutic uses. *Front. Pharmacol.* **2021**, *12*, 777804. [CrossRef]
118. Zanettini, C.; Panlilio, L.V.; Alicki, M.; Goldberg, S.R.; Haller, J.; Yasar, S. Effects of endocannabinoid system modulation on cognitive and emotional behavior. *Front. Behav. Neurosci.* **2011**, *5*, 57. [CrossRef]
119. Murillo-Rodriguez, E.; Pastrana-Trejo, J.C.; Salas-Crisóstomo, M.; de-la-Cruz, M. The endocannabinoid system modulating levels of consciousness, emotions and likely dream contents. *CNS Neurol. Disord. Drug Targets* **2017**, *16*, 370–379. [CrossRef]
120. Pauli, C.S.; Conroy, M.; Vanden Heuvel, B.D.; Park, S.H. Cannabidiol drugs clinical trial outcomes and adverse effects. *Front. Pharmacol.* **2020**, *11*, 63. [CrossRef]
121. Fraguas-Sánchez, A.I.; Torres-Suárez, A.I. Medical use of cannabinoids. *Drugs* **2018**, *78*, 1665–1703. [CrossRef]
122. Romero-Sandoval, E.A.; Fincham, J.E.; Kolano, A.L.; Sharpe, B.N.; Alvarado-Vázquez, P.A. *Cannabis* for chronic pain: Challenges and considerations. *Pharmacotherapy* **2018**, *38*, 651–662. [CrossRef]
123. Malaca, S.; Busardò, F.P.; Nittari, G.; Sirignano, A.; Ricci, G. Fourth generation of synthetic cannabinoid receptor agonists: A review on the latest insights. *Curr. Pharm. Des.* **2021**; *in press.* [CrossRef]
124. Matsuda, L.A.; Lolait, S.J.; Brownstein, M.J.; Young, A.C.; Bonner, T.I. Structure of a cannabinoid receptor and functional expression of the cloned cDNA. *Nature* **1990**, *346*, 561–564. [CrossRef]
125. Munro, S.; Thomas, K.L.; Abu-Shaar, M. Molecular characterization of a peripheral receptor for cannabinoids. *Nature* **1993**, *365*, 61–65. [CrossRef] [PubMed]
126. Pertwee, R.G.; Howlett, A.C.; Abood, M.E.; Alexander, S.P.; Di Marzo, V.; Elphick, M.R.; Greasley, P.J.; Hansen, H.S.; Kunos, G.; Mackie, K.; et al. International Union of Basic and Clinical Pharmacology. LXXIX. Cannabinoid receptors and their ligands: Beyond CB_1 and CB_2. *Pharmacol. Rev.* **2010**, *62*, 588–631. [CrossRef] [PubMed]
127. Gómez del Pulgar, T.; Velasco, G.; Guzmán, M. The CB1 cannabinoid receptor is coupled to the activation of protein kinase B/Akt. *Biochem. J.* **2000**, *347*, 369–373. [CrossRef] [PubMed]
128. Rueda, D.; Galve-Roperh, I.; Haro, A.; Guzmán, M. The CB_1 cannabinoid receptor is coupled to the activation of c-Jun N-terminal kinase. *Mol. Pharmacol.* **2000**, *58*, 814–820. [CrossRef] [PubMed]
129. Galve-Roperh, I.; Rueda, D.; Gómez del Pulgar, T.; Velasco, G.; Guzmán, M. Mechanism of extracellular signal-regulated kinase activation by the CB_1 cannabinoid receptor. *Mol. Pharmacol.* **2002**, *62*, 1385–1392. [CrossRef]
130. Blázquez, C.; Chiarlone, A.; Bellocchio, L.; Resel, E.; Pruunsild, P.; García-Rincón, D.; Sendtner, M.; Timmusk, T.; Lutz, B.; Galve-Roperh, I.; et al. The CB1 cannabinoid receptor signals striatal neuroprotection via a PI3K/Akt/mTORC1/BDNF pathway. *Cell Death Differ.* **2015**, *22*, 1618–1629. [CrossRef]
131. Molina-Holgado, E.; Vela, J.M.; Arévalo-Martín, A.; Almazán, G.; Molina-Holgado, F.; Borrell, J.; Guaza, C. Cannabinoids promote oligodendrocyte progenitor survival: Involvement of cannabinoid receptors and phosphatidylinositol-3 kinase/Akt signaling. *J. Neurosci.* **2002**, *22*, 9742–9753. [CrossRef]
132. Gomez, O.; Sanchez-Rodriguez, A.; Le, M.; Sanchez-Caro, C.; Molina-Holgado, F.; Molina-Holgado, E. Cannabinoid receptor agonists modulate oligodendrocyte differentiation by activating PI3K/Akt and the mammalian target of rapamycin (mTOR) pathways. *Br. J. Pharmacol.* **2011**, *163*, 1520–1532. [CrossRef]
133. Rhee, M.H.; Vogel, Z.; Barg, J.; Bayewitch, M.; Levy, R.; Hanus, L.; Breuer, A.; Mechoulam, R. Cannabinol derivatives: Binding to cannabinoid receptors and inhibition of adenylylcyclase. *J. Med. Chem.* **1997**, *40*, 3228–3233. [CrossRef]
134. Howlett, A.C.; Abood, M.E. CB_1 and CB_2 receptor pharmacology. *Adv. Pharmacol.* **2017**, *80*, 169–206. [CrossRef]
135. Devane, W.A.; Hanus, L.; Breuer, A.; Pertwee, R.G.; Stevenson, L.A.; Griffin, G.; Gibson, D.; Mandelbaum, A.; Etinger, A.; Mechoulam, R. Isolation and structure of a brain constituent that binds to the cannabinoid receptor. *Science* **1992**, *258*, 1946–1949. [CrossRef] [PubMed]
136. Sugiura, T.; Waku, K. 2-Arachidonoylglycerol and the cannabinoid receptors. *Chem. Phys. Lipids* **2000**, *108*, 89–106. [CrossRef]
137. Kendall, D.A.; Yudowski, G.A. Cannabinoid receptors in the central nervous system: Their signaling and roles in disease. *Front. Cell. Neurosci.* **2016**, *10*, 294. [CrossRef] [PubMed]
138. Pertwee, R.G. The diverse CB1 and CB2 receptor pharmacology of three plant cannabinoids: Delta9-tetrahydrocannabinol, cannabidiol and delta9-tetrahydrocannabivarin. *Br. J. Pharmacol.* **2008**, *153*, 199–215. [CrossRef]
139. Svízenská, I.; Dubový, P.; Sulcová, A. Cannabinoid receptors 1 and 2 (CB1 and CB2), their distribution, ligands and functional involvement in nervous system structures—A short review. *Pharmacol. Biochem. Behav.* **2008**, *90*, 501–511. [CrossRef]
140. Koch, M. Cannabinoid receptor signaling in central regulation of feeding behavior: A mini-review. *Front. Neurosci.* **2017**, *11*, 293. [CrossRef]
141. Ashton, J.C.; Wright, J.L.; McPartland, J.M.; Tyndall, J.D. Cannabinoid CB1 and CB2 receptor ligand specificity and the development of CB2-selective agonists. *Curr. Med. Chem.* **2008**, *15*, 1428–1443. [CrossRef]
142. Wei, C.; Huang, L.; Zheng, Y.; Cai, X. Selective activation of cannabinoid receptor 2 regulates Treg/Th17 balance to ameliorate neutrophilic asthma in mice. *Ann. Transl. Med.* **2021**, *9*, 1015. [CrossRef]

143. Saldaña-Shumaker, S.L.; Grenning, A.J.; Cunningham, C.W. Modern approaches to the development of synthetic cannabinoid receptor probes. *Pharmacol. Biochem. Behav.* **2021**, *203*, 173119. [CrossRef]
144. Gertsch, J.; Leonti, M.; Raduner, S.; Racz, I.; Chen, J.Z.; Xie, X.Q.; Altmann, K.H.; Karsak, M.; Zimmer, A. Beta-caryophyllene is a dietary cannabinoid. *Proc. Natl. Acad. Sci. USA* **2008**, *105*, 9099–9104. [CrossRef]
145. Kumawat, V.S.; Kaur, G. Cannabinoid 2 receptor agonist and L-arginine combination attenuates diabetic cardiomyopathy in rats via NF-kβ inhibition. *Can. J. Physiol. Pharmacol.* **2021**, *100*, 259–271. [CrossRef] [PubMed]
146. Mlost, J.; Kac, P.; Kędziora, M.; Starowicz, K. Antinociceptive and chondroprotective effects of prolonged β-caryophyllene treatment in the animal model of osteoarthritis: Focus on tolerance development. *Neuropharmacology* **2022**, *204*, 108908. [CrossRef] [PubMed]
147. Katsuyama, S.; Mizoguchi, H.; Kuwahata, H.; Komatsu, T.; Nagaoka, K.; Nakamura, H.; Bagetta, G.; Sakurada, T.; Sakurada, S. Involvement of peripheral cannabinoid and opioid receptors in β-caryophyllene-induced antinociception. *Eur. J. Pain* **2013**, *17*, 664–675. [CrossRef] [PubMed]
148. Lowin, T.; Straub, R.H. Cannabinoid-based drugs targeting CB1 and TRPV1, the sympathetic nervous system, and arthritis. *Arthritis Res. Ther.* **2015**, *17*, 226. [CrossRef]
149. Ross, R.A. Anandamide and vanilloid TRPV1 receptors. *Br. J. Pharmacol.* **2003**, *140*, 790–801. [CrossRef] [PubMed]
150. Ryberg, E.; Larsson, N.; Sjögren, S.; Hjorth, S.; Hermansson, N.O.; Leonova, J.; Elebring, T.; Nilsson, K.; Drmota, T.; Greasley, P.J. The orphan receptor GPR55 is a novel cannabinoid receptor. *Br. J. Pharmacol.* **2007**, *152*, 1092–1101. [CrossRef] [PubMed]
151. McHugh, D.; Page, J.; Dunn, E.; Bradshaw, H.B. Δ(9)-Tetrahydrocannabinol and N-arachidonyl glycine are full agonists at GPR18 receptors and induce migration in human endometrial HEC-1B cells. *Br. J. Pharmacol.* **2012**, *165*, 2414–2424. [CrossRef] [PubMed]
152. O'Sullivan, S.E. Cannabinoids go nuclear: Evidence for activation of peroxisome proliferator-activated receptors. *Br. J. Pharmacol.* **2007**, *152*, 576–582. [CrossRef]
153. Comelli, F.; Giagnoni, G.; Bettoni, I.; Colleoni, M.; Costa, B. Antihyperalgesic effect of a *Cannabis sativa* extract in a rat model of neuropathic pain: Mechanisms involved. *Phytother. Res.* **2008**, *22*, 1017–1024. [CrossRef]
154. Ibrahim, M.M.; Porreca, F.; Lai, J.; Albrecht, P.J.; Rice, F.L.; Khodorova, A.; Davar, G.; Makriyannis, A.; Vanderah, T.W.; Mata, H.P.; et al. CB2 cannabinoid receptor activation produces antinociception by stimulating peripheral release of endogenous opioids. *Proc. Natl. Acad. Sci. USA* **2005**, *102*, 3093–3098. [CrossRef]
155. Callén, L.; Moreno, E.; Barroso-Chinea, P.; Moreno-Delgado, D.; Cortés, A.; Mallol, J.; Casadó, V.; Lanciego, J.L.; Franco, R.; Lluis, C.; et al. Cannabinoid receptors CB1 and CB2 form functional heteromers in brain. *J. Biol. Chem.* **2012**, *287*, 20851–20865. [CrossRef] [PubMed]
156. Carriba, P.; Ortiz, O.; Patkar, K.; Justinova, Z.; Stroik, J.; Themann, A.; Müller, C.; Woods, A.S.; Hope, B.T.; Ciruela, F.; et al. Striatal adenosine A2A and cannabinoid CB1 receptors form functional heteromeric complexes that mediate the motor effects of cannabinoids. *Neuropsychopharmacology* **2007**, *32*, 2249–2259. [CrossRef]
157. Navarro, G.; Carriba, P.; Gandía, J.; Ciruela, F.; Casadó, V.; Cortés, A.; Mallol, J.; Canela, E.I.; Lluis, C.; Franco, R. Detection of heteromers formed by cannabinoid CB1, dopamine D2, and adenosine A2A G-protein-coupled receptors by combining bimolecular fluorescence complementation and bioluminescence energy transfer. *Sci. World J.* **2008**, *8*, 1088–1097. [CrossRef] [PubMed]
158. Tebano, M.T.; Martire, A.; Chiodi, V.; Pepponi, R.; Ferrante, A.; Domenici, M.R.; Frank, C.; Chen, J.F.; Ledent, C.; Popoli, P. Adenosine A2A receptors enable the synaptic effects of cannabinoid CB1 receptors in the rodent striatum. *J. Neurochem.* **2009**, *110*, 1921–1930. [CrossRef] [PubMed]
159. Rozenfeld, R.; Gupta, A.; Gagnidze, K.; Lim, M.P.; Gomes, I.; Lee-Ramos, D.; Nieto, N.; Devi, L.A. AT1R-CB$_1$R heteromerization reveals a new mechanism for the pathogenic properties of angiotensin II. *EMBO J.* **2011**, *30*, 2350–2363. [CrossRef] [PubMed]
160. Hojo, M.; Sudo, Y.; Ando, Y.; Minami, K.; Takada, M.; Matsubara, T.; Kanaide, M.; Taniyama, K.; Sumikawa, K.; Uezono, Y. Mu-Opioid receptor forms a functional heterodimer with cannabinoid CB1 receptor: Electrophysiological and FRET assay analysis. *J. Pharmacol. Sci.* **2008**, *108*, 308–319. [CrossRef] [PubMed]
161. López-Moreno, J.A.; López-Jiménez, A.; Gorriti, M.A.; de Fonseca, F.R. Functional interactions between endogenous cannabinoid and opioid systems: Focus on alcohol, genetics and drug-addicted behaviors. *Curr. Drug Targets* **2010**, *11*, 406–428. [CrossRef] [PubMed]
162. Ward, R.J.; Pediani, J.D.; Milligan, G. Heteromultimerization of cannabinoid CB$_1$ receptor and orexin OX$_1$ receptor generates a unique complex in which both protomers are regulated by orexin A. *J. Biol. Chem.* **2011**, *286*, 37414–37428. [CrossRef]
163. Zou, S.; Kumar, U. Cannabinoid Receptors and the endocannabinoid system: Signaling and function in the central nervous system. *Int. J. Mol. Sci.* **2018**, *19*, 833. [CrossRef]
164. Shahbazi, F.; Grandi, V.; Banerjee, A.; Trant, J.F. Cannabinoids and cannabinoid receptors: The story so far. *iScience* **2020**, *23*, 101301. [CrossRef]
165. Raïch, I.; Rivas-Santisteban, R.; Lillo, A.; Lillo, J.; Reyes-Resina, I.; Nadal, X.; Ferreiro-Vera, C.; de Medina, V.S.; Majellaro, M.; Sotelo, E.; et al. Similarities and differences upon binding of naturally occurring Δ^9-tetrahydrocannabinol-derivatives to cannabinoid CB$_1$ and CB$_2$ receptors. *Pharmacol. Res.* **2021**, *174*, 105970. [CrossRef] [PubMed]
166. Volkow, N.D.; Baler, R.D.; Compton, W.M.; Weiss, S.R. Adverse health effects of marijuana use. *N. Engl. J. Med.* **2014**, *370*, 2219–2227. [CrossRef] [PubMed]

167. Badowski, M.E. A review of oral cannabinoids and medical marijuana for the treatment of chemotherapy-induced nausea and vomiting: A focus on pharmacokinetic variability and pharmacodynamics. *Cancer Chemother. Pharmacol.* **2017**, *80*, 441–449. [CrossRef] [PubMed]
168. Ng, T.; Gupta, V. Tetrahydrocannabinol (THC). In *StatPearls*; StatPearls Publishing LLC: Treasure Island, FL, USA, 2021.
169. Pacher, P.; Kunos, G. Modulating the endocannabinoid system in human health and disease—Successes and failures. *FEBS J.* **2013**, *280*, 1918–1943. [CrossRef] [PubMed]
170. Conte, A.; Vila Silván, C. Review of available data for the efficacy and effectiveness of nabiximols oromucosal spray (Sativex®) in multiple sclerosis patients with moderate to severe spasticity. *Neurodegener. Dis.* 2021; *in press*. [CrossRef]
171. Laprairie, R.B.; Bagher, A.M.; Kelly, M.E.; Denovan-Wright, E.M. Cannabidiol is a negative allosteric modulator of the cannabinoid CB1 receptor. *Br. J. Pharmacol.* **2015**, *172*, 4790–4805. [CrossRef] [PubMed]
172. de la Harpe, A.; Beukes, N.; Frost, C.L. CBD activation of TRPV1 induces oxidative signaling and subsequent ER stress in breast cancer cell lines. *Biotechnol. Appl. Biochem.* 2021; *in press*. [CrossRef]
173. Mechoulam, R.; Peters, M.; Murillo-Rodriguez, E.; Hanus, L.O. Cannabidiol—Recent advances. *Chem. Biodivers.* **2007**, *4*, 1678–1692. [CrossRef]
174. Soares, V.P.; Campos, A.C. Evidences for the anti-panic actions of cannabidiol. *Curr. Neuropharmacol.* **2017**, *15*, 291–299. [CrossRef]
175. Zuardi, A.W.; Crippa, J.A.; Hallak, J.E.; Moreira, F.A.; Guimarães, F.S. Cannabidiol, a *Cannabis sativa* constituent, as an antipsychotic drug. *Braz. J. Med. Biol. Res.* **2006**, *39*, 421–429. [CrossRef]
176. Moltke, J.; Hindocha, C. Reasons for cannabidiol use: A cross-sectional study of CBD users, focusing on self-perceived stress, anxiety, and sleep problems. *J. Cannabis Res.* **2021**, *3*, 5. [CrossRef]
177. Jones, N.A.; Hill, A.J.; Smith, I.; Bevan, S.A.; Williams, C.M.; Whalley, B.J.; Stephens, G.J. Cannabidiol displays antiepileptiform and antiseizure properties in vitro and in vivo. *J. Pharmacol. Exp. Ther.* **2010**, *332*, 569–577. [CrossRef]
178. Carrier, E.J.; Auchampach, J.A.; Hillard, C.J. Inhibition of an equilibrative nucleoside transporter by cannabidiol: A mechanism of cannabinoid immunosuppression. *Proc. Natl. Acad. Sci. USA* **2006**, *103*, 7895–7900. [CrossRef] [PubMed]
179. Devinsky, O.; Cilio, M.R.; Cross, H.; Fernandez-Ruiz, J.; French, J.; Hill, C.; Katz, R.; Di Marzo, V.; Jutras-Aswad, D.; Notcutt, W.G.; et al. Cannabidiol: Pharmacology and potential therapeutic role in epilepsy and other neuropsychiatric disorders. *Epilepsia* **2014**, *55*, 791–802. [CrossRef] [PubMed]
180. Burstein, S. Cannabidiol (CBD) and its analogs: A review of their effects on inflammation. *Bioorg. Med. Chem.* **2015**, *23*, 1377–1385. [CrossRef] [PubMed]
181. Costa, B.; Colleoni, M.; Conti, S.; Parolaro, D.; Franke, C.; Trovato, A.E.; Giagnoni, G. Oral anti-inflammatory activity of cannabidiol, a non-psychoactive constituent of cannabis, in acute carrageenan-induced inflammation in the rat paw. *Naunyn Schmiedebergs Arch. Pharm.* **2004**, *369*, 294–299. [CrossRef] [PubMed]
182. Costa, B.; Trovato, A.E.; Comelli, F.; Giagnoni, G.; Colleoni, M. The non-psychoactive cannabis constituent cannabidiol is an orally effective therapeutic agent in rat chronic inflammatory and neuropathic pain. *Eur. J. Pharmacol.* **2007**, *556*, 75–83. [CrossRef] [PubMed]
183. Pereira, S.R.; Hackett, B.; O'Driscoll, D.N.; Sun, M.C.; Downer, E.J. Cannabidiol modulation of oxidative stress and signalling. *Neuronal Signal.* **2021**, *5*, 20200080. [CrossRef]
184. Graczyk, M.; Lewandowska, A.A.; Dzierżanowski, T. The therapeutic potential of *Cannabis* in counteracting oxidative stress and inflammation. *Molecules* **2021**, *26*, 4551. [CrossRef]
185. Jeong, S.; Jo, M.J.; Yun, H.K.; Kim, D.Y.; Kim, B.R.; Kim, J.L.; Park, S.H.; Na, Y.J.; Jeong, Y.A.; Kim, B.G.; et al. Cannabidiol promotes apoptosis via regulation of XIAP/Smac in gastric cancer. *Cell Death Dis.* **2019**, *10*, 846. [CrossRef]
186. Hamad, H.; Olsen, B.B. Cannabidiol induces cell death in human lung cancer cells and cancer stem cells. *Pharmaceuticals* **2021**, *14*, 1169. [CrossRef]
187. Shrivastava, A.; Kuzontkoski, P.M.; Groopman, J.E.; Prasad, A. Cannabidiol induces programmed cell death in breast cancer cells by coordinating the cross-talk between apoptosis and autophagy. *Mol. Cancer Ther.* **2011**, *10*, 1161–1172. [CrossRef]
188. Kovalchuk, O.; Kovalchuk, I. Cannabinoids as anticancer therapeutic agents. *Cell Cycle* **2020**, *19*, 961–989. [CrossRef] [PubMed]
189. Oláh, A.; Tóth, B.I.; Borbíró, I.; Sugawara, K.; Szöllõsi, A.G.; Czifra, G.; Pál, B.; Ambrus, L.; Kloepper, J.; Camera, E.; et al. Cannabidiol exerts sebostatic and antiinflammatory effects on human sebocytes. *J. Clin. Investig.* **2014**, *124*, 3713–3724. [CrossRef] [PubMed]
190. Hampson, A.J.; Grimaldi, M.; Lolic, M.; Wink, D.; Rosenthal, R.; Axelrod, J. Neuroprotective antioxidants from marijuana. *Ann. N. Y. Acad. Sci.* **2000**, *899*, 274–282. [CrossRef] [PubMed]
191. Di Giacomo, V.; Chiavaroli, A.; Recinella, L.; Orlando, G.; Cataldi, A.; Rapino, M.; Di Valerio, V.; Ronci, M.; Leone, S.; Brunetti, L.; et al. Antioxidant and neuroprotective effects induced by cannabidiol and cannabigerol in rat CTX-TNA2 astrocytes and isolated cortexes. *Int. J. Mol. Sci.* **2020**, *21*, 3575. [CrossRef] [PubMed]
192. Boyaji, S.; Merkow, J.; Elman, R.N.M.; Kaye, A.D.; Yong, R.J.; Urman, R.D. The role of cannabidiol (CBD) in chronic pain management: An Assessment of current evidence. *Curr. Pain Headache Rep.* **2020**, *24*, 4. [CrossRef]
193. Bonaccorso, S.; Ricciardi, A.; Zangani, C.; Chiappini, S.; Schifano, F. Cannabidiol (CBD) use in psychiatric disorders: A systematic review. *Neurotoxicology* **2019**, *74*, 282–298. [CrossRef]
194. Graczyk, M.; Łukowicz, M.; Dzierzanowski, T. Prospects for the use of cannabinoids in psychiatric disorders. *Front. Psychiatry* **2021**, *12*, 620073. [CrossRef]

195. Bergamaschi, M.M.; Queiroz, R.H.; Zuardi, A.W.; Crippa, J.A. Safety and side effects of cannabidiol, a *Cannabis sativa* constituent. *Curr. Drug Saf.* **2011**, *6*, 237–249. [CrossRef]
196. Devinsky, O.; Cross, J.H.; Laux, L.; Marsh, E.; Miller, I.; Nabbout, R.; Scheffer, I.E.; Thiele, E.A.; Wright, S. Trial of cannabidiol for drug-resistant seizures in the Dravet Syndrome. *N. Engl. J. Med.* **2017**, *376*, 2011–2020. [CrossRef]
197. Taylor, L.; Gidal, B.; Blakey, G.; Tayo, B.; Morrison, G. A Phase I, Randomized, double-blind, placebo-controlled, single ascending dose, multiple dose, and food effect trial of the safety, tolerability and pharmacokinetics of highly purified cannabidiol in healthy subjects. *CNS Drugs* **2018**, *32*, 1053–1067. [CrossRef]
198. Walsh, K.B.; Andersen, H.K. Molecular pharmacology of synthetic cannabinoids: Delineating CB1 receptor-mediated cell signaling. *Int. J. Mol. Sci.* **2020**, *21*, 6115. [CrossRef] [PubMed]
199. Gallily, R.; Yekhtin, Z. Avidekel *Cannabis* extracts and cannabidiol are as efficient as Copaxone in suppressing EAE in SJL/J mice. *Inflammopharmacology* **2019**, *27*, 167–173. [CrossRef] [PubMed]
200. Malfait, A.M.; Gallily, R.; Sumariwalla, P.F.; Malik, A.S.; Andreakos, E.; Mechoulam, R.; Feldmann, M. The nonpsychoactive cannabis constituent cannabidiol is an oral anti-arthritic therapeutic in murine collagen-induced arthritis. *Proc. Natl. Acad. Sci. USA* **2000**, *97*, 9561–9566. [CrossRef] [PubMed]
201. Elliott, D.M.; Singh, N.; Nagarkatti, M.; Nagarkatti, P.S. Cannabidiol attenuates experimental autoimmune encephalomyelitis model of multiple sclerosis through induction of myeloid-derived suppressor cells. *Front. Immunol.* **2018**, *9*, 1782. [CrossRef] [PubMed]
202. Weiss, L.; Zeira, M.; Reich, S.; Slavin, S.; Raz, I.; Mechoulam, R.; Gallily, R. Cannabidiol arrests onset of autoimmune diabetes in NOD mice. *Neuropharmacology* **2008**, *54*, 244–249. [CrossRef] [PubMed]
203. Gallily, R.; Yekhtin, Z.; Hanuš, L.O. Overcoming the bell-shaped dose-response of cannabidiol by using *Cannabis* extract enriched in cannabidiol. *Pharmacol. Pharm.* **2015**, *6*, 75. [CrossRef]
204. Gaoni, Y.; Mechoulam, R. The isolation and structure of delta-1-tetrahydrocannabinol and other neutral cannabinoids from hashish. *J. Am. Chem. Soc.* **1971**, *93*, 217–224. [CrossRef]
205. Fournier, G.; Richez-Dumanois, C.; Duvezin, J.; Mathieu, J.P.; Paris, M. Identification of a new chemotype in *Cannabis sativa*: Cannabigerol-dominant plants, biogenetic and agronomic prospects. *Planta Med.* **1987**, *53*, 277–280. [CrossRef]
206. Ioannidis, K.; Dadiotis, E.; Mitsis, V.; Melliou, E.; Magiatis, P. Biotechnological approaches on two high CBD and CBG *Cannabis sativa* L. (*Cannabaceae*) varieties: In vitro regeneration and phytochemical consistency evaluation of micropropagated plants using quantitative ^{1}H-NMR. *Molecules* **2020**, *25*, 5928. [CrossRef]
207. Navarro, G.; Varani, K.; Reyes-Resina, I.; Sánchez de Medina, V.; Rivas-Santisteban, R.; Sánchez-Carnerero Callado, C.; Vincenzi, F.; Casano, S.; Ferreiro-Vera, C.; Canela, E.I.; et al. Cannabigerol action at cannabinoid CB_1 and CB_2 receptors and at CB_1-CB_2 heteroreceptor complexes. *Front. Pharmacol.* **2018**, *9*, 632. [CrossRef]
208. Husni, A.S.; McCurdy, C.R.; Radwan, M.M.; Ahmed, S.A.; Slade, D.; Ross, S.A.; ElSohly, M.A.; Cutler, S.J. Evaluation of phytocannabinoids from high potency *Cannabis sativa* using in vitro bioassays to determine structure-activity relationships for cannabinoid receptor 1 and cannabinoid receptor 2. *Med. Chem. Res.* **2014**, *23*, 4295–4300. [CrossRef] [PubMed]
209. Zagzoog, A.; Mohamed, K.A.; Kim, H.J.J.; Kim, E.D.; Frank, C.S.; Black, T.; Jadhav, P.D.; Holbrook, L.A.; Laprairie, R.B. In vitro and in vivo pharmacological activity of minor cannabinoids isolated from *Cannabis sativa*. *Sci. Rep.* **2020**, *10*, 20405. [CrossRef] [PubMed]
210. De Petrocellis, L.; Ligresti, A.; Moriello, A.S.; Allarà, M.; Bisogno, T.; Petrosino, S.; Stott, C.G.; Di Marzo, V. Effects of cannabinoids and cannabinoid-enriched *Cannabis* extracts on TRP channels and endocannabinoid metabolic enzymes. *Br. J. Pharmacol.* **2011**, *163*, 1479–1494. [CrossRef]
211. Cascio, M.G.; Gauson, L.A.; Stevenson, L.A.; Ross, R.A.; Pertwee, R.G. Evidence that the plant cannabinoid cannabigerol is a highly potent alpha2-adrenoceptor agonist and moderately potent 5HT1A receptor antagonist. *Br. J. Pharmacol.* **2010**, *159*, 129–141. [CrossRef] [PubMed]
212. D'Aniello, E.; Fellous, T.; Iannotti, F.A.; Gentile, A.; Allarà, M.; Balestrieri, F.; Gray, R.; Amodeo, P.; Vitale, R.M.; Di Marzo, V. Identification and characterization of phytocannabinoids as novel dual PPARα/γ agonists by a computational and in vitro experimental approach. *Biochim. Biophys. Acta Gen. Subj.* **2019**, *1863*, 586–597. [CrossRef]
213. Borrelli, F.; Pagano, E.; Romano, B.; Panzera, S.; Maiello, F.; Coppola, D.; De Petrocellis, L.; Buono, L.; Orlando, P.; Izzo, A.A. Colon carcinogenesis is inhibited by the TRPM8 antagonist cannabigerol, a *Cannabis*-derived non-psychotropic cannabinoid. *Carcinogenesis* **2014**, *35*, 2787–2797. [CrossRef] [PubMed]
214. De Petrocellis, L.; Vellani, V.; Schiano-Moriello, A.; Marini, P.; Magherini, P.C.; Orlando, P.; Di Marzo, V. Plant-derived cannabinoids modulate the activity of transient receptor potential channels of ankyrin type-1 and melastatin type-8. *J. Pharmacol. Exp. Ther.* **2008**, *325*, 1007–1015. [CrossRef]
215. Nachnani, R.; Raup-Konsavage, W.M.; Vrana, K.E. The pharmacological case for cannabigerol. *J. Pharmacol. Exp. Ther.* **2021**, *376*, 204–212. [CrossRef]
216. Pagano, E.; Iannotti, F.A.; Piscitelli, F.; Romano, B.; Lucariello, G.; Venneri, T.; Di Marzo, V.; Izzo, A.A.; Borrelli, F. Efficacy of combined therapy with fish oil and phytocannabinoids in murine intestinal inflammation. *Phytother. Res.* **2021**, *35*, 517–529. [CrossRef]
217. Ruhaak, L.R.; Felth, J.; Karlsson, P.C.; Rafter, J.J.; Verpoorte, R.; Bohlin, L. Evaluation of the cyclooxygenase inhibiting effects of six major cannabinoids isolated from *Cannabis sativa*. *Biol. Pharm. Bull.* **2011**, *34*, 774–778. [CrossRef]

218. Hill, A.J.; Williams, C.M.; Whalley, B.J.; Stephens, G.J. Phytocannabinoids as novel therapeutic agents in CNS disorders. *Pharmacol. Ther.* **2012**, *133*, 79–97. [CrossRef] [PubMed]
219. Borrelli, F.; Fasolino, I.; Romano, B.; Capasso, R.; Maiello, F.; Coppola, D.; Orlando, P.; Battista, G.; Pagano, E.; Di Marzo, V.; et al. Beneficial effect of the non-psychotropic plant cannabinoid cannabigerol on experimental inflammatory bowel disease. *Biochem. Pharmacol.* **2013**, *85*, 1306–1316. [CrossRef] [PubMed]
220. Turner, C.E.; Elsohly, M.A. Biological activity of cannabichromene, its homologs and isomers. *J. Clin. Pharmacol.* **1981**, *21*, 283s–291s. [CrossRef]
221. Maione, S.; Piscitelli, F.; Gatta, L.; Vita, D.; De Petrocellis, L.; Palazzo, E.; de Novellis, V.; Di Marzo, V. Non-psychoactive cannabinoids modulate the descending pathway of antinociception in anaesthetized rats through several mechanisms of action. *Br. J. Pharmacol.* **2011**, *162*, 584–596. [CrossRef]
222. Romano, B.; Borrelli, F.; Fasolino, I.; Capasso, R.; Piscitelli, F.; Cascio, M.; Pertwee, R.; Coppola, D.; Vassallo, L.; Orlando, P.; et al. The cannabinoid TRPA1 agonist cannabichromene inhibits nitric oxide production in macrophages and ameliorates murine colitis. *Br. J. Pharmacol.* **2013**, *169*, 213–229. [CrossRef] [PubMed]
223. Izzo, A.A.; Capasso, R.; Aviello, G.; Borrelli, F.; Romano, B.; Piscitelli, F.; Gallo, L.; Capasso, F.; Orlando, P.; Di Marzo, V. Inhibitory effect of cannabichromene, a major non-psychotropic cannabinoid extracted from *Cannabis sativa*, on inflammation-induced hypermotility in mice. *Br. J. Pharmacol.* **2012**, *166*, 1444–1460. [CrossRef] [PubMed]
224. Shinjyo, N.; Di Marzo, V. The effect of cannabichromene on adult neural stem/progenitor cells. *Neurochem. Int.* **2013**, *63*, 432–437. [CrossRef]
225. Covelo, A.; Eraso-Pichot, A.; Fernández-Moncada, I.; Serrat, R.; Marsicano, G. CB1R-dependent regulation of astrocyte physiology and astrocyte-neuron interactions. *Neuropharmacology* **2021**, *195*, 108678. [CrossRef]
226. Anderson, L.L.; Ametovski, A.; Lin Luo, J.; Everett-Morgan, D.; McGregor, I.S.; Banister, S.D.; Arnold, J.C. Cannabichromene, related phytocannabinoids, and 5-fluoro-cannabichromene have anticonvulsant properties in a mouse model of Dravet Syndrome. *ACS Chem. Neurosci.* **2021**, *12*, 330–339. [CrossRef]
227. Anis, O.; Vinayaka, A.C.; Shalev, N.; Namdar, D.; Nadarajan, S.; Anil, S.M.; Cohen, O.; Belausov, E.; Ramon, J.; Mayzlish Gati, E.; et al. Cannabis-derived compounds cannabichromene and Δ^9-tetrahydrocannabinol interact and exhibit cytotoxic activity against urothelial cell carcinoma correlated with inhibition of cell migration and cytoskeleton organization. *Molecules* **2021**, *26*, 465. [CrossRef]
228. De Petrocellis, L.; Ligresti, A.; Schiano Moriello, A.; Iappelli, M.; Verde, R.; Stott, C.G.; Cristino, L.; Orlando, P.; Di Marzo, V. Non-THC cannabinoids inhibit prostate carcinoma growth in vitro and in vivo: Pro-apoptotic effects and underlying mechanisms. *Br. J. Pharmacol.* **2013**, *168*, 79–102. [CrossRef] [PubMed]
229. Navarro, G.; Varani, K.; Lillo, A.; Vincenzi, F.; Rivas-Santisteban, R.; Raïch, I.; Reyes-Resina, I.; Ferreiro-Vera, C.; Borea, P.A.; Sánchez de Medina, V.; et al. Pharmacological data of cannabidiol- and cannabigerol-type phytocannabinoids acting on cannabinoid CB_1, CB_2 and CB_1/CB_2 heteromer receptors. *Pharmacol. Res.* **2020**, *159*, 104940. [CrossRef] [PubMed]
230. Bolognini, D.; Rock, E.M.; Cluny, N.L.; Cascio, M.G.; Limebeer, C.L.; Duncan, M.; Stott, C.G.; Javid, F.A.; Parker, L.A.; Pertwee, R.G. Cannabidiolic acid prevents vomiting in *Suncus murinus* and nausea-induced behaviour in rats by enhancing 5-HT1A receptor activation. *Br. J. Pharmacol.* **2013**, *168*, 1456–1470. [CrossRef] [PubMed]
231. Rock, E.M.; Sullivan, M.T.; Collins, S.A.; Goodman, H.; Limebeer, C.L.; Mechoulam, R.; Parker, L.A. Evaluation of repeated or acute treatment with cannabidiol (CBD), cannabidiolic acid (CBDA) or CBDA methyl ester (HU-580) on nausea and/or vomiting in rats and shrews. *Psychopharmacology* **2020**, *237*, 2621–2631. [CrossRef]
232. Rock, E.M.; Limebeer, C.L.; Pertwee, R.G.; Mechoulam, R.; Parker, L.A. Therapeutic potential of cannabidiol, cannabidiolic acid, and cannabidiolic acid methyl ester as treatments for nausea and vomiting. *Cannabis Cannabinoid Res.* **2021**, *6*, 266–274. [CrossRef]
233. Pertwee, R.G.; Rock, E.M.; Guenther, K.; Limebeer, C.L.; Stevenson, L.A.; Haj, C.; Smoum, R.; Parker, L.A.; Mechoulam, R. Cannabidiolic acid methyl ester, a stable synthetic analogue of cannabidiolic acid, can produce 5-HT_{1A} receptor-mediated suppression of nausea and anxiety in rats. *Br. J. Pharmacol.* **2018**, *175*, 100–112. [CrossRef]
234. Takeda, S.; Misawa, K.; Yamamoto, I.; Watanabe, K. Cannabidiolic acid as a selective cyclooxygenase-2 inhibitory component in cannabis. *Drug Metab. Dispos.* **2008**, *36*, 1917–1921. [CrossRef]
235. Rock, E.M.; Limebeer, C.L.; Parker, L.A. Effect of cannabidiolic acid and Δ^9-tetrahydrocannabinol on carrageenan-induced hyperalgesia and edema in a rodent model of inflammatory pain. *Psychopharmacology* **2018**, *235*, 3259–3271. [CrossRef]
236. Anderson, L.L.; Low, I.K.; Banister, S.D.; McGregor, I.S.; Arnold, J.C. Pharmacokinetics of phytocannabinoid acids and anticonvulsant effect of cannabidiolic acid in a mouse model of Dravet Syndrome. *J. Nat. Prod.* **2019**, *82*, 3047–3055. [CrossRef]
237. Assareh, N.; Gururajan, A.; Zhou, C.; Luo, J.L.; Kevin, R.C.; Arnold, J.C. Cannabidiol disrupts conditioned fear expression and cannabidiolic acid reduces trauma-induced anxiety-related behaviour in mice. *Behav. Pharmacol.* **2020**, *31*, 591–596. [CrossRef]
238. Rock, E.M.; Limebeer, C.L.; Petrie, G.N.; Williams, L.A.; Mechoulam, R.; Parker, L.A. Effect of prior foot shock stress and Δ^9-tetrahydrocannabinol, cannabidiolic acid, and cannabidiol on anxiety-like responding in the light-dark emergence test in rats. *Psychopharmacology* **2017**, *234*, 2207–2217. [CrossRef] [PubMed]
239. Smeriglio, A.; Giofrè, S.V.; Galati, E.M.; Monforte, M.T.; Cicero, N.; D'Angelo, V.; Grassi, G.; Circosta, C. Inhibition of aldose reductase activity by *Cannabis sativa* chemotypes extracts with high content of cannabidiol or cannabigerol. *Fitoterapia* **2018**, *127*, 101–108. [CrossRef] [PubMed]

240. Anderson, L.L.; Heblinski, M.; Absalom, N.L.; Hawkins, N.A.; Bowen, M.T.; Benson, M.J.; Zhang, F.; Bahceci, D.; Doohan, P.T.; Chebib, M.; et al. Cannabigerolic acid, a major biosynthetic precursor molecule in cannabis, exhibits divergent effects on seizures in mouse models of epilepsy. *Br. J. Pharmacol.* **2021**, *178*, 4826–4841. [CrossRef] [PubMed]
241. Schubert, D.; Kepchia, D.; Liang, Z.; Dargusch, R.; Goldberg, J.; Maher, P. Efficacy of cannabinoids in a pre-clinical drug-screening platform for Alzheimer's disease. *Mol. Neurobiol.* **2019**, *56*, 7719–7730. [CrossRef]
242. Liang, Z.; Soriano-Castell, D.; Kepchia, D.; Duggan, B.M.; Currais, A.; Schubert, D.; Maher, P. Cannabinol inhibits oxytosis/ferroptosis by directly targeting mitochondria independently of cannabinoid receptors. *Free Radic. Biol. Med.* **2022**, *180*, 33–51. [CrossRef]
243. Aqawi, M.; Sionov, R.V.; Gallily, R.; Friedman, M.; Steinberg, D. Anti-biofilm activity of cannabigerol against *Streptococcus mutans*. *Microorganisms* **2021**, *9*, 2031. [CrossRef]
244. Aqawi, M.; Sionov, R.V.; Gallily, R.; Friedman, M.; Steinberg, D. Anti-bacterial properties of cannabigerol toward *Streptococcus mutans*. *Front. Microbiol.* **2021**, *12*, 656471. [CrossRef]
245. Van Klingeren, B.; Ten Ham, M. Antibacterial activity of delta9-tetrahydrocannabinol and cannabidiol. *Antonie Van Leeuwenhoek* **1976**, *42*, 9–12. [CrossRef]
246. Nalli, Y.; Arora, P.; Riyaz-Ul-Hassan, S.; Ali, A. Chemical investigation of *Cannabis sativa* leading to the discovery of a prenylspirodinone with anti-microbial potential. *Tetrahedron Lett.* **2018**, *59*, 2470–2472. [CrossRef]
247. Blaskovich, M.A.T.; Kavanagh, A.M.; Elliott, A.G.; Zhang, B.; Ramu, S.; Amado, M.; Lowe, G.J.; Hinton, A.O.; Pham, D.M.T.; Zuegg, J.; et al. The antimicrobial potential of cannabidiol. *Commun. Biol.* **2021**, *4*, 7. [CrossRef]
248. Aqawi, M.; Gallily, R.; Sionov, R.V.; Zaks, B.; Friedman, M.; Steinberg, D. Cannabigerol prevents quorum sensing and biofilm formation of *Vibrio harveyi*. *Front. Microbiol.* **2020**, *11*, 858. [CrossRef] [PubMed]
249. Soni, D.; Smoum, R.; Breuer, A.; Mechoulam, R.; Steinberg, D. Effect of the synthetic cannabinoid HU-210 on quorum sensing and on the production of quorum sensing-mediated virulence factors by *Vibrio harveyi*. *BMC Microbiol.* **2015**, *15*, 159. [CrossRef] [PubMed]
250. Kosgodage, U.S.; Matewele, P.; Awamaria, B.; Kraev, I.; Warde, P.; Mastroianni, G.; Nunn, A.V.; Guy, G.W.; Bell, J.D.; Inal, J.M.; et al. Cannabidiol is a novel modulator of bacterial membrane vesicles. *Front. Cell. Infect. Microbiol.* **2019**, *9*, 324. [CrossRef] [PubMed]
251. Wassmann, C.S.; Højrup, P.; Klitgaard, J.K. Cannabidiol is an effective helper compound in combination with bacitracin to kill Gram-positive bacteria. *Sci. Rep.* **2020**, *10*, 4112. [CrossRef] [PubMed]
252. Russo, C.; Lavorgna, M.; Nugnes, R.; Orlo, E.; Isidori, M. Comparative assessment of antimicrobial, antiradical and cytotoxic activities of cannabidiol and its propyl analogue cannabidivarin. *Sci. Rep.* **2021**, *11*, 22494. [CrossRef]
253. Feldman, M.; Sionov, R.V.; Mechoulam, R.; Steinberg, D. Anti-biofilm activity of cannabidiol against *Candida albicans*. *Microorganisms* **2021**, *9*, 441. [CrossRef]
254. Galletta, M.; Reekie, T.A.; Nagalingam, G.; Bottomley, A.L.; Harry, E.J.; Kassiou, M.; Triccas, J.A. Rapid Antibacterial activity of cannabichromenic acid against methicillin-resistant *Staphylococcus aureus*. *Antibiotics* **2020**, *9*, 523. [CrossRef]
255. Wood, T.K.; Knabel, S.J.; Kwan, B.W. Bacterial persister cell formation and dormancy. *Appl. Environ. Microbiol.* **2013**, *79*, 7116–7121. [CrossRef]
256. Andersson, D.I.; Hughes, D. Persistence of antibiotic resistance in bacterial populations. *FEMS Microbiol. Rev.* **2011**, *35*, 901–911. [CrossRef]
257. Yan, J.; Bassler, B.L. Surviving as a community: Antibiotic tolerance and persistence in bacterial biofilms. *Cell Host Microbe* **2019**, *26*, 15–21. [CrossRef]
258. Aslam, B.; Wang, W.; Arshad, M.I.; Khurshid, M.; Muzammil, S.; Rasool, M.H.; Nisar, M.A.; Alvi, R.F.; Aslam, M.A.; Qamar, M.U.; et al. Antibiotic resistance: A rundown of a global crisis. *Infect. Drug Resist.* **2018**, *11*, 1645–1658. [CrossRef] [PubMed]
259. Sharma, D.; Misba, L.; Khan, A.U. Antibiotics versus biofilm: An emerging battleground in microbial communities. *Antimicrob. Resist. Infect. Control* **2019**, *8*, 76. [CrossRef] [PubMed]
260. Ciofu, O.; Moser, C.; Jensen, P.; Høiby, N. Tolerance and resistance of microbial biofilms. *Nat. Rev. Microbiol.* **2022**; in press. [CrossRef]
261. Stahl, V.; Vasudevan, K. Comparison of efficacy of cannabinoids versus commercial oral care products in reducing bacterial content from dental plaque: A preliminary observation. *Cureus* **2020**, *12*, e6809. [CrossRef] [PubMed]
262. Bowler, P.; Murphy, C.; Wolcott, R. Biofilm exacerbates antibiotic resistance: Is this a current oversight in antimicrobial stewardship? *Antimicrob. Resist. Infect. Control* **2020**, *9*, 162. [CrossRef]
263. Singh, S.; Datta, S.; Narayanan, K.B.; Rajnish, K.N. Bacterial exo-polysaccharides in biofilms: Role in antimicrobial resistance and treatments. *J. Genet. Eng. Biotechnol.* **2021**, *19*, 140. [CrossRef]
264. Raj, V.; Park, J.G.; Cho, K.H.; Choi, P.; Kim, T.; Ham, J.; Lee, J. Assessment of antiviral potencies of cannabinoids against SARS-CoV-2 using computational and in vitro approaches. *Int. J. Biol. Macromol.* **2021**, *168*, 474–485. [CrossRef]
265. van Breemen, R.B.; Muchiri, R.N.; Bates, T.A.; Weinstein, J.B.; Leier, H.C.; Farley, S.; Tafesse, F.G. Cannabinoids block cellular entry of SARS-CoV-2 and the emerging variants. *J. Nat. Prod.* **2022**, *85*, 176–184. [CrossRef]
266. Paland, N.; Pechkovsky, A.; Aswad, M.; Hamza, H.; Popov, T.; Shahar, E.; Louria-Hayon, I. The immunopathology of COVID-19 and the *Cannabis* paradigm. *Front. Immunol.* **2021**, *12*, 631233. [CrossRef]

267. Crippa, J.A.S.; Pacheco, J.C.; Zuardi, A.W.; Guimarães, F.S.; Campos, A.C.; Osório, F.L.; Loureiro, S.R.; Dos Santos, R.G.; Souza, J.D.S.; Ushirohira, J.M.; et al. Cannabidiol for COVID-19 patients with mild to moderate symptoms (CANDIDATE Study): A randomized, double-blind, placebo-controlled clinical trial. *Cannabis Cannabinoid Res.* 2021; in press. [CrossRef]
268. Reiss, C.S. Cannabinoids and viral infections. *Pharmaceuticals* 2010, *3*, 1873–1886. [CrossRef]
269. Zaami, S.; Sirignano, A.; García-Algar, Ó.; Marinelli, E. COVID-19 pandemic, substance use disorders and body image issues, a worrisome correlation. *Eur. Rev. Med. Pharmacol. Sci.* 2022, *26*, 291–297. [CrossRef]
270. Vidot, D.C.; Islam, J.Y.; Marlene, C.-R.; Harrell, M.B.; Rao, D.R.; Chavez, J.V.; Lucas, G.O.; Hlaing, W.M.; Weiner, M.; Messiah, S.E. The COVID-19 cannabis health study: Results from an epidemiologic assessment of adults who use cannabis for medicinal reasons in the United States. *J. Addict. Dis.* 2021, *39*, 26–36. [CrossRef] [PubMed]
271. Hatoum, A.S.; Morrison, C.L.; Colbert, S.M.C.; Winiger, E.A.; Johnson, E.C.; Agrawal, A.; Bogdan, R. Genetic liability to Cannabis use disorder and COVID-19 hospitalization. *Biol. Psychiatry Glob. Open Sci.* 2021, *1*, 317–323. [CrossRef] [PubMed]
272. Pinzi, L.; Lherbet, C.; Baltas, M.; Pellati, F.; Rastelli, G. In silico repositioning of cannabigerol as a novel inhibitor of the enoyl acyl carrier protein (ACP) reductase (InhA). *Molecules* 2019, *24*, 2567. [CrossRef] [PubMed]
273. Toyofuku, M.; Nomura, N.; Eberl, L. Types and origins of bacterial membrane vesicles. *Nat. Rev. Microbiol.* 2019, *17*, 13–24. [CrossRef]
274. Mukherjee, S.; Bassler, B.L. Bacterial quorum sensing in complex and dynamically changing environments. *Nat. Rev. Microbiol.* 2019, *17*, 371–382. [CrossRef]
275. Burkey, T.H.; Quock, R.M.; Consroe, P.; Ehlert, F.J.; Hosohata, Y.; Roeske, W.R.; Yamamura, H.I. Relative efficacies of cannabinoid CB1 receptor agonists in the mouse brain. *Eur. J. Pharmacol.* 1997, *336*, 295–298. [CrossRef]
276. Howlett, A.C.; Barth, F.; Bonner, T.I.; Cabral, G.; Casellas, P.; Devane, W.A.; Felder, C.C.; Herkenham, M.; Mackie, K.; Martin, B.R.; et al. International Union of Pharmacology. XXVII. Classification of cannabinoid receptors. *Pharmacol. Rev.* 2002, *54*, 161–202. [CrossRef]
277. Klein, T.W.; Newton, C.; Larsen, K.; Lu, L.; Perkins, I.; Nong, L.; Friedman, H. The cannabinoid system and immune modulation. *J. Leukoc. Biol.* 2003, *74*, 486–496. [CrossRef]
278. Mackie, K.; Stella, N. Cannabinoid receptors and endocannabinoids: Evidence for new players. *AAPS J.* 2006, *8*, E298–E306. [CrossRef]
279. Murillo-Rodríguez, E.; Budde, H.; Veras, A.B.; Rocha, N.B.; Telles-Correia, D.; Monteiro, D.; Cid, L.; Yamamoto, T.; Machado, S.; Torterolo, P. The endocannabinoid system may modulate sleep disorders in aging. *Curr. Neuropharmacol.* 2020, *18*, 97–108. [CrossRef]
280. Ashton, C.H.; Moore, P.B. Endocannabinoid system dysfunction in mood and related disorders. *Acta Psychiatr. Scand.* 2011, *124*, 250–261. [CrossRef] [PubMed]
281. Gallego-Landin, I.; García-Baos, A.; Castro-Zavala, A.; Valverde, O. Reviewing the role of the endocannabinoid system in the pathophysiology of depression. *Front. Pharmacol.* 2021, *12*, 762738. [CrossRef] [PubMed]
282. Braile, M.; Marcella, S.; Marone, G.; Galdiero, M.R.; Varricchi, G.; Loffredo, S. The interplay between the immune and the endocannabinoid systems in cancer. *Cells* 2021, *10*, 1282. [CrossRef] [PubMed]
283. Rahman, S.M.K.; Uyama, T.; Hussain, Z.; Ueda, N. Roles of endocannabinoids and endocannabinoid-like molecules in energy homeostasis and metabolic regulation: A nutritional perspective. *Annu. Rev. Nutr.* 2021, *41*, 177–202. [CrossRef] [PubMed]
284. Marsicano, G.; Lutz, B. Neuromodulatory functions of the endocannabinoid system. *J. Endocrinol. Investig.* 2006, *29*, 27–46.
285. Cani, P.D.; Plovier, H.; Van Hul, M.; Geurts, L.; Delzenne, N.M.; Druart, C.; Everard, A. Endocannabinoids—At the crossroads between the gut microbiota and host metabolism. *Nat. Rev. Endocrinol.* 2016, *12*, 133–143. [CrossRef]
286. Ahmed, I.; Rehman, S.U.; Shahmohamadnejad, S.; Zia, M.A.; Ahmad, M.; Saeed, M.M.; Akram, Z.; Iqbal, H.M.N.; Liu, Q. Therapeutic attributes of endocannabinoid system against neuro-inflammatory autoimmune disorders. *Molecules* 2021, *26*, 3389. [CrossRef]
287. Jackson, A.R.; Hegde, V.L.; Nagarkatti, P.S.; Nagarkatti, M. Characterization of endocannabinoid-mediated induction of myeloid-derived suppressor cells involving mast cells and MCP-1. *J. Leukoc. Biol.* 2014, *95*, 609–619. [CrossRef]
288. Osafo, N.; Yeboah, O.K.; Antwi, A.O. Endocannabinoid system and its modulation of brain, gut, joint and skin inflammation. *Mol. Biol. Rep.* 2021, *48*, 3665–3680. [CrossRef]
289. Pandey, R.; Mousawy, K.; Nagarkatti, M.; Nagarkatti, P. Endocannabinoids and immune regulation. *Pharmacol. Res.* 2009, *60*, 85–92. [CrossRef]
290. Sido, J.M.; Nagarkatti, P.S.; Nagarkatti, M. Production of endocannabinoids by activated T cells and B cells modulates inflammation associated with delayed-type hypersensitivity. *Eur. J. Immunol.* 2016, *46*, 1472–1479. [CrossRef] [PubMed]
291. Rahaman, O.; Ganguly, D. Endocannabinoids in immune regulation and immunopathologies. *Immunology* 2021, *164*, 242–252. [CrossRef] [PubMed]
292. Aguado, T.; Monory, K.; Palazuelos, J.; Stella, N.; Cravatt, B.; Lutz, B.; Marsicano, G.; Kokaia, Z.; Guzmán, M.; Galve-Roperh, I. The endocannabinoid system drives neural progenitor proliferation. *FASEB J.* 2005, *19*, 1704–1706. [CrossRef]
293. Paraíso-Luna, J.; Aguareles, J.; Martín, R.; Ayo-Martín, A.C.; Simón-Sánchez, S.; García-Rincón, D.; Costas-Insua, C.; García-Taboada, E.; de Salas-Quiroga, A.; Díaz-Alonso, J.; et al. Endocannabinoid signalling in stem cells and cerebral organoids drives differentiation to deep layer projection neurons via CB_1 receptors. *Development* 2020, *147*, dev192161. [CrossRef] [PubMed]

294. Veldhuis, W.B.; van Der Stelt, M.; Wadman, M.W.; van Zadelhoff, G.; Maccarrone, M.; Fezza, F.; Veldink, G.A.; Vliegenthart, J.F.; Bär, P.R.; Nicolay, K.; et al. Neuroprotection by the endogenous cannabinoid anandamide and arvanil against in vivo excitotoxicity in the rat: Role of vanilloid receptors and lipoxygenases. *J. Neurosci.* **2003**, *23*, 4127–4133. [CrossRef] [PubMed]
295. Palazuelos, J.; Aguado, T.; Egia, A.; Mechoulam, R.; Guzmán, M.; Galve-Roperh, I. Non-psychoactive CB2 cannabinoid agonists stimulate neural progenitor proliferation. *FASEB J.* **2006**, *20*, 2405–2407. [CrossRef] [PubMed]
296. Jin, K.; Xie, L.; Kim, S.H.; Parmentier-Batteur, S.; Sun, Y.; Mao, X.O.; Childs, J.; Greenberg, D.A. Defective adult neurogenesis in CB1 cannabinoid receptor knockout mice. *Mol. Pharmacol.* **2004**, *66*, 204–208. [CrossRef]
297. Lu, H.C.; Mackie, K. An Introduction to the endogenous cannabinoid system. *Biol. Psychiatry* **2016**, *79*, 516–525. [CrossRef]
298. Iannotti, F.A.; Di Marzo, V. The gut microbiome, endocannabinoids and metabolic disorders. *J. Endocrinol.* **2021**, *248*, R83–R97. [CrossRef]
299. Kreitzer, A.C. Neurotransmission: Emerging roles of endocannabinoids. *Curr. Biol.* **2005**, *15*, R549–R551. [CrossRef]
300. Chevaleyre, V.; Takahashi, K.A.; Castillo, P.E. Endocannabinoid-mediated synaptic plasticity in the CNS. *Annu. Rev. Neurosci.* **2006**, *29*, 37–76. [CrossRef] [PubMed]
301. Mackie, K. Mechanisms of CB1 receptor signaling: Endocannabinoid modulation of synaptic strength. *Int. J. Obes.* **2006**, *30* (Suppl. S1), S19–S23. [CrossRef] [PubMed]
302. Heifets, B.D.; Castillo, P.E. Endocannabinoid signaling and long-term synaptic plasticity. *Annu. Rev. Physiol.* **2009**, *71*, 283–306. [CrossRef] [PubMed]
303. Jung, K.M.; Astarita, G.; Zhu, C.; Wallace, M.; Mackie, K.; Piomelli, D. A key role for diacylglycerol lipase-alpha in metabotropic glutamate receptor-dependent endocannabinoid mobilization. *Mol. Pharmacol.* **2007**, *72*, 612–621. [CrossRef]
304. Tong, J.; Liu, X.; Vickstrom, C.; Li, Y.; Yu, L.; Lu, Y.; Smrcka, A.V.; Liu, Q.S. The Epac-phospholipase Cε pathway regulates endocannabinoid signaling and cocaine-induced disinhibition of ventral tegmental area dopamine neurons. *J. Neurosci.* **2017**, *37*, 3030–3044. [CrossRef]
305. Jing, H.; Reed, A.; Ulanovskaya, O.A.; Grigoleit, J.S.; Herbst, D.M.; Henry, C.L.; Li, H.; Barbas, S.; Germain, J.; Masuda, K.; et al. Phospholipase Cγ2 regulates endocannabinoid and eicosanoid networks in innate immune cells. *Proc. Natl. Acad. Sci. USA* **2021**, *118*, e2112971118. [CrossRef]
306. Okamoto, Y.; Wang, J.; Morishita, J.; Ueda, N. Biosynthetic pathways of the endocannabinoid anandamide. *Chem. Biodivers.* **2007**, *4*, 1842–1857. [CrossRef]
307. Fride, E. Endocannabinoids in the central nervous system—An overview. *Prostaglandins Leukot. Essent. Fat. Acids* **2002**, *66*, 221–233. [CrossRef]
308. Stella, N.; Schweitzer, P.; Piomelli, D. A second endogenous cannabinoid that modulates long-term potentiation. *Nature* **1997**, *388*, 773–778. [CrossRef]
309. Mechoulam, R.; Ben-Shabat, S.; Hanus, L.; Ligumsky, M.; Kaminski, N.E.; Schatz, A.R.; Gopher, A.; Almog, S.; Martin, B.R.; Compton, D.R.; et al. Identification of an endogenous 2-monoglyceride, present in canine gut, that binds to cannabinoid receptors. *Biochem. Pharmacol.* **1995**, *50*, 83–90. [CrossRef]
310. Yang, H.Y.; Karoum, F.; Felder, C.; Badger, H.; Wang, T.C.; Markey, S.P. GC/MS analysis of anandamide and quantification of N-arachidonoylphosphatidylethanolamides in various brain regions, spinal cord, testis, and spleen of the rat. *J. Neurochem.* **1999**, *72*, 1959–1968. [CrossRef] [PubMed]
311. Staiano, R.I.; Loffredo, S.; Borriello, F.; Iannotti, F.A.; Piscitelli, F.; Orlando, P.; Secondo, A.; Granata, F.; Lepore, M.T.; Fiorelli, A.; et al. Human lung-resident macrophages express CB1 and CB2 receptors whose activation inhibits the release of angiogenic and lymphangiogenic factors. *J. Leukoc. Biol.* **2016**, *99*, 531–540. [CrossRef] [PubMed]
312. Di Marzo, V. New approaches and challenges to targeting the endocannabinoid system. *Nat. Rev. Drug Discov.* **2018**, *17*, 623–639. [CrossRef] [PubMed]
313. Pestonjamasp, V.K.; Burstein, S.H. Anandamide synthesis is induced by arachidonate mobilizing agonists in cells of the immune system. *Biochim. Biophys. Acta* **1998**, *1394*, 249–260. [CrossRef]
314. Mecha, M.; Feliú, A.; Carrillo-Salinas, F.J.; Rueda-Zubiaurre, A.; Ortega-Gutiérrez, S.; de Sola, R.G.; Guaza, C. Endocannabinoids drive the acquisition of an alternative phenotype in microglia. *Brain Behav. Immun.* **2015**, *49*, 233–245. [CrossRef]
315. Lam, P.M.; Marczylo, T.H.; Konje, J.C. Simultaneous measurement of three N-acylethanolamides in human bio-matrices using ultra performance liquid chromatography-tandem mass spectrometry. *Anal. Bioanal. Chem.* **2010**, *398*, 2089–2097. [CrossRef]
316. Hillard, C.J. Circulating endocannabinoids: From whence do they come and where are they going? *Neuropsychopharmacology* **2018**, *43*, 155–172. [CrossRef]
317. Opitz, C.A.; Rimmerman, N.; Zhang, Y.; Mead, L.E.; Yoder, M.C.; Ingram, D.A.; Walker, J.M.; Rehman, J. Production of the endocannabinoids anandamide and 2-arachidonoylglycerol by endothelial progenitor cells. *FEBS Lett.* **2007**, *581*, 4927–4931. [CrossRef]
318. Liu, J.; Batkai, S.; Pacher, P.; Harvey-White, J.; Wagner, J.A.; Cravatt, B.F.; Gao, B.; Kunos, G. Lipopolysaccharide induces anandamide synthesis in macrophages via CD14/MAPK/phosphoinositide 3-kinase/NF-kappaB independently of platelet-activating factor. *J. Biol. Chem.* **2003**, *278*, 45034–45039. [CrossRef]
319. Walter, L.; Franklin, A.; Witting, A.; Moller, T.; Stella, N. Astrocytes in culture produce anandamide and other acylethanolamides. *J. Biol. Chem.* **2002**, *277*, 20869–20876. [CrossRef]

320. Hillard, C.J.; Weinlander, K.M.; Stuhr, K.L. Contributions of endocannabinoid signaling to psychiatric disorders in humans: Genetic and biochemical evidence. *Neuroscience* **2012**, *204*, 207–229. [CrossRef] [PubMed]
321. Leweke, F.M.; Piomelli, D.; Pahlisch, F.; Muhl, D.; Gerth, C.W.; Hoyer, C.; Klosterkötter, J.; Hellmich, M.; Koethe, D. Cannabidiol enhances anandamide signaling and alleviates psychotic symptoms of schizophrenia. *Transl. Psychiatry* **2012**, *2*, e94. [CrossRef] [PubMed]
322. Felder, C.C.; Briley, E.M.; Axelrod, J.; Simpson, J.T.; Mackie, K.; Devane, W.A. Anandamide, an endogenous cannabimimetic eicosanoid, binds to the cloned human cannabinoid receptor and stimulates receptor-mediated signal transduction. *Proc. Natl. Acad. Sci. USA* **1993**, *90*, 7656–7660. [CrossRef] [PubMed]
323. Gonsiorek, W.; Lunn, C.; Fan, X.; Narula, S.; Lundell, D.; Hipkin, R.W. Endocannabinoid 2-arachidonyl glycerol is a full agonist through human type 2 cannabinoid receptor: Antagonism by anandamide. *Mol. Pharmacol.* **2000**, *57*, 1045–1050. [PubMed]
324. Luk, T.; Jin, W.; Zvonok, A.; Lu, D.; Lin, X.Z.; Chavkin, C.; Makriyannis, A.; Mackie, K. Identification of a potent and highly efficacious, yet slowly desensitizing CB1 cannabinoid receptor agonist. *Br. J. Pharmacol.* **2004**, *142*, 495–500. [CrossRef]
325. Sugiura, T.; Kondo, S.; Sukagawa, A.; Nakane, S.; Shinoda, A.; Itoh, K.; Yamashita, A.; Waku, K. 2-Arachidonoylglycerol: A possible endogenous cannabinoid receptor ligand in brain. *Biochem. Biophys. Res. Commun.* **1995**, *215*, 89–97. [CrossRef]
326. Muller, C.; Lynch, D.L.; Hurst, D.P.; Reggio, P.H. TRPV1 activation by anandamide via a unique lipid pathway. *J. Chem. Inf. Model.* **2021**, *61*, 5742–5746. [CrossRef]
327. Muller, C.; Lynch, D.L.; Hurst, D.P.; Reggio, P.H. A closer look at anandamide interaction with TRPV1. *Front. Mol. Biosci.* **2020**, *7*, 144. [CrossRef]
328. Li, Y.; Chen, X.; Nie, Y.; Tian, Y.; Xiao, X.; Yang, F. Endocannabinoid activation of the TRPV1 ion channel is distinct from activation by capsaicin. *J. Biol. Chem.* **2021**, *297*, 101022. [CrossRef]
329. Di Marzo, V.; De Petrocellis, L. Endocannabinoids as regulators of transient receptor potential (TRP) channels: A further opportunity to develop new endocannabinoid-based therapeutic drugs. *Curr. Med. Chem.* **2010**, *17*, 1430–1449. [CrossRef]
330. Al-Hayani, A.; Wease, K.N.; Ross, R.A.; Pertwee, R.G.; Davies, S.N. The endogenous cannabinoid anandamide activates vanilloid receptors in the rat hippocampal slice. *Neuropharmacology* **2001**, *41*, 1000–1005. [CrossRef]
331. Smart, D.; Gunthorpe, M.J.; Jerman, J.C.; Nasir, S.; Gray, J.; Muir, A.I.; Chambers, J.K.; Randall, A.D.; Davis, J.B. The endogenous lipid anandamide is a full agonist at the human vanilloid receptor (hVR1). *Br. J. Pharmacol.* **2000**, *129*, 227–230. [CrossRef] [PubMed]
332. Lauckner, J.E.; Jensen, J.B.; Chen, H.Y.; Lu, H.C.; Hille, B.; Mackie, K. GPR55 is a cannabinoid receptor that increases intracellular calcium and inhibits M current. *Proc. Natl. Acad. Sci. USA* **2008**, *105*, 2699–2704. [CrossRef] [PubMed]
333. Gootjes, E.C.; Bakkerus, L.; Ten Tije, A.J.; Witteveen, P.O.; Buffart, T.E.; Bridgewater, J.A.; Primrose, J.N.; Verhoef, C.; Verheul, H.M.W. The value of tumour debulking for patients with extensive multi-organ metastatic colorectal cancer. *Eur. J. Cancer* **2018**, *103*, 160–164. [CrossRef]
334. De Petrocellis, L.; Schiano Moriello, A.; Imperatore, R.; Cristino, L.; Starowicz, K.; Di Marzo, V. A re-evaluation of 9-HODE activity at TRPV1 channels in comparison with anandamide: Enantioselectivity and effects at other TRP channels and in sensory neurons. *Br. J. Pharmacol.* **2012**, *167*, 1643–1651. [CrossRef]
335. Cristino, L.; Bisogno, T.; Di Marzo, V. Cannabinoids and the expanded endocannabinoid system in neurological disorders. *Nat. Rev. Neurol.* **2020**, *16*, 9–29. [CrossRef]
336. Zygmunt, P.M.; Petersson, J.; Andersson, D.A.; Chuang, H.; Sørgård, M.; Di Marzo, V.; Julius, D.; Högestätt, E.D. Vanilloid receptors on sensory nerves mediate the vasodilator action of anandamide. *Nature* **1999**, *400*, 452–457. [CrossRef]
337. Lawton, S.K.; Xu, F.; Tran, A.; Wong, E.; Prakash, A.; Schumacher, M.; Hellman, J.; Wilhelmsen, K. N-arachidonoyl dopamine modulates acute systemic inflammation via nonhematopoietic TRPV1. *J. Immunol.* **2017**, *199*, 1465–1475. [CrossRef]
338. Smaga, I.; Bystrowska, B.; Gawliński, D.; Przegaliński, E.; Filip, M. The endocannabinoid/endovanilloid system and depression. *Curr. Neuropharmacol.* **2014**, *12*, 462–474. [CrossRef]
339. Kasatkina, L.A.; Rittchen, S.; Sturm, E.M. Neuroprotective and immunomodulatory action of the endocannabinoid system under neuroinflammation. *Int. J. Mol. Sci.* **2021**, *22*, 5431. [CrossRef]
340. Lin, Y.F. Potassium channels as molecular targets of endocannabinoids. *Channels* **2021**, *15*, 408–423. [CrossRef] [PubMed]
341. Alger, B.E. Endocannabinoids: Getting the message across. *Proc. Natl. Acad. Sci. USA* **2004**, *101*, 8512–8513. [CrossRef] [PubMed]
342. Diana, M.A.; Marty, A. Endocannabinoid-mediated short-term synaptic plasticity: Depolarization-induced suppression of inhibition (DSI) and depolarization-induced suppression of excitation (DSE). *Br. J. Pharmacol.* **2004**, *142*, 9–19. [CrossRef] [PubMed]
343. Araque, A.; Castillo, P.E.; Manzoni, O.J.; Tonini, R. Synaptic functions of endocannabinoid signaling in health and disease. *Neuropharmacology* **2017**, *124*, 13–24. [CrossRef]
344. Kano, M.; Ohno-Shosaku, T.; Hashimotodani, Y.; Uchigashima, M.; Watanabe, M. Endocannabinoid-mediated control of synaptic transmission. *Physiol. Rev.* **2009**, *89*, 309–380. [CrossRef]
345. Di Scala, C.; Fantini, J.; Yahi, N.; Barrantes, F.J.; Chahinian, H. Anandamide Revisited: How cholesterol and ceramides control receptor-dependent and receptor-independent signal transmission pathways of a lipid neurotransmitter. *Biomolecules* **2018**, *8*, 31. [CrossRef]
346. Di Pasquale, E.; Chahinian, H.; Sanchez, P.; Fantini, J. The insertion and transport of anandamide in synthetic lipid membranes are both cholesterol-dependent. *PLoS ONE* **2009**, *4*, e4989. [CrossRef]

347. Di Scala, C.; Mazzarino, M.; Yahi, N.; Varini, K.; Garmy, N.; Fantini, J.; Chahinian, H. Ceramide binding to anandamide increases its half-life and potentiates its cytotoxicity in human neuroblastoma cells. *Chem. Phys. Lipids* **2017**, *205*, 11–17. [CrossRef]
348. Castagnet, P.I.; Golovko, M.Y.; Barceló-Coblijn, G.C.; Nussbaum, R.L.; Murphy, E.J. Fatty acid incorporation is decreased in astrocytes cultured from alpha-synuclein gene-ablated mice. *J. Neurochem.* **2005**, *94*, 839–849. [CrossRef]
349. Kaczocha, M.; Glaser, S.T.; Deutsch, D.G. Identification of intracellular carriers for the endocannabinoid anandamide. *Proc. Natl. Acad. Sci. USA* **2009**, *106*, 6375–6380. [CrossRef]
350. Chivet, M.; Hemming, F.; Pernet-Gallay, K.; Fraboulet, S.; Sadoul, R. Emerging role of neuronal exosomes in the central nervous system. *Front. Physiol.* **2012**, *3*, 145. [CrossRef] [PubMed]
351. Huo, L.; Du, X.; Li, X.; Liu, S.; Xu, Y. The emerging role of neural cell-derived exosomes in intercellular communication in health and neurodegenerative diseases. *Front. Neurosci.* **2021**, *15*, 738442. [CrossRef] [PubMed]
352. Gabrielli, M.; Battista, N.; Riganti, L.; Prada, I.; Antonucci, F.; Cantone, L.; Matteoli, M.; Maccarrone, M.; Verderio, C. Active endocannabinoids are secreted on extracellular membrane vesicles. *EMBO Rep.* **2015**, *16*, 213–220. [CrossRef] [PubMed]
353. Carrier, E.J.; Kearn, C.S.; Barkmeier, A.J.; Breese, N.M.; Yang, W.; Nithipatikom, K.; Pfister, S.L.; Campbell, W.B.; Hillard, C.J. Cultured rat microglial cells synthesize the endocannabinoid 2-arachidonylglycerol, which increases proliferation via a CB2 receptor-dependent mechanism. *Mol. Pharmacol.* **2004**, *65*, 999–1007. [CrossRef]
354. Stella, N. Endocannabinoid signaling in microglial cells. *Neuropharmacology* **2009**, *56* (Suppl. S1), 244–253. [CrossRef]
355. Navarrete, M.; Araque, A. Endocannabinoids mediate neuron-astrocyte communication. *Neuron* **2008**, *57*, 883–893. [CrossRef]
356. Karwad, M.A.; Macpherson, T.; Wang, B.; Theophilidou, E.; Sarmad, S.; Barrett, D.A.; Larvin, M.; Wright, K.L.; Lund, J.N.; O'Sullivan, S.E. Oleoylethanolamine and palmitoylethanolamine modulate intestinal permeability in vitro via TRPV1 and PPARα. *FASEB J.* **2017**, *31*, 469–481. [CrossRef]
357. Couch, D.G.; Cook, H.; Ortori, C.; Barrett, D.; Lund, J.N.; O'Sullivan, S.E. Palmitoylethanolamide and cannabidiol prevent inflammation-induced hyperpermeability of the human gut in vitro and in vivo—A randomized, placebo-controlled, double-blind controlled trial. *Inflamm. Bowel Dis.* **2019**, *25*, 1006–1018. [CrossRef]
358. Fezza, F.; Bari, M.; Florio, R.; Talamonti, E.; Feole, M.; Maccarrone, M. Endocannabinoids, related compounds and their metabolic routes. *Molecules* **2014**, *19*, 17078–17106. [CrossRef]
359. Muccioli, G.G.; Stella, N. Microglia produce and hydrolyze palmitoylethanolamide. *Neuropharmacology* **2008**, *54*, 16–22. [CrossRef]
360. Stella, N.; Piomelli, D. Receptor-dependent formation of endogenous cannabinoids in cortical neurons. *Eur. J. Pharmacol.* **2001**, *425*, 189–196. [CrossRef]
361. Koch, M.; Kreutz, S.; Böttger, C.; Benz, A.; Maronde, E.; Ghadban, C.; Korf, H.W.; Dehghani, F. Palmitoylethanolamide protects dentate gyrus granule cells via peroxisome proliferator-activated receptor-α. *Neurotox. Res.* **2011**, *19*, 330–340. [CrossRef] [PubMed]
362. Skaper, S.D.; Facci, L.; Giusti, P. Glia and mast cells as targets for palmitoylethanolamide, an anti-inflammatory and neuroprotective lipid mediator. *Mol. Neurobiol.* **2013**, *48*, 340–352. [CrossRef] [PubMed]
363. Clayton, P.; Subah, S.; Venkatesh, R.; Hill, M.; Bogoda, N. Palmitoylethanolamide: A potential alternative to cannabidiol. *J. Diet. Suppl.* 2021; in press. [CrossRef]
364. Vaia, M.; Petrosino, S.; De Filippis, D.; Negro, L.; Guarino, A.; Carnuccio, R.; Di Marzo, V.; Iuvone, T. Palmitoylethanolamide reduces inflammation and itch in a mouse model of contact allergic dermatitis. *Eur. J. Pharmacol.* **2016**, *791*, 669–674. [CrossRef]
365. Borrelli, F.; Romano, B.; Petrosino, S.; Pagano, E.; Capasso, R.; Coppola, D.; Battista, G.; Orlando, P.; Di Marzo, V.; Izzo, A.A. Palmitoylethanolamide, a naturally occurring lipid, is an orally effective intestinal anti-inflammatory agent. *Br. J. Pharmacol.* **2015**, *172*, 142–158. [CrossRef]
366. Keppel Hesselink, J.M.; Kopsky, D.J. Palmitoylethanolamide, a neutraceutical, in nerve compression syndromes: Efficacy and safety in sciatic pain and carpal tunnel syndrome. *J. Pain Res.* **2015**, *8*, 729–734. [CrossRef]
367. Calignano, A.; La Rana, G.; Giuffrida, A.; Piomelli, D. Control of pain initiation by endogenous cannabinoids. *Nature* **1998**, *394*, 277–281. [CrossRef]
368. Facci, L.; Dal Toso, R.; Romanello, S.; Buriani, A.; Skaper, S.D.; Leon, A. Mast cells express a peripheral cannabinoid receptor with differential sensitivity to anandamide and palmitoylethanolamide. *Proc. Natl. Acad. Sci. USA* **1995**, *92*, 3376–3380. [CrossRef]
369. Ueda, N.; Yamanaka, K.; Yamamoto, S. Purification and characterization of an acid amidase selective for N-palmitoylethanolamine, a putative endogenous anti-inflammatory substance. *J. Biol. Chem.* **2001**, *276*, 35552–35557. [CrossRef]
370. Di Marzo, V.; Melck, D.; Orlando, P.; Bisogno, T.; Zagoory, O.; Bifulco, M.; Vogel, Z.; De Petrocellis, L. Palmitoylethanolamide inhibits the expression of fatty acid amide hydrolase and enhances the anti-proliferative effect of anandamide in human breast cancer cells. *Biochem. J.* **2001**, *358*, 249–255. [CrossRef]
371. Guida, F.; Luongo, L.; Boccella, S.; Giordano, M.E.; Romano, R.; Bellini, G.; Manzo, I.; Furiano, A.; Rizzo, A.; Imperatore, R.; et al. Palmitoylethanolamide induces microglia changes associated with increased migration and phagocytic activity: Involvement of the CB2 receptor. *Sci. Rep.* **2017**, *7*, 375. [CrossRef] [PubMed]
372. Lo Verme, J.; Fu, J.; Astarita, G.; La Rana, G.; Russo, R.; Calignano, A.; Piomelli, D. The nuclear receptor peroxisome proliferator-activated receptor-alpha mediates the anti-inflammatory actions of palmitoylethanolamide. *Mol. Pharmacol.* **2005**, *67*, 15–19. [CrossRef] [PubMed]
373. Piomelli, D. A fatty gut feeling. *Trends Endocrinol. Metab.* **2013**, *24*, 332–341. [CrossRef]

374. Schwartz, G.J.; Fu, J.; Astarita, G.; Li, X.; Gaetani, S.; Campolongo, P.; Cuomo, V.; Piomelli, D. The lipid messenger OEA links dietary fat intake to satiety. *Cell Metab.* **2008**, *8*, 281–288. [CrossRef] [PubMed]
375. Fu, J.; Oveisi, F.; Gaetani, S.; Lin, E.; Piomelli, D. Oleoylethanolamide, an endogenous PPAR-alpha agonist, lowers body weight and hyperlipidemia in obese rats. *Neuropharmacology* **2005**, *48*, 1147–1153. [CrossRef] [PubMed]
376. Sihag, J.; Jones, P.J.H. Oleoylethanolamide: The role of a bioactive lipid amide in modulating eating behaviour. *Obes. Rev.* **2018**, *19*, 178–197. [CrossRef] [PubMed]
377. Shoemaker, J.L.; Joseph, B.K.; Ruckle, M.B.; Mayeux, P.R.; Prather, P.L. The endocannabinoid noladin ether acts as a full agonist at human CB2 cannabinoid receptors. *J. Pharmacol. Exp. Ther.* **2005**, *314*, 868–875. [CrossRef]
378. Porter, A.C.; Sauer, J.M.; Knierman, M.D.; Becker, G.W.; Berna, M.J.; Bao, J.; Nomikos, G.G.; Carter, P.; Bymaster, F.P.; Leese, A.B.; et al. Characterization of a novel endocannabinoid, virodhamine, with antagonist activity at the CB1 receptor. *J. Pharmacol. Exp. Ther.* **2002**, *301*, 1020–1024. [CrossRef]
379. Sharir, H.; Console-Bram, L.; Mundy, C.; Popoff, S.N.; Kapur, A.; Abood, M.E. The endocannabinoids anandamide and virodhamine modulate the activity of the candidate cannabinoid receptor GPR55. *J. Neuroimmune Pharmacol.* **2012**, *7*, 856–865. [CrossRef]
380. Huang, S.M.; Bisogno, T.; Trevisani, M.; Al-Hayani, A.; De Petrocellis, L.; Fezza, F.; Tognetto, M.; Petros, T.J.; Krey, J.F.; Chu, C.J.; et al. An endogenous capsaicin-like substance with high potency at recombinant and native vanilloid VR1 receptors. *Proc. Natl. Acad. Sci. USA* **2002**, *99*, 8400–8405. [CrossRef] [PubMed]
381. Bisogno, T.; Melck, D.; Bobrov, M.; Gretskaya, N.M.; Bezuglov, V.V.; De Petrocellis, L.; Di Marzo, V. N-acyl-dopamines: Novel synthetic CB(1) cannabinoid-receptor ligands and inhibitors of anandamide inactivation with cannabimimetic activity in vitro and in vivo. *Biochem. J.* **2000**, *351 Pt 3*, 817–824. [CrossRef] [PubMed]
382. Arnold, W.R.; Carnevale, L.N.; Xie, Z.; Baylon, J.L.; Tajkhorshid, E.; Hu, H.; Das, A. Anti-inflammatory dopamine- and serotonin-based endocannabinoid epoxides reciprocally regulate cannabinoid receptors and the TRPV1 channel. *Nat. Commun.* **2021**, *12*, 926. [CrossRef] [PubMed]
383. Grabiec, U.; Dehghani, F. N-Arachidonoyl Dopamine: A novel endocannabinoid and endovanilloid with widespread physiological and pharmacological activities. *Cannabis Cannabinoid Res.* **2017**, *2*, 183–196. [CrossRef] [PubMed]
384. Chu, C.J.; Huang, S.M.; De Petrocellis, L.; Bisogno, T.; Ewing, S.A.; Miller, J.D.; Zipkin, R.E.; Daddario, N.; Appendino, G.; Di Marzo, V.; et al. N-oleoyldopamine, a novel endogenous capsaicin-like lipid that produces hyperalgesia. *J. Biol. Chem.* **2003**, *278*, 13633–13639. [CrossRef]
385. Kino, T.; Tomori, T.; Abutarboush, R.; Castri, P.; Chen, Y.; Lenz, F.A.; McCarron, R.M.; Spatz, M. Effect of N-arachidonoyl-L-serine on human cerebromicrovascular endothelium. *Biochem. Biophys. Rep.* **2016**, *8*, 254–260. [CrossRef]
386. Milman, G.; Maor, Y.; Abu-Lafi, S.; Horowitz, M.; Gallily, R.; Batkai, S.; Mo, F.M.; Offertaler, L.; Pacher, P.; Kunos, G.; et al. N-arachidonoyl L-serine, an endocannabinoid-like brain constituent with vasodilatory properties. *Proc. Natl. Acad. Sci. USA* **2006**, *103*, 2428–2433. [CrossRef]
387. Zhang, X.; Maor, Y.; Wang, J.F.; Kunos, G.; Groopman, J.E. Endocannabinoid-like N-arachidonoyl serine is a novel pro-angiogenic mediator. *Br. J. Pharmacol.* **2010**, *160*, 1583–1594. [CrossRef]
388. Cohen-Yeshurun, A.; Willner, D.; Trembovler, V.; Alexandrovich, A.; Mechoulam, R.; Shohami, E.; Leker, R.R. N-arachidonoyl-L-serine (AraS) possesses proneurogenic properties in vitro and in vivo after traumatic brain injury. *J. Cereb. Blood Flow Metab.* **2013**, *33*, 1242–1250. [CrossRef]
389. Sionov, R.V.; Feldman, M.; Smoum, R.; Mechoulam, R.; Steinberg, D. Anandamide prevents the adhesion of filamentous Candida albicans to cervical epithelial cells. *Sci. Rep.* **2020**, *10*, 13728. [CrossRef]
390. Fornelos, N.; Franzosa, E.A.; Bishai, J.; Annand, J.W.; Oka, A.; Lloyd-Price, J.; Arthur, T.D.; Garner, A.; Avila-Pacheco, J.; Haiser, H.J.; et al. Growth effects of N-Acylethanolamines on gut bacteria reflect altered bacterial abundances in inflammatory bowel disease. *Nat. Microbiol.* **2020**, *5*, 486–497. [CrossRef] [PubMed]
391. Balaban, N.Q.; Merrin, J.; Chait, R.; Kowalik, L.; Leibler, S. Bacterial persistence as a phenotypic switch. *Science* **2004**, *305*, 1622–1625. [CrossRef] [PubMed]
392. Lee, A.J.; Wang, S.; Meredith, H.R.; Zhuang, B.; Dai, Z.; You, L. Robust, linear correlations between growth rates and β-lactam-mediated lysis rates. *Proc. Natl. Acad. Sci. USA* **2018**, *115*, 4069–4074. [CrossRef] [PubMed]
393. Ferrer-González, E.; Huh, H.; Al-Tameemi, H.M.; Boyd, J.M.; Lee, S.H.; Pilch, D.S. Impact of FtsZ inhibition on the localization of the penicillin binding proteins in methicillin-resistant *Staphylococcus aureus*. *J. Bacteriol.* **2021**, *203*, e0020421. [CrossRef]
394. Periasamy, S.; Joo, H.S.; Duong, A.C.; Bach, T.H.; Tan, V.Y.; Chatterjee, S.S.; Cheung, G.Y.; Otto, M. How *Staphylococcus aureus* biofilms develop their characteristic structure. *Proc. Natl. Acad. Sci. USA* **2012**, *109*, 1281–1286. [CrossRef]
395. Schwartz, K.; Syed, A.K.; Stephenson, R.E.; Rickard, A.H.; Boles, B.R. Functional amyloids composed of phenol soluble modulins stabilize *Staphylococcus aureus* biofilms. *PLoS Pathog.* **2012**, *8*, e1002744. [CrossRef]
396. Schwartz, K.; Ganesan, M.; Payne, D.E.; Solomon, M.J.; Boles, B.R. Extracellular DNA facilitates the formation of functional amyloids in *Staphylococcus aureus* biofilms. *Mol. Microbiol.* **2016**, *99*, 123–134. [CrossRef]
397. Russo, R.; Cristiano, C.; Avagliano, C.; De Caro, C.; La Rana, G.; Raso, G.M.; Canani, R.B.; Meli, R.; Calignano, A. Gut-brain axis: Role of lipids in the regulation of inflammation, pain and CNS diseases. *Curr. Med. Chem.* **2018**, *25*, 3930–3952. [CrossRef]

398. Lacroix, S.; Pechereau, F.; Leblanc, N.; Boubertakh, B.; Houde, A.; Martin, C.; Flamand, N.; Silvestri, C.; Raymond, F.; Di Marzo, V.; et al. Rapid and concomitant gut microbiota and endocannabinoidome response to diet-induced obesity in mice. *MSystems* **2019**, *4*, e00407-19. [CrossRef]
399. Sihag, J.; Di Marzo, V. (Wh)olistic (E)ndocannabinoidome-Microbiome-Axis modulation through (N)utrition (WHEN) to curb obesity and related disorders. *Lipids Health Dis.* **2022**, *21*, 9. [CrossRef]
400. Lian, J.; Casari, I.; Falasca, M. Modulatory role of the endocannabinoidome in the pathophysiology of the gastrointestinal tract. *Pharmacol. Res.* **2022**, *175*, 106025. [CrossRef] [PubMed]
401. Bisogno, T.; Lauritano, A.; Piscitelli, F. The endocannabinoid system: A bridge between Alzheimer's disease and gut microbiota. *Life* **2021**, *11*, 934. [CrossRef] [PubMed]
402. Khan, R.N.; Maner-Smith, K.; AOwens, J.; Barbian, M.E.; Jones, R.M.; RNaudin, C. At the heart of microbial conversations: Endocannabinoids and the microbiome in cardiometabolic risk. *Gut Microbes* **2021**, *13*, 1911572. [CrossRef] [PubMed]
403. Berg, G.; Rybakova, D.; Fischer, D.; Cernava, T.; Vergès, M.C.; Charles, T.; Chen, X.; Cocolin, L.; Eversole, K.; Corral, G.H.; et al. Microbiome definition re-visited: Old concepts and new challenges. *Microbiome* **2020**, *8*, 103. [CrossRef] [PubMed]
404. Allin, K.H.; Tremaroli, V.; Caesar, R.; Jensen, B.A.H.; Damgaard, M.T.F.; Bahl, M.I.; Licht, T.R.; Hansen, T.H.; Nielsen, T.; Dantoft, T.M.; et al. Aberrant intestinal microbiota in individuals with prediabetes. *Diabetologia* **2018**, *61*, 810–820. [CrossRef] [PubMed]
405. Valles-Colomer, M.; Falony, G.; Darzi, Y.; Tigchelaar, E.F.; Wang, J.; Tito, R.Y.; Schiweck, C.; Kurilshikov, A.; Joossens, M.; Wijmenga, C.; et al. The neuroactive potential of the human gut microbiota in quality of life and depression. *Nat. Microbiol.* **2019**, *4*, 623–632. [CrossRef]
406. Sorboni, S.G.; Moghaddam, H.S.; Jafarzadeh-Esfehani, R.; Soleimanpour, S. A comprehensive review on the role of the gut microbiome in human neurological disorders. *Clin. Microbiol. Rev.* **2022**, *35*, e0033820. [CrossRef]
407. Dicks, L.M.T.; Hurn, D.; Hermanus, D. Gut bacteria and neuropsychiatric disorders. *Microorganisms* **2021**, *9*, 2583. [CrossRef]
408. Kelly, J.R.; Minuto, C.; Cryan, J.F.; Clarke, G.; Dinan, T.G. The role of the gut microbiome in the development of schizophrenia. *Schizophr. Res.* **2021**, *234*, 4–23. [CrossRef]
409. Giloteaux, L.; Goodrich, J.K.; Walters, W.A.; Levine, S.M.; Ley, R.E.; Hanson, M.R. Reduced diversity and altered composition of the gut microbiome in individuals with myalgic encephalomyelitis/chronic fatigue syndrome. *Microbiome* **2016**, *4*, 30. [CrossRef]
410. Minichino, A.; Jackson, M.A.; Francesconi, M.; Steves, C.J.; Menni, C.; Burnet, P.W.J.; Lennox, B.R. Endocannabinoid system mediates the association between gut-microbial diversity and anhedonia/amotivation in a general population cohort. *Mol. Psychiatry* **2021**, *26*, 6269–6276. [CrossRef] [PubMed]
411. Chevalier, G.; Siopi, E.; Guenin-Macé, L.; Pascal, M.; Laval, T.; Rifflet, A.; Boneca, I.G.; Demangel, C.; Colsch, B.; Pruvost, A.; et al. Effect of gut microbiota on depressive-like behaviors in mice is mediated by the endocannabinoid system. *Nat. Commun.* **2020**, *11*, 6363. [CrossRef] [PubMed]
412. Li, H.; Liu, F.; Lu, J.; Shi, J.; Guan, J.; Yan, F.; Li, B.; Huo, G. Probiotic mixture of *Lactobacillus plantarum* strains improves lipid metabolism and gut microbiota structure in high fat diet-fed mice. *Front. Microbiol.* **2020**, *11*, 512. [CrossRef] [PubMed]
413. Xie, N.; Cui, Y.; Yin, Y.N.; Zhao, X.; Yang, J.W.; Wang, Z.G.; Fu, N.; Tang, Y.; Wang, X.H.; Liu, X.W.; et al. Effects of two *Lactobacillus* strains on lipid metabolism and intestinal microflora in rats fed a high-cholesterol diet. *BMC Complement. Altern. Med.* **2011**, *11*, 53. [CrossRef]
414. Rousseaux, C.; Thuru, X.; Gelot, A.; Barnich, N.; Neut, C.; Dubuquoy, L.; Dubuquoy, C.; Merour, E.; Geboes, K.; Chamaillard, M.; et al. *Lactobacillus acidophilus* modulates intestinal pain and induces opioid and cannabinoid receptors. *Nat. Med.* **2007**, *13*, 35–37. [CrossRef]
415. Alhouayek, M.; Muccioli, G.G. Harnessing the anti-inflammatory potential of palmitoylethanolamide. *Drug Discov. Today* **2014**, *19*, 1632–1639. [CrossRef]
416. Coppola, M.; Mondola, R. Is there a role for palmitoylethanolamide in the treatment of depression? *Med. Hypotheses* **2014**, *82*, 507–511. [CrossRef]
417. Zimmermann, T.; Bartsch, J.C.; Beer, A.; Lomazzo, E.; Guggenhuber, S.; Lange, M.D.; Bindila, L.; Pape, H.C.; Lutz, B. Impaired anandamide/palmitoylethanolamide signaling in hippocampal glutamatergic neurons alters synaptic plasticity, learning, and emotional responses. *Neuropsychopharmacology* **2019**, *44*, 1377–1388. [CrossRef]
418. Guida, F.; Boccella, S.; Belardo, C.; Iannotta, M.; Piscitelli, F.; De Filippis, F.; Paino, S.; Ricciardi, F.; Siniscalco, D.; Marabese, I.; et al. Altered gut microbiota and endocannabinoid system tone in vitamin D deficiency-mediated chronic pain. *Brain Behav. Immun.* **2020**, *85*, 128–141. [CrossRef]
419. Cristiano, C.; Pirozzi, C.; Coretti, L.; Cavaliere, G.; Lama, A.; Russo, R.; Lembo, F.; Mollica, M.P.; Meli, R.; Calignano, A.; et al. Palmitoylethanolamide counteracts autistic-like behaviours in BTBR T+tf/J mice: Contribution of central and peripheral mechanisms. *Brain Behav. Immun.* **2018**, *74*, 166–175. [CrossRef]
420. Sultan, M.; Wilson, K.; Abdulla, O.A.; Busbee, P.B.; Hall, A.; Carter, T.; Singh, N.; Chatterjee, S.; Nagarkatti, P.; Nagarkatti, M. Endocannabinoid anandamide attenuates acute respiratory distress syndrome through modulation of microbiome in the gut-lung axis. *Cells* **2021**, *10*, 3305. [CrossRef] [PubMed]
421. Muccioli, G.G.; Naslain, D.; Bäckhed, F.; Reigstad, C.S.; Lambert, D.M.; Delzenne, N.M.; Cani, P.D. The endocannabinoid system links gut microbiota to adipogenesis. *Mol. Syst. Biol.* **2010**, *6*, 392. [CrossRef] [PubMed]
422. Storr, M.A.; Yüce, B.; Andrews, C.N.; Sharkey, K.A. The role of the endocannabinoid system in the pathophysiology and treatment of irritable bowel syndrome. *Neurogastroenterol. Motil.* **2008**, *20*, 857–868. [CrossRef] [PubMed]

423. Camilleri, M. Cannabinoids and gastrointestinal motility: Pharmacology, clinical effects, and potential therapeutics in humans. *Neurogastroenterol. Motil.* **2018**, *30*, e13370. [CrossRef]
424. Abalo, R.; Vera, G.; López-Pérez, A.E.; Martínez-Villaluenga, M.; Martín-Fontelles, M.I. The gastrointestinal pharmacology of cannabinoids: Focus on motility. *Pharmacology* **2012**, *90*, 1–10. [CrossRef]
425. Osei-Hyiaman, D.; DePetrillo, M.; Pacher, P.; Liu, J.; Radaeva, S.; Bátkai, S.; Harvey-White, J.; Mackie, K.; Offertáler, L.; Wang, L.; et al. Endocannabinoid activation at hepatic CB1 receptors stimulates fatty acid synthesis and contributes to diet-induced obesity. *J. Clin. Investig.* **2005**, *115*, 1298–1305. [CrossRef]
426. Osei-Hyiaman, D.; Liu, J.; Zhou, L.; Godlewski, G.; Harvey-White, J.; Jeong, W.I.; Bátkai, S.; Marsicano, G.; Lutz, B.; Buettner, C.; et al. Hepatic CB1 receptor is required for development of diet-induced steatosis, dyslipidemia, and insulin and leptin resistance in mice. *J. Clin. Investig.* **2008**, *118*, 3160–3169. [CrossRef]
427. Ravinet Trillou, C.; Delgorge, C.; Menet, C.; Arnone, M.; Soubrié, P. CB1 cannabinoid receptor knockout in mice leads to leanness, resistance to diet-induced obesity and enhanced leptin sensitivity. *Int. J. Obes. Relat. Metab. Disord.* **2004**, *28*, 640–648. [CrossRef]
428. Hoareau, L.; Buyse, M.; Festy, F.; Ravanan, P.; Gonthier, M.P.; Matias, I.; Petrosino, S.; Tallet, F.; D'Hellencourt, C.L.; Cesari, M.; et al. Anti-inflammatory effect of palmitoylethanolamide on human adipocytes. *Obesity* **2009**, *17*, 431–438. [CrossRef]
429. Di Marzo, V.; Bisogno, T.; De Petrocellis, L.; Melck, D.; Orlando, P.; Wagner, J.A.; Kunos, G. Biosynthesis and inactivation of the endocannabinoid 2-arachidonoylglycerol in circulating and tumoral macrophages. *Eur. J. Biochem.* **1999**, *264*, 258–267. [CrossRef]
430. Maccarrone, M.; De Petrocellis, L.; Bari, M.; Fezza, F.; Salvati, S.; Di Marzo, V.; Finazzi-Agrò, A. Lipopolysaccharide downregulates fatty acid amide hydrolase expression and increases anandamide levels in human peripheral lymphocytes. *Arch. Biochem. Biophys.* **2001**, *393*, 321–328. [CrossRef] [PubMed]
431. Di Patrizio, N.V. Endocannabinoids in the gut. *Cannabis Cannabinoid Res.* **2016**, *1*, 67–77. [CrossRef] [PubMed]
432. Mehrpouya-Bahrami, P.; Chitrala, K.N.; Ganewatta, M.S.; Tang, C.; Murphy, E.A.; Enos, R.T.; Velazquez, K.T.; McCellan, J.; Nagarkatti, M.; Nagarkatti, P. Blockade of CB1 cannabinoid receptor alters gut microbiota and attenuates inflammation and diet-induced obesity. *Sci. Rep.* **2017**, *7*, 15645. [CrossRef] [PubMed]
433. Gross, A.; Terraza, A.; Marchant, J.; Bouaboula, M.; Ouahrani-Bettache, S.; Liautard, J.P.; Casellas, P.; Dornand, J. A beneficial aspect of a CB1 cannabinoid receptor antagonist: SR141716A is a potent inhibitor of macrophage infection by the intracellular pathogen *Brucella suis*. *J. Leukoc. Biol.* **2000**, *67*, 335–344. [CrossRef] [PubMed]
434. Zhang, M.; Lu, J.; Duan, X.; Chen, J.; Jin, X.; Lin, Z.; Pang, Y.; Wang, X.; Lou, H.; Chang, W. Rimonabant potentiates the antifungal activity of amphotericin B by increasing cellular oxidative stress and cell membrane permeability. *FEMS Yeast Res.* **2021**, *21*, foab016. [CrossRef]
435. Kim, H.Y.; Spector, A.A. N-Docosahexaenoylethanolamine: A neurotrophic and neuroprotective metabolite of docosahexaenoic acid. *Mol. Asp. Med.* **2018**, *64*, 34–44. [CrossRef]
436. Di Paola, M.; Bonechi, E.; Provensi, G.; Costa, A.; Clarke, G.; Ballerini, C.; De Filippo, C.; Passani, M.B. Oleoylethanolamide treatment affects gut microbiota composition and the expression of intestinal cytokines in Peyer's patches of mice. *Sci. Rep.* **2018**, *8*, 14881. [CrossRef]
437. Hryhorowicz, S.; Kaczmarek-Ryś, M.; Zielińska, A.; Scott, R.J.; Słomski, R.; Pławski, A. Endocannabinoid system as a promising therapeutic target in inflammatory bowel disease—A systematic review. *Front. Immunol.* **2021**, *12*, 790803. [CrossRef]
438. Esposito, G.; Capoccia, E.; Turco, F.; Palumbo, I.; Lu, J.; Steardo, A.; Cuomo, R.; Sarnelli, G.; Steardo, L. Palmitoylethanolamide improves colon inflammation through an enteric glia/toll like receptor 4-dependent PPAR-α activation. *Gut* **2014**, *63*, 1300–1312. [CrossRef]
439. Engel, M.A.; Kellermann, C.A.; Rau, T.; Burnat, G.; Hahn, E.G.; Konturek, P.C. Ulcerative colitis in AKR mice is attenuated by intraperitoneally administered anandamide. *J. Physiol. Pharmacol.* **2008**, *59*, 673–689.
440. D'Argenio, G.; Valenti, M.; Scaglione, G.; Cosenza, V.; Sorrentini, I.; Di Marzo, V. Up-regulation of anandamide levels as an endogenous mechanism and a pharmacological strategy to limit colon inflammation. *FASEB J.* **2006**, *20*, 568–570. [CrossRef] [PubMed]
441. Storr, M.A.; Keenan, C.M.; Emmerdinger, D.; Zhang, H.; Yüce, B.; Sibaev, A.; Massa, F.; Buckley, N.E.; Lutz, B.; Göke, B.; et al. Targeting endocannabinoid degradation protects against experimental colitis in mice: Involvement of CB1 and CB2 receptors. *J. Mol. Med.* **2008**, *86*, 925–936. [CrossRef] [PubMed]
442. Louis, P.; Hold, G.L.; Flint, H.J. The gut microbiota, bacterial metabolites and colorectal cancer. *Nat. Rev. Microbiol.* **2014**, *12*, 661–672. [CrossRef] [PubMed]
443. Vijay, A.; Kouraki, A.; Gohir, S.; Turnbull, J.; Kelly, A.; Chapman, V.; Barrett, D.A.; Bulsiewicz, W.J.; Valdes, A.M. The anti-inflammatory effect of bacterial short chain fatty acids is partially mediated by endocannabinoids. *Gut Microbes* **2021**, *13*, 1997559. [CrossRef]
444. Redlich, S.; Ribes, S.; Schütze, S.; Czesnik, D.; Nau, R. Palmitoylethanolamide stimulates phagocytosis of *Escherichia coli* K1 and *Streptococcus pneumoniae* R6 by microglial cells. *J. Neuroimmunol.* **2012**, *244*, 32–34. [CrossRef]
445. Redlich, S.; Ribes, S.; Schütze, S.; Nau, R. Palmitoylethanolamide stimulates phagocytosis of *Escherichia coli* K1 by macrophages and increases the resistance of mice against infections. *J. Neuroinflammation* **2014**, *11*, 108. [CrossRef]
446. Heide, E.C.; Bindila, L.; Post, J.M.; Malzahn, D.; Lutz, B.; Seele, J.; Nau, R.; Ribes, S. Prophylactic palmitoylethanolamide prolongs survival and decreases detrimental inflammation in aged mice with bacterial meningitis. *Front. Immunol.* **2018**, *9*, 2671. [CrossRef]

447. Lloyd-Price, J.; Arze, C.; Ananthakrishnan, A.N.; Schirmer, M.; Avila-Pacheco, J.; Poon, T.W.; Andrews, E.; Ajami, N.J.; Bonham, K.S.; Brislawn, C.J.; et al. Multi-omics of the gut microbial ecosystem in inflammatory bowel diseases. *Nature* **2019**, *569*, 655–662. [CrossRef]
448. Franzosa, E.A.; Sirota-Madi, A.; Avila-Pacheco, J.; Fornelos, N.; Haiser, H.J.; Reinker, S.; Vatanen, T.; Hall, A.B.; Mallick, H.; McIver, L.J.; et al. Gut microbiome structure and metabolic activity in inflammatory bowel disease. *Nat. Microbiol.* **2019**, *4*, 293–305. [CrossRef]
449. Wahlström, A.; Sayin, S.I.; Marschall, H.U.; Bäckhed, F. Intestinal crosstalk between bile acids and microbiota and its impact on host metabolism. *Cell Metab.* **2016**, *24*, 41–50. [CrossRef]
450. Rémy, B.; Mion, S.; Plener, L.; Elias, M.; Chabrière, E.; Daudé, D. Interference in bacterial quorum sensing: A biopharmaceutical perspective. *Front. Pharmacol.* **2018**, *9*, 203. [CrossRef] [PubMed]

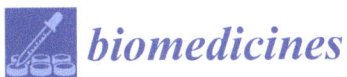

Brief Report

Impaired Ghrelin Signaling Does Not Lead to Alterations of Anxiety-like Behaviors in Adult Mice Chronically Exposed to THC during Adolescence

Matija Sestan-Pesa [1,2], Marya Shanabrough [1,2], Tamas L. Horvath [1,2] and Maria Consolata Miletta [1,2,3,*]

1. Department of Comparative Medicine, Yale University School of Medicine, New Haven, CT 06520, USA
2. Program in Integrative Cell Signaling and Neurobiology of Metabolism, Yale University School of Medicine, New Haven, CT 06520, USA
3. Larsson-Rosenquist Foundation Center for Neurodevelopment, Growth and Nutrition of the Newborn, Department of Neonatology, University of Zurich and University Hospital Zurich, 8006 Zurich, Switzerland
* Correspondence: maria.miletta@uzh.ch

Abstract: As marijuana use during adolescence has been increasing, the need to understand the effects of its long-term use becomes crucial. Previous research suggested that marijuana consumption during adolescence increases the risk of developing mental illnesses, such as schizophrenia, depression, and anxiety. Ghrelin is a peptide produced primarily in the gut and is important for feeding behavior. Recent studies have shown that ghrelin and its receptor, the growth hormone secretagogue receptor (GHSR), play important roles in mediating stress, as well as anxiety and depression-like behaviors in animal models. Here, we investigated the effects of chronic tetrahydrocannabinol (THC) administration during late adolescence (P42–55) in GHSR (GHSR $^{-/-}$) knockout mice and their wild-type littermates in relation to anxiety-like behaviors. We determined that continuous THC exposure during late adolescence did not lead to any significant alterations in the anxiety-like behaviors of adult mice, regardless of genotype, following a prolonged period of no exposure (1 month). These data indicate that in the presence of intact or impaired ghrelin/GHSR signaling, THC exposure during late adolescence has limited if any long-term impact on anxiety-like behaviors in mice.

Keywords: ghrelin; tetrahydrocannabinol (THC); GHSR signaling; late adolescence; endocannabinoid system

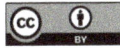

1. Introduction

Adolescence is the developmental period of transition between childhood and adulthood, on average starting at age 12 and ending at age 18 [1,2]. This period is marked by significant neuroplasticity in the prefrontal cortex and limbic regions, two brain regions involved in development of adult behavior and cognitive functions [1,3].

Cannabis use among adolescents is very high, with 9.4% of 8th graders, 23.9% of 10th graders, and 36.5% of 12th graders reporting cannabis use in the last 12 months in 2016 [4]. This event is concerning as cannabis abuse can lead to persistent cognitive impairments in learning, attention and memory [5–10]. Moreover, early cannabis use before 16 years of age increases the risk of developing psychiatric disorders, including anxiety-related symptoms [11–13]. Anxiety appears to be the most common complication arising from heavy cannabis use, with up to 20% of cannabis users experiencing anxiety [14] while the prevalence of anxiety in the general population is estimated to be around 6–17% [15].

The primary psychoactive component of cannabis is delta-9-tetrahydrocannabinol (THC). The biological effects of THC are mainly mediated by members of the G protein-coupled receptor (GPCR) family, such as cannabinoid receptors (CB1R and CB2R).

The cannabinoid receptors together with their naturally occurring ligands (anandamide and 2-arachidonoyl glycerol) and the enzymes responsible for their biosynthesis constitute the endocannabinoid system [16,17]. This system plays a critical role in the maturation of brain circuits during adolescence by regulating excitatory and inhibitory neurotransmission [18]. Further, CB1R expression increases dramatically in regions such as the prefrontal cortex, striatum, and hippocampus [19]. Imaging studies have shown decreased cortical thickness in the right superior prefrontal cortex (PFC), bilateral insula and bilateral superior cortices in adolescent cannabis users compared to adolescents who do not use cannabis [20], as well as a decrease in volume of the right medial orbitofrontal cortex [21] and bilateral hippocampus [22,23].

Ghrelin is a hormone mainly produced in the gut [24]. It stimulates potent orexigenic effects through metabolic homeostatic regulatory mechanisms in the hypothalamus and by increasing food reward and motivation through mesolimbic activation [25,26]. Ghrelin mediates both peripheral and central physiological functions through the growth hormone secretagogue receptor (GHSR) [27]. Ghrelin's role in regulating mood is very complex and it has a dual role in regulating anxiety. In some cases, injecting ghrelin centrally increased anxiety-like behaviors assessed by elevated plus maze [28], while other reports suggest the opposite effect, with ghrelin injections showing a decrease in anxiety-like behaviors as assessed by elevated plus maze [29]. This discrepancy might be related to the timing of the behavioral experiments. Another factor that contributes to modulateing ghrelin's effect on behavior is food availability, with ghrelin increasing locomotion in the absence of food [30] and decreasing locomotion in the presence of food [31]. Findings in ghrelin knockout mice also demonstrate the controversial relationship between ghrelin and anxiety. Ghrelin knockout (Ghr$^{-/-}$) mice appear to be less anxious than their wild-type counterparts under non-stressed conditions, but display more anxious behavior under mild stress conditions (15 min restraint) [32]. Of note is that stress increases ghrelin and corticosterone concurrently. GHSR and ghrelin knockout mice showed decreased plasma levels of corticosterone after chronic social defeat stress and acute restraint stress, as well as increased anxiety-like behavior [32,33]. Taken together, these findings suggest that ghrelin and GHSR are important for the ability of animals to cope with anxiety-inducing stressors. GHSR and the cannabinoid CB1R are expressed within overlapping brain regions that are crucial for feeding (hypothalamus), reward and motivation (Ventral tegmental area/VTA, nucleus accubens/NAC). Both systems mutually interact to a significant extent in the regulation of homeostatic as well as hedonic food intake [34–37]. Further, systemic pretreatment with the CB1R antagonist rimonabant significantly reduced intracerebroventricular ghrelin-induced NAC dopamine release and hyperlocomotion in mice [38]. Despite this knowledge, there are limited data on the mutual role of cannabis and ghrelin in promoting anxiety-like behaviors. Therefore, we aim to test the way in which GHSR$^{-/-}$ mice (and their wild-type counterparts) would respond to chronic THC administration during adolescence. To investigate the long-term effects of THC on behavior relating to anxiety, we exposed the animals to 10 mg of THC daily (via pulmonary route) during sexual maturation (6–8 weeks old mice), which roughly corresponds to adolescence in humans. After 14 days of THC administration, animals (male and female mice) could recover for additional 4 weeks. At 12 weeks of age, behavioral testing was performed to evaluate any long-term effects from THC administration (Figure 1A).

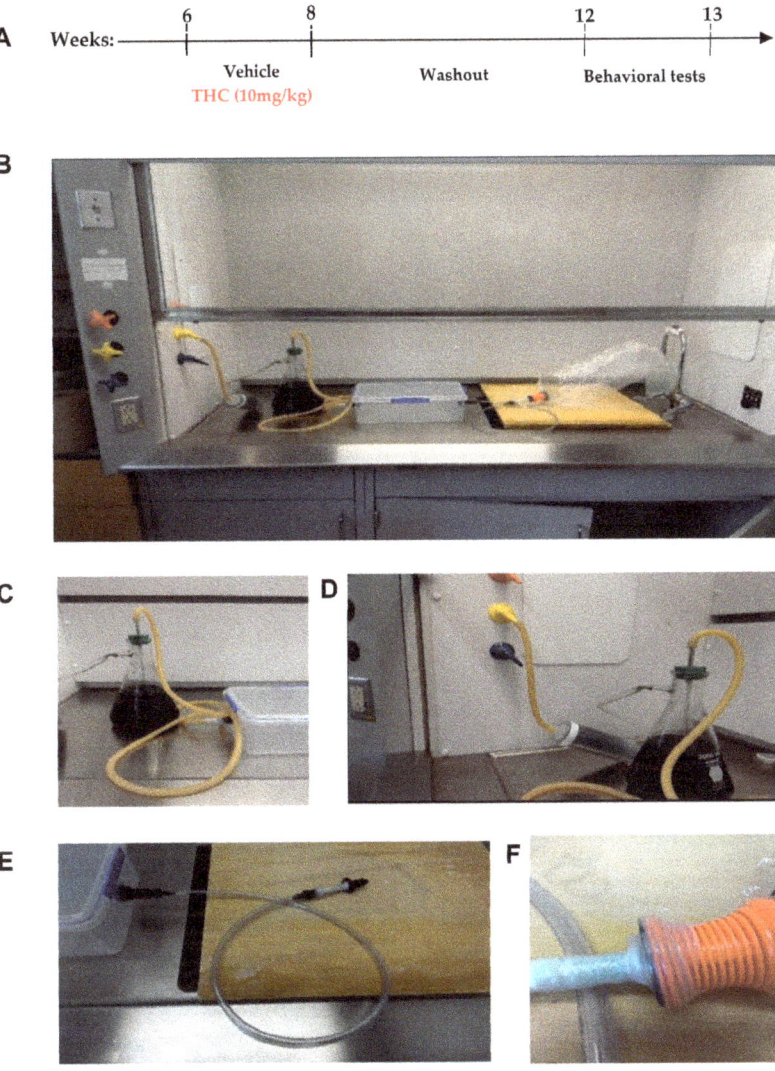

Figure 1. Experiment design and equipment for THC administration. (**A**) Experimental design, time course for THC (or vehicle) administration and behavioral testing. (**B**) Entire apparatus used to administer THC and vehicle under a chemical hood. (**C**) Tubing leading from administration box to activated charcoal trap. (**D**) Tubing leading from activated charcoal trap to the activated charcoal filter, which then leads to the vacuum line. (**E**) Open-ended tube with Volcano mouthpiece attached. (**F**) Balloon attached to the open-ended mouthpiece, sealed with parafilm.

2. Materials and Methods

2.1. Materials

To closely mimic human THC consumption, we used a formulation of THC (3.62% THC, 6.47% tetrahydrocannabinolic acid (THCA), a total of 101 mg/ml of THC) with a minimal content of terpenes (β-myrcene 0.06%, β-caryophyllene 0.64%, humulene 0.39%; a total of 1.09% terpenes) dissolved in Polyethylenglycol (PEG 400), designed for use with a commercially available vaporization apparatus.

PEG 400 with terpenes was used as the vehicle for the control group. Connecticut Pharmaceutical Solutions, LLC, Portland, CT, USA (a state-licensed grower) provided the compounds through the Connecticut Medical Marijuana Research Program.

2.2. Animals

The Institutional Animal Care and Use Committee of Yale University approved all experiments (protocol code 2019-07942). Mice were kept under standard laboratory conditions with free access to standard chow food and water except during behavioral testing. Mice were generated by breeding C57BL/6J (n. 000664 Jackson Lab) with GHSR $^{-/+}$ mice in order to obtain an F1 generation of heterozygous GHSR knock-out animals. These progenies were subsequently used to generate GHSR $^{+/+}$ (WT) and GHSR $^{-/-}$ (KO) animals used in this study. All animals were generated, bred and weaned by our laboratory and housed in the same animal room. Further details can be obtained from our previous publication [39]. THC was administered to animals from 6 to 8 weeks of age and behavioral testing was performed at 12 to 13 weeks of age (Figure 1A). Animals were placed into 2 treatment groups (vehicle and 10 mg THC) for each genotype (wild type and knock-out). Since we did not have a strict hypothesis of what sort of difference we can expect, we used the "resource equation" method for defining our sample size, a commonly used way of establishing sample size in exploratory studies [40]. We did not control for the estrous cycle in female mice.

2.3. THC Administration

Most adolescents smoke cannabis; therefore, we decided to mimic smoking as a method of administration of THC. We used commercially available vaporization equipment for marijuana administration, commonly used by marijuana consumers. Previously described experiments used the Volcano® Vapourization device (Storz and Bickel, GmbH and Co., Tuttlingen, Germany) to administer ethanol-dissolved THC to lab animals in a consistent and reproducible manner, and presented similar dose-dependent and time-dependent changes for both pulmonary and parenteral administration [41,42]. We followed their procedure, except for the following modifications. In our study, the THC containing formulation and vehicle were vaporized at 175 °C in order to avoid excessive formation and vaporization of cannabinol (CBN, a psychoactive metabolite of THC which may confound results) and reaching the flashpoint of the vehicle (PEG400, 250 °C).

THC and vehicle were administered under a chemical hood to prevent cross-contamination due to leakage of vapor, as well as maintaining a consistent experimental environment (Figure 1B). Mice were placed, in groups of 2–4, inside a closed chamber (33 cm × 20.3 cm × 10.2 cm) with valves and tubing on two of the narrower sides. To further minimize vapor escaping, on one side the tubing led to an improvised activated charcoal trap, leading to an activated charcoal filter, leading to the vacuum line (Figure 1C,D). On the other side, tubing was open-ended with a Volcano Vaporizer mouthpiece fixed to it (Figure 1E). The mouthpiece was used to release the seal on the balloons, which were filled with a vapor containing THC (or vehicle; note that the content of the balloons is mostly air so that the animal was always normoxic while in the chamber). Parafilm was used to seal the connection making it airtight (Figure 1F). Animals were exposed to the vapor for 5 min, with half of the balloon being emptied at the beginning and the other half being emptied after 2 or 3 minutes of exposure. We separated the evacuation of the vapor-filled balloon into 2 parts to prevent excessive leaking of vapors caused by increasing pressure inside of the box which exacerbates cracks in the boxes' seal during balloon evacuation. The vacuum pump line was not efficient enough at maintaining a stable pressure to avoid side leakage and posed a danger to the animals inside the box if activated when they were still inside. The leakage was minimized to our satisfaction by splitting the balloon evacuation into 2 parts. After the exposure, animals were quickly removed from the chamber, and the vacuum line was turned on to remove any residual vapor. The inside of the box was cleaned with 70% ethanol between each group of animals.

2.4. Behavioral Assessments

Open field and elevated zero maze were used to establish behavioral phenotypes induced by THC administration. Behavioral testing was performed during the light phase of the cycle from 1 pm to 7 pm.

2.4.1. Open Field

The open field apparatus (Stoelting Company, Wood Dale, IL, USA) is a square, polyurethane box (35.5 cm × 35.5 cm × 30 cm). The animal was placed in the center of the apparatus. General locomotion parameters (distance traveled, locomotion speed, time mobile) and parameters relating to anxiety (freezing time; time spent, distance travelled, and entries into central and periphery zones) were recorded for 10 min. The apparatus was cleaned with 70% ethanol after each animal's exposure. ANY-Maze software (Stoelting Company, Wood Dale, IL, USA) was used to record and analyze the behavioral data.

2.4.2. Elevated Zero Maze

The elevated zero maze apparatus is an elevated (60 cm high) ring-shaped runway (5 cm wide), with 2 equally sized (25% of the runway length) sections closed off by walls (40 cm high) opposite each other. The other two sections are open (Stoelting Company, Wood Dale, IL, USA). The maze was equally illuminated in all four sections. Mice were placed in the center of one of the open sections, facing one of the closed sections, and allowed to explore the maze for 5 min. The apparatus was cleaned with 70% ethanol after each animal's exposure. ANY-Maze SoftwareTM (Stoelting Company, Wood Dale, IL, USA) was used to record and analyze the behavioral data.

2.5. Statistics

GraphPad Prism 8.0 and Microsoft Excel 14.4.2 were used to analyze data and plot figures. Since our goal was to compare the means of more than two groups of animals, while controlling for two variables (genotype and THC treatment), two-way ANOVA was used to analyze the results. When results were significant, a multiple comparison test was performed, comparing the means of all groups, regardless of the variable in question. Data are expressed as the mean ± standard error of the mean (SEM), and a p value ≤ 0.5. was considered statistically significant.

3. Results

3.1. Open Field

The open field exploration test represents a unique opportunity to systematically assess novel environment exploration and general locomotor activity and provides initial screening for anxiety-related behaviors in rodents [43]. Two factors influence anxiety-like behaviors in the open field. The first is social isolation resulting from the physical separation from cage mates when performing the test. The second is the stress created by the brightly lit, unprotected, novel test environment [44,45]. To assess the behavioral effects of adolescent exposure to THC, we treated female and male mice of two different genotypes (GHSR $^{+/+}$ WT) and GHSR $^{-/-}$ (KO) during adolescence. We assessed anxiety-like behaviors in young adulthood (Figure 1A).

In our experimental setting, parameters that evaluate general locomotion showed no differences amongst the groups, suggesting locomotion was unaffected by THC exposure (Figure 2A–E). Further, we did not observe significant differences in the in the open field parameters indicative of anxiety-like behaviors in all groups independently of genotype and/or treatment (Figure 3A–E). For all main effects and interaction, $p \geq 0.05$.

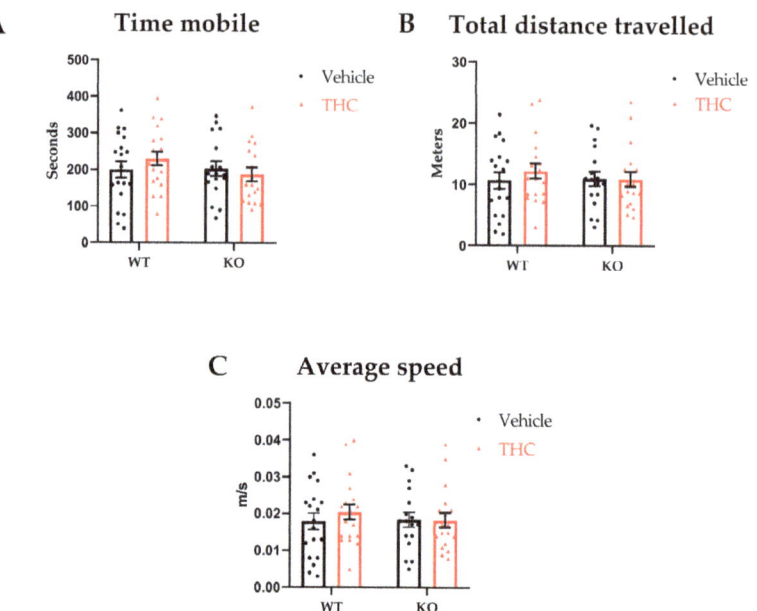

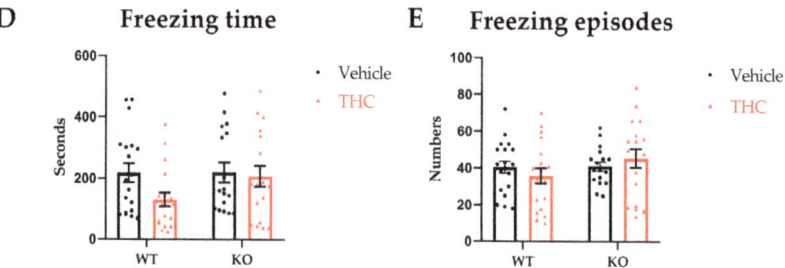

Figure 2. Open field, general locomotion. WT-vehicle n = 19, WT-THC n = 18, KO-vehicle n = 19, KO-THC n = 18; Male and female mice were included. (**A**) Time mobile. (**B**) Total distance travelled. (**C**) Average speed. (**D**) Freezing time. (**E**) Number of freezing episodes. Data are expressed as mean ± SEM Two-way ANOVA plus post hoc comparison test.

3.2. Elevated Zero Maze

Elevated zero maze is the master test for assessing anxiety-like behaviors in mice. The test exploits the natural tendencies of mice to explore novel environments [46].

We did not observe significant differences in the willingness of mice to explore open environments in all groups independently of genotype and/or treatment. For all main effects and interaction, $p \geq 0.05$ Figure 4A–E.

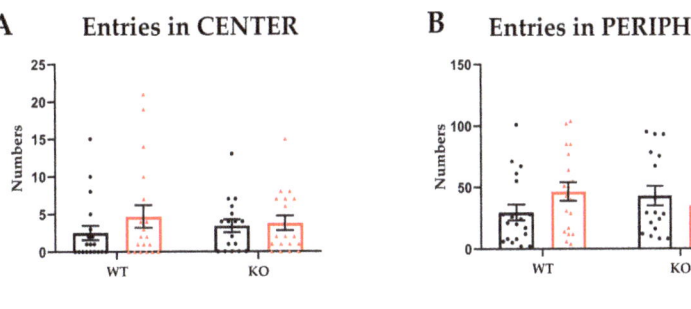
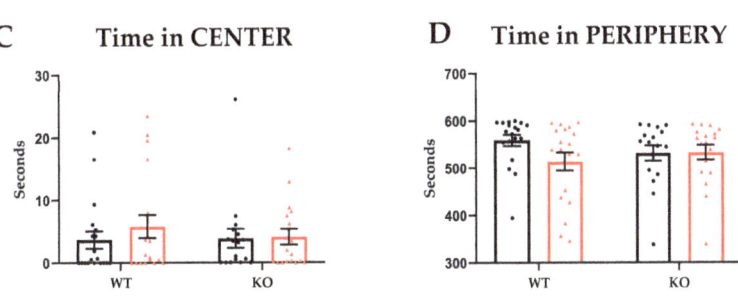
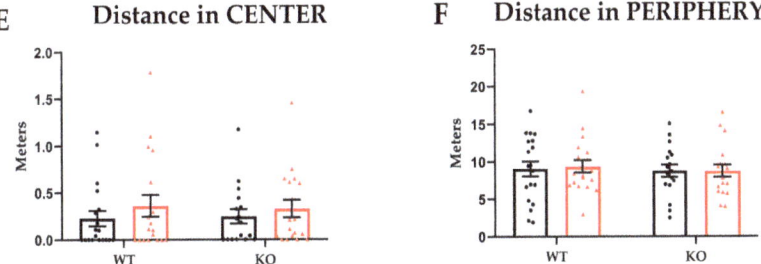

Figure 3. Open field, anxiety-related parameters. WT-vehicle n = 19, WT-THC n = 18, KO-vehicle n = 19, KO-THC n = 18; Male and female mice were included. (**A,B**) Number of entries in the central or peripheral zone. (**C,D**) Time spent in central or peripheral zone. (**E,F**) Total distance traveled in central or peripheral zone. Data are expressed as mean ± SEM. Two-way ANOVA plus post hoc comparison tests.

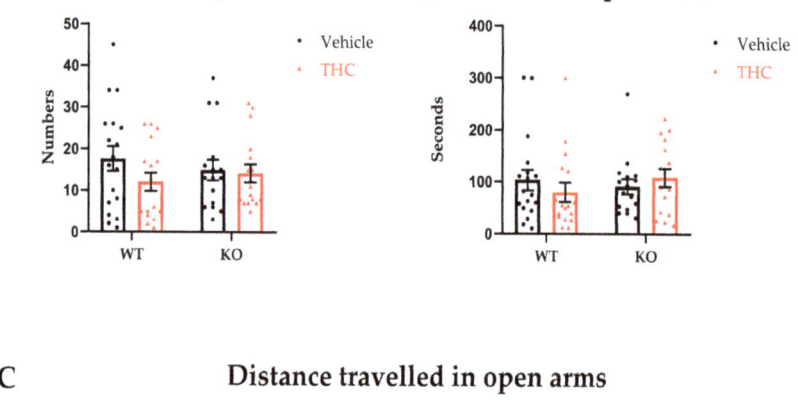
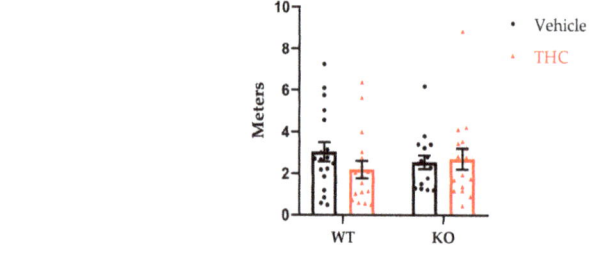
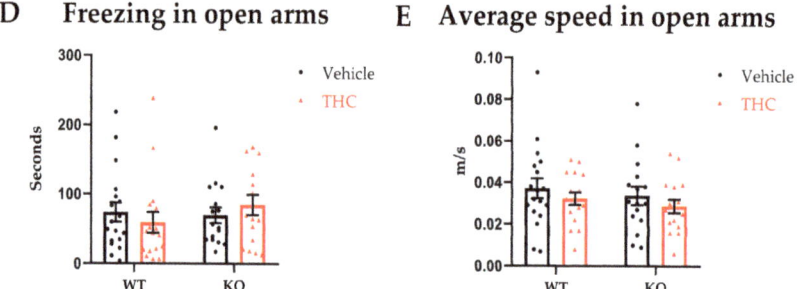

Figure 4. Elevated Zero Maze. WT-vehicle n = 19, WT-THC n = 18, KO-vehicle n = 19, KO-THC n = 18. Male and female mice were included. (**A**) Entries in open arms. (**B**) Time spent in open arms. (**C**) Distance travelled in open arms. (**D**) Average speed in open arms. (**E**) Time spent freezing in open arms. Data are expressed as mean ± SEM. Two-way ANOVA plus post hoc comparison test.

4. Discussion

In this study, we demonstrated that administration of THC to adolescent mice does not cause anxiety-like behavior in adult mice nor affect basic locomotor activity. Further, we showed that impairment of the ghrelin signaling through the knockout of the GHRS does not confer an increased risk of developing THC induced anxiety in adult mice. Our results are consistent with previous reports in rodent models that concluded that prolonged adolescent THC exposure in mice does not have substantive negative impacts on several mPFC-mediated behaviors [47–50]. In particular, Chen et al. [49] treated 28-day-old C57BL6/J mice of both sexes for three weeks with 3 mg/kg THC (daily intraperitoneal injections i.p.). One week after recovery, they analyzed several cognitive behaviors and detected little effect on anxiety-like behaviors. In another study, Zuo et al. [48] treated female and male mice with 10 mg/kg of THC in early adolescence (1 i.p. for 21 consecutive days during postnatal weeks 5–7) and assessed the impact on anxiety-like behaviors two weeks later. Their behavioral analysis demonstrated that adolescent exposure to THC in mice led to long-term impairments in object recognition, memory and social interaction, but not in anxiety-like behaviors. The experimental evidence on long-term effect of cannabis exposure during adolescence includes cannabidiol (CBD) as well, a non-intoxicating phytocannabinoid. Prolonged adolescent CBD exposure had no detrimental effects on locomotor activity in the open field and anxiety-like behaviors on the elevated plus maze in male and female C57BL/6J mice treated for 20 days mg/kg with two daily i.p. injections of CBD (20 mg/kg) [47].

Our exposure period starting at postnatal day (PND) 42 and ending at PND 55 represents the mouse brain development period similar to human adolescence [51]. Earlier findings identified this period as the critical time window for persistent detrimental effects of cannabis misuse [52,53]. Cannabis mainly acts on the developing cerebral cortex, especially the medial prefrontal cortex, a late-developing brain region whose volume decreases dramatically during adolescence as it undergoes synaptic refinement [54].

Interestingly, our results show that impairing ghrelin signaling through GHSR knockout does not affect the long-term outcome of the THC treatment. Since ghrelin and THC often act synergistically in many pathways [37], the results on GHRS KO mice further corroborate the lack of significant long-term alterations of anxiety-like behavior induced by THC in our experimental setting.

Preclinical studies collectively suggest that ghrelin/GHSR reinforces the action of cannabinoids and CB1 agonists [55,56].

These studies imply the potential interaction of the ghrelin signaling with other neurotransmitter systems (the endocannabinoid, and GABA systems) within the NAC in the reinforcing effects of cannabinoids [57].

For example, the GHSR antagonist JMV2959 significantly reduced several parameters of cannabinoid reward and attenuated cannabinoid intake and drug-seeking behavior [56].

The ghrelin receptor can interact with the CB2 cannabinoid receptor in both heterologous cells and cells of the central nervous system [58].

Overall, the long-term outcomes of cannabis exposure during adolescence are complex and can result from multiple factors. Early life interferences such as maternal deprivation or immune system activation could increase the vulnerability to cannabis-related developmental insults [59,60]. Investigations into the neurodevelopmental exposure to THC in translational animal models could provide insights into various neural pathways and biomarkers involved in THC-related pathological outcomes, identifying potential molecular targets for novel pharmacotherapeutic approaches [61].

Limitations and Future Studies

In this study, we used the vaporization method to administer THC. Compared to i.p. injections, the pharmacodynamics of the THC following vaporization is less known. Future research should establish the dose and plasma level relationship for the vaporization method using the liquid chromatography–mass spectrometry (LC/MS) method, as performed before [41,42]. Moreover, we used a lower temperature for the vaporizations, thus we should assume that less of the material was vaporized compared to the original papers [41,42]. Most of our animals exposed to THC displayed instant changes in behavior, such as headshakes (similar to hallucinogen-induced headshakes), hyperactivity, or mild somnolence. Considering that the experiments on rats, from the original study, showed a hyperactivity phenotype at 1 mg and hypomobility/somnolence with 10 mg of vaporized THC, we assumed that in our experiments, active THC reached levels between these two reported doses.

Changing conditions such as dose, the time of THC exposure, concomitant stress exposure, and presence/lack of food could clarify if there are any relevant conditions under which THC can significantly alter long-term anxiety-like behaviors with or without an intact Ghrelin/GHRS signaling. Male and female mice might be affected differently by THC exposure since the literature suggests that females may be more vulnerable to THC's effect on anxiety [62,63]. To address the possible sex differences and ghrelin's role in them, THC exposure should be coupled with a variety of adjunct treatments, such as sex hormone inhibitors and ghrelin. Lastly, additional behavioral tests, such as pre-pulse inhibition, marble burying, and tail suspension, should be employed to investigate whether THC exposure in late adolescence affects behaviors related to sensory gating, compulsiveness, and mood regulation.

Author Contributions: T.L.H. developed the concept; M.C.M. supervised the work; M.C.M. and M.S.-P. developed the experimental strategy with input from T.L.H.; M.S. provided throughout technical support; M.C.M. and M.S.-P. conducted experiments and analyzed data; M.S.-P., M.C.M. and T.L.H. wrote the paper with input from all authors. All the experiment were performed in Tamas L. Horvath's laboratory, Yale University School of Medicine, CT-06520 New Haven USA. All authors have read and agreed to the published version of the manuscript.

Funding: This work was partly funded by the Swiss National Science Foundation (Early Postdoc. Mobility P2BEP3_172252 to M.C.M.).

Institutional Review Board Statement: The study was conducted according to the guidelines of the Declaration of Helsinki, and approved by the Institutional Animal Are and Use Committee of Yale University (protocol code 2019-07942).

Informed Consent Statement: Not applicable.

Data Availability Statement: The data that support the findings of this study are available from the corresponding author upon reasonable request.

Acknowledgments: We would like to thank Connecticut Pharmaceutical Solutions, LLC for providing us with the compounds used in this study.

Conflicts of Interest: The authors declare no conflict of interest.

References

1. Spear, L.P. The adolescent brain and age-related behavioral manifestations. *Neurosci. Biobehav. Rev.* **2000**, *24*, 417–463. [CrossRef] [PubMed]
2. Dahl, R.E. Adolescent development and the regulation of behavior and emotion: Introduction to part VIII. *Ann. N. Y. Acad. Sci.* **2004**, *1021*, 294–295. [CrossRef] [PubMed]
3. Andersen, S.L. Trajectories of brain development: Point of vulnerability or window of opportunity? *Neurosci. Biobehav. Rev.* **2003**, *27*, 3–18. [CrossRef] [PubMed]
4. Miech, R.; Johnston, L.; O'Malley, P.M. Prevalence and Attitudes Regarding Marijuana Use Among Adolescents Over the Past Decade. *Pediatrics* **2017**, *140*, e20170982. [CrossRef]
5. Curran, H.V.; Freeman, T.P.; Mokrysz, C.; Lewis, D.A.; Morgan, C.J.; Parsons, L.H. Keep off the grass? Cannabis, cognition and addiction. *Nat. Rev. Neurosci.* **2016**, *17*, 293–306. [CrossRef] [PubMed]
6. Silins, E.; Horwood, L.J.; Patton, G.C.; Fergusson, D.M.; Olsson, C.A.; Hutchinson, D.M.; Spry, E.; Toumbourou, J.W.; Degenhardt, L.; Swift, W.; et al. Young adult sequelae of adolescent cannabis use: An integrative analysis. *Lancet Psychiatry* **2014**, *1*, 286–293. [CrossRef]
7. Volkow, N.D. Effects of Cannabis Use on Human Behavior-Reply. *JAMA Psychiatry* **2016**, *73*, 996. [CrossRef]
8. Castellanos-Ryan, N.; Pingault, J.B.; Parent, S.; Vitaro, F.; Tremblay, R.E.; Seguin, J.R. Adolescent cannabis use, change in neurocognitive function, and high-school graduation: A longitudinal study from early adolescence to young adulthood. *Dev. Psychopathol.* **2017**, *29*, 1253–1266. [CrossRef]
9. Volkow, N.D.; Swanson, J.M.; Evins, A.E.; DeLisi, L.E.; Meier, M.H.; Gonzalez, R.; Bloomfield, M.A.; Curran, H.V.; Baler, R. Effects of Cannabis Use on Human Behavior, Including Cognition, Motivation, and Psychosis: A Review. *JAMA Psychiatry* **2016**, *73*, 292–297. [CrossRef]
10. Crean, R.D.; Crane, N.A.; Mason, B.J. An evidence based review of acute and long-term effects of cannabis use on executive cognitive functions. *J Addict. Med.* **2011**, *5*, 1. [CrossRef]
11. Simpson, A.K.; Magid, V. Cannabis Use Disorder in Adolescence. *Child Adolesc. Psychiatr. Clin. N. Am.* **2016**, *25*, 431–443. [CrossRef]
12. Connor, J.P.; Stjepanovic, D.; Le Foll, B.; Hoch, E.; Budney, A.J.; Hall, W.D. Cannabis use and cannabis use disorder. *Nat. Rev. Dis. Prim.* **2021**, *7*, 16. [CrossRef]

13. Portugalov, A.; Akirav, I. Do Adolescent Exposure to Cannabinoids and Early Adverse Experience Interact to Increase the Risk of Psychiatric Disorders: Evidence from Rodent Models. *Int. J. Mol. Sci.* **2021**, *22*, 730. [CrossRef]
14. Reilly, D.; Didcott, P.; Swift, W.; Hall, W. Long-term cannabis use: Characteristics of users in an Australian rural area. *Addiction* **1998**, *93*, 837–846. [CrossRef]
15. Kedzior, K.K.; Laeber, L.T. A positive association between anxiety disorders and cannabis use or cannabis use disorders in the general population–a meta-analysis of 31 studies. *BMC Psychiatry* **2014**, *14*, 136. [CrossRef]
16. Mechoulam, R.; Parker, L.A. The endocannabinoid system and the brain. *Annu. Rev. Psychol.* **2013**, *64*, 21–47. [CrossRef]
17. Lu, H.C.; Mackie, K. An Introduction to the Endogenous Cannabinoid System. *Biol. Psychiatry* **2016**, *79*, 516–525. [CrossRef]
18. Viveros, M.P.; Llorente, R.; Suarez, J.; Llorente-Berzal, A.; Lopez-Gallardo, M.; de Fonseca, F.R. The endocannabinoid system in critical neurodevelopmental periods: Sex differences and neuropsychiatric implications. *J. Psychopharmacol.* **2012**, *26*, 164–176. [CrossRef]
19. Mato, S.; Del Olmo, E.; Pazos, A. Ontogenetic development of cannabinoid receptor expression and signal transduction functionality in the human brain. *Eur. J. Neurosci.* **2003**, *17*, 1747–1754. [CrossRef]
20. Lopez-Larson, M.P.; Bogorodzki, P.; Rogowska, J.; McGlade, E.; King, J.B.; Terry, J.; Yurgelun-Todd, D. Altered prefrontal and insular cortical thickness in adolescent marijuana users. *Behav. Brain Res.* **2011**, *220*, 164–172. [CrossRef]
21. Churchwell, J.C.; Lopez-Larson, M.; Yurgelun-Todd, D.A. Altered frontal cortical volume and decision making in adolescent cannabis users. *Front. Psychol.* **2010**, *1*, 225. [CrossRef] [PubMed]
22. Yucel, M.; Solowij, N.; Respondek, C.; Whittle, S.; Fornito, A.; Pantelis, C.; Lubman, D.I. Regional brain abnormalities associated with long-term heavy cannabis use. *Arch. Gen. Psychiatry* **2008**, *65*, 694–701. [CrossRef] [PubMed]
23. Ashtari, M.; Avants, B.; Cyckowski, L.; Cervellione, K.L.; Roofeh, D.; Cook, P.; Gee, J.; Sevy, S.; Kumra, S. Medial temporal structures and memory functions in adolescents with heavy cannabis use. *J. Psychiatry Res.* **2011**, *45*, 1055–1066. [CrossRef] [PubMed]
24. Kojima, M.; Hosoda, H.; Date, Y.; Nakazato, M.; Matsuo, H.; Kangawa, K. Ghrelin is a growth-hormone-releasing acylated peptide from stomach. *Nature* **1999**, *402*, 656–660. [CrossRef] [PubMed]
25. Mason, B.L.; Wang, Q.; Zigman, J.M. The central nervous system sites mediating the orexigenic actions of ghrelin. *Annu. Rev. Physiol.* **2014**, *76*, 519–533. [CrossRef]
26. Naleid, A.M.; Grace, M.K.; Cummings, D.E.; Levine, A.S. Ghrelin induces feeding in the mesolimbic reward pathway between the ventral tegmental area and the nucleus accumbens. *Peptides* **2005**, *26*, 2274–2279. [CrossRef]
27. Abizaid, A.; Hougland, J.L. Ghrelin Signaling: GOAT and GHS-R1a Take a LEAP in Complexity. *Trends Endocrinol. Metab.* **2020**, *31*, 107–117. [CrossRef]
28. Carlini, V.P.; Monzon, M.E.; Varas, M.M.; Cragnolini, A.B.; Schioth, H.B.; Scimonelli, T.N.; de Barioglio, S.R. Ghrelin increases anxiety-like behavior and memory retention in rats. *Biochem. Biophys. Res. Commun.* **2002**, *299*, 739–743. [CrossRef]
29. Lutter, M.; Sakata, I.; Osborne-Lawrence, S.; Rovinsky, S.A.; Anderson, J.G.; Jung, S.; Birnbaum, S.; Yanagisawa, M.; Elmquist, J.K.; Nestler, E.J.; et al. The orexigenic hormone ghrelin defends against depressive symptoms of chronic stress. *Nat. Neurosci.* **2008**, *11*, 752–753. [CrossRef]
30. Jerlhag, E.; Egecioglu, E.; Dickson, S.L.; Andersson, M.; Svensson, L.; Engel, J.A. Ghrelin stimulates locomotor activity and accumbal dopamine-overflow via central cholinergic systems in mice: Implications for its involvement in brain reward. *Addict. Biol.* **2006**, *11*, 45–54. [CrossRef]
31. Tang-Christensen, M.; Vrang, N.; Ortmann, S.; Bidlingmaier, M.; Horvath, T.L.; Tschop, M. Central administration of ghrelin and agouti-related protein (83–132) increases food intake and decreases spontaneous locomotor activity in rats. *Endocrinology* **2004**, *145*, 4645–4652. [CrossRef]
32. Spencer, S.J.; Xu, L.; Clarke, M.A.; Lemus, M.; Reichenbach, A.; Geenen, B.; Kozicz, T.; Andrews, Z.B. Ghrelin regulates the hypothalamic-pituitary-adrenal axis and restricts anxiety after acute stress. *Biol. Psychiatry* **2012**, *72*, 457–465. [CrossRef]
33. Chuang, J.C.; Perello, M.; Sakata, I.; Osborne-Lawrence, S.; Savitt, J.M.; Lutter, M.; Zigman, J.M. Ghrelin mediates stress-induced food-reward behavior in mice. *J. Clin. Investig.* **2011**, *121*, 2684–2692. [CrossRef]
34. Alen, F.; Crespo, I.; Ramirez-Lopez, M.T.; Jagerovic, N.; Goya, P.; de Fonseca, F.R.; de Heras, R.G.; Orio, L. Ghrelin-induced orexigenic effect in rats depends on the metabolic status and is counteracted by peripheral CB1 receptor antagonism. *PLoS ONE* **2013**, *8*, e60918. [CrossRef]
35. Tucci, S.A.; Rogers, E.K.; Korbonits, M.; Kirkham, T.C. The cannabinoid CB1 receptor antagonist SR141716 blocks the orexigenic effects of intrahypothalamic ghrelin. *Br. J. Pharmacol.* **2004**, *143*, 520–523. [CrossRef]
36. Edwards, A.; Abizaid, A. Driving the need to feed: Insight into the collaborative interaction between ghrelin and endocannabinoid systems in modulating brain reward systems. *Neurosci. Biobehav. Rev.* **2016**, *66*, 33–53. [CrossRef]
37. Sustkova-Fiserova, M.; Charalambous, C.; Khryakova, A.; Certilina, A.; Lapka, M.; Slamberova, R. The Role of Ghrelin/GHS-R1A Signaling in Nonalcohol Drug Addictions. *Int. J. Mol. Sci.* **2022**, *23*, 761. [CrossRef]
38. Kalafateli, A.L.; Vallof, D.; Jornulf, J.W.; Heilig, M.; Jerlhag, E. A cannabinoid receptor antagonist attenuates ghrelin-induced activation of the mesolimbic dopamine system in mice. *Physiol. Behav.* **2018**, *184*, 211–219. [CrossRef]

39. Abizaid, A.; Liu, Z.W.; Andrews, Z.B.; Shanabrough, M.; Borok, E.; Elsworth, J.D.; Roth, R.H.; Sleeman, M.W.; Picciotto, M.R.; Tschop, M.H.; et al. Ghrelin modulates the activity and synaptic input organization of midbrain dopamine neurons while promoting appetite. *J. Clin. Investig.* **2006**, *116*, 3229–3239. [CrossRef]
40. Charan, J.; Kantharia, N.D. How to calculate sample size in animal studies? *J. Pharmacol. Pharmacother.* **2013**, *4*, 303–306. [CrossRef]
41. Manwell, L.A.; Charchoglyan, A.; Brewer, D.; Matthews, B.A.; Heipel, H.; Mallet, P.E. A vapourized Delta(9)-tetrahydrocannabinol (Delta(9)-THC) delivery system part I: Development and validation of a pulmonary cannabinoid route of exposure for experimental pharmacology studies in rodents. *J. Pharmacol. Toxicol. Methods* **2014**, *70*, 120–127. [CrossRef] [PubMed]
42. Manwell, L.A.; Ford, B.; Matthews, B.A.; Heipel, H.; Mallet, P.E. A vapourized Delta(9)-tetrahydrocannabinol (Delta(9)-THC) delivery system part II: Comparison of behavioural effects of pulmonary versus parenteral cannabinoid exposure in rodents. *J. Pharmacol. Toxicol. Methods* **2014**, *70*, 112–119. [CrossRef] [PubMed]
43. Bailey, K.R.; Crawley, J.N. *Anxiety-Related Behaviors in Mice Methods of Behavior Analysis in Neuroscience*; Taylor & Francis Group, LLC.: Boca Raton, FL, USA, 2009.
44. File, S.E. The use of social interaction as a method for detecting anxiolytic activity of chlordiazepoxide-like drugs. *J. Neurosci. Methods* **1980**, *2*, 219–238. [CrossRef] [PubMed]
45. Prut, L.; Belzung, C. The open field as a paradigm to measure the effects of drugs on anxiety-like behaviors: A review. *Eur. J. Pharmacol.* **2003**, *463*, 3–33. [CrossRef] [PubMed]
46. Rodgers, R.J.; Dalvi, A. Anxiety, defence and the elevated plus-maze. *Neurosci. Biobehav. Rev.* **1997**, *21*, 801–810. [CrossRef]
47. Kaplan, J.S.; Wagner, J.K.; Reid, K.; McGuinness, F.; Arvila, S.; Brooks, M.; Stevenson, H.; Jones, J.; Risch, B.; McGillis, T.; et al. Cannabidiol Exposure During the Mouse Adolescent Period Is Without Harmful Behavioral Effects on Locomotor Activity, Anxiety, and Spatial Memory. *Front. Behav. Neurosci.* **2021**, *15*, 711639. [CrossRef]
48. Zuo, Y.; Iemolo, A.; Montilla-Perez, P.; Li, H.R.; Yang, X.; Telese, F. Chronic adolescent exposure to cannabis in mice leads to sex-biased changes in gene expression networks across brain regions. *Neuropsychopharmacology* **2022**, *47*, 2071–2080. [CrossRef]
49. Chen, H.T.; Mackie, K. Adolescent Delta(9)-Tetrahydrocannabinol Exposure Selectively Impairs Working Memory but Not Several Other mPFC-Mediated Behaviors. *Front. Psychiatry* **2020**, *11*, 576214. [CrossRef]
50. Hamidullah, S.; Lutelmowski, C.D.; Creighton, S.D.; Luciani, K.R.; Frie, J.A.; Winters, B.D.; Khokhar, J.Y. Effects of vapourized THC and voluntary alcohol drinking during adolescence on cognition, reward, and anxiety-like behaviours in rats. *Prog. Neuropsychopharmacol. Biol. Psychiatry* **2021**, *106*, 110141. [CrossRef]
51. Brust, V.; Schindler, P.M.; Lewejohann, L. Lifetime development of behavioural phenotype in the house mouse (Mus musculus). *Front. Zool.* **2015**, *12* (Suppl. S1), S17. [CrossRef]
52. Bilkei-Gorzo, A.; Albayram, O.; Draffehn, A.; Michel, K.; Piyanova, A.; Oppenheimer, H.; Dvir-Ginzberg, M.; Racz, I.; Ulas, T.; Imbeault, S.; et al. A chronic low dose of Delta(9)-tetrahydrocannabinol (THC) restores cognitive function in old mice. *Nat. Med.* **2017**, *23*, 782–787. [CrossRef]
53. Renard, J.; Szkudlarek, H.J.; Kramar, C.P.; Jobson, C.E.L.; Moura, K.; Rushlow, W.J.; Laviolette, S.R. Adolescent THC Exposure Causes Enduring Prefrontal Cortical Disruption of GABAergic Inhibition and Dysregulation of Sub-Cortical Dopamine Function. *Sci. Rep.* **2017**, *7*, 11420. [CrossRef]
54. Mills, K.L.; Lalonde, F.; Clasen, L.S.; Giedd, J.N.; Blakemore, S.J. Developmental changes in the structure of the social brain in late childhood and adolescence. *Soc. Cogn. Affect. Neurosci.* **2014**, *9*, 123–131. [CrossRef]
55. Zbucki, R.L.; Sawicki, B.; Hryniewicz, A.; Winnicka, M.M. Cannabinoids enhance gastric X/A-like cells activity. *Folia Histochem. Cytobiol.* **2008**, *46*, 219–224. [CrossRef]
56. Charalambous, C.; Havlickova, T.; Lapka, M.; Puskina, N.; Slamberova, R.; Kuchar, M.; Sustkova-Fiserova, M. Cannabinoid-Induced Conditioned Place Preference, Intravenous Self-Administration, and Behavioral Stimulation Influenced by Ghrelin Receptor Antagonism in Rats. *Int. J. Mol. Sci.* **2021**, *22*, 2397. [CrossRef]
57. Charalambous, C.; Lapka, M.; Havlickova, T.; Syslova, K.; Sustkova-Fiserova, M. Alterations in Rat Accumbens Dopamine, Endocannabinoids and GABA Content During WIN55,212-2 Treatment: The Role of Ghrelin. *Int. J. Mol. Sci.* **2020**, *22*, 210. [CrossRef]
58. Lillo, J.; Lillo, A.; Zafra, D.A.; Miralpeix, C.; Rivas-Santisteban, R.; Casals, N.; Navarro, G.; Franco, R. Identification of the Ghrelin and Cannabinoid CB(2) Receptor Heteromer Functionality and Marked Upregulation in Striatal Neurons from Offspring of Mice under a High-Fat Diet. *Int. J. Mol. Sci.* **2021**, *22*, 8928. [CrossRef]
59. Zamberletti, E.; Prini, P.; Speziali, S.; Gabaglio, M.; Solinas, M.; Parolaro, D.; Rubino, T. Gender-dependent behavioral and biochemical effects of adolescent delta-9-tetrahydrocannabinol in adult maternally deprived rats. *Neuroscience* **2012**, *204*, 245–257. [CrossRef]
60. Lecca, S.; Luchicchi, A.; Scherma, M.; Fadda, P.; Muntoni, A.L.; Pistis, M. Delta(9)-Tetrahydrocannabinol During Adolescence Attenuates Disruption of Dopamine Function Induced in Rats by Maternal Immune Activation. *Front. Behav. Neurosci.* **2019**, *13*, 202. [CrossRef]
61. De Felice, M.; Laviolette, S.R. Reversing the Psychiatric Effects of Neurodevelopmental Cannabinoid Exposure: Exploring Pharmacotherapeutic Interventions for Symptom Improvement. *Int. J. Mol. Sci.* **2021**, *22*, 7861. [CrossRef]

62. Patton, G.C.; Coffey, C.; Carlin, J.B.; Degenhardt, L.; Lynskey, M.; Hall, W. Cannabis use and mental health in young people: Cohort study. *BMJ* **2002**, *325*, 1195–1198. [CrossRef] [PubMed]
63. Hayatbakhsh, M.R.; Najman, J.M.; Jamrozik, K.; Mamun, A.A.; Alati, R.; Bor, W. Cannabis and anxiety and depression in young adults: A large prospective study. *J. Am. Acad. Child Adolesc. Psychiatry* **2007**, *46*, 408–417. [CrossRef] [PubMed]

Disclaimer/Publisher's Note: The statements, opinions and data contained in all publications are solely those of the individual author(s) and contributor(s) and not of MDPI and/or the editor(s). MDPI and/or the editor(s) disclaim responsibility for any injury to people or property resulting from any ideas, methods, instructions or products referred to in the content.

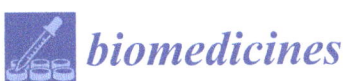

Systematic Review

A Review on the Bioactivity of Cannabinoids on Zebrafish Models: Emphasis on Neurodevelopment

Rosario Licitra [1], Maria Marchese [1,*], Valentina Naef [1], Asahi Ogi [1], Marco Martinelli [2], Claudia Kiferle [2], Baldassare Fronte [3] and Filippo Maria Santorelli [1,*]

1. Molecular Medicine and Neurobiology—ZebraLab, IRCCS Fondazione Stella Maris, 56128 Pisa, Italy; rosario.licitra@fsm.unipi.it (R.L.); valentina.naef@fsm.unipi.it (V.N.); a.ogi@hotmail.com (A.O.)
2. PlantLab, Institute of Life Sciences, Scuola Superiore Sant'Anna, 56124 Pisa, Italy; marco.martinelli@santannapisa.it (M.M.); claudia.kiferle@santannapisa.it (C.K.)
3. Department of Veterinary Science, University of Pisa, 56124 Pisa, Italy; baldassare.fronte@unipi.it
* Correspondence: maria.marchese@fsm.unipi.it (M.M.); filippo3364@gmail.com (F.M.S.)

Abstract: For centuries, the cannabis plant has been used as a source of food, fiber, and medicine. Recently, scientific interest in cannabis has increased considerably, as its bioactive compounds have shown promising potential in the treatment of numerous musculoskeletal and neurological diseases in humans. However, the mechanisms that underlie its possible effects on neurodevelopment and nervous-system functioning remain poorly understood and need to be further investigated. Although the bulk of research on cannabis and cannabinoids is based on in vitro or rodent models, the zebrafish has now emerged as a powerful in vivo model for drug-screening studies and translational research. We here review the available literature on the use of cannabis/cannabinoids in zebrafish, and particularly in zebrafish models of neurological disorders. A critical analysis suggests that zebrafish could serve as an experimental tool for testing the bioactivity of cannabinoids, and they could thus provide important insights into the safety and efficacy of different cannabis-extract-based products. The review showed that zebrafish exhibit similar behaviors to rodents following cannabinoid exposure. The authors stress the importance of analyzing the full spectrum of naturally occurring cannabinoids, rather than just the main ones, THC and CBD, and they offer some pointers on performing behavioral analysis in zebrafish.

Keywords: zebrafish; cannabis; cannabinoids; phytocannabinoids; ∆9-tetrahydrocannabinol; THC; cannabidiol; CBD

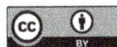

1. Introduction

For centuries, the cannabis plant (*Cannabis sativa* and *Cannabis indica*) has been used as a source of food, fiber, and medicine [1–4]. In recent decades, scientific interest in cannabis has increased considerably, as its bioactive compounds have shown promising potential in the treatment of numerous musculoskeletal and neurological diseases in humans [5,6]. Among young people, cannabis is the illicit substance that is most commonly used for recreational purposes [5,7,8], thanks to its anxiolytic effect and the associated sense of euphoria [9]. It is also widely used among pregnant women, mainly to reduce morning sickness, nausea, and vomiting [3,10]. However, because cannabinoids can readily cross the placenta and reach the fetus, they may impact the development of the embryo, which increases the risk of neurological disorders in newborns [3]. The mechanistic pathways by which cannabis and its metabolites affect neurodevelopment and nervous-system functioning remain poorly understood and need to be further investigated. To date, around 500 compounds have been identified in the cannabis plant; these include more than 150 cannabinoids, which generate more than 2000 compounds when smoked [11]. The plant also contains other bioactive compounds of medical and industrial interest, such as phenolics and flavonoids [12]. Cannabinoids and terpenes are abundant in the viscous resin that is produced by the glandular structures of the cannabis flowers, called trichromes [4]. The quantitative and qualitative characteristics of the plant are quite variable, with its composition, concentration, and yield greatly affected by the growing conditions, processing, and storage [13,14]. Biochemically, cannabinoids are highly lipophilic substances that are soluble in alcohols, fats, and other nonpolar organic solvents. They can remain associated with cell membranes long after the actual exposure to the substance [10].

In human medicine, cannabinoids are already considered to be antiemetic, antispastic, analgesic, and appetite-stimulating compounds [2,5]. Their therapeutic effects have also been examined in a series of syndromes, including multiple sclerosis [15], Dravet syndrome [16,17], epilepsy [18], fibromyalgia [19], anxiety [20], schizophrenia [21], chronic pain [22], and cancer [23,24]. Many people look to naturally derived compounds, such as cannabinoids, to treat illness and disease because they wish to avoid the strong side effects of synthetic drugs [25]. However, the literature suggests that cannabinoids may unfortunately have serious and undesirable effects, such as dependency, as well as a possible causative association with psychotic illness and cognitive impairment, including deleterious effects on memory [15]. Cannabinoids, for instance, have pronounced effects on the recognition memory and social behavior in pubertal rats, which suggests that the developing brain is sensitive to cannabinoid exposure [26]. Moreover, some studies link cannabis use to adverse birth outcomes, including low birthweights and preterm births, while other studies do not report any negative effects on children [27]. Cannabinoid use is still subject to uncertainty over aspects such as the dosing and side-effect profiles, and there is an overall lack of knowledge of their underlying mechanism of action; clinicians are therefore often reluctant to prescribe cannabis [25,28]. However, cannabis shows a lower potential to cause dependence (8.9%) than do other common substances of abuse, such as cocaine (20.9%), alcohol (22.7%), and nicotine (67.5%) [29]; moreover, it has recently been suggested that susceptibility to psychosis-like symptoms varies between cannabis consumers, as it involves a complex interplay between environmental factors and genetic predispositions [2]. Cannabinoids aside, it is also worth noting that potentially synergistic effects of phytocannabinoids and terpenoids have been reported in the treatment of pain, inflammation, depression, and anxiety [12].

Although the use of cannabis is still illegal in most countries, the cannabis world market is now approaching USD 30 billion, and the profits from illicit trafficking are certainly higher than that [30]. Currently, medications based on both synthetic cannabinoids (e.g., Nabilone® and Dronabinol®) and cannabis extracts (e.g., Sativex® and Epidiolex®) are approved for human use [14,16,24,31]. It is therefore very important for patients, doctors, and the entire scientific community to better understand the effects of cannabis/cannabinoid exposure on health [32].

The two main cannabinoids found in cannabis are Δ9-tetrahydrocannabinol (THC) and cannabidiol (CBD) [33]. THC is considered a psychoactive component, while CBD lacks psychotropic activity [10]. THC and CBD are present in the flowers and leaves of the female plants at concentrations ranging between 0.1 and 25% and 0.1 and 2.89% (w/w), respectively [30]. In addition to CBD and THC, cannabis contains numerous other cannabinoids with known or potential bioactivity [34]. For instance, cannabinol (CBN), the main metabolite of THC, was considered to be an inactive cannabinoid until studies shed light on its biological activities [30,35]. The typical concentration of CBN in cannabis inflorescences ranges between 0.1 and 1.6% (w/w of dry weight). It forms primarily through the degradation of THC that occurs as the plant ages and as an effect of storage conditions [36]. Other minor cannabinoids present in cannabis are Δ9-tetrahydrocannabivarin (THCV), cannabichromene (CBC), cannabigerol (CBG), cannabigerovarin (CBGV), cannabidivarin (CBDV), and 11-hydroxy-Δ9-tetrahydrocannabivarin (THCV−OH) [14,37]. A novel Δ9-tetrahydrocannabiphorol (THCP) was isolated and reported to have higher in vivo "cannabimimetic" activity than normal THC [38]. Figure 1 shows the molecular structures of the aforementioned cannabis phytocannabinoids.

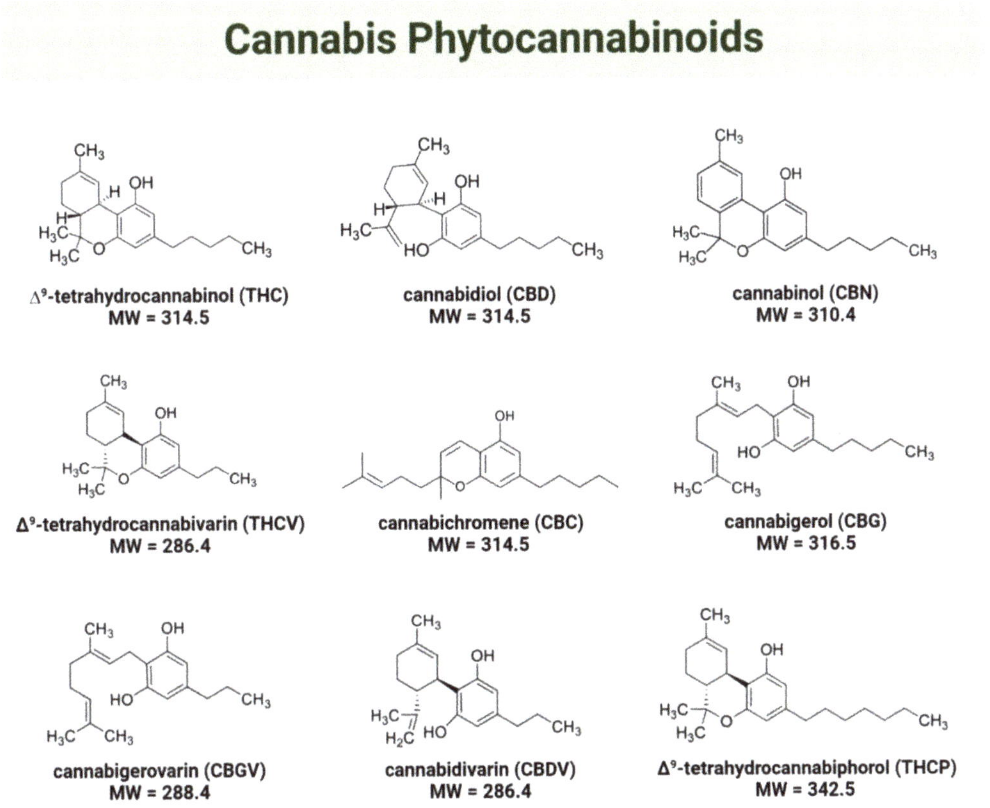

Cannabis Phytocannabinoids

Δ⁹-tetrahydrocannabinol (THC)
MW = 314.5

cannabidiol (CBD)
MW = 314.5

cannabinol (CBN)
MW = 310.4

Δ⁹-tetrahydrocannabivarin (THCV)
MW = 286.4

cannabichromene (CBC)
MW = 314.5

cannabigerol (CBG)
MW = 316.5

cannabigerovarin (CBGV)
MW = 288.4

cannabidivarin (CBDV)
MW = 286.4

Δ⁹-tetrahydrocannabiphorol (THCP)
MW = 342.5

Figure 1. Molecular structures of phytocannabinoids found in cannabis.

THC and its derivatives are studied mainly for their psychotropic properties and other pharmacological activities, including their possible anticonvulsant, antidepressant, hypotensive, bronchodilator, and analgesic actions, as well as their ability to lower intraocular pressure [15]. However, there is also evidence that THC may increase the resilience to certain stressors, as it has been observed that low doses of THC protect against a wide range of neuronal insults, including 3,4 methylene-dioxymethamphetamine (MDMA) and carbon monoxide exposure [27]. In addition, researchers have shown an increasing interest in determining whether THC or other cannabinoids can positively affect neurological health and neurodegenerative disease development in advanced age. This hypothesis is supported by a study that reports that cannabinoids protect against neurodegenerative diseases in many animal models when they are administered in adulthood or advanced age [39]. The anti-inflammatory properties of THC may help to protect the brain against neurodegenerative diseases [40]. Indeed, while high doses of THC can cause memory deficits [41], low doses of THC have been shown to slow or halt Alzheimer's disease (AD) progression by reducing the amyloid beta, which is the main component of the amyloid plaques found in the brains of people affected by AD [42,43], and to restore cognitive function in old mice [44]. Taken together, these findings reinforce the suggestion that the THC doses and patient age determine the beneficial versus detrimental effects of THC on neuronal health [27]. Moreover, the dose seems to influence the resultant behavioral phenotype, as low doses may induce anxiolytic effects, whereas high THC doses generally cause the opposite responses [45]. Some researchers suggest that the plant produces this molecule in order to protect it from ultraviolet radiation. Indeed, ultraviolet radiation can stimulate cannabinoid biosynthesis [46], and, apparently, the higher the altitude at which cannabis grows, the more THC it produces. Current evidence indicates that even visible LED light can enhance the THC, CBG, and terpene accumulation in the flowers, but not the accumulation of CBD [47].

CBD has been used to reduce bouts of nausea and vomiting, and as an anxiolytic, antipsychotic, antirheumatic, appetite stimulant, and analgesic, as well as a natural remedy for multiple sclerosis and epilepsy [10,25,48]. Moreover, CBD possesses antioxidative and antiapoptotic properties, and it exerts anti-inflammatory effects [7]. It has well-recognized behavioral effects of clinical interest, especially with regard to its anxiolytic properties, and an inverted U-shaped dose–response curve has been reported in several animal models featuring anxiety [48]. In general, CBD does not appear to affect memory formation and may protect against memory impairment [49], but research is still ongoing. Surprisingly, it has been reported that CBD degrades into THC in gastric fluid [50]. As observed with THC, the therapeutic potential of CBD is related to its interaction with the central nervous system (CNS) via several pathways, including the endocannabinoid-system (ECS) pathway, serotonin receptors, and intracellular mechanisms [25,51]. Finally, the CBD:THC ratio also seems to play an important role in determining the symptomatic effects of cannabis [6].

1.1. The Endocannabinoid System

In 1988, Devane and colleagues [52] discovered a specific brain receptor for cannabinoids. Subsequently, it was understood that the cells equipped with these receptors constitute part of a network of neurons, analogous to that involving dopamine, serotonin, and endorphins, and capable of triggering cognitive, behavioral, or physiological changes. Cannabinoid receptors were found to be particularly expressed in brain areas involved in the control of learning and memory (cortex and hippocampus), motor behavior (basal ganglia, cerebellum), emotions (amygdala), and autonomic and endocrine functions (hypothalamus, pons, and medulla), and they may therefore be involved in the control of numerous neurobiological processes [53,54]. Four years after the discovery of cannabinoid receptors, the same research group [55] isolated an endocannabinoid produced by the human brain. It was named "anandamide" (AEA), after the Hindu term "Ananda", meaning "happiness or bliss". Specifically, there is evidence of a role for AEA in social facilitation, which is closely related to the action of oxytocin [56]. Indeed, the oxytocinergic system is known to regulate social and maternal behavior in mammals [57], and AEA, mediating the action of oxytocin, has been considered crucial for social behavior, and even a possible therapeutic compound for autism-related social impairment [58]. Although the scientific literature on the relationship between zebrafish social behavior and isotocin (teleost homolog of mammalian oxytocin) is quite limited, the effects of bioactive fatty acid amide derivatives on zebrafish bone metabolism [59], growth, and lipid metabolism [60] have been described.

In vertebrates, the ECS involves the cannabinoid receptors 1 and 2 (CB^1 and CB^2, re-spectively), endogenous ligands (such as anandamide and 2-arachidonoylglycerol), and the mechanism responsible for receptor and ligand synthesis and degradation [10]. CB^1 has been found to be the most abundant G-protein-coupled receptor within the CNS [5]. CB^1 and CB^2 are activated both by endogenous ligands and exogenous phytocannabinoids, such as THC and CBD [10]. These receptors are typically located presynaptically, and they work as retrograde messengers to decrease the synaptic output. By activating the G_α subunit, cannabinoids are able to inhibit voltage-gated calcium channels and potentiate inwardly rectifying potassium channels [61]. Even though CBD interacts with both cannabinoid receptors, it shows lower affinity compared with THC [3]. Indeed, CBD seems to be 10 times less active than THC on both CB^1 and CB^2 [48]. CB_1 controls the vesicular release of gamma aminobutyric acid (GABA) or glutamate by inhibiting voltage-gated Ca^{2+} channels [62]. Moreover, CB_1 is also present in the external membrane of mitochondria [63], where it regulates memory processes via the modulation of the mitochondrial energy metabolism [64].

In addition, several findings have shown that the ECS, through CB_1 receptor activation, is associated with the neuronal differentiation and maturation of adult progenitor stem cells into neurons or astrocytes [65], which is a role that could be relevant in the treatment of neurodegenerative diseases. Conversely, although CB_2 expression was initially described only in the immune system, more recently, it was also detected in particular brain regions [66], and previous studies in rodents have already reported schizophrenia-related behaviors [67,68], altered cognitive function [69], modified drug-reward behaviors [70], and increased aggressiveness and anxiety [68] in CB_2-knock-out mice. By contrast, CB_2 overexpression was associated with reduced anxiety-like behaviors and higher resistance to depression in a murine model [71,72]. In this context, it has been suggested that CB_2 can regulate the synaptic transmission in hippocampal pyramidal cells and modulate both the gamma oscillation and activity of the sodium–bicarbonate co-transporter, which leads to a hyperpolarization of the neurons [73]. The ECS has also been shown to modulate the expression of neurotransmitters in the basal ganglia that is involved in coordinated movement [74], and it has the ability to control neuronal migration and differentiation by regulating growth-factor activities [10,75]. Through the activation of their receptors, cannabinoids can regulate synaptic neurotransmission, playing a key role in AD, anxiety, epilepsy, multiple sclerosis, Huntington's, and pain perception [39,53,66,76]. While most actions of cannabinoids are mediated through the activation of CB_1 and CB_2, cannabinoids can produce effects completely or partially independent of the aforementioned receptors, acting instead through other G-protein-coupled receptors, such as GPR18 and GPR55, serotonin receptors (5HT1Rs), and vanilloid transient receptor potential cation channel receptors [10,24], as well as receptors of the dopaminergic, glutamatergic, cholinergic, and opioidergic systems [2,45].

1.2. Zebrafish as a Model System to Test the Bioactivity of Cannabinoids

Although the bulk of the literature published to date on cannabis and cannabinoids consists of experiments performed using in vitro or rodent models, the zebrafish (*Danio rerio*) has recently gained attention as a powerful in vivo model, combining the experimental efficiency of cell cultures and organoids with the opportunity to study whole living vertebrate organisms [77]. Over the past three decades, the use of zebrafish has helped to further the knowledge and understanding of the neurobiological basis of vertebrate behavior and the pathogeneses of human neurological diseases [2,25,78–80]. Zebrafish show high genetic homology to mammals; the sequencing of the zebrafish genome revealed that 70% of human genes have at least one zebrafish ortholog, and that 84% of genes known to be associated with human disease have a zebrafish counterpart [17]. Many zebrafish genes are duplicated, making the investigation of their functions particularly challenging [81]. One advantage of zebrafish as a model species is that their embryos develop externally, which facilitates the study of embryo development [15]. Zebrafish development progresses quite quickly, with most organs developed within the first hours postfertilization (hpf); muscle activity starts from 17 hpf [81]. Pharmacological screening is among the most common applications of zebrafish [45,77]. At all stages of development, zebrafish can absorb through the skin's small molecules from the surrounding water, and this makes them ideal for performing studies on drug bioavailability and metabolites in a multiorgan system [24]. Moreover, numerous genetic tools, in vivo imaging techniques, and electrophysiological and neurobehavioral assays can be used to study the consequences of drug administration in zebrafish [82–85]. The ECS is highly conserved between zebrafish and mammals—this is not a characteristic of common high-throughput invertebrate model organisms—and ontogenetic analysis has revealed that ECS gene expression begins early during zebrafish development [79]. Recently, the zebrafish ECS has been well characterized: it comprises the same receptors, ligands, and enzymes as its mammalian equivalent [86,87]. Zebrafish larvae begin to express *CB₁* mRNA at the three-somite stage; expression is widespread in the CNS (preoptic area, telencephalon, hypothalamus, tegmentum, and anterior hindbrain) at 48 hpf, with the highest expression occurring in the telencephalon at 96 hpf [31,86,88]. In addition,

CB_1 protein has been observed in larval zebrafish brain homogenates from 48 hpf through 15 days postfertilization (dpf) [88]. A high level of sequence conservation of CB_1 has been shown between zebrafish and mammals. Indeed, the receptor shows 65–69% similarity at the nucleotide level, and 66–75% at the amino acid level [89]. One study showed that the morpholino knockdown of the *cnr1* gene (encoding CB_1) led to aberrant patterns of axonal growth and the fasciculation of reticulospinal neurons [90]. These data support the idea that CB_1 is needed for brain and locomotor behavior development, even in fish larvae [88]. Less is known regarding the CB_2 expression patterns throughout zebrafish development, but a comparison of the zebrafish CB_2 revealed a 39% amino acid similarity with its human counterpart [17]. Elsewhere, after the generation of a CB_2-knock-out zebrafish, the resulting homozygote (*cnr2* $^{upr1/upr1}$) larvae were shown to be characterized by lower swimming performances and increased anxiety-like behaviors [66]. These findings suggest that zebrafish could be a suitable model for investigating individual ECS gene functions, and for identifying novel genetic modifiers of cannabinoid signaling. Recently, zebrafish were used to test the effects of cannabinoids, administered alone, in combination, and as part of a complex, and were found to offer certain distinct advantages over mammalian models for drug studies [91,92]. The exposure of zebrafish to cannabinoids has been shown to alter a range of behaviors, physiological processes, and gene-expression pathways that are closely related to the ECS [75]. A broad range of behaviors can be analyzed in zebrafish larvae, including multiple swimming parameters, optokinetic and optomotor responses, prey tracking, phototaxis and thigmotaxis, and even learning and memory [93,94]. Due to the rapid development of larvae, these behaviors can be studied within the first week after fertilization. To evaluate the behavioral effects of cannabinoids on zebrafish larvae, most researchers have used the visual-motor-response (VMR) test, which is a validated behavioral assay that measures larval activity first in a light environment, and then in darkness, to study a single transition or dark–light cycles [15,25,31,32]. Typically, zebrafish larvae make frequent low-amplitude movements when exposed to a stable light condition, but an abrupt transition from light to dark causes an immediate increase in their motor activity for 10–15 min, after which it slowly declines to baseline levels [78,86,95,96]. The VMR test has been used to evaluate the sensory-motor function of zebrafish mutants/transgenic lines, and to assess the neurobehavioral responses to nutraceuticals and drugs [78,91]. This behavioral assay thus makes it possible to assess the effects of each compound both on baseline activity and after a standardized stimulus.

To assess the zebrafish anxiety state, and the related efficacy of anxiolytics, two behavioral assays are commonly used: the thigmotaxis paradigm, which is based on an analysis of the preference to swim in close proximity to the tank walls [32], or the light–dark preference test, which is based on the known marked preference of zebrafish larvae for the dark compartment [97]. In the latter test, an increase in activity and time spent in the white/light compartment is considered to reflect anxiolytic behavior, whereas increased activity in the dark compartment indicates anxiety-promoting behavior. Adult zebrafish, due to their size and low housing costs, also provide a cost-effective model for molecular-screening purposes. The most popular, sensitive, and reliable behavioral test in adult zebrafish is the novel tank paradigm, in which the fish locomotor activity and anxiety can be monitored at the same time [98]. Behavioral phenotypes in adult zebrafish are already well characterized [94] and include social, aggressive, affective, and cognitive behaviors [99–101], which are all highly sensitive to a wide range of CNS drugs [102].

We here review the available literature on the use of cannabis/cannabinoids in zebrafish models in order to establish, through a critical analysis of the articles, whether zebrafish might serve as a powerful experimental tool for testing the bioactivity of cannabinoids, and thus for gaining important insights into the safety and efficacy of different cannabis-extract-based products.

2. Materials and Methods

Data Sources and Searches

We followed the Preferred Reporting Items for Systematic Reviews and Meta-Analyses (PRISMA) guidelines. The study was registered in PROSPERO; registration number was 344190. The search was conducted by a medical librarian in MEDLINE (via PubMed up to 20 December 2021) using the keyworks "cannabis" (all fields) AND "cannabinoids" (all fields) AND "zebrafish" (all fields). The search yielded 25 matches, but 2 articles were excluded: one because the authors did not discuss the effects of cannabis on zebrafish, and the other because it did not concern zebrafish. The reference lists of these publications were examined, and a further 11 papers were identified. Overall, 34 articles were included in this review. Figure 2 shows a PRISMA flow diagram summarizing the methodology, which was created following the recent indications of Page et al. [103].

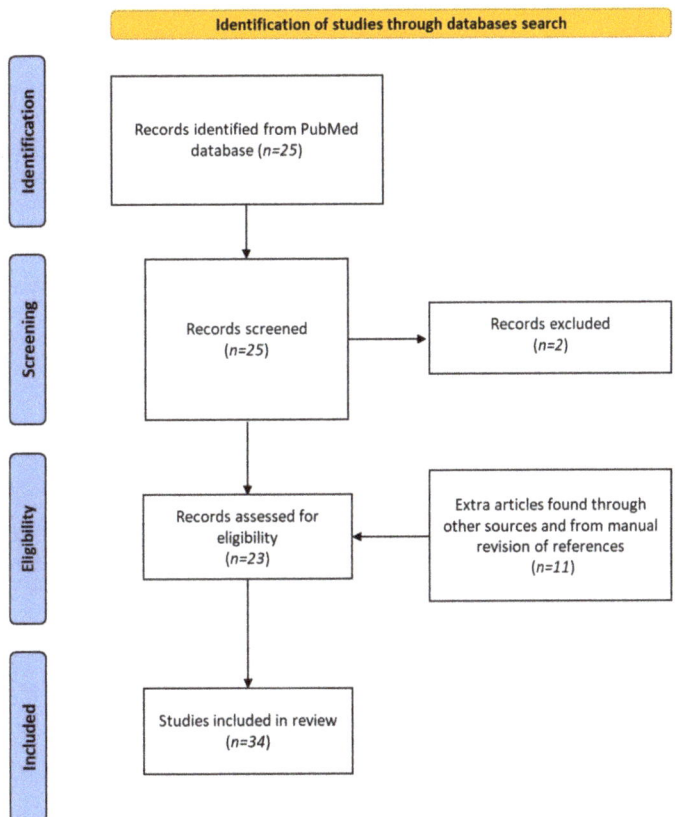

Figure 2. PRISMA 2020 flow diagram of the literature-search process.

Table 1 gives details of the experimental protocols of all the studies included in the review. It must be emphasized that the single cannabinoids tested were purified standard chemicals, which were used in all the studies, except for one, where THC was purified by using centrifugal partition chromatography [15]. Whereas in the two studies in which the whole-plant cannabis extract was employed, the analytical determination of the main cannabinoids was performed by gas or liquid chromatography coupled with high-resolution mass spectrometry.

3. Discussion

3.1. Effects of Phytocannabinoids in Wild-Type Zebrafish

The use of zebrafish to test the toxicity of phytocannabinoids dates back to a 1975 study in which THC was dissolved in aquarium water (acute exposure), and its median lethal dose (LD_{50}) calculated in zebrafish embryos was found to range between 2 and 5 mg/L [104]. Interest in studying cannabis/cannabinoids in the zebrafish model, however, has grown only in the past 10–15 years. The harmful effects of cannabinoid administration during zebrafish embryonic development have been well studied: embryos treated with THC and/or CBD exhibited shorter body lengths and mild deformities, reduced survival and basal heart rates, decreased synaptic activity and red-muscle-fiber thickness, alterations in the branching patterns of secondary motor neurons and Mauthner cells, changes in the expressions of postsynaptic nicotinic acetylcholine receptors in skeletal muscle, and reduced hatching rates [10,15,75]. In these studies, THC and CBD were used at concentrations believed to mimic the physiological range of cannabis use in humans (0.3–10 mg/L and 3–4 mg/L, respectively). In this regard, blood-plasma concentrations of THC and CBD caused by the consumption of a single cannabis cigarette have been found to reach peaks as high as 0.162 and 0.056 mg/L, respectively [105,106]. Table 1 summarizes studies on this topic.

Considering the deleterious effects of THC and CBD on developing embryos, the impact of these compounds on neural activity has recently been investigated through a novel in vivo assay based on a calcium-modulated photoactivatable ratiometric integrator (CaMPARI) system, which is able to provide a practical read-out of the neural activity in freely swimming larvae [3].

In acute regimens, both THC and CBD, if administered at high concentrations (6 and 3 mg/L, respectively), dramatically reduced the neural activity and locomotor activity of larvae at 4–5 dpf. Interestingly, the neuro-locomotor decrease was more pronounced when CBD and THC were combined. When treating embryos and 4 dpf larvae with low concentrations of CBD (up to 0.3–0.6 mg/L), no significant differences in the morphological parameters were observed, although the CBD significantly delayed the hatching of the embryos at the highest concentration used [32,51]. In most behavioral studies on the effects of cannabinoids in zebrafish, larvae were used at 5 dpf because, at this stage, they have fully developed digestive systems and inflated swim bladders, show mature swimming, and actively search for food [81,107]. In wild-type larvae at 5 dpf, the LD_{50} for THC, measured after chronic exposure (96 h beginning at age 24 hpf), was 3.37 mg/L [15]. In a study using zebrafish larvae with different characteristics and considering different drug-exposure times, a similar THC LD_{50} (3.65 mg/L) was found in fluorescent zebrafish of the Tg(fli1: EGFP) transgenic line at 4 dpf [86]. In acute regimens, the exposure of wild-type larvae to THC prompted a biphasic behavioral response consisting of increasing hyperactivity at concentrations ranging from 0.6 to 1.2 mg/L (2–4 µM), followed by the suppression of activity as the dose increased to 3.4 mg/L (10.8 µM) [15]. In line with these results, younger larvae (4 dpf) exposed to 0.3 mg/L THC exhibited a significantly increased duration of movement, while doses in the 0.6–1.25 mg/L range reduced the locomotor activity [32,86]. Evidence for the sedative effect of high doses of THC is also provided by Thornton et al. [14] and Amin et al. [75], who showed that THC at concentrations of 4–6 mg/L reduced swimming performances. These findings are consistent with results reported in rodents (i.e., dose-dependent hyperactivity followed by suppression at higher concentrations), as well as with the well-reported "stoning" action of THC in humans [45,108]. In chronic regimens, THC showed habituation, which is the development of tolerance to many of the acute effects in chronic exposition. Nevertheless, THC at 1.2 mg/L increased the distance traveled by fish [15]. This phenomenon has been associated with the downregulation of cannabinoid receptors after long-term exposure to cannabinoids [109]. In addition, the observation of reduced larval basal activity in response to exposure to THC at doses of up to 0.625 mg/L (2 µM) [31] suggests that THC produces a calming effect on larval locomotor activity up to this concentration, as opposed to hyperactivity at concentrations ranging from 0.6 to 2.4 mg/L, and sedation at concentrations higher than 2.4 mg/L (see Figure 3). In this context, psychoactive drugs, such as THC or its analog WIN55,212-2, by activating cannabinoid receptors, can induce hypothermia and hypoactivity, increase tremors and startle behaviors, and, in severe cases, induce catalepsy-like immobilization [110,111].

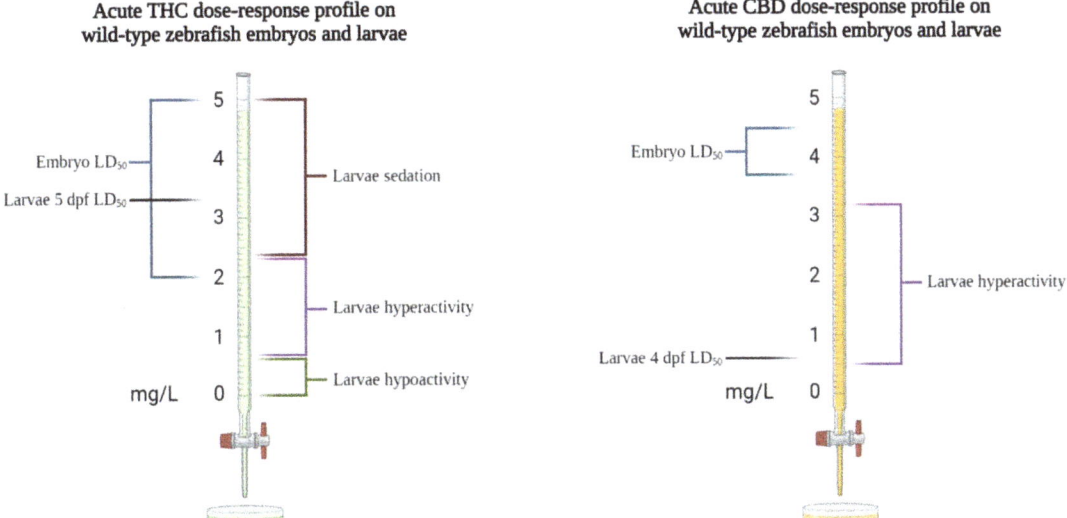

Figure 3. Toxicological and behavioral effects of acute THC and CBD administration on wild-type zebrafish embryos and larvae.

Zebrafish treated with WIN55,212-2 at 0.5 and 1 µg/mL showed no activity, even in darkness, whereas this was lethal if applied at 10 µg/mL [111]. Chronic early-life treatment with THC (0.6 mg/L) did not affect the locomotor abilities in 30-month-old zebrafish, which suggests that this psychoactive cannabinoid has no long-term effects on swimming behavior if used at low doses [27].

As for CBD, embryonic exposure to concentrations of up to 0.15 mg/L did not cause notable morphological abnormalities [32]. The LD_{50} values for CBD, calculated in zebrafish, are 4.4 mg/L at 2 dpf, 3.7 mg/L at 3 dpf [112], and 0.53 mg/L at 4 dpf [86]. In this latter study, larvae chronically exposed to low concentrations of CBD showed a biphasic locomotor response pattern, similar to that previously reported for THC [15]. In detail, 0.07 mg/L CBD produced a significantly increased duration of larval movement, while concentrations of 0.1–0.3 mg/L had a hypolocomotor effect. The acute administration of CBD at doses of up to 0.3 mg/L did not alter the locomotor behavior of 5 dpf zebrafish larvae, whereas higher concentrations caused larval hyperactivity [31]. In support of these findings, a study using auditory/mechanical tests to evaluate fish behavioral responses to unexpected sound and touch stimuli showed that THC and CBD concentrations of 6 mg/L and 3 mg/L, respectively, reduced their responses to sound [10]. An inhibitory effect on locomotion of low doses of CBD, ranging from 0.5 to 10 µg/mL, has been reported, but without a dose-dependent mechanism [111]. The same research evaluated larval responses to CBD after an initial exposure to WIN55,212-2. The results indicated that CBD could attenuate the WIN55,212-2-induced abnormal immobilization. Differences between the control and CBD-treated groups were no longer detected after 24 h of recovery in clean water, and this recovery trend was observed even after exposure to toxic levels of WIN55,212-2. Another study tested the analgesic properties of THC and CBD in a zebrafish larval model of nociception [25]. In detail, larvae, while recovering from acute exposure to low levels (0.1–0.5%) of acetic acid (nociception stimulus), were exposed to low levels of

THC or CDB (0.15 mg/L). The THC-exposed larvae showed reduced activity compared with that of both the acetic acid-treated and control groups, which is in line with the proposed calming effect of THC at doses of up to 0.6 mg/L (Figure 3). Notably, however, CBD appeared to increase the larval locomotor activity after acetic acid exposure, and it also had a nominal effect on the control-group locomotion, seemingly confirming its nociceptive properties. In other research analyzing both the immediate and long-term effects of THC (up to 0.6 mg/L) and CBD (up to 0.15 mg/L) on larval locomotor behavior, it was observed that THC exposure reduced the swimming behavior in the treated larvae (F0), as previously reported, whereas the locomotor parameters in their offspring (F1) were increased in comparison with the controls. Instead, CBD had no effect on F0 larvae, and it decreased activity in unexposed F1 larvae [32]. Furthermore, in 3 dpf larvae, 1.25 mg/L of CBD extract accelerated the caudal-fin regeneration and reduced apoptosis after amputation [112].

Several different cannabinoids have been tested on 5 dpf wild-type zebrafish larvae. In particular, exposure to CBN and CBDV at concentrations higher than 0.75 mg/L led to malformations and bradycardia, and the calculated LD_{50} for CBN was 1.12 mg/L [14,30]. A behavioral analysis suggested that the locomotion of the treated larvae remained unaltered up to 0.043 mg/L of CBN [14], but was significantly reduced at higher concentrations, in both dark and light conditions, which also affected their anxiety status. Conversely, CBDV administration had no significant effect on zebrafish [30]. In another study, a novel dihydrophenanthrene derivative, isolated from commercial cannabis, exhibited behavioral dose effects similar to those previously described with CBD [12]. Evaluating the toxicity and antitumor effects of abnormal CBD and its analog O-1602 (which have no or only little affinity for CB_1 and CB_2), Tomko et al. [24] found that both atypical cannabinoids significantly reduced tumor growth, but concentrations greater than 0.8 mg/L caused higher levels of toxicity to the larvae. Finally, data from another study indicated that THCV and THCV−OH have significant effects on the skeletal ossification of larvae at 8 dpf [37].

Recently, two similar behavioral studies, conducted independently in Canada and Italy, evaluated the effects induced by full-spectrum cannabis extracts, as opposed to purified major cannabinoids, on the zebrafish model. Research data on these extracts are scarce, and because cannabis consumers use the entire inflorescences, more scientific evidence is needed to clarify the bioactivity of all the cannabinoids, including their simultaneous interactions. In the study by Nixon et al. [92], acute exposure to the extracts produced similar complex concentration-dependent activity patterns to those observed by the group when using pure THC and CBD in a previous study [31]. However, distinct concentration-dependent differences were found both between the extracts (characterized by different ratios of THC:CBD) and versus the purified THC and CBD, which suggests that these differences might be related to the activity of other minor cannabinoids (specifically CBC, CBG, and CBDA). In the study by Licitra et al. [91], an excitatory effect on the locomotor activity was observed in larvae exposed to cannabis extract derived from CBD-rich-strain plants (containing about 0.5 and 7 µg/L of THC and CBD, respectively), without leading to toxicity effects. These studies underlined that the precise bioactivity of the single compounds in cannabis extracts and their interaction with the ECS pathway are highly complex issues that require further work.

Research on acute exposure to the cannabis receptor agonists WIN55,212-2 and CP55,940 indicated that both compounds reduce the locomotor activity in a dose-dependent fashion, in both light and dark phases, while the specific CB_2 agonists HU-910 and JWH-133 had no effect on locomotion, in any circadian phase [87]. Using $cnr1^{-/-}$ larvae, the authors found no inhibitory effect of WIN55,212-2 or CP55,940 on the average swimming velocity. The CB_1 antagonist AM251 did not affect locomotor activity, but blocked the effect of WIN55,212-2, which indicates that these endocannabinoids are not active in regulating the locomotor activity in zebrafish larvae at 5 dpf.

Another gene-expression analysis, performed on 4 dpf fluorescent larval zebrafish exposed at 96 hpf to THC or CBD, focused on the differential expressions of 10 key morphogenic or neurogenic genes [86]. The authors found the c-fos expression to be differentially upregulated in a concentration-dependent manner following both THC (1.25 and 2.5 mg/L) and CBD (0.07 and 0.1 mg/L) exposure, and it was correlated with increased neural activity and hyperlocomotor behavior in the zebrafish. In addition, the same concentrations of THC resulted in deleted in azoospermia-like (dazl)-gene upregulation, while the expressions of vasa, sox2, sox3, sox9a, bdnf, reln, krit1, and the CB_1-expressing gene cnr1 were similar to the control values. Along the same lines, during the key developmental stages (14, 24, 48, 72, and 96 hpf), THC and CBD caused the differential expressions of c-fos, bdnf, and dazl [32]. Contrary to the findings on cnr1 gene expression reported by Carty et al. [86], treatment with a full-spectrum cannabis extract (THC-poor strain) induced the overexpression of both cnr1 and cnr2 cannabinoid receptors in 5 dpf zebrafish larvae [91]. Additionally, CBD was found to reduce the gene- and protein-expression levels of cxcl8, tnf-α, and il-1β, and of IL-1β, caspase 3, and PARP [112]. Pandelides and colleagues observed that treatment with cannabinoids can alter the expression of proinflammatory cytokines in aged fish, which suggests a possible reduction in inflammation over the course of the lifespan [27]. In particular, exposure to low levels of THC during zebrafish development led to a significant reduction in tnf-α and il-1β at an advanced age, but this was not observed at higher doses, which indicates a biphasic or hormetic effect. Furthermore, the differential effect on the pparγ expression of exposure to cannabinoids in adult male vs. female zebrafish suggests that cannabinoid exposure could have long-term effects on reproduction, growth, and survival during early development [27].

In addition to larval locomotor activity, Achenbach et al. [31] assessed the uptake kinetics of THC and CBD, and their possible metabolism by larvae, suggesting that both cannabinoids are bioaccumulated in the living organism, but at concentrations that are substantially lower than their levels in test media. Studies involving liquid chromatography–tandem mass spectrometry analysis have shown that, when a test compound is dissolved in the embryo water, only 0.1–10% of it typically crosses the chorion and actually reaches the embryo [3,10], which limits the effectiveness of the treatment. In support of this, Carty et al. [87] found that, despite the best laboratory efforts, the actual THC concentrations in water corresponded to between 64% and 88% of the expected values at time 0, and the THC detection rate fell to between 16% and 32% at 96 hpf. Similarly, the actual CBD concentrations were only 33–40% of the nominal at time 0, and decreased to either not detected or 3% of baseline after 96 h. Indeed, in pharmacological and toxicological research with aquatic species, where the test compounds are usually diluted in the incubation water, it is essential to consider the relationship between the drug concentration in the medium and its adsorption and degradation rates.

Behavioral data from adult wild-type zebrafish indicate that a sedative effect was evoked following acute exposure to high doses of THC (30 and 50 mg/L) [45]. Moreover, reduced top swimming behavior was observed during the THC exposure, which indicated an anxiogenic effect. In another study, low doses of THC (up to 0.6 mg/L) did not cause significant behavioral effects in treated adults, but a significant reduction in thigmotaxis was seen in F1-generation fishes [32]. Other authors, however, have found these THC doses (0.3–0.6 mg/L) to induce repetitive swimming patterns in adult zebrafish [2]. In the same study, N-methyl-D-aspartate (NMDA), GABA antagonist pentylenetetrazol (PTZ), selective CB_2 inverse agonist AM630, and sulpiride (an antipsychotic) attenuated a THC-induced behavioral stereotypy, while the selective CB_1 inverse agonist AM251 did not. These results support a possible role for CB_2 as a mediator of abnormal behavioral patterns induced by THC [2]. In terms of cognitive abilities, it has been reported that the acute administration of tiny doses of THC (0.03 mg/L) did not lead to any observable effect on color-discrimination learning, but heavily impaired the fish spatial-memory retrieval [113]. Conversely, in studies of possible CBD effects, acute exposure to 40 mg/L reduced the swimming speed and distance [7], while no changes in these parameters were reported when using concentrations ranging from 0.1 to 10 mg/L [48]. These latter lower doses showed an anxiolytic effect on zebrafish in the novel tank test, which is in line with the findings in acute regimens in mammalian models [114]. However, CBD at 5 mg/L caused memory impairment in an avoidance task, while the same dose did not affect aggressive behavior and social interaction [48].

Studies exploring the reproductive effects of cannabinoids suggest that developmental exposure to THC can cause persistent sex-specific alterations to the reproductive system, particularly in male fish [32], and even across generations [27]. Similarly, THC treatment significantly reduced the ATP levels in mammal spermatozoa [115], and altered ECS signaling is linked to infertility in human semen [116]. Thus, the reproductive effects could be a result of altered metabolism [27]. In rodents, greater tolerance to THC in female rats than in male rats has been observed; this is probably due to the presence of hormones that are able to modulate the THC effects [117]. However, both in rats and zebrafish, maternal exposure to THC has been linked to altered locomotor and exploratory behavior in the offspring [32,118]. Unexpectedly, treating embryos with a low dose of THC (0.024 mg/L) increased the survival in aged males (30 months old), while, in aged females, the same dose improved egg production and reduced body mass [27].

3.2. Effects of Phytocannabinoids in Zebrafish Models of Neurological Disorders

The observed neuromodulatory effects of cannabinoids on the CNS have led neuropharmacological researchers to increasingly focus on the clinical potential of these molecules for use in the treatment of neurological disorders. Several zebrafish lines characterized by neuro-hyperactivity, seizures, bipolar disorder, and anxiety/stress and addiction behaviors have already been developed [17,31,119]. Epilepsy is a common neurological disorder that affects over 70 million people worldwide [120]. Approximately one-third of patients show multidrug resistance [121]. Therefore, research efforts are aimed at developing new drug treatments. Seizure treatment is one of the oldest reported uses of cannabis, and recently, the use of pure cannabinoids has been suggested as a means to treat severe forms of refractory childhood epilepsy (i.e., Dravet syndrome) [122,123]. Several zebrafish models of epilepsy, and more generally of psychiatric and muscular disorders linked to neuro-hyperactivity, have already been created and offer several specific key advantages, as explained below [14,17,119]. A number of small molecules targeting different receptors or ion channels can be used to induce seizures or neural hyperactivity in zebrafish larvae. The best characterized chemically induced model is PTZ exposure. Zebrafish larvae exposed to PTZ show a concentration-dependent abnormal pattern of behavior: increased locomotion followed by fast darting activity, and finally, clonic convulsions accompanied by a loss of posture [119]. In addition, PTZ administration leads to electrophysiological changes in the zebrafish optic tectum [124]. For instance, homozygous scn1Lab$^{-/-}$ mutants display significant phenotypic similarity to humans with Dravet syndrome, including spontaneous seizures, resistance to many available antiepileptic drugs, and early death [14,17]. The zebrafish knock-out model of neuro-hyperactivity, obtained by loss-of-function mutations in the GABA receptor subunit alpha 1 (gabra1$^{-/-}$), offers a unique advantage for drug-screening purposes because seizures (in addition to the sporadic ones) can be triggered by exposure to light [119]. In this context, CBD and THC significantly reduced the seizure-induced total distance moved, both in chemically induced and genetic models [14,119]. Although the exact mechanisms by which cannabinoids exert their antiseizure effects are not well understood, a number of molecular targets are known to be modulated by cannabinoids. Because CBD is a positive allosteric modulator of GABA receptors, it could, for example, be capable of reducing seizure events through this mechanism. This might hold true despite the fact that THC has been associated with GABA-release inhibition [14], as, even in this case, the THC properties depend, at least in part, on the seizure-model characteristics and cannabinoid dose. Furthermore, as previously indicated, the ability of these phytocannabinoids to reduce seizures could also be mediated by the transient receptor potential vanilloid 1 (TRPV1) channel: THC, CBD, CBN, and CBDV are all transient receptor potential cation channel subfamily A member 1 agonists. Finally, NMDA receptor, glycolysis, and fatty acid amide hydrolase may be potential cannabinoid targets, participating in seizure-effect modulation [14]. Recently, a commercially available library containing

370 synthetic cannabinoids (compounds engineered to bind cannabinoid receptors with high affinity) was screened [17] in 5 dpf homozygous scn1Lab$^{-/-}$ zebrafish larvae in order to identify molecules with the ability to reduce seizure-like behaviors. Five compounds exerting significant antiseizure activity during acute exposure were identified. It is essential to note that synthetic cannabinoids are not FDA-approved "for human or veterinary use", and substantial evidence of serious adverse effects has been reported for some of them [17]. Further research using the above models could be of great help in discerning the true therapeutic potential of various cannabinoids for the treatment of epilepsy.

Table 1. An overview of cannabis-exposure effects in zebrafish.

Compound Concentration and Exposure	Strain	Age	Studies Carried Out on Embryos/Larvae		Results	References
			Nonbehavioral Analysis	Behavioral Analysis		
THC (0.016, 0.031, 0.156, 0.469, and 0.625 mg/L) and **CBD** (0.225, 0.3, 0.525, 0.75, and 1.125 mg/L). **Acute exposure** (3–4 min before analysis).	AB/TU [1]	5 dpf	/	VMR test: 150 min of light followed by a 5 min dark–light cycle for 30 min.	**Locomotion:** THC: decreased locomotor activity at all concentrations tested; CBD: increased locomotor activity at concentrations above 0.525 mg/L.	Achenbach et al., 2018 [34]
THC (2, 4, 6, 8, and 10 mg/L) and **CBD** (1, 2, 3, and 4 mg/L). **Acute exposure** (5 h during gastrulation stage).	TL [2]	5 dpf	Survival, hatching rate, morphology, basal heart rate, and synaptic activity at neuromuscular junctions	Auditory/mechanical escape response test	**Survival:** Embryos exposed to 8–10 mg/L THC and 3–4 mg/L CBD had reduced survival rates. **Hatching rate:** Reduced with both THC and CBD, at all concentrations tested. **Morphology and basal heart rate:** Dose-dependent reductions in both body length and heart rate. **Synaptic activity:** Reduced with 6 mg/L THC and 3 mg/L CBD. **Escape response:** No reduction in touch response but decreases in sound response with 6 mg/L of THC and 3 mg/L of CBD.	Ahmed et al., 2018 [10]
THC (0.3–3.4 mg/L), **CP 55,940** (2.25–18 mg/L), and **WIN 55,212-2** (0.3–1.8 mg/L). **Acute exposure** (1, 4, and 12 min before analysis) and **chronic exposure** (96 h: from 24 to 120 hpf).	/	5 dpf	LD$_{50}$ determination and morphology	VMR test: 4 min of light followed by 4 min of dark.	LD$_{50}$: A total of 3.37 mg/L for THC, 1.8 mg/L for WIN 55,212-2, and 16.92 mg/L for CP 55,940. **Morphology:** THC caused malformations at all concentrations tested, while CP 55,940 and WIN 55,212-2 did not significantly increase the frequency of malformations. **Locomotion:** In acute exposure conditions, a biphasic response (stimulation at low concentrations and suppression at high concentrations) was observed; in chronic exposure, only 1.2 mg/L THC had a significant effect (increased distance traveled).	Akhtar et al., 2013 [15]

Table 1. Cont.

			Studies Carried Out on Embryos/Larvae			
Compound Concentration and Exposure	Strain	Age	Nonbehavioral Analysis	Behavioral Analysis	Results	References
THC (6 mg/L). **Acute exposure** (5 h during gastrulation stage).	TL [2]	2 and 5 dpf	Morphology of Mauthner cells and immunohistochemical analysis of the trunk muscles	Mechanical escape response test at 2 dpf and VMR test at 5 dpf (60 min).	**Morphology:** THC exposure reduced axonal diameter of Mauthner cells. **Escape response:** No reduction in C-bend response rate, but C-bend angle was increased in THC-treated embryos. **Immunohistochemistry:** White and red muscle fibers appeared thinner and slightly disorganized in THC-treated embryos. **Locomotion:** THC impaired locomotor performance.	Amin et al., 2020 [75]
Dihydrophenanthrene derivative (1–5 µM). **Acute exposure** (3–4 min before analysis).	AB/TU [1]	5 dpf	/	VMR test: 150 min of light followed by 5-min dark–light cycles (for 30 min).	**Locomotion:** Locomotor activity was increased at concentrations from 2.5 to 5 µM during the first 50 min, but normally increased larval locomotor activity was reduced during the dark phases.	Banskota et al., 2021 [12]
THC (0.3125, 0.625, 1.25, 2.5, 5 mg/) and **CBD** (0.0075, 0.15, 0.3, 0.6, 1.2 mg/L). **Chronic exposure** (94 h: from 2 to 96 hpf).	Tg(fli1:egfp)	4 dpf	Toxicity and morphology	Touch response and VMR test: 10 min light–dark cycles (for 30 min).	**Morphology:** THC and CBD displayed concentration-dependent morphological toxicities. **Locomotion:** Larvae exposed to 0.3 mg/L THC, or 0.07 mg/L CBD, exhibited a significantly increased duration of movement during dark phases compared with control. By contrast, 1.25 mg/L THC and 0.1–0.3 mg/L CBD significantly reduced duration of movement compared with control.	Carty et al., 2018 [86]
THC (0.024, 0.12, and 0.6 mg/L) and **CBD** (0.006, 0.03, and 0.15 mg/L). **Chronic exposure** (90 h: from 6 to 96 hpf).	Tg(fli1:egfp)	4 dpf	Survival and fertility rate	VMR test: 10 min dark–light cycles (for 30 min).	**Survival and fertility:** Not affected by treatments. **Locomotion:** Hypoactivity observed in larvae exposed to the lowest concentration of THC, and only during the dark phases.	Carty et al., 2019 [32]

Table 1. Cont.

Compound Concentration and Exposure	Strain	Age	Studies Carried Out on Embryos/Larvae		Results	References
			Nonbehavioral Analysis	Behavioral Analysis		
CBN (0.25, 0.75, 1.0, 1.125, 1.2, 1.25, and 2 mg/L). Chronic exposure (96 h: from 24 to 120 hpf).	AB	5–7 dpf	Survival, morphology, LD$_{50}$, and basal heart rate	VMR test: 10 min dark–light cycles (for 30 min). Mechanical escape response test: 2 min in dark conditions.	LD$_{50}$: 1.12 mg/L. **Morphology:** Concentrations higher than 0.75 mg/L led to malformations. **Basal heart rate:** At concentrations higher than 0.75 mg/l, heart rate decreased significantly, exhibiting characteristic bradycardia. **Locomotion:** Distance was significantly reduced as CBN concentration increased in both dark and light conditions; velocity increased with increasing CBN concentration under dark conditions and decreased under light conditions. **Escape response:** No differences.	Chousidis et al., 2020 [30]
Acute exposure to acetic acid solution (0.1–0.5%) (nociception stimulus), followed by exposure to THC (0.15625 mg/L) or CBD (0.15 mg/L). Acute exposure (2 h before analysis).	AB/TU [1]	5 dpf	/	VMR test: 2.5 h exposure to light followed by 5 min dark–light cycles (for 30 min).	**Locomotion:** THC-exposed larvae showed reduced activity compared with both acetic acid-exposed and control-group larvae, while CBD elevated the activity level of the larvae compared with acetic acid-exposed group. There was no significant reduction in the light–dark transition response in any of the test groups.	Ellis et al., 2018 [25]
20 synthetic cannabinoids (1, 10, and 100 µM). Acute exposure (20 min before analysis).	scn1lab$^{-/-}$	5 dpf	Electrophysiology	VMR test: 10 min	**Electrophysiology:** Five synthetic cannabinoids decreased the frequency of spontaneous epileptiform events. **Locomotion:** Five synthetic cannabinoids decreased seizure-like swims in a concentration-dependent manner.	Griffin et al., 2020 [17]

Table 1. Cont.

Compound Concentration and Exposure	Strain	Age	Studies Carried Out on Embryos/Larvae		Results	References
			Nonbehavioral Analysis	Behavioral Analysis		
CBD (0.5, 1, 5, and 10 mg/L) and WIN55,212-2 (0.5, 1, 5, and 10 mg/L). Acute exposure (30 min).	/	4–6 dpf	/	VMR test: 15 min dark–light cycle for 180 min.	**Locomotion:** CBD reduced the movement velocity and total distance moved. Moreover, CBD at 10 mg/L attenuated the responses of larvae exposed to darkness. No differences were detected between the control and CBD-treated groups after 24 h in fresh water. Fish treated with WIN55,212-2 at 0.5 and 1 mg/L showed virtually no activity, even in darkness, whereas a concentration of 10 mg/L induced mortality. A 24 h period in fresh water had the effect of reversing most of the drug-induced immobilization, even in the WIN55,212-2-treated groups. Finally, treatment with CBD attenuated WIN55,212-2-induced abnormal immobilization, whereas equivalent doses of CBD and WIN55,212-2 produced a mixed response.	Hasumi et al., 2020 [111]
THCV (0.286 and 0.859 mg/L) and THCV–OH (0.859 mg/L). Chronic exposure (5 days: from 3 to 8 dpf).	/	8 dpf	Number of ossified vertebral centers	/	**Morphology:** THCV reduced the number of ossified vertebral centers, whereas THCV–OH increased it.	Janssens et al., 2018 [37]
THC (2, 3, 4, and 6 μg/mL) and CBD (1.5, 2, and 3 mg/L). Acute exposure (9.5 h: from 0.5 to 10 hpf).	CaMPARI transgenic/Casper	4–5 dpf	Neural activity	VMR test: 60 min	**Neural activity:** Reduced in embryos exposed to 2–3 mg/L of CBD and 4–6 mg/L of THC. **Locomotion:** Reduced in embryos exposed to 3 mg/L CBD and 6 mg/L THC.	Kanyo et al., 2021 [3]
Whole-plant cannabis extract. Chronic exposure (96 h of exposition starting at 24 hpf).	AB	5 dpf	Gene expression	VMR test: 150 min of light followed by 5 min dark–light cycles (for 30 min).	**Locomotion:** During both the first 150 min of light and the remaining 30 min of light–dark cycles, larvae treated with cannabis at the highest dose (200 μL) showed increased locomotor activity. **Gene expression:** Both zebrafish cannabinoid receptors ($cnr1$ and $cnr2$) were overexpressed at the highest dose (200 μL).	Licitra et al., 2021 [91]

Table 1. Cont.

Compound Concentration and Exposure	Strain	Age	Studies Carried Out on Embryos/Larvae		Results	References
			Nonbehavioral Analysis	Behavioral Analysis		
WIN55,212-2 (0.014–3.412 mg/L) and CP55,940 (0.188–3.013 mg/L), and specific cnr2 agonists HU-910 and JWH-133. Acute exposure (1 h before analysis).	AB/TU [1] and cnr1−/−	5 dpf	/	VMR test: 4 min of light, 4 min of dark, and 30 min of light.	**Locomotion:** WIN55,212-2 and CP55,940 produced a dose-dependent reduction in locomotor activity in both the light and dark phases. HU-910 and JWH-133 have no effect on locomotion. In the cnr1−/− larvae, no inhibitory effect of WIN55,212-2 or CP55,940 on the average swimming velocity was found. The cnr1 antagonist AM251 did not affect locomotor activity, but blocked the effect of WIN55,212-2, which suggests that endocannabinoids are not active in regulating locomotor activity in zebrafish larvae at 5 dpf.	Luchtenburg et al., 2019 [87]
Whole-plant cannabis extracts. Acute exposure (2 h).	AB/TU [1]	5 dpf	/	VMR test: 90 min of light followed by 5 min dark-light cycles (for 30 min).	**Locomotion:** During the first 30 min of light, exposure to high THC extracts led to reduced activity at 0.25 mg/L and higher activity at 1 and 2 mg/L. Instead, exposure to high CBD extracts led to hyperactivity at 0.5 and 1 mg/L. During the final 30 min of the light cycle, high THC extracts significantly decreased activity at all concentrations tested, while high CBD extracts led to a reduction in activity only at 2 mg/L. During light-dark transitions, the locomotor response was abolished at 2 mg/L (in the dark phase).	Nixon et al., 2021 [92]
THC (0.156–2.1875 mg/L), CBD (0.3–2.1 mg/L), and THC–CBD combination. Acute exposure (1 h before analysis).	AB/TU + PTZ and GABRA1 knock-out	5 dpf	/	VMR test: 30 min	**Locomotion:** THC, CBD, and their combination reduced PTZ-induced neuro-hyperactivity and alleviated GABRA1−/− seizures.	Samarut et al., 2019 [119]
THC (1, 2, 5, and 10 mg/L). Acute exposure (19.5 h: from 4.5 to 24 hpf).	/	1–9 dpf	Survival and morphology	Tail twitches	**Survival:** After 24 h of exposure, no effects of THC on survival were recorded, but after between 2 and 9 days of exposure, survival was greatly reduced. **Morphology:** At levels above 2 mg/L THC, larvae showed curved trunks and/or bulbous-tipped tails. **Coiling:** At 26–28 hpf, the number of twitches following exposure to 5 or 10 mg/L THC was significantly reduced.	Thomas, 1975 [104]

Table 1. Cont.

Studies Carried Out on Embryos/Larvae

Compound Concentration and Exposure	Strain	Age	Nonbehavioral Analysis	Behavioral Analysis	Results	References
CBD (0.075–0.3 mg/L), **THC** (0.3125–1.25 mg/L), **CBDV** (0.072, 0.172, 0.286, and 1.146 mg/L), **CBN** (0.078, 0.186, 0.310, and 1.242 mg/L), or **LN** (0.107, 0.256, 0.427, and 1.707 mg/L). **Acute exposure** (24 h: from 120 to 144 hpf).	$scn1lab^{-/-}$ and WT ($scn1lab^{+/+}$ or $scn1lab^{+/-}$ + PTZ)	6 dpf	Morphology	VMR test: 15 min	**Morphology:** CBN and CBDV led to a high incidence of deformities. **Locomotion:** THC (1.25 mg/L) significantly reduced total distance traveled. In wild-type specimens, PTZ-induced hyperlocomotion was significantly reduced following exposure to CBD or THC, but no changes were observed following CBDV, CBN, or LN exposure. In the $scn1lab^{-/-}$ mutants, the total distance traveled was significantly reduced following exposure to CBD (0.15 mg/L), THC (0.3125 mg/L), CBN, and LN.	Thornton et al., 2020 [14]
O-1602 and abnormal CBD (up to 3.14 mg/L). **Chronic exposure** (3 days: from 2 to 5 dpf).	AB/TU [1]	5 dpf	Toxicity and antitumor effects	/	**Toxicity:** Concentrations greater than 2.5 μM led to higher levels of toxicity to the larvae. **Antitumor:** Both atypical cannabinoids significantly reduced the presence of injected cancer cells in the zebrafish larvae, by approximately 50%.	Tomko et al., 2019 [24]
CBD (5, 20, 70, 150, and 300 μg/L). **Chronic exposure** (4 days: from 0 to 4 dpf).	/	3–4 dpf	Toxicity and morphological analysis	Motor activity calculated as number of active events for 3 min.	**Toxicity and morphology:** CBD did not show significant differences in the morphological parameters at any dose, but at the highest concentration, CBD significantly delayed the hatching time of embryos. **Locomotion:** Above 20 μg/L, CBD increases the motor activity at 24 hpf, but not at 48 hpf.	Valim Brigante et al., 2018 [52]

Studies carried out in adult fish

Compound Concentration and Exposure	Strain	Age	Nonbehavioral Analysis	Behavioral Analysis	Results	References
THC (0.024, 0.12, and 0.6 mg/L) and **CBD** (0.006, 0.03, and 0.15 mg/L). **Chronic exposure** (90 h: from 6 to 96 hpf).	Tg(fli1:egfp)	12–18 months	Reproductive parameters	Open field test: 6 min	**Reproduction:** Reduced fecundity in adults exposed to CBD (0.15 mg/L) and THC (0.024 and 0.12 mg/L). **Locomotion:** No significant effects.	Carty et al., 2019 [32]
WIN55,212-2 (0.5, 5, or 50 mg/L). **Acute aqueous exposure** (10 min) and **dietary exposure** (1 μg/day/fish for 1 week).	/	/	/	Light–dark cross-maze test: 5 min	**Locomotion:** Altered behavioral anxiolytic responses and reduced locomotor activity at all tested doses. A 1-week dietary exposure promoted zebrafish exploration.	Connors et al., 2014. [125]
THC (0.0125, 0.3125, and 0.625 mg/L). **Acute exposure** (2 min prior to starting analysis).	EK	9–12 months	/	Locomotion: 20 min	**Locomotion:** THC (0.3125 mg/L) reduced velocity and induced repetitive swimming patterns.	Dahlén et al., 2021 [2]

Table 1. Cont.

Compound Concentration and Exposure	Strain	Age	Studies Carried Out on Embryos/Larvae		Results	References
			Nonbehavioral Analysis	Behavioral Analysis		
CBD (40 mg/L). **Acute exposure** (30 min).	/	6 months	Gene expression	Locomotion: 3 min	**Locomotion:** CBD reduced distance traveled and velocity. **Gene expression:** CBD activated genes encoding proinflammatory cytokines (il-$1b$ and il-$17af2$).	Jensen et al., 2018 [7]
CBD (0.1 0.5, 5.0, or 10 mg/kg) via intraperitoneal injection (1 h before analysis).	TU	4 months	/	Locomotion, anxiety, aggressive behavior (1 min), and social interaction (10 min). Memory-assessment task.	**Locomotion:** Not affected. **Anxiety:** Inverted U-shaped dose-response curve with 0.5 mg/kg reducing the anxiety. **Aggressive behavior and social interaction:** Not affected by 5 mg/kg CBD. **Memory:** CBD (5 mg/kg) caused memory impairment.	Nazario et al., 2015 [48]
THC (0.024, 0.12, and 0.6 mg/L). **Chronic exposure** (90 h: from 6 to 96 hpf).	Tg(fli1:egfp)	12–30 months	Survival, reproductive and growth parameters, and gene expression	Open field: 5 min	**Survival:** Increased at 0.024 mg/L THC in male fish. A significant reduction in survival of F1 THC-treated male fish by 30 months of age. **Reproduction:** THC exposition did not significantly alter sperm production, and exposure to 0.024 mg/L THC improved egg production in aged females; the resulting offspring at 96 hpf showed similar survival to both young and aged control fish. The F1 fish parentally exposed to 0.6 mg/L THC were completely unable to reproduce, unlike the aged controls. **Growth:** No difference in body length or mass was observed in male fish exposed to vehicle or THC, while exposure to the lowest concentration of THC (0.024 mg/L) resulted in significant reductions in mass in advanced aged females. **Locomotion:** With the exception of increased mobility in 0.12 mg/L-THC-exposed males, early-life treatment with THC did not affect locomotor abilities in 30-month-old male or female fish. **Gene expression:** Significant reductions in tnf-α and il-1β, and increases in il-6, $ppar\alpha$ and $ppar\gamma$.	Pandelides et al., 2020 [27]

Table 1. Cont.

Compound Concentration and Exposure	Strain	Age	Studies Carried Out on Embryos/Larvae			References
			Nonbehavioral Analysis	Behavioral Analysis	Results	
THC (0.03125 mg/L). **Acute exposure** (1 h).	/	12 months	/	Color-discrimination learning and spatial-cognition task.	**Color-discrimination learning:** THC administration did not lead to any observable effect on color-discrimination learning. **Spatial cognition:** Impaired.	Ruhl et al., 2014 [113]

[1] Tübingen; [2] Tübingen longfin.

4. Pointers on Behavioral Analysis

Behavioral analysis was performed in 18 of the 21 studies dealing with zebrafish larvae. The age of the larvae ranged from 1 to 7 dpf. Two tests were applied: the VMR test and the mechanical escape response; the latter was used in three of the 18 studies and was combined with an auditory stimulus in only one of them [10]. The VMR test normally involves several phases of light–dark succession, and it aims to stimulate an unconscious defensive response initiated by a drastic change in lighting [126]. In wild-type larvae without sight impediments, the locomotor activity increases at light onset, before decreasing to the baseline level after ca. 30 s. The wild type also shows increased locomotor activity at light offset, but they need more time (ca. 30 min.) to return to the baseline level of locomotion [127]. During embryogenesis, mechanical stimulus to the tail of the zebrafish embryo can be used to elicit the coiling behavior (touch response) [128]. Similarly, the escape response can be stimulated in larvae using mechanical, acoustic, electrical, or optical stimuli [129]. The escape response mimics predator-avoidance behavior, which is usually mediated by the Mauthner cells [130] located in the hindbrain [125,131].

Of the five studies carried out in zebrafish adults, four evaluated locomotion, one of these also explored social behavior and memory [48], and the other was conducted on color-discrimination learning and spatial cognition [113].

Overall, the results on the locomotion, both in larvae and adult fish, showed significant differences between studies. Cannabinoids, depending on the concentrations used, could either increase or decrease locomotor activity. As we stated in a recent systematic review on social-preference tests in zebrafish [101], the lack of a standardized approach to behavioral assessment makes it difficult to compare studies. Furthermore, in view of the heterogeneity in terms of the administered cannabinoids, doses, and exposure times of the current research, the standardization of behavioral tests could help to allow inferences to be drawn from findings in zebrafish species and provide more consistent data for translational-medicine purposes. The age of larvae used to perform the VMR test could, ideally, be set at 5 dpf: at this age, the larvae show limited (but sufficient) physiological development [132], but they are not yet independently feeding and are therefore subject to the EU directive on the protection of animals used for scientific purposes (Directive 2010/63/EU). Moreover, the exposure time could be set at 24 hpf, or 120 hpf to evaluate the effects of prolonged exposure. It should be highlighted that the daily replacement of the drug was performed in only one of the studies reviewed [37]. Although the adsorption of the medication can be considered minimal, and especially in the case of cannabinoids [3,10], we still believe that an approach that keeps the drug concentration constant over time, and that also considers the possible evaporation of egg water or medical compound, if volatile, will be the most accurate. The approach could be further standardized by introducing a standard duration of locomotor experiments and choosing the preferred drug-administration route for studies in adult zebrafish. We think the duration should be 30 min, and that drugs could be optimally administered through food. Furthermore, with regard to the method used to analyze the behavioral effects of cannabinoid treatments in adults, it may be useful to elect the novel tank test as the major read-out, considering that behavioral experiments should ideally last 10 min, after 5 min of habituation time.

5. Conclusions

This review showed that the zebrafish may prove a useful model for cannabinoid translational research because it displays similar behaviors to rodents following cannabinoid exposure. Moreover, it is clearly necessary to pay more attention to the full spectrum of naturally occurring cannabinoids, rather than focusing on the main ones: THC and CBD. These results indicate a need for additional cannabis-based studies to shed light on the mechanistic properties of cannabinoids, and to provide insight into the potential risks of its therapeutic application. At the same time, it is necessary to consider the long-term consequences of early-life exposure to cannabinoids.

Author Contributions: Conceptualization, R.L.; methodology, R.L. and V.N.; software, R.L.; investigation, R.L., V.N., M.M. (Maria Marchese), and A.O.; resources, M.M. (Maria Marchese) and M.M. (Marco Martinelli); data curation, R.L. and A.O.; writing—original draft preparation, R.L.; writing—review and editing, R.L., V.N., M.M. (Maria Marchese), A.O., C.K., and F.M.S.; visualization, M.M. (Marco Martinelli); supervision, B.F. and F.M.S.; project administration, R.L.; funding acquisition, B.F. and F.M.S. All authors have read and agreed to the published version of the manuscript.

Funding: This research was funded by the Italian Ministry of Health, Ricerca Corrente 2021, Fondo 5X1000.

Institutional Review Board Statement: Not applicable.

Informed Consent Statement: Not applicable.

Data Availability Statement: Not applicable.

Acknowledgments: We are thankful to Catherine J. Wrenn for the expert text editing and advice.

Conflicts of Interest: The authors declare no conflict of interest.

References

1. Bonini, S.A.; Premoli, M.; Tambaro, S.; Kumar, A.; Maccarinelli, G.; Memo, M.; Mastinu, A. Cannabis sativa: A comprehensive eethnopharmacological review of a medicinal plant with a long history. *J. Ethnopharmacol.* **2018**, *5*, 300–315. [CrossRef] [PubMed]
2. Dahlén, A.; Zarei, M.; Melgoza, A.; Wagle, M.; Guo, S. THC-induced behavioral stereotypy in zebrafish as a model of psychosis-like behavior. *Sci. Rep.* **2021**, *11*, 15693. [CrossRef]
3. Kanyo, R.; Amin, M.R.; Locskai, L.F.; Bouvier, D.D.; Olthuis, A.M.; Allison, W.T.; Ali, D.W. Medium-throughput zebrafish optogenetic platform identifies deficits in subsequent neural activity following brief early exposure to cannabidiol and Δ^9-tetrahydrocannabinol. *Sci. Rep.* **2021**, *11*, 11515. [CrossRef] [PubMed]
4. Lazarjani, M.P.; Young, O.; Kebede, L.; Seyfoddin, A. Processing and extraction methods of medicinal cannabis: A narrative review. *J. Cannabis Res.* **2021**, *3*, 32. [CrossRef] [PubMed]
5. Chiarlone, A.; Börner, C.; Martín-Gómez, L.; Jiménez-González, A.; García-Concejo, A.; García-Bermejo, M.L.; Lorente, M.; Blázquez, C.; García-Taboada, E.; de Haro, A.; et al. MicroRNA let-7d is a target of cannabinoid CB_1 receptor and controls cannabinoid signaling. *Neuropharmacology* **2016**, *108*, 345–352. [CrossRef] [PubMed]
6. Khurshid, H.; Qureshi, I.A.; Jahan, N.; Went, T.R.; Sultan, W.; Sapkota, A.; Alfonso, M. A Systematic Review of Fibromyalgia and Recent Advancements in Treatment: Is Medicinal Cannabis a New Hope? *Cureus* **2021**, *13*, e17332. [CrossRef] [PubMed]
7. Jensen, H.M.; Korbut, R.; Kania, P.W.; Buchmann, K. Cannabidiol effects on behaviour and immune gene expression in zebrafish (*Danio rerio*). *PLoS ONE* **2018**, *31*, e0200016. [CrossRef] [PubMed]
8. Goodwin, R.D.; Kim, J.H.; Cheslack-Postava, K.; Weinberger, A.H.; Wu, M.; Wyka, K.; Kattan, M. Trends in cannabis use among adults with children in the home in the United States, 2004–2017: Impact of state-level legalization for recreational and medical use. *Addiction* **2021**, *116*, 2770–2778. [CrossRef]
9. Crippa, J.A.; Derenusson, G.N.; Ferrari, T.B.; Wichert-Ana, L.; Duran, F.L.; Martin-Santos, R.; Simões, M.V.; Bhattacharyya, S.; Fusar-Poli, P.; Atakan, Z.; et al. Neural basis of anxiolytic effects of cannabidiol (CBD) in generalized social anxiety disorder: A preliminary report. *J. Psychopharmacol.* **2011**, *25*, 121–130. [CrossRef]
10. Ahmed, K.T.; Amin, M.R.; Shah, P.; Ali, D.W. Motor neuron development in zebrafish is altered by brief (5-hr) exposures to THC (Δ^9-tetrahydrocannabinol) or CBD (cannabidiol) during gastrulation. *Sci. Rep.* **2018**, *8*, 10518. [CrossRef]
11. Omare, M.O.; Kibet, J.K.; Cherutoi, J.K.; Kengara, F.O. Current Trends in the Use of *Cannabis sativa*: Beyond Recreational and Medicinal Applications. *Open Access Libr.* **2021**, *8*, 6. [CrossRef]
12. Banskota, A.H.; Stefanova, R.; Hui, J.P.M.; Berrué, F.; Achenbach, J.C.; Ellis, L. 9,10-Dihydro-5-hydroxy-2,3,6-trimethoxyphenanthrene-1,4-dione: A new dihydrophenanthrene from commercial cannabis and its effect on zebrafish larval behaviour. *Nat. Prod. Res.* **2021**, *36*, 3553–3558. [CrossRef] [PubMed]
13. Fu, J.; Gong, Z.; Kelly, B.C. Metabolomic profiling of zebrafish (*Danio rerio*) embryos exposed to the antibacterial agent triclosan. *Environ. Toxicol. Chem.* **2019**, *38*, 240–249. [CrossRef]
14. Thornton, C.; Dickson, K.E.; Carty, D.R.; Ashpole, N.M.; Willett, K.L. Cannabis constituents reduce seizure behavior in chemically-induced and *scn1a*-mutant zebrafish. *Epilepsy Behav.* **2020**, *110*, 107152. [CrossRef] [PubMed]
15. Akhtar, M.T.; Ali, S.; Rashidi, H.; van der Kooy, F.; Verpoorte, R.; Richardson, M.K. Developmental effects of cannabinoids on zebrafish larvae. *Zebrafish* **2013**, *10*, 283–293. [CrossRef]
16. Devinsky, O.; Cross, J.H.; Laux, L.; Marsh, E.; Miller, I.; Nabbout, R.; Scheffer, I.E.; Thiele, E.A.; Wright, S. Trial of cannabidiol for drug-resistant seizures in the dravet syndrome. *N. Engl. J. Med.* **2017**, *376*, 2011–2020. [CrossRef]
17. Griffin, A.; Anvar, M.; Hamling, K.; Baraban, S.C. Phenotype-Based Screening of Synthetic Cannabinoids in a Dravet Syndrome Zebrafish Model. *Front. Pharmacol.* **2020**, *11*, 464. [CrossRef]
18. Kerr, A.; Walston, V.; Wong, V.S.S.; Kellogg, M.; Ernst, L. Marijuana use among patients with epilepsy at a tertiary care center. *Epilepsy Behav.* **2019**, *97*, 144–148. [CrossRef]

19. Sagdeo, A.; Askari, A.; Ball, P.; Morrissey, H. Exploring the efficacy and safety of cannabis in the management of fibromyalgia. *Int. J. Curr. Pharm. Rev. Res.* **2022**, *14*, 27–30. [CrossRef]
20. Kosiba, J.D.; Maisto, S.A.; Ditre, J.W. Patient-reported use of medical cannabis for pain, anxiety, and depression symptoms: Systematic review and metaanalysis. *Soc. Sci. Med.* **2019**, *233*, 181–192. [CrossRef]
21. Hamilton, I.; Monaghan, M. Cannabis and psychosis: Are we any closer to understanding the relationship. *Curr. Psychiatr. Rep.* **2019**, *21*, 21–48. [CrossRef] [PubMed]
22. Boehnke, K.F.; Scott, J.R.; Litinas, E.; Sisley, S.; Williams, D.A.; Clauw, D.J. Pills to pot: Observational analyses of cannabis substitution among medical cannabis users with chronic pain. *J. Pain* **2019**, *20*, 830–841. [CrossRef] [PubMed]
23. Guzmàn, M. Cannabis for the management of cancer symptoms: THC version 2.0? *Cannabis Cannabinoid. Res.* **2018**, *3*, 117–119. [CrossRef] [PubMed]
24. Tomko, A.; O'Leary, L.; Trask, H.; Achenbach, J.C.; Hall, S.R.; Goralski, K.B.; Ellis, L.D.; Dupré, D.J. Antitumor Activity of Abnormal Cannabidiol and Its Analog O-1602 in Taxol-Resistant Preclinical Models of Breast Cancer. *Front. Pharmacol.* **2019**, *10*, 1124. [CrossRef]
25. Ellis, L.D.; Berrue, F.; Morash, M.; Achenbach, J.C.; Hill, J.; McDougall, J.J. Comparison of cannabinoids with known analgesics using a novel high throughput zebrafish larval model of nociception. *Behav. Brain Res.* **2018**, *337*, 151–159. [CrossRef]
26. Schneider, M.; Schomig, E.; Leweke, F.M. Acute and chronic cannabinoid treatment differentially affects recognition memory and social behavior in pubertal and adult rats. *Addict. Biol.* **2008**, *13*, 345–357. [CrossRef]
27. Pandelides, Z.; Thornton, C.; Lovitt, K.G.; Faruque, A.S.; Whitehead, A.P.; Willett, K.L.; Ashpole, N.M. Developmental exposure to Δ^9-tetrahydrocannabinol (THC) causes biphasic effects on longevity, inflammation, and reproduction in aged zebrafish (*Danio rerio*). *Geroscience* **2020**, *42*, 923–926. [CrossRef]
28. Carlini, B.H.; Garrett, S.B.; Carter, G.T. Medicinal Cannabis: A Survey Among Health Care Providers in Washington State. *Am. J. Hosp. Palliat. Care* **2017**, *34*, 85–91. [CrossRef]
29. Lopez-Quintero, C.; Hasin, D.S.; de Los Cobos, J.P.; Pines, A.; Wang, S.; Grant, B.F.; Blanco, C. Probability and predictors of remission from life-time nicotine, alcohol, cannabis or cocaine dependence: Results from the National Epidemiologic Survey on Alcohol and Related Conditions. *Addiction* **2011**, *106*, 657–669. [CrossRef]
30. Chousidis, I.; Chatzimitakos, T.; Leonardos, D.; Filiou, M.D.; Stalikas, C.D.; Leonardos, I.D. Cannabinol in the spotlight: Toxicometabolomic study and behavioral analysis of zebrafish embryos exposed to the unknown cannabinoid. *Chemosphere* **2020**, *252*, 126417. [CrossRef]
31. Achenbach, J.C.; Hill, J.; Hui, J.P.M.; Morash, M.G.; Berrue, F.; Ellis, L.D. Analysis of the Uptake, Metabolism, and Behavioral Effects of Cannabinoids on Zebrafish Larvae. *Zebrafish* **2018**, *15*, 349–360. [CrossRef] [PubMed]
32. Carty, D.R.; Miller, Z.S.; Thornton, C.; Pandelides, Z.; Kutchma, M.L.; Willett, K.L. Multigenerational consequences of early-life cannabinoid exposure in zebrafish. *Toxicol. Appl. Pharmacol.* **2019**, *364*, 133–143. [CrossRef]
33. Borgelt, L.M.; Franson, K.L.; Nussbaum, A.M.; Wang, G.S. The pharmacologic and clinical effects of medical cannabis. *Pharmacotherapy* **2013**, *33*, 195–209. [CrossRef] [PubMed]
34. Pisanti, S.; Malfitano, A.M.; Ciaglia, E.; Lamberti, A.; Ranieri, R.; Cuomo, G.; Abate, M.; Faggiana, G.; Proto, M.C.; Fiore, D.; et al. Cannabidiol: State of the art and new challenges for therapeutic applications. *Pharmacol. Ther.* **2017**, *175*, 133–150. [CrossRef] [PubMed]
35. Trofin, I.G.; Dabija, G.; Vaireanu, D.I.; Filipescu, L. Long term storage and cannabis oil stability. *Rev. Chim.* **2012**, *63*, 293–297.
36. Herring, A.C.; Faubert Kaplan, B.L.; Kaminski, N.E. Modulation of CREB and NFκB signal transduction by cannabinol in activated thymocytes. *Cell. Signal.* **2001**, *13*, 241–250. [CrossRef]
37. Janssens, A.; Silvestri, C.; Martella, A.; Vanoevelen, J.M.; Di Marzo, V.; Voets, T. Δ^9-tetrahydrocannabivarin impairs epithelial calcium transport through inhibition of TRPV5 and TRPV6. *Pharmacol. Res.* **2018**, *136*, 83–89. [CrossRef]
38. Citti, C.; Linciano, P.; Russo, F.; Luongo, L.; Iannotta, M.; Maione, S.; Lagana, A.; Capriotti, A.L.; Forni, F.; Vandelli, M.A.; et al. A novel phytocannabinoid isolated from *Cannabis sativa* L. with an in vivo cannabimimetic activity higher than Δ^9-tetrahydrocannabinol: Δ^9-tetrahydrocannabiphorol. *Sci. Rep.* **2019**, *9*, 20335. [CrossRef]
39. Fernández-Ruiz, J.; Gómez-Ruiz, M.; García, C.; Hernández, M.; Ramos, J.A. Modeling Neurodegenerative Disorders for Developing Cannabinoid-Based Neuroprotective Therapies. *Meth. Enzymol.* **2017**, *593*, 175–198. [CrossRef]
40. Ramírez, B.G.; Blázquez, C.; Gómez del Pulgar, T.; Guzmán, M.; de Ceballos, M.L. Prevention of Alzheimer's disease pathology by cannabinoids: Neuroprotection mediated by blockade of microglial activation. *J Neurosci.* **2005**, *25*, 1904–1913. [CrossRef]
41. Varvel, S.; Hamm, R.; Martin, B.; Lichtman, A. Differential effects of Δ^9-THC on spatial reference and working memory in mice. *Psychopharmacology* **2001**, *157*, 142–150. [CrossRef]
42. Hamley, I.W. The amyloid beta peptide: A chemist's perspective. Role in Alzheimer's and fibrillization. *Chem. Rev.* **2012**, *112*, 5147–5192. [CrossRef] [PubMed]
43. Cao, C.; Li, Y.; Liu, H.; Bai, G.; Mayl, J.; Lin, X.; Sutherland, K.; Nabar, N.; Cai, J. The potential therapeutic effects of THC on Alzheimer's disease. *J. Alzheimers Dis.* **2014**, *42*, 973–984. [CrossRef] [PubMed]
44. Bilkei-Gorzo, A.; Albayram, O.; Draffehn, A.; Michel, K.; Piyanova, A.; Oppenheimer, H.; Dvir-Ginzberg, M.; Rácz, I.; Ulas, T.; Imbeault, S.; et al. A chronic low dose of Δ^9-tetrahydrocannabinol (THC) restores cognitive function in old mice. *Nat. Med.* **2017**, *23*, 782–787. [CrossRef] [PubMed]

45. Stewart, A.M.; Kalueff, A.V. The behavioral effects of acute Δ^9-tetrahydrocannabinol and heroin (diacetylmorphine) exposure in adult zebrafish. *Brain Res.* **2014**, *1543*, 109–119. [CrossRef]
46. Magagnini, G.; Grassi, G.; Kotiranta, S. The effect of light spectrum on the morphology and cannabinoid content of *Cannabis sativa* L. *Med. Cannabis Cannabinoids* **2018**, *1*, 19–27. [CrossRef]
47. Desaulniers Brousseau, V.; Wu, B.S.; MacPherson, S.; Morello, V.; Lefsrud, M. Cannabinoids and Terpenes: How Production of Photo-Protectants Can Be Manipulated to Enhance *Cannabis sativa* L. Phytochemistry. *Front. Plant. Sci.* **2021**, *12*, 620021. [CrossRef]
48. Nazario, L.R.; Antonioli, R.; Capiotti, K.M.; Hallak, J.E.; Zuardi, A.W.; Crippa, J.A.; Bonan, C.D.; da Silva, R.S. Caffeine protects against memory loss induced by high and non-anxiolytic dose of cannabidiol in adult zebrafish (*Danio rerio*). *Pharmacol. Biochem. Behav.* **2015**, *135*, 210–216. [CrossRef]
49. Barichello, T.; Ceretta, R.A.; Generoso, J.S.; Moreira, A.P.; Simões, L.R.; Comim, C.M.; Quevedo, J.; Vilela, M.C.; Zuardi, A.W.; Crippa, J.A.; et al. Cannabidiol reduces host immune response and prevents cognitive impairments in Wistar rats submitted to pneumococcal meningitis. *Eur. J. Pharmacol.* **2012**, *697*, 158–164. [CrossRef]
50. Merrick, J.; Lane, B.; Sebree, T.; Yaksh, T.; O'Neill, C.; Banks, S.L. Identification of Psychoactive Degradants of Cannabidiol in Simulated Gastric and Physiological Fluid. *Cannabis Cannabinoid Res.* **2016**, *1*, 102–112. [CrossRef] [PubMed]
51. Valim Brigante, T.A.; Abe, F.R.; Zuardi, A.W.; Hallak, J.E.C.; Crippa, J.A.S.; de Oliveira, D.P. Cannabidiol did not induce teratogenicity or neurotoxicity in exposed zebrafish embryos. *Chem. Biol. Interact.* **2018**, *291*, 81–86. [CrossRef] [PubMed]
52. Devane, W.A.; Dysarz, F.A.; Johnson, M.R.; Melvin, L.S.; Howlett, A.C. Determination and characterization of a cannabinoid receptor in rat brain. *Mol. Pharmacol.* **1988**, *34*, 605–613. [PubMed]
53. Piomelli, D. The molecular logic of endocannabinoid signalling. *Nat. Rev. Neurosci.* **2003**, *4*, 873–884. [CrossRef]
54. Katona, I.; Freund, T.F. Endocannabinoid signaling as a synaptic circuit breaker in neurological disease. *Nat. Med.* **2008**, *14*, 923–930. [CrossRef] [PubMed]
55. Devane, W.A.; Hanus, L.; Breuer, A.; Pertwee, R.G.; Stevenson, L.A.; Griffin, G.; Gibson, D.; Mandelbaum, A.; Etinger, A.; Mechoulam, R. Isolation and structure of a brain constituent that binds to the cannabinoid receptor. *Science* **1992**, *258*, 1946–1949. [CrossRef] [PubMed]
56. Wei, D.; Lee, D.; Cox, C.D.; Karsten, C.A.; Peñagarikano, O.; Geschwind, D.H.; Gall, C.M.; Piomelli, D. Endocannabinoid signaling mediates oxytocin-driven social reward. *Proc. Natl. Acad. Sci. USA* **2015**, *112*, 14084–14089. [CrossRef] [PubMed]
57. Ogi, A.; Mariti, C.; Pirrone, F.; Baragli, P.; Gazzano, A. The Influence of Oxytocin on Maternal Care in Lactating Dogs. *Animals* **2021**, *11*, 1130. [CrossRef]
58. Wei, D.; Dinh, D.; Lee, D.; Li, D.; Anguren, A.; Moreno-Sanz, G.; Gall, C.M.; Piomelli, D. Enhancement of Anandamide-Mediated Endocannabinoid Signaling Corrects Autism-Related Social Impairment. *Cannabis Cannabinoid Res.* **2016**, *1*, 81–89. [CrossRef]
59. Carnovali, M.; Ottria, R.; Pasqualetti, S.; Banfi, G.; Ciuffreda, P.; Mariotti, M. Effects of bioactive fatty acid amide derivatives in zebrafish scale model of bone metabolism and disease. *Pharmacol. Res.* **2016**, *104*, 1–8. [CrossRef] [PubMed]
60. Migliarini, B.; Carnevali, O. Anandamide modulates growth and lipid metabolism in the zebrafish Danio rerio. *Mol. Cell. Endocrinol.* **2008**, *286*, S12–S16. [CrossRef] [PubMed]
61. Baker, D.; Pryce, G.; Visintin, C.; Sisay, S.; Bondarenko, A.I.; Vanessa Ho, W.S.; Jackson, S.J.; Williams, T.E.; Al-Izki, S.; Sevastou, I.; et al. Big conductance calcium-activated potassium channel openers control spasticity without sedation. *Br. J. Pharmacol.* **2017**, *174*, 2662–2681. [CrossRef] [PubMed]
62. Farkas, I.; Kalló, I.; Deli, L.; Vida, B.; Hrabovszky, E.; Fekete, C.; Moenter, S.M.; Watanabe, M.; Liposits, Z. Retrograde endocannabinoid signaling reduces GABAergic synaptic transmission to gonadotropin-releasing hormone neurons. *Endocrinology* **2010**, *151*, 5818–5829. [CrossRef]
63. Bénard, G.; Massa, F.; Puente, N.; Lourenço, J.; Bellocchio, L.; Soria-Gómez, E.; Matias, I.; Delamarre, A.; Metna-Laurent, M.; Cannich, A.; et al. Mitochondrial CB_1 receptors regulate neuronal energy metabolism. *Nat. Neurosci.* **2012**, *15*, 558–564. [CrossRef] [PubMed]
64. Hebert-Chatelain, E.; Desprez, T.; Serrat, R.; Bellocchio, L.; Soria-Gomez, E.; Busquets-Garcia, A.; Pagano Zottola, A.C.; Delamarre, A.; Cannich, A.; Vincent, P.; et al. A cannabinoid link between mitochondria and memory. *Nature* **2016**, *539*, 555–559. [CrossRef] [PubMed]
65. Compagnucci, C.; Di Siena, S.; Bustamante, M.B.; Di Giacomo, D.; Di Tommaso, M.; Maccarrone, M.; Grimaldi, P.; Sette, C. Type-1 (CB1) cannabinoid receptor promotes neuronal differentiation and maturation of neural stem cells. *PLoS ONE* **2013**, *8*, e54271. [CrossRef] [PubMed]
66. Acevedo-Canabal, A.; Colón-Cruz, L.; Rodriguez-Morales, R.; Varshney, G.K.; Burgess, S.; González-Sepúlveda, L.; Yudowski, G.; Behra, M. Altered Swimming Behaviors in Zebrafish Larvae Lacking Cannabinoid Receptor 2. *Cannabis Cannabinoid Res.* **2019**, *4*, 88–101. [CrossRef]
67. Ortega-Alvaro, A.; Aracil-Fernández, A.; García-Gutiérrez, M.S.; Navarrete, F.; Manzanares, J. Deletion of CB2 cannabinoid receptor induces schizophrenia-related behaviors in mice. *Neuropsychopharmacology* **2011**, *36*, 1489–1504. [CrossRef]
68. Liu, Q.R.; Canseco-Alba, A.; Zhang, H.Y.; Tagliaferro, P.; Chung, M.; Dennis, E.; Sanabria, B.; Schanz, N.; Escosteguy-Neto, J.C.; Ishiguro, H.; et al. Cannabinoid type 2 receptors in dopamine neurons inhibits psychomotor behaviors, alters anxiety, depression and alcohol preference. *Sci. Rep.* **2017**, *7*, 17410. [CrossRef]

69. Li, Y.; Kim, J. CB₂ cannabinoid receptor knockout in mice impairs contextual long-term memory and enhances spatial working memory. *Neural. Plast.* **2016**, *2016*, 9817089. [CrossRef] [PubMed]
70. Xi, Z.X.; Peng, X.Q.; Li, X.; Song, R.; Zhang, H.Y.; Liu, Q.R.; Yang, H.J.; Bi, G.H.; Li, J.; Gardner, E.L. Brain cannabinoid CB_2 receptors modulate cocaine's actions in mice. *Nat. Neurosci.* **2011**, *14*, 1160–1166. [CrossRef]
71. Garcia-Gutierrez, M.S.; Manzanares, J. Overexpression of CB₂ cannabinoid receptors decreased vulnerability to anxiety and impaired anxiolytic action of alprazolam in mice. *J. Psychopharmacol.* **2011**, *25*, 111–120. [CrossRef] [PubMed]
72. García-Gutiérrez, M.S.; Pérez-Ortiz, J.M.; Gutiérrez-Adán, A.; Manzanares, J. Depression-resistant endophenotype in mice overexpressing cannabinoid CB(2) receptors. *Br. J. Pharmacol.* **2010**, *160*, 1773–1784. [CrossRef] [PubMed]
73. Stempel, A.V.; Stumpf, A.; Zhang, H.Y.; Özdoğan, T.; Pannasch, U.; Theis, A.K.; Otte, D.M.; Wojtalla, A.; Rácz, I.; Ponomarenko, A.; et al. Cannabinoid Type 2 Receptors Mediate a Cell Type-Specific Plasticity in the Hippocampus. *Neuron* **2016**, *90*, 795–809. [CrossRef]
74. Benarroch, E. Endocannabinoids in basal ganglia circuits: Implications for Parkinson disease. *Neurology* **2007**, *69*, 306–309. [CrossRef] [PubMed]
75. Amin, M.R.; Ahmed, K.T.; Ali, D.W. Early Exposure to THC Alters M-Cell Development in Zebrafish Embryos. *Biomedicines* **2020**, *8*, 5. [CrossRef] [PubMed]
76. Basavarajappa, B.S.; Shivakumar, M.; Joshi, V.; Subbanna, S. Endocannabinoid system in neurodegenerative disorders. *J. Neurochem.* **2017**, *142*, 624–648. [CrossRef] [PubMed]
77. Van Wijk, R.C.; Krekels, E.H.J.; Kantae, V.; Harms, A.C.; Hankemeier, T.; van der Graaf, P.H.; Spaink, H.P. Impact of post-hatching maturation on the pharmacokinetics of paracetamol in zebrafish larvae. *Sci. Rep.* **2019**, *9*, 2149. [CrossRef] [PubMed]
78. Burton, C.E.; Zhou, Y.; Bai, Q.; Burton, E.A. Spectral properties of the zebrafish visual motor response. *Neurosci. Let.* **2017**, *646*, 62–67. [CrossRef]
79. Krug, R.G.; Clark, K.J. Elucidating cannabinoid biology in zebrafish (*Danio rerio*). *Gene* **2015**, *570*, 168–179. [CrossRef]
80. Oltrabella, F.; Melgoza, A.; Nguyen, B.; Guo, S. Role of the endocannabinoid system in vertebrates: Emphasis on the zebrafish model. *Dev. Growth Differ.* **2017**, *59*, 194–210. [CrossRef]
81. Vaz, R.; Hofmeister, W.; Lindstrand, A. Zebrafish Models of Neurodevelopmental Disorders: Limitations and Benefits of Current Tools and Techniques. *Int. J. Mol. Sci.* **2019**, *20*, 1296. [CrossRef] [PubMed]
82. Cozzolino, O.; Sicca, F.; Paoli, E.; Trovato, F.; Santorelli, F.M.; Ratto, G.M.; Marchese, M. Evolution of Epileptiform Activity in Zebrafish by Statistical-Based Integration of Electrophysiology and 2-Photon Ca^{2+} Imaging. *Cells* **2020**, *9*, 769. [CrossRef] [PubMed]
83. Cassar, S.; Adatto, I.; Freeman, J.L.; Gamse, J.T.; Iturria, I.; Lawrence, C.; Muriana, A.; Peterson, R.T.; Van Cruchten, S.; Zon, L.I. Use of Zebrafish in Drug Discovery Toxicology. *Chem. Res. Toxicol.* **2020**, *33*, 95–118. [CrossRef] [PubMed]
84. Brogi, L.; Marchese, M.; Cellerino, A.; Licitra, R.; Naef, V.; Mero, S.; Bibbiani, C.; Fronte, B. β-Glucans as Dietary Supplement to Improve Locomotion and Mitochondrial Respiration in a Model of Duchenne Muscular Dystrophy. *Nutrients* **2021**, *13*, 1619. [CrossRef] [PubMed]
85. Naef, V.; Marchese, M.; Ogi, A.; Fichi, G.; Galatolo, D.; Licitra, R.; Doccini, S.; Verri, T.; Argenton, F.; Morani, F.; et al. Efficient Neuroprotective Rescue of Sacsin-Related Disease Phenotypes in Zebrafish. *Int. J. Mol. Sci.* **2021**, *22*, 8401. [CrossRef] [PubMed]
86. Carty, D.R.; Thornton, C.; Gledhill, J.H.; Willett, K.L. Developmental Effects of Cannabidiol and Δ9-Tetrahydrocannabinol in Zebrafish. *Toxicol. Sci.* **2018**, *162*, 137–145. [CrossRef] [PubMed]
87. Luchtenburg, F.J.; Schaaf, M.J.M.; Richardson, M.K. Functional characterization of the cannabinoid receptors 1 and 2 in zebrafish larvae using behavioral analysis. *Psychopharmacology* **2019**, *236*, 2049–2058. [CrossRef]
88. Migliarini, B.; Carnevali, O. A novel role for the endocannabinoid system during zebrafish development. *Mol. Cell. Endocrinol.* **2009**, *299*, 172–177. [CrossRef]
89. Lam, C.S.; Rastegar, S.; Strahle, U. Distribution of cannabinoid receptor 1 in the CNS of zebrafish. *Neuroscience* **2006**, *138*, 83–95. [CrossRef]
90. Watson, S.; Chambers, D.; Hobbs, C.; Doherty, P.; Graham, A. The endocannabinoid receptor, CB1, is required for normal axonal growth and fasciculation. *Mol. Cell. Neurosci.* **2008**, *38*, 89–97. [CrossRef]
91. Licitra, R.; Martinelli, M.; Petrocchi, J.L.; Marchese, M.; Kiferle, C.; Fronte, B. In Vivo Evaluation of *Cannabis sativa* Full Extract on Zebrafish Larvae Development, Locomotion Behavior and Gene Expression. *Pharmaceuticals* **2021**, *14*, 1224. [CrossRef] [PubMed]
92. Nixon, J.; Abramovici, H.; Cabecinha, A.; Martinez-Farina, C.; Hui, J.; Ellis, L. Assessing the bioactivity of cannabis extracts in larval zebrafish. *J. Cannabis Res.* **2021**, *3*, 44. [CrossRef] [PubMed]
93. Gerlai, R. Using zebrafish to unravel the genetics of complex brain disorders. *Curr. Top. Behav. Neurosci.* **2012**, *12*, 3–24. [CrossRef] [PubMed]
94. Kalueff, A.V.; Gebhardt, M.; Stewart, A.M.; Cachat, J.M.; Brimmer, M.; Chawla, J.S.; Craddock, C.; Kyzar, E.J.; Roth, A.; Landsman, S.; et al. Towards a comprehensive catalog of zebrafish behavior 1.0 and beyond. *Zebrafish* **2013**, *10*, 70–86. [CrossRef] [PubMed]
95. Kirla, K.T.; Groh, K.J.; Steuer, A.E.; Poetzsch, M.; Banote, R.K.; Stadnicka-Michalak, J.; Eggen, R.I.; Schirmer, K.; Kraemer, T. From the Cover: Zebrafish Larvae Are Insensitive to Stimulation by Cocaine: Importance of Exposure Route and Toxicokinetics. *Toxicol. Sci.* **2016**, *154*, 183–193. [CrossRef]
96. MacPhail, R.C.; Brooks, J.; Hunter, D.L.; Padnos, B.; Irons, T.D.; Padilla, S. Locomotion in larval zebrafish: Influence of time of day, lighting and ethanol. *Neurotoxicology* **2009**, *30*, 52–58. [CrossRef]

97. Maximino, C.; De Brito, T.M.; de Mattos Dias, C.A.G.; Gouveia, A., Jr.; Morato, S. Scototaxis as anxiety-like behavior in fish. *Nat. Protoc.* **2010**, *5*, 209. [CrossRef] [PubMed]
98. Stewart, A.M.; Kaluyeva, A.A.; Poudel, M.K.; Nguyen, M.; Song, C.; Kalueff, A.V. Building Zebrafish Neurobehavioral Phenomics: Effects of Common Environmental Factors on Anxiety and Locomotor Activity. *Zebrafish* **2015**, *12*, 339–348. [CrossRef]
99. de Abreu, M.S.; Friend, A.J.; Demin, K.A.; Amstislavskaya, T.G.; Bao, W.; Kalueff, A.V. Zebrafish models: Do we have valid paradigms for depression? *J. Pharmacol. Toxicol. Methods* **2018**, *94*, 16–22. [CrossRef]
100. Audira, G.; Sampurna, B.P.; Juniardi, S.; Liang, S.-T.; Lai, Y.-H.; Hsiao, C.-D. A Versatile Setup for Measuring Multiple Behavior Endpoints in Zebrafish. *Inventions* **2018**, *3*, 75. [CrossRef]
101. Ogi, A.; Licitra, R.; Naef, V.; Marchese, M.; Fronte, B.; Gazzano, A.; Santorelli, F.M. Social Preference Tests in Zebrafish: A Systematic Review. *Front. Vet. Sci.* **2021**, *7*, 590057. [CrossRef] [PubMed]
102. De Abreu, M.S.; Giacomini, A.; Genario, R.; Dos Santos, B.E.; da Rosa, L.G.; Demin, K.A.; Wappler-Guzzetta, E.A.; Kalueff, A.V. Neuropharmacology, pharmacogenetics and pharmacogenomics of aggression: The zebrafish model. *Pharmacol. Res.* **2019**, *141*, 602–608. [CrossRef] [PubMed]
103. Page, M.J.; McKenzie, J.E.; Bossuyt, P.M.; Boutron, I.; Hoffmann, T.C.; Mulrow, C.D.; Shamseer, L.; Tetzlaff, J.M.; Akl, E.A.; Brennan, S.E.; et al. The PRISMA 2020 statement: An updated guideline for reporting systematic reviews. *BMJ* **2021**, *372*, 71. [CrossRef] [PubMed]
104. Thomas, R.J. The toxicologic and teratologic effects of delta-9-tetrahydrocannabinol in the zebrafish embryo. *Toxicol. Appl. Pharmacol.* **1975**, *32*, 184–190. [CrossRef]
105. Huestis, M.A. Human cannabinoid pharmacokinetics. *Chem. Biodivers.* **2007**, *4*, 1770–1804. [CrossRef] [PubMed]
106. Pacifici, R.; Pichini, S.; Pellegrini, M.; Rotolo, M.C.; Giorgetti, R.; Tagliabracci, A.; Busardò, F.P.; Huestis, M.A. THC and CBD concentrations in blood, oral fluid and urine following a single and repeated administration of "light cannabis". *Clin. Chem. Lab. Med.* **2020**, *58*, 682–689. [CrossRef]
107. Clift, D.; Richendrfer, H.; Thorn, R.J.; Colwill, R.M.; Creton, R. High-throughput analysis of behavior in zebrafish larvae: Effects of feeding. *Zebrafish* **2014**, *11*, 455–461. [CrossRef]
108. Grisham, M.G.; Ferraro, D.P. Biphasic effects of 9-tetrahydrocannabinol on variable interval schedule performance in rats. *Psychopharmacology* **1972**, *27*, 163–169. [CrossRef] [PubMed]
109. Howlett, A.C.; Breivogel, C.S.; Childers, S.R.; Deadwyler, S.A.; Hampson, R.E.; Porrino, L.J. Cannabinoid physiology and pharmacology: 30 years of progress. *Neuropharmacology* **2004**, *47*, 345–358. [CrossRef]
110. Morris, C.V.; DiNieri, J.A.; Szutorisz, H.; Hurd, Y.L. Molecular mechanisms of maternal cannabis and cigarette use on human neurodevelopment. *Eur. J. Neurosci.* **2011**, *34*, 1574–1583. [CrossRef]
111. Hasumi, A.; Maeda, H.; Yoshida, K. Analyzing cannabinoid-induced abnormal behavior in a zebrafish model. *PLoS ONE* **2020**, *15*, e0236606. [CrossRef] [PubMed]
112. Xu, S.; Zhang, H.; Li, C.-Z.; Lai, P.-S.; Wang, G.; Chan, Y.S.; Cheng, S.H.; Chen, X. Cannabidiol promotes fin regeneration and reduces apoptosis in zebrafish embryos. *J. Funct. Foods* **2021**, *86*, 104694. [CrossRef]
113. Ruhl, T.; Prinz, N.; Oellers, N.; Seidel, N.I.; Jonas, A.; Albayram, O.; Bilkei-Gorzo, A.; Von Der Emde, G. Acute administration of THC impairs spatial but not associative memory function in zebrafish. *Psychopharmacology* **2014**, *231*, 3829–3842. [CrossRef] [PubMed]
114. Moreira, F.A.; Aguiar, D.C.; Guimaraes, F.S. Anxiolytic-like effect of cannabidiol in the rat Vogel conflict test. *Prog. Neuropsychopharmacol. Biol. Psychiatry* **2006**, *30*, 1466–1471. [CrossRef] [PubMed]
115. Morgan, D.J.; Muller, C.H.; Murataeva, N.A.; Davis, B.J.; Mackie, K. Δ 9-tetrahydrocannabinol (Δ 9-THC) attenuates mouse sperm motility and male fecundity. *Br. J. Pharmacol.* **2012**, *165*, 2575–2583. [CrossRef] [PubMed]
116. Lewis, S.E.M.; Rapino, C.; Di Tommaso, M.; Pucci, M.; Battista, N.; Paro, R.; Simon, L.; Lutton, D.; Maccarrone, M. Differences in the endocannabinoid system of sperm from fertile and infertile men. *PLoS ONE* **2012**, *7*, e47704. [CrossRef] [PubMed]
117. Bara, A.; Manduca, A.; Bernabeu, A.; Borsoi, M.; Serviado, M.; Lassalle, O.; Murphy, M.; Wager-Miller, J.; Mackie, K.; Pelissier-Alicot, A.-L.; et al. Sex-dependent effects of in utero cannabinoid exposure on cortical function. *eLife* **2018**, *7*, e36234. [CrossRef]
118. Navarro, M.; Rubio, P.; de Fonseca, F.R. Behavioural consequences of maternal exposure to natural cannabinoids in rats. *Psychopharmacology* **1995**, *122*, 226. [CrossRef] [PubMed]
119. Samarut, É.; Nixon, J.; Kundap, U.P.; Drapeau, P.; Ellis, L.D. Single and Synergistic Effects of Cannabidiol and Δ-9-Tetrahydrocannabinol on Zebrafish Models of Neuro-Hyperactivity. *Front. Pharmacol.* **2019**, *10*, 226. [CrossRef]
120. Tang, F.; Hartz, A.M.S.; Bauer, B. Drug-Resistant Epilepsy: Multiple Hypotheses, Few Answers. *Front. Neurol.* **2017**, *8*, 301. [CrossRef]
121. Zaheer, S.; Kumar, D.; Khan, M.T.; Giyanwani, P.R.; Kiran, F. Epilepsy and Cannabis: A Literature Review. *Cureus* **2018**, *10*, e3278. [CrossRef] [PubMed]
122. De Caro, C.; Leo, A.; Citraro, R.; De Sarro, C.; Russo, R.; Calignano, A.; Russo, E. The potential role of cannabinoids in epilepsy treatment. *Expert Rev. Neurother.* **2017**, *17*, 1069–1079. [CrossRef] [PubMed]
123. Silvestro, S.; Mammana, S.; Cavalli, E.; Bramanti, P.; Mazzon, E. Use of Cannabidiol in the Treatment of Epilepsy: Efficacy and Security in Clinical Trials. *Molecules* **2019**, *24*, 1459. [CrossRef] [PubMed]
124. Baraban, S.C.; Taylor, M.R.; Castro, P.A.; Baier, H. Pentylenetetrazole induced changes in zebrafish behavior, neural activity and c-fos expression. *Neuroscience* **2005**, *131*, 759–768. [CrossRef] [PubMed]

125. Connors, K.A.; Valenti, T.W.; Lawless, K.; Sackerman, J.; Onaivi, E.S.; Brooks, B.W.; Gould, G.G. Similar anxiolytic effects of agonists targeting serotonin 5-HT1A or cannabinoid CB receptors on zebrafish behavior in novel environments. *Aquat. Toxicol.* **2014**, *151*, 105–113. [CrossRef]
126. Emran, F.; Rihel, J.; Dowling, J.E. A Behavioral Assay to Measure Responsiveness of Zebrafish to Changes in Light Intensities. *J. Vis. Exp.* **2008**, *20*, 923. [CrossRef]
127. Ganzen, L.; Venkatraman, P.; Pang, C.P.; Leung, Y.F.; Zhang, M. Utilizing Zebrafish Visual Behaviors in Drug Screening for Retinal Degeneration. *Int. J. Mol. Sci.* **2017**, *18*, 1185. [CrossRef]
128. Knafo, S.; Wyart, C. Active mechanosensory feedback during locomotion in the zebrafish spinal cord. *Curr. Opin. Neurobiol.* **2018**, *52*, 48–53. [CrossRef]
129. El-Daher, F.; Becker, C.G. Neural circuit reorganisation after spinal cord injury in zebrafish. *Curr. Opin. Genet. Dev.* **2020**, *64*, 44–51. [CrossRef]
130. Danos, N.; Lauder, G.V. Challenging zebrafish escape responses by increasing water viscosity. *J. Exp. Biol.* **2012**, *215*, 1854–1862. [CrossRef]
131. Sillar, K.T. Mauthner cells. *Curr. Biol.* **2009**, *19*, 353–355. [CrossRef] [PubMed]
132. Liu, Y.; Carmer, R.; Zhang, G.; Venkatraman, P.; Brown, S.A.; Pang, C.-P.; Zhang, M.; Ma, P.; Leung, Y.F. Statistical Analysis of Zebrafish Locomotor Response. *PLoS ONE* **2015**, *10*, e0139521. [CrossRef] [PubMed]

MDPI
St. Alban-Anlage 66
4052 Basel
Switzerland
Tel. +41 61 683 77 34
Fax +41 61 302 89 18
www.mdpi.com

Biomedicines Editorial Office
E-mail: biomedicines@mdpi.com
www.mdpi.com/journal/biomedicines

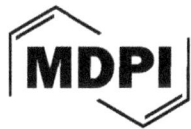